# EMBALMING
History, Theory, and Practice

**NOTICE**

Medicine is an ever-changing science. As new research and clinical experience broaden our knowledge, changes in treatment and drug therapy are required. The author and the publisher of this work have checked with sources believed to be reliable in their efforts to provide information that is complete and generally in accord with the standards accepted at the time of publication. However, in view of the possibility of human error or changes in medical sciences, neither the author nor the publisher nor any other party who has been involved in the preparation or publication of this work warrants that the information contained herein is in every respect accurate or complete, and they disclaim all responsibility for any errors or omissions or for the results obtained from use of the information contained in this work. Readers are encouraged to confirm the information contained herein with other sources. For example and in particular, readers are advised to check the product information sheet included in the package of each drug they plan to administer to be certain that the information contained in this work is accurate and that changes have not been made in the recommended dose or in the contraindications for administration. This recommendation is of particular importance in connection with new or infrequently used drugs.

# EMBALMING
## History, Theory, and Practice
### Sixth Edition

**Sharon L. Gee-Mascarello, CFSP, MBIE**
*Licensed Embalmer and Funeral Director*
Saint Clair Shores, Michigan
Adjunct Professor
Mortuary Science Program
Wayne State University
Detroit, Michigan

*With a Foreword by*

**Robert G. Mayer, FBIE**
*Licensed Embalmer and Funeral Director*
Pittsburgh, Pennsylvania
Adjunct Professor
Pittsburgh Institute of Mortuary Science
Pittsburgh, Pennsylvania

New York   Chicago   San Francisco   Athens   London   Madrid
Mexico City   New Delhi   Milan   Singapore   Sydney   Toronto

**Embalming: History, Theory, and Practice, Sixth Edition**

Copyright © 2022 by McGraw Hill. All rights reserved. Printed in the United States of America. Except as permitted under the United States Copyright Act of 1976, no part of this publication may be reproduced or distributed in any form or by any means, or stored in a data base or retrieval system, without the prior written permission of the publisher.

3 4 5 6 7 LBC 28 27 26 25 24

ISBN 978-1-260-01007-7
MHID 1-260-01007-4

This book was set in Minion Pro by KnowledgeWorks Global Ltd.
The editors were Michael Weitz, Sydney Keen, and Kim J. Davis.
The production supervisor was Catherine H. Saggese.
Project management was provided by Warishree Pant, KnowledgeWorks Global Ltd.
The cover designer was Tim Lawlis.

This book is printed on acid-free paper.

Library of Congress Cataloging-in-Publication Data

Names: Gee-Mascarello, Sharon L. author.
Title: Embalming: History, Theory, and Practice / Sharon L. Gee-Mascarello; with a foreword by Robert G. Mayer.
Description: Sixth edition. | New York: McGraw Hill Education [2022] |
  Preceded by Embalming / Robert G. Mayer. 5th ed. c2012. | Includes
  bibliographical references and index. | Summary: "This book covers
  embalming as no other book ever has and is useful as a teaching text,
  historical, or technical reference for the funeral service practitioner
  or the lay reader"-- Provided by publisher.
Identifiers: LCCN 2021026531 (print) | LCCN 2021026532 (ebook) | ISBN
  9781260010077 (hardcover; alk. paper) | ISBN 9781260010084 (ebook)
Subjects: MESH: Embalming
Classification: LCC GT3340 (print) | LCC GT3340 (ebook) | NLM WA 844 |
  DDC 393/.3--dc23
LC record available at https://lccn.loc.gov/2021026531
LC ebook record available at https://lccn.loc.gov/2021026532

McGraw Hill books are available at special quantity discounts to use as premiums and sales promotions or for use in corporate training programs. To contact a representative, please visit the Contact Us pages at www.mhprofessional.com.

The sixth edition is dedicated in remembrance of
the more than 4.5 million souls worldwide
who lost their lives from complications of SARS-CoV-2.
We honor their memory and console all who mourn them.

An abundance of gratitude to the first responders;
emergency technicians, firefighters, police officers,
health care professionals,
and countless essential frontline workers.

In heartfelt appreciation of the last responders;
embalmers and funeral directors,
organ and tissue recovery teams,
coroners and medical examiners,
cemetery, crematory, and livery personnel,
bereavement care specialists,
and countless essential support staff.

# Contents

*Editorial Consultants* ................................................................. ix
*Contributors* ............................................................................... xi
*Foreword* ................................................................................... xv
*Preface* ..................................................................................... xvii
*Acknowledgments* ................................................................... xix

## PART I. The Theory and Practice of Embalming .......... 1

1. Origins of Embalming and Reverent Care of the Dead. ........................................................... 3
2. Fundamentals of Embalming. ........................... 11
3. Personal Health and Regulatory Standards .......... 33
4. The Preparation Room ..................................... 61
5. Death: Agonal and Postmortem Changes. ........... 83
6. Embalming Chemicals ..................................... 95
7. Use of Embalming Chemicals ......................... 109
8. Anatomical Considerations. ............................ 121
9. Embalming Vessel Sites and Selections ........... 139
10. Embalming Analysis ..................................... 149
11. Preparation of the Body Prior to Arterial Injection ..... 159
12. Injection and Drainage Techniques ................. 179
13. Distribution and Diffusion of Arterial Solution ...... 193
14. Cavity Embalming ........................................ 209
15. Treatments after Arterial Injection .................. 223
16. General Age Considerations. ......................... 237
17. Preparation of Autopsied Bodies .................... 249
18. Preparation of Organ and Tissue Donors .......... 263
19. Delayed Embalming ...................................... 277
20. Discolorations .............................................. 287
21. Moisture Considerations ............................... 303
22. Vascular Considerations. ............................... 315
23. Effect of Drugs on the Embalming Process ...... 323
24. Selected Conditions ..................................... 329
25. Viewing without Embalming, Delayed Viewing, Re-embalming, and Human Remains Shipping ..... 341

## PART II. The Origin and History of Embalming ....... 345

*Edward C. Johnson, Gail R. Johnson, and Melissa Johnson*

## PART III. History of Modern Restorative Art. ......... 385

*Edward C. Johnson, Gail R. Johnson, and Melissa J. Williams*

## PART IV. Selected Readings ..................... 401

1. Summary of Guidelines Submitted to OSHA from the National Funeral Directors Association Committee on Infectious Disease, Summer, 1989. ... 402
2. Mortuary Care of Armed Forces Service Members. From: Standards for Department of Defense (DOD) Mortuary Facilities and for Drafting a Performance Work Statement (PWS) for DOD Contracted Mortuary Services, March 2019. .................... 405
3. Identification: An Essential Part of What We Do ..... 409
   *Michael Kubasak*
4. The Mathematics of Embalming Chemistry: Part I. A Critical Evaluation of "One-Bottle" Embalming Chemical Claims ...................... 412
   *Jerome F. Frederick, PhD*
5. The Measurement of Formaldehyde Retention in the Tissues of Embalmed Bodies ............... 414
   *John Kroshus, Joseph McConnell, and Jay Bardole*
6. The Two-Year Fix: Long-Term Preservation for Delayed Viewing ................................. 416
   *Kerry Don Peterson*
7. Occupational Exposure to Formaldehyde in Mortuaries ......................................... 419
   *L. Lamont Moore, CIH, CSP and Eugene C. Ogrodnik, MS*
8. The Strange Case of Dr. Jekyll and Formaldehyde (Is It Good or Is It Evil?) ........................... 423
   *Maureen Robinson*
9. The Preparation Room: Ventilation ................. 430
   *Jack Adams, CFSP*
10. Risk of Infection and Tracking of Work-related Infectious Diseases in the Funeral Industry. ..... 432
    *Susan Salter Davidson, MS, MT (ASCP) and William H. Benjamin, Jr., PhD*
11. Creutzfeldt-Jakob Disease: A Comprehensive Guide for Healthcare Personnel, Section 3: Information for Embalmers .............. 436
    *Curtis D. Rostad, CFSP*
12. Hepatitis from A to G ................................. 447
    *Kim Collison*

13. The Increase in MRSA and VRE......................450
    *Mike Cloud, Jr.*
14. The Antimicrobial Activity of Embalming Chemicals and Topical Disinfectants on the Microbial Flora of Human Remains .................451
    *Peter A. Burke* and *A. L. Sheffner*
15. The Microbiologic Evaluation and Enumeration of Postmortem Specimens from Human Remains...453
    *Gordon W. Rose, PhD* and *Robert N. Hockett, MS*
16. Professional Hair Care for Human Remains..........456
    *Darla A. Tripoli, CO, LFD, CFSP*
17. Restricted Cervical Injection as a Primary Injection Method ..................................459
    *Ben Whitworth*
18. Enhance Emaciated Features Arterially Using Split Injection and Restricted Drainage .............461
    *Sharon L. Gee*
19. Embalming—United Kingdom and European.......462
    *Peter J. Ball, FBIE*
20. The Art of Embalming and its Purpose..............464
    *Ron Hast*
21. Embalming COVID-19: Infection Control and Storage .......................................465
    *Jzyk S. Ennis, PhD*
22. Cosmetic Airbrushing of Un-embalmed Decedents........................................467
    *Daryl M. Hammond*

*Glossary* .....................................................469
*Index* .......................................................485

# Editorial Consultants

**Jeffrey P. Bellefleur, MD**
Attending Physician
William Beaumont Hospital
Royal Oak, Michigan

**Gary J. Brown, MA, LFD**
Instructor, Funeral Services Program
St. Petersburg College
Pinellas Park, Florida

**Duff D. Chamberlain**
Licensed Embalmer and Funeral Director
Taylor, Michigan

**Jzyk S. Ennis, PhD**
Instructor, Funeral Service Education
Jefferson State Community College
Birmingham, Alabama

**Dedrick A. Gantt, CFSP**
Instructor, Funeral Service Education
Piedmont Technical College
Greenwood, South Carolina

**Roger Husband, CFSP**
Licensed Embalmer and Funeral Director
Husband Family Funeral Home
Westland, Michigan

**Barry T. Lease, PhD**
Program Director
Pittsburgh Institute of Mortuary Science
Pittsburgh, Pennsylvania

**Stephanie Bookout Sommer**
Funeral Director and Medical Examiner Liaison
Gift of Life Michigan
Ann Arbor, Michigan

# Contributors

**Brytany Bailey, RN, BSN**
Tissue Recovery Manager
Gift of Life Michigan
Ann Arbor, Michigan

**Thomas J. Buist, MBIE**
Mortuary Science Licensee
The Dodge Company
USA

**Mike Cloud, CFSP**
Licensed Embalmer
Cloud Mortuary Services
Whitesburg, Georgia

**Melissa A. Cyfers, BS, MS, MA**
Program Director
Fine Mortuary College
Norwood, Massachusetts

**Christopher L. Donhost**
Donor Recovery Liaison
Sierra Donor Services
Sacramento, California

**Kevin A. Drobish, BS, CFC**
Administrative Coordinator
Pittsburgh Institute of Mortuary Science
Pittsburgh, Pennsylvania

**Jzyk S. Ennis, PhD**
Instructor, Funeral Service Education
Jefferson State Community College
Birmingham, Alabama

**Dave Gifford**
Licensed Funeral Director - Class 1
Department of Anatomy and Cell Biology
The University of Western Ontario
London, Ontario, Canada

**Daryl M. Hammond**
Licensed Funeral Director and Embalmer
Jefferson, GA

**Kendra E. Harris**
Funeral Home/Medical Examiner Liaison
The Living Legacy Foundation of Maryland
Baltimore, Maryland

**Christina Tursi Holmes, CFSP**
Clinical Instructor, Piedmont Technical College
Greenwood, South Carolina
Funeral Home Liaison, We Are Sharing Hope SC
Charleston, South Carolina

**Edward Karber**
General Manager
Denver Personal Care Center
Denver, Colorado

**Alain Koninckx, MBIE, CFSP**
Licensed Embalmer
Namur, Belgium

**Haley Linklater**
Body Bequeathal Coordinator/Lab Supervisor
Department of Anatomy and Cell Biology
Schulich School of Medicine & Dentistry
The University of Western Ontario
London, Ontario, Canada

**Cody L. Lopasky, MA, CFSP**
Associate Dean of Academics and Distance Education Coordinator
Commonwealth Institute of Funeral Service
Houston, Texas

**Andrew Palombella**
Prosector and Lab Demonstrator
Education Program in Anatomy
McMaster University
Hamilton, Ontario, Canada

**Jasmine Rockarts**
Prosector and Lab Demonstrator
Education Program in Anatomy
McMaster University
Hamilton, Ontario, Canada

**Shawna R. Rodabaugh, MBA**
Program Coordinator of Embalming and Anatomical
  Laboratories
Fayetteville Technical Community College
Fayetteville, North Carolina

**Curpri Sanders, MPH, CTBS**
Referral Intake Manager
Funeral Director and Medical Examiner Liaison
Gift of Life Michigan
Ann Arbor, Michigan

**Gabriel Schauf**
Program Coordinator and Instructor
Milwaukee Area Technical College
Milwaukee, Wisconsin

**Ben Whitworth, CFSP, Dip FD, LMBIFD, MBIE, MEAE, MNZEA**
Education & Technical Support
The MazWell Group Ltd
Whitchurch, Hampshire, United Kingdom

**Rickey Williams II, BSEE, MBA**
Instructor and Clinical Coordinator
Gupton-Jones College of Funeral Service
Decatur, Georgia

# Past Contributors, 1990-2012

*The following individuals contributed to the development of this textbook, either at its inception or throughout the five editions.*

John Alsobrooks, MS
R. Stanley Barnes
Daniel Buchanan, MA
Jeff Chancellor
Paul Cimiluca, BS, MA
William Counce, PhD
Emmet Crahan
Kenneth Curl, PhD
James M. Dorn, MS
Donald E. Douthit, MS
Dan Flory, PhD
Vernie R. Fountain
Jerome F. Fredrick, PhD
Sharon L. Gee, BS
Arthur Grabowski
Marvin E. Grant, Med
David G. Hicks, MSEd
Barbara M. Hopkins, PhD
Patty S. Hutcheson
Edward C. Johnson
Gail R. Johnson
Melissa Johnson, CFSP
Ralph Klicker, MSEd
John M. Kroshus, PhD
Michael Kubasak
Michael Landon
Daniel Lawlor
Terry McEnany, MA
Michael C. Mathews, MA

Robert G. Mayer, CFSP, FBIE
Nathan Minnich
Louis Misantone
Stuart E. Moen, MA
Frank P. Nagy, PhD
Shun Newbern
Robert W. Ninker
Eugene C. Ogrodnik
John B. Pludeman
George H. Poston, PhD
Leandro Rendon, MS
N. Thomas Rogness, MA
Gordon W. Rose, PhD
Curtis D. Rostad
Shelly J. Roy
C. Richard Sanders
Donald W. Sawyer
Dale E. Stroud
Brenda L. Tersine, MA
John R. Trout
Todd W. Van Beck, MA
Michael Weakland
Karl Wenzel
Larry Whitaker
Kenneth R. Whittaker
Alta Williams

# Foreword

*"You must express your grief at the death of a loved one, and then you must move on. The eyes of the dead must be gently closed and the eyes of the living must be gently opened."*

Jan Brugler, 1973

October 1990, the National Funeral Directors Association 109th convention was held in Louisville, Kentucky. On the opening day, a book signing was held for three primary authors/editors who had published new books relevant to funeral service. Included was Howard C. Raether, Michael Kubasak, and myself, Robert Mayer. As the line formed in front of me by persons who had purchased, *Embalming: History, Theory and Practice*, the thought suddenly struck me, *What is appropriate to write as greeting in a book whose subject is embalming?*

Dr. Gordon Bigelow, Executive Director of the American Board of Funeral Service Education, had agreed, at my insisting, to place the Jan Brugler quote above in his foreword in that first 1990 edition. At the signings what to say was simple . . . .it was merely a matter of drawing the purchaser's attention to the quote, for indeed, it states the purpose and mission of funeral service. That Brugler quote was later included in all four editions that would follow during my time as primary author/editor. In addition, I usually added the statement "the learning never ends!"

This sixth edition of *Embalming: History, Theory and Practice,* is the culmination of a joint project first begun by the American Board of Funeral Service Education and the National Funeral Directors Association in 1984. These groups identified the need for a completely new instructional and reference work on embalming. Start-up *seed monies* were provided by the Heritage Club of the NFDA. Three dozen funeral service educators, practitioners and suppliers made an early draft of twenty-five chapters, portions of which were later incorporated in the final 1990 first edition. In 2012, the fifth edition contained the names of over fifty contributors! The text has grown from a national to an internationally recognized definitive teaching and reference work.

Dr. Bigelow's foreword in that first edition also stated, "This book covers embalming as no other book ever has . . . useful as a teaching text, historical or technical reference for the funeral service practitioner or the lay reader." All six editions have contained the core curriculum and glossary of the subject of embalming, drafted by the American Board of Funeral Service Education. Course content is reviewed on a set cycle of every seven years. Initial drafts of this uniform curriculum originated as early as the Second Teachers Institute held in 1947 in Pittsburgh. This latest edition continues to include the histories of embalming and restorative arts written and updated over the years by Edward and Gail Johnson and their daughter Melissa Johnson-Williams. Each edition has included a library of *Selected Readings* - current topics and in-depth studies with relevance to embalming and the mortuary arts and sciences representing a diverse group of authors.

This edition returns to the original format of the first two editions which covered only the topic of embalming. Both sections on restorative art treatments and mortuary cosmetology have been removed. These subjects are best covered in greater depth within available texts related directly to these topics.

Those who are familiar with previous editions of this textbook will find a new look in many respects. A fresh new look begins with all new color photographs. This is the first full color edition. The first four editions contained only black-and-white photographs, the fifth edition had simply a color center insert of ten pages. The chapter objectives have been revised. Additional questions and terminology have been added to Concepts for Study in each chapter. Instrumentation and OSHA materials have been updated. A greater emphasis has been placed on the use of personal protective equipment. Alternative methods of body disposition are presented. Finally, a completely new chapter on the preparation of organ and tissue donors.

The preparation of this sixth edition has been in the capable hands of Sharon Gee-Mascarello, licensed embalmer and funeral director in Michigan for 35 years, and instructor for nearly a quarter of a century with Wayne State University Mortuary Science Program; teaching embalming theory and practice her entire tenure. She has also taught in the areas of mortuary cosmetology and presentation of the body, world religions and coordinated student practicum rotations. Numerous times Professor Gee-Mascarello has received the Part-Time Faculty Award, nominated by her students as their outstanding instructor and by the University. Her classroom experience makes her thoroughly familiar with the American Board embalming syllabus and curriculum and current literature in the funeral service profession.

Since 1985, she has been associated with several Michigan funeral homes serving in the capacity of funeral director, manager, and OSHA compliance officer. She continues in the capacity of consultant, funeral director and embalmer for several funeral establishments. This allows her contact with families, firm employees, and student interns, as well as hundreds of former students.

She is a recognized name in funeral service continuing education circles being called for presentations by a diverse number of funeral organizations in a number of states. She is an engaging and informative presenter and a skilled writer, having contributed technical articles to a variety of professional journals. She served on the editorial committee for the fourth and fifth editions of this textbook. Most recently, she produced and was principal demonstrator for video materials used for the distance learning program at Wayne State, including a 15-minute "Introduction to Embalming" video.

Her curriculum vitae lists memberships in local, state, national and international funeral service organizations; including membership in the nationally recognized Academy of Professional Funeral Service Practitioners (APFSP), carrying the recognized status acronym CFSP (Certified Funeral Service Professional).

Education is obtained by various disciplines, those who practice the mortuary art and science of embalming and its related subjects become educated and skilled by a variety of sources – classroom instruction – mentors – practical experience – seminars – internet discussion groups – virtual seminars – written journal articles – tutors – preceptor/intern/apprentice relationships and of course textbooks. Education is a shared experience, as each of the aforesaid demonstrate. Textbooks contain the principles and standards of a particular subject. This revised sixth edition of *Embalming: History, Theory and Practice,* under the authorship and editorial direction of Sharon Gee-Mascarello gives funeral service practitioners and *future* funeral service practitioners a valuable tool in the mortuary art and science in the care of the deceased human body as practiced in the early years of the twenty-first century.

**Robert G. Mayer**
Pittsburgh, Pennsylvania
February 2021

# Preface

*Embalming: History, Theory, and Practice* is considered the gold standard in embalming education. The previous five volumes of work by Robert G. Mayer formed an indelible impression upon generations of embalmers, myself included. I am honored to serve as primary author and editor of this sixth edition by appointment of the American Board of Funeral Service Education.

Preparation for the sixth edition of this textbook began *pre-pandemic*, a phrase now deeply rooted in our collective experience. Before any of us could fathom the devastating impact of the novel coronavirus, we planned for future events and lived our daily lives in the usual fashion. When death occurred, we engaged the funeral home, planned the memorial event, and invited the attendance of family and friends. But COVID-19 upended plans for honoring our dead and derailed timelines for fulfilling final disposition. Public health concerns questioned the feasibility of indoor public gatherings and imposed attendance limitations for funerals and homegoing celebrations. Physical distancing measures further restricted human contact. All gestures of consolation were discouraged in favor of contactless greetings. The hand shaking and hand holding, extended bear hugs, and tearful embraces reduced to a swift bump of an elbow or fist. Touch became something to avoid. The lowering of heads and closing of eyes conveyed healing emotions that defied being stifled.

Initially, even the embalming of the dead seemed taboo. As we yearned for physical connection with the ones we love, we also longed to be present with the ones we had lost. Adaptation and resilience in the face of adversity prevails. The funeral professionals found a way. The embalmers understand how embalming chemistry supports the inactivation of viral pathogens and slows the progression of natural postmortem changes. Personal protective equipment coupled with infectious embalming protocols provided safeguards. Embalming paused time so that necessary decisions could be made for the dead. Poet W.H. Auden ordered, *"stop all the clocks...bring out the coffin, let the mourners come"*. Perhaps Auden's lament to pause time and gather together for one final moment with the deceased punctuates this significant benefit of embalming. Time is an elusive commodity in ordinary times. During a pandemic, time shared for any reason is priceless. Gathering for somber or celebratory farewells and time afforded for one last look upon the faces of the beloved is both priceless and essential.

Completion of this manuscript surpassed two years. During the sanctioned quarantine I consumed the daily barrage of virus updates. There were few opportunities to leave the house. Sporadic getaways were confined to the essential work of directing funerals, embalming, and periodic quests to find needed provisions. A self-imposed sequestering followed the quarantine. I reviewed all five previous editions of this textbook, poured over curriculum outlines, read countless journal articles, attended webinars, and kept contact with colleagues. Total immersion in matters of death care definitively set my belief in the merits of embalming and in the significance of ceremony.

Pandemic aftershocks appear inexhaustible. Global mourning is palpable. Life and death rituals may be altered indefinitely. Yet, allied death care professionals continue to honor those lives lived and function with resilience beyond the challenges. The embalmers continue to care for the dead; to bathe and groom them, provide minimal care and embalming care, and restore a comforting expression to each of the quieted faces. The funeral directors continue to facilitate the final events of memorialization and faithfully lay the dead to rest. I have never been so proud of Funeral Service.

**Sharon L. Gee-Mascarello**
Saint Clair Shores, Michigan
April 2021

# Acknowledgments

I am indebted to so many people who have given valued counsel and made worthy recommendations during the preparation of the sixth edition of *Embalming: History, Theory, and Practice*. Without your input and unwavering support of this project, the final outcome would not have been possible. Accepting the role of editor for a textbook that is revered by embalmers around the globe is a daunting task that has proven more rewarding than I could have ever imagined. I am honored to follow in the footsteps of Robert G. Mayer who is widely admired and considered a legendary figure in embalming education. Bob, the privilege of stewarding your collection of work means more to me than I can properly express.

To the members of the American Board of Funeral Service Education who granted me this unparalleled career opportunity, I am grateful to each of you. A special mention to Mark Evely for encouraging me to apply for the position. My sincerest thanks to Robert C. Smith, III for your unwavering patience when a number of unexpected curveballs temporarily affected the book's progress. Special appreciation to Deb Tolboom who fielded my phone calls and emails and forwarded updates to the membership. With utmost admiration I recognize the members of the Editorial Committee: Jzyk S. Ennis, Gary J. Brown, Dedrick A. Gantt, and Barry T. Lease. These fine educators volunteered countless hours to review the final manuscript. Your comments were helpful and your contributions enhance the overall narrative.

My heartfelt thank you to Melissa Johnson Williams for adding new content to *The Origin and History of Embalming* and *History of Modern Restorative Art* chapters. These historical accounts were written in collaboration with Melissa's parents, Edward C. and Gail R. Johnson, both former educators. These works have continued as a mainstay of the book since the second edition.

I am indebted to Dr. Jeffrey Bellefleur for his medical perspective and for climbing aboard and staying for the duration of this wild ride. Dr. Jeff's deep appreciation of funeral directors and embalmers prompted him to read the fifth edition cover to cover. Many engaging conversations ultimately shaped some areas of the narrative to better suit student readers.

Special thanks to the following individuals who made worthwhile suggestions: James Omar Clea, James Norris, and Sandra Zampogna of Pittsburgh Institute of Mortuary Science (Class of 2019); Emily Allera, Skyler Barnett, Jessica Hoover, Andrew "Owen" Lorence, Geoffrey Muir, Kayden Nachtyr, Haley Simpson, and Jillian Thompson of Wayne State University Mortuary Science Program (Class of 2019); and Amanda Chanske, Kylie Strong, and Paige Williams (Class of 2020).

I am very appreciative of the following individuals who created original artwork for this edition: Tim Lawlis for the outstanding cover design, Kristine Miller for color renditions of various suturing methods, Darryl G. Shreve for updating the body outline in the decedent care report, and Cherie Mascarello for illustrating the longitudinal vessel incision. Adding a full complement of new color photographs involved an enormous collaborative effort. Abundant thanks to Kevin A. Drobish and Barry T. Lease of Pittsburgh Institute of Mortuary Science; to Kevin for supplying needed photos on demand and to Dr. Lease for sharing your library of images. Photos of the Denver Personal Care Center were made possible by Vern Pixley and Edward Karber of Dignity Memorial. Thank you to Chris Janowiak, Fred Voran, Jr., and the late Dick Kaatz for allowing me access to photograph your newly-appointed preparation rooms.

Thank you to Tim Collison of the Dodge Company and Alicia Carr of Kelco Supply Company for supplying the embalming instrument images. And to the following companies for providing images of the various embalming machines: the Dodge Company, Frigid Fluid Company, Pierce Chemical/The Wilbert Group, The Embalmers Supply Company (ESCO), NoAyr Funeral Supply, Inc., and Radical Scientific Pvt. Ltd.

A warm expression of gratitude to the individuals who invited us to share in their personal loss through the images appearing in the first chapter: Roger Husband, Keith Humes, ShaQuita Johnson, and Chris Belcher; Duff Chamberlain in memory of his wife, Roxane Benavides; Dr. Jeff Wilner in memory of his mother, Marjorie Wilner; and Aftyn (D'Anthony) Carroll in memory of her father, Charles Vallette.

A very special thank you to Stephanie Sommer and Curpri Sanders of Gift of Life Michigan. Many of the organ and tissue recovery photos are credited to Curpri. Stephanie contributed updated information regarding the donation process, reviewed seemingly endless drafts of the chapter, and regularly checked in with me for progress updates. I am also grateful for contributions from Duff D. Chamberlain, Christopher L. Donhost, Kendra E. Harris, and Christina Tursi Holmes.

I am grateful to the Ohio Embalmers Association for supporting my trip to Chicago for the 2019 National Funeral Directors Association International Convention and Expo. I attended every technical seminar and engaged in conversation with each of the presenters. Listening to colleagues share experiences and offer best practices has yielded great benefit in the preparation of this sixth edition.

The team at McGraw Hill deserves accolades. Thank you to my editors, Michael Weitz, Kim Davis, and Sydney Keen for expertly navigating a first-timer through the textbook publishing process. And to Becky Hainz-Baxter for securing permissions from a myriad of contributors and serving as yet another pair of eyes to review this manuscript. I am grateful to Warishree Pant for endless patience during the compositing amidst numerous edits.

I am blessed with the truest friends. Thank you for an endless supply of encouragement and inspiration. Your words nourished me. I crossed the finish line in large part because of my wife, Cherie. I am so fortunate to share my life with the person I adore and admire most. And I feel so proud to share this significant accomplishment with you.

**Sharon L. Gee-Mascarello**
Saint Clair Shores, Michigan
May 2021

# PART I

## The Theory and Practice of Embalming

# CHAPTER 1

# Origins of Embalming and Reverent Care of the Dead

## CHAPTER OVERVIEW

- Definition of Embalming
- Origins of Burial and Embalming
- Reverent Care of the Dead
- Universal Customs and Rituals
- Viewing of the Body
- Ethical Performance Standards

## EMBALMING DEFINED

Embalming is defined by the American Board of Funeral Service Education (ABFSE) as:

*"the chemical treatment of the dead human body to reduce the presence and growth of microorganisms, to temporarily inhibit organic decomposition, and to restore the dead human body to an acceptable physical appearance."*

Embalming suspends the natural decomposition processes in the deceased human body by creating a temporary state of preservation. Embalming also suspends time for completion of the necessary and numerous details that follow a death. Author and Editor Ron Hast stated, "Embalming is the best-known method of presenting the decedent well through the memorial event."

## BURIAL AND EMBALMING

Anthropological studies demonstrate that burial of the dead is the oldest of all religious customs.

According to Edward C. Johnson, embalming and funeral practice historian, "Embalming as a means of artificially preserving the dead human body is one of humankind's longest practiced arts."[1] Reverence for the dead is deeply ingrained in human nature and is the basic ethical axiom of the funeral service profession. Current mourning customs, cultural practices, and religious ceremonies observe varying forms of preparation and presentation of the dead body.

The earliest known Homo sapiens performed deliberate, ritualistic burials. Reverent care is suggested in the practices of **Homo sapiens neanderthalensis.** Researchers discovered the remains of eight adult and two infant Neanderthals in the Shanidar Cave of northern Iraq. Some of the dead were adorned with elk antlers and shoulder blades. Whole clumps of flower pollen found in the cave suggest the placement of entire flowering plants. Flowers likely served two purposes: as medicinal offerings and to mask unpleasant corpse odors. Stone tools were also discovered. Neanderthal behavior is linked to an instinctual drive to provide care for the dead.

In ancient Egypt, the dead were embalmed according to religious custom. An exhibit at the National Archeological Museum in Athens, Greece, describes the care of the dead: "The ancient Egyptians did not regard death as the end of life, but as an intermediary stage towards a better eternal life. Eternity was achieved by those who had lived a virtuous life and were able to furnish their tombs and receive funerary offerings from their relatives. The poor attained immortality through the mercy of the gods. Released after death, the spiritual elements continued to exist so long as the body remained in a recognizable state, hence the development of mummification." Resting within those ancient tombs of stone, the embalmed and mummified dead, just as old as the pyramids themselves, await eternal life. From ancient Arab proverb, "All the world fears Time, but Time fears the Pyramids."

The funeral has always been an essential ritual of world religions. Specific references to embalming appear twice in the Old Testament of the Christian Bible. *Genesis 50:2–3* recounts the death of Jacob (also known as Israel): "And Joseph commanded his servants the physicians to embalm his father. So the physicians embalmed Israel." *Genesis 50:26* refers to the embalming of Joseph: "So Joseph died, being one hundred and ten years old and they embalmed him, and he was put in a coffin in Egypt." References to the reverent care of the dead are also found in the New Testament. *John 11:44* describes burial preparations for Lazarus: the use of grave straps to bind the

---
[1] See *The Origin and History of Embalming.*

arms, feet, and chin. Similarity is drawn to modern methods of mouth closure and positioning devices used to create natural appearance. The funerary preparations of Jesus describe the binding of his body, dressing in fine white linens, and anointing with spices, fragrant oils, and myrrh. Numerous cultures in the transcontinental region of the Middle East practice ceremonial bathing and shrouding.

Dr. Thomas G. Long, Professor Emeritus, writes, "Rituals of death rest on the basic need, recognized by all societies, to remove the bodies of the dead from among the living. A corpse must be taken fairly quickly from here, the place of death, to somewhere else. But no healthy society has ever treated this as a perfunctory task, a matter of mere disposal. Indeed, from the beginning, humans have used poetry, song, and prayer to describe the journey of the dead from 'here' to 'there' in symbolic, even sacred, terms. The dead are not simply being carted to the pit, the fire, or the river; they are traveling toward the next world or the Mystery or the Great Beyond or heaven or the communion of the saints. And we are accompanying them the last mile of the way. Every generation reimagines these images of what lies beyond this life, but what persists is the conviction that the dead are not refuse to be discarded; they are human treasures traveling somewhere and it is our holy responsibility to go with them all the way to the place of farewell."

The tradition of treating the dead with great reverence and respect is an age-old custom, as old as humanity itself. Funeral service professionals maintain the dignity of all decedents in their care through the consistent application and practice of showing respect and honor for the dead.

## REVERENT CARE OF THE DEAD

Care of the dead is both privilege and responsibility. All who care for the dead are charged with the maintenance of moral and ethical duty. Every profession has a primary and supreme ethic in the discharge of its duties. Medicine, for example, bases professional practice on the Hippocratic Oath, which articulates the ethic of healing. Law bases its practice on the ethic of justice. The supreme ethic for the funeral service profession has come to be known as *reverence for the dead*.

Former British Prime Minister William Evart Gladstone (1809–1898) is cited extensively in funeral service publications. A great ethical truth about reverence for the dead is revealed in his timeless words. Repetition does not lessen the impact.

> *"Show me the manner in which a nation or community cares for its dead and I will measure with mathematical exactness the tender sympathies of its people, their respect for the laws of the land, and their loyalty to high ideals."*

History suggests that the decline of governmental and sociological order can be partly attributed to neglect of the dead. A common denominator in the collapse of powerful regimes and the downfall of civilizations is the rise in apathy toward reverent care of their dead. Ancient Rome, Greece, and the Nazi Germany serve as examples. The lack of proper care for the dead was commonplace. The annals of history depict how the rites, rituals, and ceremonies for mourning the dead serve as barometers to measure the *tender sympathies of its people*.

In her book, *Advice for Future Corpses (and Those Who Love Them)*, Sallie Tisdale shares enlightenment she received as a student of anatomy, "Working with cadavers makes it clear what death *is*. A subject becomes an object. A person becomes a body. And, miraculously, turns *back*: this body, this firm, immobile object, is, was, a person, a warm, breathing person. A body is not an ordinary object—can never be an ordinary object. This particular object had once been awake."

## UNIVERSAL CUSTOMS AND RITUALS

Customs and rituals concerning care and commemoration of the dead are widely diverse. The world over, all cultures attend to some form of care for their dead. Each has developed unique rituals to implement this care. Anthropological, archaeological, and religious literature describes the importance of honoring, mourning, even celebrating the dead. The significance of having the dead present for the memorial event demonstrates a need to maintain a connection with the dead body. The Neanderthals made memorials with elk antlers and shoulder blades; today, we use granite and marble. The ethic is the same; the materials are different. We have an innate ethical drive to care for the dead.

Studies of past civilizations have yielded discoveries of sacred locations where bodies and relics of the dead were placed. Ancient cemeteries, mausoleums, and columbaria suggest a need to maintain a connection with the dead. Present cultures observe sacred resting places and, like their predecessors, erect monuments, and memorials to honor and remember the dead. Through the ages the dead have been commemorated with the creation of art, music, and literature, requiem masses and funeral hymns, and biographies and elegies. This universal ethic of reverence for the dead is ingrained in the human psyche. Different cultures manifest this reverence in widely varying ways. Reverence for the dead is a basic thread binding all of humanity.

### Events That Shaped Public Sentiment

Viewing the dead body is one way of confronting the stark reality of death. Seeing and touching the deceased for one last time can bring comfort. Being physically present with them can foster acceptance of the otherwise unimaginable.

The year was 1955, and the brutal murder of a 14-year-old boy exposed deeply rooted racial injustices and tensions in the American South. The young man's grief-stricken mother defied an order forbidding the casket to be opened. Mamie Till-Mobley insisted that her son's mutilated body be publicly viewed so that everyone could see what his attackers had done. Fifty thousand people in Chicago viewed the lifeless body of Emmett Till. Witnessing the unthinkable can profoundly shape societal views and attitudes.

In 1963, Jessica Mitford published *The American Way of Death*, a relentless attack on the funeral profession. The book caused an immediate uproar among funeral directors. Within months of the book's release, President John F. Kennedy was assassinated. The shocking murder of a beloved president was an event that rocked the entire nation. The funeral of the president was a public event viewed worldwide through media outlets. Over the span of 18 hours, nearly 250,000 people personally paid their respects as former President Kennedy's body lay in state; some are waiting for as long as 10 hours in a line that stretched 40 blocks. Universal grief was palpable. Mourners did not feel comfortable criticizing funeral directors, symbols of compassionate and dignified care when the nation was in the throes of mourning a slain President. To refer to President Kennedy's body merely as *dead tissue,* as Mitford described a dead body, was blasphemous. To dispose of his body without ceremony would have been morally irresponsible.

When a body is missing or unrecovered during military conflict or war, enormous effort and cost go into search and recovery efforts. Anxiety and remorse result when these efforts fail. Without the body, an essential element to the grieving process is missing.

## Psychosocial Model

Human beings are basically social creatures. We talk, live, work, and play with other people. Our social interactions take on many different dimensions. We can have shallow or very deep interactions; we can act with indifference or with profound sympathy. In the course of a single day, we may exhibit these and a thousand other characteristics. It is through this complex web of daily interactions that we experience life and creates attachments to others. The quality of these attachments varies from one relationship to another; some are deep, some shallow, others indifferent, joyful, or painful. Here, we shall explore the role that embalming plays in the process of helping us separate from these attached relationships in a healthy manner.

Within the realm of attachments between people are attachments known as deep links. Deep-link attachments are strong and profoundly interwoven psychological bonds that are extremely powerful. In these circumstances, our needs for security and devotion are satisfied, and virtually every part of the human psyche is involved. Through daily visual and interactive reinforcement of these deep attachments, our relationships with significant persons undergo a kind of layering process in our brains. The thoughts and feelings create perceptual patterns of recognition. These patterns of recognition that develop between people become so familiar that there are instances in which the individual involved is frequently unaware of the depth of these attachments until the relationship is terminated through separation by death, or physical, or emotional distance.

The how and why of attachments are baffling. Attachments are among our most rudimentary attributes, they flourish throughout our lives, and they can be so powerful as to continue even beyond the grave. The magnitude of these attachments are often unrealized by the person, and individuals are often unaware of how deeply their behaviors and attitudes are affected. Attachments arise from countless life experiences. They are created by the sound of a voice, the color of someone's eyes, the texture of someone's hair, and in their style and manner of dress and movement. It is fortunate indeed that humans have the capacity to develop these attachments because they often culminate in deeply cherished, singular relationships with others; feelings of love. It is from this type of deep relationship that we experience the joy of love, but it is equally true that from these same deep attachments, we also experience the inevitable anguish of separation and loss. As painful as it is at times, a fact of human existence is that attachments cannot exist without grief.

It is through continual life experiences shared with significant others that our attachments become rooted. As the theories of attachment demonstrate, our ability to connect with our fellow humans goes very deep. Through this process, familiarity with the characteristics of the significant other is imprinted in our minds. This imprinting is caused by constant exposure to the attached person, and a mental photograph develops in our hearts and minds. In funeral service, this mental photograph is referred to as the **body image**.

The body image that develops is reinforced unconsciously and consciously through our personal interactions with the attached person; we relate and respond to their created sensory image. The sightless is particularly talented at creating a body image using sensory data derived from the senses other than sight, and their verbal descriptions of what they imagine with their mind's eye are remarkably accurate.

We habitually relate to, recognize, and identify our significant others based on the familiar body image to which our perceptions have become attached. Due to this constant exposure to the body image, people often form an unrealistic expectation of permanency in the attached relationship.

It becomes simple for individuals who are profoundly attached to one another to feel confident that the relationship will last forever, irrational as this may seem. Although we know subconsciously that such permanence in even the strongest relationship is simply not possible, many prefer to live under the blissful misconception that death will not end the attachment. Human relationships, however, are not limitless; they too must die, either through physical or psychological separation or ultimately, through death.

It is crucial that the funeral service practitioner appreciates the complex processes behind the separation of human attachment. It is these psychological processes on which the ethic of reverence for the dead is based and which necessitate the need for ceremony. Without human attachments, there would be little, if any, need for funerals. A funeral is, in its most elementary form, a social function that reflects the reality of our capacity to form deep attachments and serves to reinforce that most human beings need to grieve and mourn the dead. Types of memorial events are as diverse as the people who practice them (**Fig. 1–1 A–D**).

Death brings with it a finality that challenges our coping skills. The realization that life once thought to be permanent and everlasting is, in truth, temporary and finite. The bereaved are challenged to divest themselves of their close attachments to the deceased person and redirect emotional energy into relationships with others. This begins the long and often painful process of grief and mourning.

Grieving begins in the bereaved psyche by sensory confrontation with the dead person's retained body image. It is often said that it is better to remember the dead as they were when they were alive. The comment, *I would rather remember them alive,* is a coping mechanism triggered by an inability to accept death. In its purest form, it is a denial of death. For honest confrontation of the reality of death, it is necessary for the mourners to see the deceased person, or a symbol of the deceased person, to fully accept the reality of death. Through the actions of seeing or

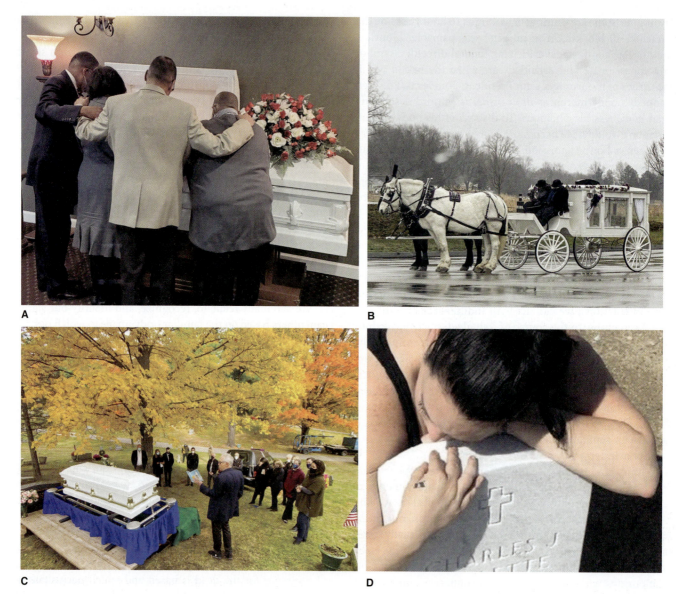

**Figure 1-1.** **A.** Friends embrace at first viewing. **B.** A horse-drawn carriage silently waits before the last ride. **C.** A family member reads at a graveside committal. **D.** A daughter hugs her father's headstone. *(Photo contributors are listed in the Acknowledgements section.)*

touching the deceased, the mourners have a visual and physical opportunity to verify the stark reality of death. When the body of the deceased is unrecoverable, no chance exists to establish the reality of death. There is a risk that mourners will experience complicated grief that lacks resolution.

## Viewing the Body

Emotional confrontation of the reality of death can be achieved when mourners can physically approach the deceased or a symbol of the deceased. Viewing and touching a dead human body is an effective way for the bereaved to accept the finality of death. Grief studies observe the process of complicated grief and find that bereaved persons will deny the significance of the death of someone to whom they were strongly attached. The process of denial takes many forms. American fiction writer Madeleine L'Engle remarked, "I rebel against death, yet I know that it is how I respond to death's inevitability that is going to make me less or more fully alive."

Denial can manifest as avoidance of contact with the reality of death, namely, the dead person's body. At first glance, this avoidance may appear as the bereaved trying to simply maintain composure. Bereavement is not a simple process that can be managed by rational thought alone. Grief is an emotional, not a rational, process.

The comprehension of human separation can never fully be accomplished through intellectual rationalizations. Often, those who are most aggrieved by the death are the ones who would most benefit from accepting the reality of the death.

Dr. Erich Lindemann, a pioneer in the study of grief management, has suggested that there is really *no escaping the slow wisdom of grief*. Lindemann postulates that avoidance of the dead body is always done at the psychological peril of the aggrieved and that this avoidance may appear at first to be consoling in the initial phase of acute grief. *But in truth, consolation is just an illusion. In time, the necessity to view the body becomes a major issue in postbereavement care.*

Lindemann offers that a common characteristic in persons experiencing complicated bereavement is an *inability to recall a clear mental image of the body in death*. Establishment of this mental image is an essential ingredient in creating a strong foundation for subsequent steps in the grieving process. *An unclear image of the deceased person or no image at all fosters a lack of full acceptance of the reality of death.*

Lindemann believed that *the most significant benefit of the funeral and embalming is achieved at that moment when the finality of the death is fully comprehended by the bereaved person. It is this moment of truth, this awareness of the reality of death that serves as the psychological framework for the validation of embalming.* The embalmed body is a stark confrontation; nevertheless, there is no denying the finality of death.

Author, Poet, and Funeral Director, Thomas Lynch, in his book *Bodies in Motion and at Rest*, "…'but remembering him the way he was,' I say, slowly, deliberately, as if the listener were breakable, 'begins by denying the way he is.' I'm an apostle of the present tense. After years and years of directing funerals, I've come to the conclusion that seeing is the hardest and most helpful part. The truth, even when it hurts, has a healing in it, better than fiction or fantasy. When someone dies, it is not them we fear seeing, it is **them dead**. It is the death. We fear that seeing will be believing."

Reverend Paul Irion believes that the function of embalming is to *make the body presentable for viewing*. This is expressed in other life situations. For example, a person prepares for social activity by performing grooming rituals, bathing, and combing the hair before greeting people in public. The ethical concepts of reverence for the dead require the same considerations during care of the dead body for viewing. In this way, the dignity of the deceased is also preserved after death.

## RITUALS AND CEREMONIES

We see the need to be social in order to live a happy, balanced life in the rituals and rites performed by human beings. Entrenched in the makeup of humankind is a ritualistic behavior that a breakdown or corruption of these life rituals may result in a human cataclysm.

Dr. Carl Jung, a pioneer in psychology, saw human psychological life as a universal phenomenon whereby identification with what he termed the *collective unconscious* linked all humanity together. Collectively, we differ by ethnicity, culture, religion, social attitudes, and so on, yet some shared constants exist that we can all identify with and understand. An archetype of our collective unconscious is the funeral event.

### Practical Model of Embalming

The practical purpose of embalming is to slow the degenerative changes that occur naturally after death. This allows the bereaved the time to make important decisions. Embalming permits time for family and friends to engage in the emotionally healing process of *leave-taking*. To fully implement the ethical, psychological, and sociological benefits of the funeral, people require time for assimilation. People need time to organize funerals, think about them, participate in them, and make decisions about how they should be carried out. Time is also required for the bereaved to assimilate all that has happened, and acknowledge the ramifications in their own lives.

Lynda Cheldelin Fell, the author of the award-winning Grief Diaries series, speaks in support of healthy grieving, "The bereaved need more than just space to grieve the loss. They also need the space to grieve the transition."

## THE ETHICAL PERFORMANCE STANDARD

Ethics is the science of rectitude and duty. Its subject is morality, and its sphere is virtuous conduct. It is concerned with the various aspects of rights and obligations. In essence, ethics is a set of principles that governs conduct for the purpose of establishing harmony in all human relations. For practical purposes, ethics is fair play. Ethical practice serves as a guide in promoting professional attitudes and ensuring ethical conduct. Sound and practical judgment are exercised in all professional interactions. This may be called judicious counsel. Funeral service professionals maintain a neutral position in serving the public at large. Courtesy, tact, and discretion should characterize all of the embalmer's professional actions.

### Misrepresentation

When the performance of duty requires licensure, the embalmer must never aid or abet an unlicensed person who engages in the unlicensed activity.

### Confidentiality

All personal information must be regarded as confidential. The embalmer is privy to information that must never be shared outside of the performance of duty. For example, the cause and manner of death and condition of the body are strictly confidential.

### Defamation of Character

Insinuations, nonfactual statements, or overplay of facts that have the intent or effect of harming another professional are unethical and must be avoided.

### Identification

The embalmer is responsible for maintaining the proper identification of the body throughout the various stages of preparation and until the time of final disposition. (see Selected Readings, *Identification: An Essential Part of What We Do*, by Michael Kubasak).

### Observing Laws, Rules, and Regulations

The embalmer must observe all legal and regulatory requirements; federal, state, or local governments and municipalities.

### Maintaining Competence in Professional Practice

The embalmer has a moral and ethical duty to maintain skills commensurate with professional practice. Opportunities for continuing education are numerous and readily accessible both in-person and remotely. Many states require a minimum number of continuing education credits or hours to maintain licensure.

### Health and Sanitation

It is the ethical responsibility to maintain a clean and sanitary work environment, offer personal protective equipment to any person allowed access to the preparation room, restrict entry to unauthorized persons, and maintain coverage of sheltered human remains.

### Documentation

Embalming must be authorized by expressed or written permission prior to the performance of the procedure. An Embalming and

Decedent Care Report should be completed for every decedent. Personal effects should be documented and securely maintained.

## Photographs

Photographs may only be taken in the performance of duty. Authorized photographs must be safeguarded, both digitally and physically, to ensure confidentiality. It is wise and prudent for the embalmer to secure permission from the authorizing agent prior to taking photographs.

## Handling Human Remains

Funeral practitioners must ensure the dignity of human remains at all times. Transferring practices from the place of death are accomplished in a manner that is respectful and involves the same level of care afforded a living patient. All mortuary equipment is maintained in a clean and sanitary condition. The modesty of the deceased person is maintained while coverings are removed. Universal precautions are strictly observed.

## Professional Embalming Standards

The Chicago-based American Society for Embalmers created a document of best practices to support the exemplary practice of embalming.

**American Society of Embalmers**

**Best Practice Embalming Tenets©**

- Treat all deceased human remains with thoughtful care, maintain dignity, and show respect at all times.
- Be knowledgeable of and in compliance with all regulatory authorities (federal, state, and local) that govern the preparation and disposition of deceased human remain.
- Prioritize the use of excellent communications among all funeral professionals involved with the decedent and family.
  - Authorizations for embalming and restorative art procedures must be shared with the embalmer, preferably in writing.
  - Confirm the identity of the deceased prior to the commencement of any procedures.
  - The Preparation Room should be kept private, and all local, state and federal laws should be observed as to its use.
  - Share information regarding the care of the deceased between the director and embalmer.
    - Obtain information about the overall condition of the remains.
    - Obtain information about the cause or nature of death.
    - Obtain the time of services to optimize the best presentation.
      - Ensure that adequate time is given to the embalming process.
      - Address and remedy problem embalming and shipping situations immediately.
- All documents, photographs, and personal information about the deceased must be kept in strict confidence and under secure storage.
  - Only those persons designated and authorized by the funeral establishment or family may be allowed attendance during the preparation of remains.
  - Photographs of deceased remains must never be placed on social media sites or shown in public places to nonfuneral professionals outside the educational setting.
- Respect and comply, without comment, with the wishes of the family or the deceased requesting organ/tissue donation, hospital or forensic autopsy, or full body donation to science.
- Professional conduct will ensure that embalmers will not knowingly allow nonlicensed embalmers (except students or apprentices, under supervision) to practice embalming and that they will not participate in derogatory public comments about other embalmers.
- Pursue ongoing and continuing education opportunities for the embalmer.
- Practice thorough and complete preservation of the entire remains.
  - Use all available embalming methods necessary: arterial, hypodermic, surface.
- Document all remains to enter the funeral facility on a Preparation Care Form.
  - Include remains for: identification only, storage, embalming, shipped-in, or shipped-out.
- Be knowledgeable of multiple methods of treating all types of embalming cases, regardless of their condition.
  - Practice custodial care; monitor remains until final disposition and makes corrections as needed.
  - Be willing to ask for assistance when needed.
- Protect yourself from all potential hazards: infectious, chemical, and physical.
- The establishment ownership and the embalming practitioner agree to have available all the necessary supplies, chemicals, dry goods, and equipment to prepare every type of embalming case.
- The preparation room and adjoining facilities will be maintained in a clean and sanitary condition.

### CONCEPTS FOR STUDY

1. State the definition of embalming accepted by the American Board of Funeral Service Education.
2. Explain the meaning of reverent care of the dead.
3. Repeat the quote by William Evart Gladstone.
4. List the benefits of viewing the dead human body as it relates to the grieving process.
5. How can funerals and memorial events confront the reality of death as well as celebrate the life of the person who has died?
6. Express the importance of ethical conduct.
7. Relate a way for the embalmer to maintain professional competence.
8. Explain ways to assure the dignity of the dead human body.

# BIBLIOGRAPHY

Duncan L. Funerals are for the living. *Women's Health* March 1986:28.

Federal Trade Commission: Funeral Rule: 16CFR Part 453.

Gladstone WE. *Dictionary of Thoughts.* New York: Standard Books, Inc., 1974:213.

Hast R. *The Art of Embalming and its Purpose*, Mortuary Management, September 2006.

*Holy Bible,* Revised Standard Version. New York: Thomas Nelson and Sons, 1952.

Irion PE. *The Funeral: Vestige or Value?* Nashville, TN: The Parthenon Press, 1966.

Lindemann E. Psychological aspects of mourning. Cited in: Jackson E. *For the Living.* Des Moines, IA: The Channel Press, 1963.

Long Thomas G. *Chronicle of a Death We Can't Accept*, The New York Times, 31 Oct. 2009.

Lynch T. *Bodies in Motion and at Rest.* New York: W.W. Norton, 2000.

*Organ and Tissue Procurement Manual.* Pittsburgh, PA: Pittsburgh Transplant Foundation, 1987.

*Resource Manual.* Brookfield, WI: National Funeral Directors Association, 1979.

Roach M. *Stiff: The Curious Lives of Human Cadavers.* New York: W.W. Norton, 2003.

Solecki RS, Leroi-Gourhan A. Paleoclimatology and archeology in the Near East. *Ann N Y Acad Sci* 1961; Vol. XCV (Art. 1):729–739.

Tisdale, Sallie. *Advice for Future Corpses (and Those Who Love Them): A Practical Perspective on Death and Dying.* Simon and Schuster, 2018.

*Undertaking Ethics.* Springfield, IL: Funeral Ethics Association, 1994.

# CHAPTER 2

# Fundamentals of Embalming

## CHAPTER OVERVIEW

- Preservation, Sanitation, and Restoration
- Expectations of Embalming
- Classifications of Embalming
  - Arterial Embalming
  - Cavity Embalming
  - Hypodermic Embalming
  - Surface Embalming
- Embalming Fundamentals
- Anatomical and Soft Embalming Methods
- APPENDIX—Embalming and Decedent Care Forms

Embalming is both science and art. Embalming is the applied chemical process concerned with sanitation and the temporary preservation of the dead body. Embalming is also a restorative process. Restoration focuses on creating and maintaining the acceptable, natural appearance of the deceased. Both elements are combined with stabilizing the body and suspend further putrefactive changes. Temporary preservation slows organic decomposition for a time. At the least, until the final disposition of the body. Embalming is customarily requested when the funeral, celebration of life, or other types of the memorial event involves public viewing of the body. The entirety of all embalming processes, in combination, serve to maintain the integrity of the body throughout the memorial event. Slowing the progression of postmortem changes purchases time so that the living can make substantive final decisions; an infinite number of them. Planning and preparation require time.

Embalming for the anatomical study of the dead human body, for medical research, and for attaining competency in clinical skills is essential to the advancement of medical science. Virtual methods reproduce human anatomy with accuracy. Virtual reality is an impressive and effective substitution. However, a true, complete reproduction of an actual human body defies replication.

Without some form of chemical intervention, decomposition will continue. Decomposition is defined as *the separation of compounds into simpler substances by the action of microbial enzymes and/or autolytic enzymes.* Decomposition begins at death. Embalming inhibits the cycle of decomposition. Indefinite preservation requires methods beyond embalming practices performed for memorialization. Indefinite preservation can negatively alter the appearance of the deceased. The length of time a body will remain preserved and recognizable is dependent upon numerous factors both within the body (intrinsic) and outside of the body (extrinsic). Intrinsic factors include pathologic processes, circulatory conditions, degree of body moisture, distribution of the preservative chemicals, and many others. Extrinsic factors include the type of preservatives used, strength and volume of embalming solutions, and environmental factors surrounding the interment or entombment (casket, vault, crypt), such as the amount of moisture, molds, bacteria, insects, and air. Under ideal conditions, embalming may be so thorough and unaffected that recognition of the face is possible many, many years later. Conversely, under unfavorable conditions, the preservation may be as brief as few days. Variables too numerous prevent assurances regarding the degree or length of time that preservation of the embalmed body can be maintained.

## PRESERVATION AND SANITATION

Embalming preservatives and germicides interact primarily with body proteins. The colloidal nature of the protein changes by establishing many cross-linkages that were not formerly present between adjacent proteins. The chemicals and the proteins combine to form a latticework of inert firm material—the **embalmed tissue**—that can no longer be easily broken down by bacterial or autolytic body enzymes.

Body proteins have many reactive centers and a great affinity to hold water. Embalming destroys these reactive centers, and the new protein-like substance no longer has the ability to retain water. As a result, these new (embalmed) protein structures are more stable and longer-lasting. Thus, the tissues are temporarily preserved. The inability of the embalmed tissue to hold water results in dryness to the embalmed tissue.

Enzymes have the ability to react with the body's proteins, fats, and carbohydrates and cause the decomposition of these body substrates. Enzymes are proteins, and they originate from body cells (autolytic enzymes) or bacteria (bacterial enzymes). Chemicals such as germicides, and preservatives in embalming fluids inactivate the body's enzymes. These same chemicals also destroy bacteria (pathogenic and nonpathogenic) through reactions with the proteins that are a part of these organisms. The likelihood of the body remaining a source of disease-producing microbes or their products is greatly reduced. Through conversion or inactivation (embalming) of (1) protein of the tissues, (2) protein of enzymes, and (3) protein of microbes, the body is sanitized and temporarily preserved. The degree of preservation depends on the number of contacts made between the preservative chemicals and the proteins of the body and the bacteria.

# RESTORATION

Restoration of the deceased to an acceptable appearance is a function of embalming. Restoration of the dead human body is not to reproduce life but rather to lessen the effects of illness, trauma, and the myriad of naturally occurring postmortem changes. Long-term illnesses and diseases, extended drug therapies, surgeries, tumors, traumas, disfigurements, and a host of postmortem changes all can adversely affect appearance. Injection of the proper embalming chemicals can (1) restore the contour of facial features, (2) decrease facial swelling, (3) remove postmortem intravascular discolorations, (4) reduce extravascular blood discolorations, and (5) restore the natural facial complexion.

## Summary and Expectations of the Embalming Process

In 1928, Professor Charles O. Dhonau, dean of the Cincinnati College of Embalming, defined the functions of embalming fluid and the process by which the fluid reaches the cells of the body. Professor Dhonou explained the function of embalming fluids to achieve sanitation, preservation, and restoration of the body's tissues. His definition remains relevant.

*An embalming fluid is a chemical substance*

*which when given physical application (or injection)*

*at the right time*

*at the right temperature*

*in the right quantity*

*of the right quality, strength dilution, concentration*

*so as to receive a complete distribution in arteries, capillaries and veins*

*will diffuse (spread) from the capillaries*

*to the lymph spaces and to the intercellular spaces*

*and to the cellular tissues*

*to unite with the cellular substances*

*so as to normalize their water content*

*restore their colors*

*and so to fix and preserve them that they will be preserved against organized (bacterial)*

*and unorganized (enzymatic) decompositions*

*and will be preserved against other kinds of changes such as in water content; oxidation; from soil chemicals*

*just so long as the after-care provides the necessary means to protect*

*what has been embalmed.*

*A part which has been embalmed will not discolor from any cause within several weeks; it will not become*

*blood discolored; or show dehydration changes;*

*or show greenish colors from protein decompositions;*

*or become malodorous from protein decompositions;*

*by proteolytic bacterial enzymes by which spore forming anaerobes, seeking (bound) oxygen, break up compounds containing it and release odorous gasses such as hydrogen sulfide;*

*or become gas distended from the gaseous decomposition of proteins*

*or carbohydrates (tissue gas); nor will the tissues soften and finally liquefy*

*through the work of organized or unorganized ferments;*

*nor will the tissues of the body pass through the cycle of changes which at the end converts the hundred or more body compounds into*

*water, nitrogen, methane and carbon dioxide, as a result of all the*

*oxidations through which decompositions proceed. A part which has*

*not been properly embalmed should be thought of by the embalmer*

*as an unsolved embalming problem, to which he or she has contributed either by lack of understanding, by carelessness or by both.*

**Cincinnati College of Mortuary Science, 1928. From Dhonau, CO, Defining Embalming Fluid.**

# CLASSIFICATIONS OF EMBALMING

There are four classifications of embalming. Each embalming treatment is applied separately. Temporary preservation, sanitation, and restoration of the dead human body are the most effective when embalming treatments are used in combination.

- **Arterial embalming.** *Also called vascular embalming.*
- **Cavity embalming.**
- **Hypodermic embalming.** *Also called subcuticular embalming.*
- **Surface embalming.**

**Arterial embalming** utilizes the blood vascular system to deliver preservative solutions to all areas of the body at once. The chemical solutions circulate throughout the blood vascular system and make contact with the tissues and cells of the body. A rudimentary explanation is the embalming solution is injected into an artery of the body while blood products are evacuated from a vein. Embalming solution is customarily delivered by a motorized **embalming machine.** An instrument called an **arterial tube** is attached to the hosing of the machine; the arterial tube is then placed into an artery. The solution in the machine replaces the blood in the vascular system.

**Cavity embalming** is the direct treatment of the contents of three body cavities: thoracic, abdominal, and pelvic as well as the lumina of the hollow viscera. Cavity embalming is applied in two phases: **aspiration** of the cavity contents and **injection** of undiluted cavity fluid. Both aspiration and injection are accomplished by an instrument called a **trocar**. Cavity embalming routinely follows arterial embalming.

**Hypodermic embalming** is the subcuticular injection of embalming chemicals directly into the tissues using a hypodermic syringe and needle (for smaller areas) or a hypovalve trocar (for larger areas). Hypodermic embalming is considered a supplemental embalming procedure.

**Surface embalming** is the preservation of tissues by direct contact. Preservative chemicals are applied to a cotton compress or inlay that makes contact with the tissues, or the chemical is applied directly to the skin surface. Surface embalming is considered a supplemental embalming procedure.

## Arterial and Cavity Embalming Combined

The primary mechanism in arterial embalming involves the replacement of body fluids with embalming fluids. The embalming procedure is conducted in two stages. The first stage is arterial embalming; the second stage is cavity embalming. Arterial embalming of the average adult body (males 200 pounds; females 171 pounds) is essentially the injection of several gallons of preservative solution under pressure into the circulatory system through a large artery, such as the common carotid or femoral. Blood and tissue fluids are concurrently removed to create room for the preservative solution from a large vein. The internal jugular vein is customarily selected as the primary source of blood drainage. The selection of embalming vessels is determined by a process used to evaluate postmortem body conditions, called **embalming analysis**.

The preservative solution flows through the arterial, capillary, and venous routes, similar to the blood circulation in the living body. The basic difference is that the embalming solution does not pass through the chambers of the heart in the same way that it does in the living body. Instead, when the solution reaches the ascending aorta, it places pressure against the aortic semilunar valves and forces them to close. Once the valves are tightly shut, the ascending aorta, arch of the aorta, and the entire aorta fill with the preservative solution and flow into the numerous branches of the circulatory system.

The capillary is the simplest division of the blood vascular system; it is the structural mediator through which the injected preservative chemicals are delivered to the receptive tissue sites. In this sense, arterial embalming might be referred to as **capillary embalming**. The capillaries are responsible for a large part of the distribution process throughout the body. Capillaries are simple tubes that connect the terminal arterioles and the venules. Capillary walls are comprised of a single layer of endothelial cells. They have an average diameter of 7–9 μm. The surface area of the capillary network in the human body approaches 6000 $m^2$ or 64,585 $ft^2$. This vast membrane comprises 1.5 acres and is the permeable barrier that controls the delivery of preserving and disinfecting chemicals to deep and superficial body tissues. The circulatory system of humans contains approximately 5–6 quarts of blood, or 8% of the body weight. Nearly 85% of blood is contained within the capillaries. Thorough profusion of the soft tissue sites with appropriate concentrations of injection chemicals involves far more than filling the aorta and its primary branches. A portion of the embalming solution passes through the capillaries and enters the tissue spaces. At the tissue level, the preservative solution makes contact with the cells of the tissues and the body proteins.

Cavity embalming is the second stage of embalming. The direct function is the treatment of the visceral organs of the body cavities. Many of these organs are hollow and their contents are not reached by the preservative solutions vascularly. The contents of hollow organs must be removed to make room for the introduction of cavity fluid. The process is called **aspiration.** A trocar is inserted through the abdominal wall near the umbilicus, also called the *belly button*. The trocar pierces the **hollow organs** to withdraw the contents and the **solid organs** to drain accumulated fluids and makes channels in these organs. Cavity aspiration also removes fluids and gases from between the organs that have accumulated ante- or postmortem, such as ascites. Once the liquids, gases, and semisolids are aspirated, the process of **injection** begins. The bottle of cavity fluid is directly attached to the trocar for injection, as in the **Evolution injector,** or is attached to a separate **cavity fluid injector** that reaches the trocar by a length of tubing. The trocar is introduced into each of the aspirated and channeled organs to deliver concentrated cavity fluid. Cavity chemical is *not diluted* for use. The accumulated waste products in the body cavities will dilute the cavity fluid upon contact. Customarily, a total of 32 to 48 ounces of cavity fluid is introduced into the three cavities: thoracic, abdominal, and pelvic. Certain conditions necessitate reaspiration of the cavities and reinjection of cavity fluid.

## Supplemental Hypodermic and Surface Embalming

Supplemental embalming methods include hypodermic and surface embalming treatments. Hypodermic embalming is the subcuticular injection of a suitable preservative chemical directly into the tissues. The chemical may be injected by a hypodermic syringe and needle or a hypovalve trocar. Trocars and needles are available in a variety of lengths and sizes of the opening or the *bore*. The area of treatment may be localized, such as a finger or area of the cheek, or maybe extensive, as in the abdominal and chest walls of the autopsied body or an entire lower extremity. Hypodermic treatment is employed when sufficient preservation is not achieved by arterial embalming and to perform restorative treatments such as tissue bleaching or contouring.

Surface embalming is the application of an embalming chemical directly to the surface of the tissues. Embalming chemicals are applied as a spray, brushed onto the surface in liquid or gel form, or applied on cotton as a surface compress. The preservative can also be applied beneath the skin in areas such as the eyelids and the mouth. In the case of an autopsy, surface embalming of the cavity walls and beneath the cranial scalp is routine.

## ANATOMICAL EMBALMING

The process of anatomical embalming varies from the embalming customary to funeral service. When the body is desired to be present for the funeral or memorial event, arterial embalming is ordinarily allowed prior to body donation. Communication with the Willed Body Program will substantiate the allowable procedures for body preparation. In general, cavity embalming is not permitted; any hypodermic treatment by hypovalve trocar should be avoided. Hypodermic treatments by needle and syringe, exclusive to facial features and fingertips, and surface embalming treatments are allowed.

Anatomical donation to medical science requires legal documentation for the donation. *Bequeathal* of the body, or *giving by will* after death, is considered a will and is legally binding. Body donation is considered a final disposition for the legal certificate of death and associated transit permits; customarily, body donation terminates in cremation.

The time of use for a cadaver spans up to 2 years. Embalming for long-term preservation of the body takes precedence over the appearance of the body. Very large volumes of solution, 8–12 gallons, are injected from a single site. Blood drainage is restricted to allow the tissues to greatly expand and to create deep diffusion of the embalming solution. Cavity aspiration is not performed; the internal organs must remain intact and undamaged for anatomical study. Concentrated embalming formulations are commonly a mixture of formalin, phenol, alcohol, wetting agents, and ethylenediaminetetraacetic acid (EDTA). During dissection, wetting agents and other chemicals may be topically applied to prevent dehydration and mold formation.

## SOFT EMBALMING METHOD FOR CADAVERS

Anatomical dissection and study frequently call for cadavers that retain muscle and joint flexibility and have the feel of living tissue. Manipulation of the tissue is paramount when performing clinical skills and mock surgeries. The pliability of these specimens is integral for accuracy in teaching. Soft embalmed cadavers do not have the longevity that traditionally embalmed cadavers do but have many important benefits as anatomical specimens. The desired outcome is to produce overall tissue firmness without gross distension. However, deliberate abdominal distension is required to completely saturate the internal organs for cadaveric research and study. The following protocol was provided by McMaster University, Hamilton, Ontario, Canada; The University of Western Ontario, London, Ontario, Canada; and Wayne State University, Detroit, Michigan.

The soft embalming fluid used in each of the anatomy programs is formaldehyde-free, comprised mainly of alcohol, phenol, and glycerin. Donors receive a total of 5 gallons (approximately 15–21 L), including the volume used for hypodermic treatments. Injection pressure is high, 60–70 psi, and the rate of flow is rapid. The first 2 gallons are injected from the right common carotid artery only. Soft embalming necessitates a six-point injection for the most successful outcome. All arteries are clamped during arterial and hypodermic injection to maintain intravascular pressure and to prevent fluid loss. No blood drainage; blood remains in the veins to allow easy vessel identification during the anatomical study.

Hypodermic treatments utilize the fewest points of entry. Hypodermic injection by hypovalve trocar includes the abdominal wall to enhance vascular embalming without risk of damage to the internal organs; the buttocks, lower back, shoulders, feet, and tissues surrounding the femoral injection sights, thighs, and pubic region. Hypodermic injection by needle and syringe is used for the fingers and the toes.

Vessels are ligated after embalming; incisions are not sutured. The donor is placed under mortuary refrigeration for a period of 2–4 weeks to *cure* before first use. Prior to each lab session, the donor is towel-dried for aesthetics and donor respect. Lab sessions are limited to a few hours. Donors remain viable for study for a period of 4–5 months and are refrigerated when not in use.

## EMBALMING AND DECEDENT CARE REPORTS

Documentation is completed for each decedent brought into the custody of a funeral home or embalming facility. When the body is being prepared for shipment to a different location, a copy of the care report should accompany the remains. Select the appropriate care form based upon the nature of decedent care provided. Separate embalming reports and decedent care reports are currently available. These two forms may soon merge to become one form called the *Embalming and Decedent Care Report*. Numerous forms are included as examples in the appendix at the conclusion of this chapter.

Decedent care reports should be filled out in detail and kept as a permanent record of the funeral home or the embalming facility. The report should provide information to accurately describe (1) the condition of the body before preparation; (2) manner and methods of preparation; (3) any postembalming or postcare treatments; and (4) date and time of arrival of the body into the custody of the funeral home or the embalming facility, starting and ending times of the preparation, and the full name and license number of the embalmer and others authorized to assist in the preparation.

Embalming and Decedent Care Reports are a critical component of any legal proceeding alleging improper decedent care; the report is the first document requested and will be scrutinized. "Documentation is essential in every circumstance … document, document, document!"*

## EMBALMING FUNDAMENTALS

- The practice of universal precautions is applied in all decedent care activities.
- The use of personal protective equipment is applied in all decedent care activities.
- Confirm the identity of all bodies and maintain the identity throughout all phases of care. Compare all forms of identification on the body and body bag, such as wristbands and toe tags, with funeral home records (**Fig. 2–1A–C**). The funeral home or the embalming facility should generate and affix its own method of identification to the body.
- Complete and maintain a decedent care report for each body brought into the funeral home or the embalming facility.
- Perform periodic monitoring of the body while in the custody of the funeral facility. Make necessary adjustments and provide treatments for adverse conditions.

---

*Kubasak, M., **Traversing the Minefield Best Practice: Reducing the Risk in Funeral-Cremation Service,** Malibu, CA: LMG Publishing, 2007.

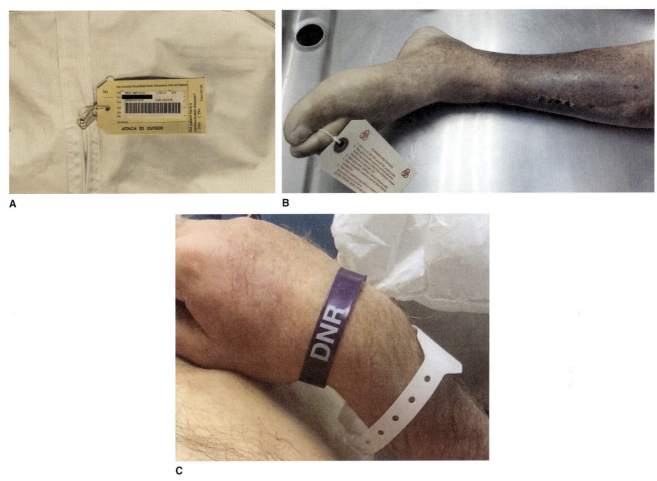

**Figure 2–1. A.** Identification tag affixed to zipper of body bag. **B.** Toe tag secured to decedent. **C.** I.D. wristband secured by the funeral home shown below the DNR (do not rescusitate) wristband from the medical facility.

- Cover the body at all times to maintain the dignity of the deceased (**Fig. 2–2**). Place a modesty cloth to cover the genitals during embalming and when providing decedent care.
- Engage the room ventilation system during the embalming process and whenever chemicals are used.
- Dispose of contaminated items such as medical waste and body bags in an approved biohazard waste container.
- Dispose of contaminated sharps, such as scalpel blades, broken cutting instruments, hypodermic needles, and needle injector wires in an approved biohazard sharps container.

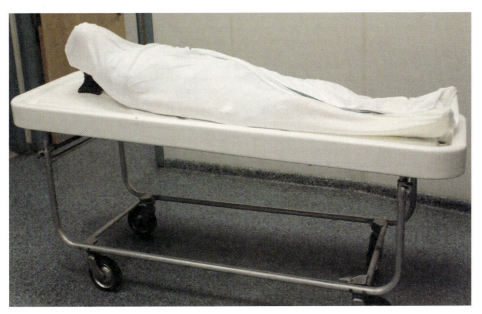

**Figure 2–2.** Full coverage of the deceased.

# Appendix

## EMBALMING AND DECEDENT CARE FORMS

*Forms are shown for the purpose of example only.*

**Embalming Authorization (Fig. 2–3),** provides permission for embalming the body and indemnification of the funeral home. Note the following:

- Expands who may assist in the embalming—funeral service students and resident trainees.
- Provides for the contract employment of a trade embalmer (independent contractor).
- Allows the body to be embalmed at the funeral home or at a separate embalming facility.

**EMBALMING AUTHORIZATION**

1. **PARTIES:**

   "FUNERAL HOME": _____
   (Name of Funeral Home)

   "REPRESENTATIVE": _____
   (Use Reverse Side for Additional Names) (Name of Representative)

   "DECEDENT": _____
   (Name of Decedent)

2. **RELATIONSHIP OF REPRESENTATIVE:** The REPRESENTATIVE warrants and represents to the FUNERAL HOME that the relationship between the REPRESENTATIVE and the DECEDENT is as follows: (Check the appropriate box)

   ☐ Spouse
   ☐ Next-of-Kin (Closest Living Relative)
   ☐ Personal Representative of the Next-of-Kin with written authorization of Next-of-Kin to act on his or her behalf.
   ☐ Other: _____

3. **AUTHORITY OF REPRESENTATIVE:** The REPRESENTATIVE warrants and represents to FUNERAL HOME that the REPRESENTATIVE is the person or the appointed agent of the person who by law has the paramount right to arrange and direct the disposition of the remains of the DECEDENT and that no other person(s) has a superior right over the right of the REPRESENTATIVE.

4. **EMBALMING AUTHORIZATION:** The REPRESENTATIVE authorizes and directs the FUNERAL HOME, its employees, independent contractors, and agents (including apprentices and/or mortuary students under the direct supervision of a licensed embalmer), to care for, embalm, perform restorative measures, and prepare the body of the DECEDENT. The REPRESENTATIVE acknowledges that this authorization encompasses permission to embalm at the FUNERAL HOME facility or at another facility equipped for embalming. In providing this authorization, REPRESENTATIVE acknowledges that embalming is not an exact science and that results are dependent upon a number of factors, including, but not limited to the conditions under which the death occurred, time lapse between death and the onset of the embalming procedure, physical condition at the time of death, medications, especially analgesics administered prior to death, life-saving procedures, cause of death, storage procedures of the releasing institution, natural elements, tissue/organ donations, and post-mortem (autopsy) examinations.

5. **PHOTOGRAPHS:** Unless the box at the end of this paragraph is checked by the REPRESENTATIVE, the FUNERAL HOME has authorization to take photographs of the remains to document the condition of the remains prior to or during embalming. These photographs will be maintained in the internal records of the FUNERAL HOME. ☐ Permission is denied.

6. **INDEMNIFICATION:** The REPRESENTATIVE agrees to indemnify and hold harmless the FUNERAL HOME from any claims or causes of action arising or related in any respect to this embalming authorization or the FUNERAL HOME's reliance thereon.

**DATE:** _____  **SIGNATURE OF REPRESENTATIVE:** _____

**Figure 2–3.** Embalming Authorization.

**SAMPLE ONLY**

---

**AUTHORIZATION FOR RESTORATIVE AND COSMETIC CARE**

I/we _____, hereby authorize the

_____ Funeral Home to perform cosmetic and

restorative work on the remains of _____,

who is related to me a as _____. I/we

hereby acknowledge full responsibility for results of same and do not hold harmless

_____ Funeral Home, its owners, employees and

agents for results herewith performed.

I/we hereby represent that I/we are of same and nearest degree of relationship to the

deceased:


_____ (seal)

_____ (seal)      _____ witness

_____ Date        _____ witness

---

**Figure 2–4.** Authorization for restorative and cosmetic care.

- Allows for restorative treatments.
- Protects the funeral home if the body has been misidentified.

**Authorization for Restorative and Cosmetic Care (Fig. 2–4),** gives necessary permission when extensive or operative restoration work may be necessary in the preparation of the body.

**Authorization for Minimum Care Services (Fig. 2–5),** authorizes minimum care when embalming is not requested. It gives the funeral facility permission to perform certain tasks to prepare the body for identification, viewing, or immediate cremation.

**Minimum Care Authorization When Embalming is Declined (Fig. 2–6),** authorizes minimum care of the body. It provides a detailed description of "minimum care" that can be performed.

**Authorization to Prepare Donation Cases for Viewing (Fig. 2–7),** is used when a funeral facility prepares a body where organs and/or tissues have been donated.

**Green Funeral Release and Indemnification (Fig. 2–8),** gives direction for disposition of the dead human body when a green burial (natural burial) is requested.

**Identification of Remains of the Decedent (Fig. 2–9),** verifies the identification of a decedent. Note the following with respect to this form:

- States who is making the identification
- States that the body was viewed and identified
- States that the next of kin refuses to identify the remains but authorizes final disposition without positive identification
- Indemnifies the funeral facility if the body is incorrectly identified

## SAMPLE ONLY
### AUTHORIZATION FOR MINIMUM CARE SERVICES

**1. PARTIES:**

FUNERAL HOME: _____
(Name of Funeral Home)

REPRESENTATIVE: _____
(Name of Representative)

DECEDENT: _____
(Name of Decedent)

**2. Relationship of Representative:** The representative warrants and represents to FUNERAL HOME that the relationship between the REPRESENTATIVE and the DECEDENT is as follows (check the appropriate item):

☐ Spouse

☐ Next of Kin (Closest Living Relative)

☐ Personal Representative

☐ Other: _____

**3. Authority of the Representative:** The REPRESENTATIVE warrants and represents to FUNERAL HOME that the REPRESENTSTIVE is the person or the appointed agent of the person who by law has the paramount right to arrange and direct the disposition of the remains of the DECEDENT and that no other person(s) has a superior right over the right of the REPRESENTATIVE.

**4. Minimum Care Services:** If the REPRESENTATIVE has directed that the remains of the DECEDENT are not to be embalmed or if a decision on embalming has not yet been made, there are services that the REPRESENTATIVE may wish to authorize so that the remains may be privately viewed, identified or reposed in a dignified and respectful manner. Below is a list of Minimum Care Services. Please check the box next to these Minimum Care Services that you authorize the FUNERAL HOME to provide for the DECEDENT'S remains:

☐ Removal of exterior medical devices (hearing aids, dentures, IV tubing, etc.)

☐ Removal of internal medical devices (pacemakers, pumps, defibrillators, etc.)

☐ Shaving the face and/or trimming beard and moustache

☐ Manicuring finger nails

☐ Trimming hair of the head

☐ Closing incisions by sutures

☐ Closing the mouth (may require sutures)

☐ Aspirating internal cavities and injecting preservative cavity fluids

☐ Application of cosmetics

☐ Other: _____

**5. Indemnification:** The REPRESENTATIVE agrees to indemnify and hold harmless the FUNERAL HOME from any claims or causes of action from or related in any respect to this decision to authorize the MINIMUM CARE SERVICES from the FUNERAL HOME.

_____     _____
**DATE**                                                                **SIGNATURE OF REPRESENTATIVE**

**Figure 2–5.** Authorization for minimum care services.

**Trauma Viewing Without Embalming (Fig. 2–10),** used when the funeral home advises against viewing the body due to severe conditions such as trauma, fire, or decomposition, but the family wishes to view.

**Attention Funeral Director (Fig. 2–11),** a form for bodies being shipped to another funeral facility. It describes the condition of the body at the shipping location and requests notification of any problems encountered by the receiving funeral facility. It is to be accompanied by a copy of the Decedent Care Report.

**Decedent Care Report (Fig. 2–12A and B),** this form must be completed in lieu of an embalming report for each deceased human body brought into the care of a funeral or an embalming facility. A copy of the report must accompany the body being shipped or transported to another funeral facility.

**Embalming Report (Fig. 2–13A–D),** this form must be completed for each deceased human body brought into a funeral or an embalming facility for the purpose of embalming. A copy of the report must accompany the body being shipped or transported to another funeral facility.

**Sample Only**

**Minimum Care Authorization When Embalming is Declined**

Name of the deceased: _____ Date of death: _____

The undersigned represents and warrants to be the next of kin to the deceased or the person(s) with the right and authority by law to control the disposition of the above-named decedent.

The undersigned has declined embalming of the above-named decedent and authorizes the funeral home, or its designated agent, to provide shelter to the body and minimum care.

The undersigned understands minimum care may include, but not be limited to sheltering the body in a clean, private environment; type of environment: refrigerated or non-refrigerated ; positioning the body; removing exterior tubes, catheters, or other medical devices deemed necessary; closing of eyes and mouth by accepted mortuary practices; aspiration of excess fluids and gasses from the body; inventory of personal effects from the body; use of surface disinfectants or deodorants; wrapping or covering the body in a suitable material. Minimum care does not include chemically treating the body by arterial injection of chemicals and does not retard organic decomposition . Minimum care will not ensure any time for presentation of the body for viewing or preservation as a replacement for arterial embalming.

The undersigned have been provided with the opportunity to ask any questions pertaining to minimum care.

The undersigned releases and discharges the funeral home, its affiliates, officers, directors, employees and agents from any and all liabilities claim, losses, damages, costs, or causes of action arising from the decision to not embalm the body, or arising out of any other decision indicated by this authorization which may result in mental or physical distress or anguish or harm or financial loss to the undersigned or others.

Signature: _____
Relationship to deceased:_____

Signature: _____
Relationship to deceased:_____

Funeral Home Representative: _____

Date signed: _____

adopted from M. Kubasak / Lamers , LMG Publishing, 2007.

**Figure 2–6.** Minimum care authorization when embalming is declined.

SAMPLE ONLY

**AUTHORIZATION TO PREPARE DONATION CASES FOR VIEWING**

1. **PARTIES:**
   FUNERAL HOME: _____

   REPRESENTATIVE: _____

   DECEDENT: _____

   PROCUREMENT ORGANIZATION: _____

2. **RELATIONSHIP OF REPRESENTATIVE:** The REPRESENTATIVE warrants and represents to the FUNERAL HOME that the relationship between the REPRESENTATIVE and the DECEDENT is as follows: (Check appropriate box).
   - [ ] Spouse
   - [ ] Next of Kin (Closest Living Relative)
   - [ ] Personal Representative of the Next of Kin with written authorization of Next of Kin to act on his/her behalf.
   - [ ] Other:

3. **DONATION:** The DEDEDENT and/or the REPRESENTATIVE has authorized the PROCUREMENT ORGANIZATION to carry out the donation specified below:
   - [ ] Organs
   - [ ] Organs and Tissues
   - [ ] Organs, Tissues and Bone
   - [ ] All Body Parts

4. **Viewing:** The REPRESENTATIVE instructs the FUNERAL HOME to prepare the remains of the DECEDENT for viewing. The REPRESENTATIVE understands and acknowledges that the appearance of the DECEDENT and the benefits of the embalming and restorative services provided by the FUNERAL HOME can be adversely impacted by donation procedures and resulting delays. The REPRESENTATIVE hereby releases and agrees to hold FUNERAL HOME, its owners, employees and agents harmless from any claims or causes of action arising or relating to the embalming and restoration of DECEDENT'S remains or the viewing thereof.

5. **RESTORATION COSTS:** The REPRESENTATIVE acknowledges and agrees that additional cost of restoration may be incurred due to the donation and that such costs will be:
   - [ ] Paid solely by the PROCUREMENT ORGANIZATION
   - [ ] Paid by those responsible for the funeral bill

6. **RELEASE:** The REPRESENTATIVE acknowledges and agrees that FUNERAL HOME, its owners, employees and agents have no legal relationship with the PROCUREMENT ORGANIZATION and are under no obligation or responsibility to insure that the PROCUREMENT ORGANIZATION has obtained informed consent to the donation, has conducted donation procedures in a lawful and ethical manner, and/or will use the donated body parts as required by law and the donation authorization.

SIGNATURE OF REPRESENTATIVE: _____

DATE: _____

**Figure 2–7.** Authorization to prepare donation cases for viewing.

## SAMPLE ONLY

### GREEN FUNERAL RELEASE AND INDEMNIFICATION

1. **Parties:**
   Funeral Home _____

   Representative of decedent _____

   Decedent _____

2. **Relationship of Representative:** The REPRESENTATIVE warrants and represents to the FUNERAL HOME that the relationship between the REPRESENTATIVE and the DECEDENT is as follows:

   ☐ Spouse

   ☐ Next of Kin (closest living relative)

   ☐ Personal Representative of Next of Kin with written authorization of Next of Kin at act on his or her behalf

   ☐ Other: _____

3. **AUTHORITY OF REPRESENTATIVE:** The REPRESENTATIVE warrants and represents to FUNERAL HOME that the REPRESENTATIVE is the person or the appointed agent of the person who by law has the paramount right to arrange and direct the disposition of the remains of the DECEDENT and that no other person(s) has a superior right over that right of the REPRESENTATIVE

4. **GREEN FUNERAL:** While the details involved in a disposition known as a "Green Funeral" may vary, they usually involve minimal preparation of the DECEDENT'S remains; no embalming or preservation services; use of a wood, cardboard, wicker, bamboo or cloth container to hold, transport and bury the body; no use of a vault or outer burial container to encase the remains in the grave; and burial in a woodland or open field setting with grave marked by rocks, trees or flowers as opposed to a permanent marker or monument.

5. **ADVISORY:** The Green Funeral choice is usually made for environmental reasons and a desire for a simpler disposition. It is an appropriate and meaningful choice for certain families. However, it does preclude certain options and poses several risks that the REPRESENTATIVE has been advised of and is now acknowledging. The REPRESENTATIVE has been advised by the FUNERAL HOME that with a Green Funeral, the FUNERAL HOME can provide no assurances regarding the appearance or the condition of the DECEDENT'S remains; that there will not be a public visitation or viewing of the DECEDENT; that there are possible health risks posed by handling an unembalmed body; that there can be substantial risks of physical injury to pallbearers from holding, carrying and transporting a body in a container that may not be designed to hold the weight or to be safely lifted and carried; that burial of the body in a grave or plot without an outer burial container may lead to the ground settling and sinking over the grave; that the body may not be able to be disinterred and moved at a later date; and that, in later years, it may be difficult or impossible to locate the grave due to the lack of a permanent marker or monument.

6. **DRECTION TO ARRANGE AND CARRY OUT GREEN FUNERAL:** The REPRESENTATIVE directs and authorizes the FUNERAL HOME to arrange and carry out the Green Funeral described above. In directing and authorizing the Green Funeral, the REPRESENTATIVE understands and appreciates the risks explained in Paragraph 5 above and other risks that may have been described by the FUNERAL HOME to the REPRESENTATIVE. Despite these risks, the REPRESENTATIVE directs the FUNERAL HOME to carry out the REPRESENTATIVE'S directions with regard to the Green Funeral for the DECEDENT.

7. **INDEMNIFICATION:** The REPRESENTATIVE hereby releases FUNERAL HOME fully from all claims and agrees to indemnify and hold harmless the FUNERAL HOME from any claims or causes of action arising from or related in any respect to the direction of the REPRESENTATIVE to carry out the Green Funeral.

**DATE:** _____

**SIGNATURE OF REPRESENTATIVE:** _____

**Figure 2–8.** Green funeral release and indemnification.

**IDENTIFICATION OF REMAINS OF THE DECEDENT**

SAMPLE ONLY

1. Parties:
   Funeral Home: _____
   (Name of Funeral Home)

   Representative: _____
   (Name of Representative – Use Reverse side for additional Names)

   Decedent: _____

2. Relationship of Representative: The REPRESENTATIVE warrants and represents to the Funeral Home that the relationship between the REPRESENTATIVE and the DECEDENT is as follows:
   (Check appropriate box)

   [ ] Spouse
   [ ] Next of Kin (Closest Living Relative)
   [ ] Personal Representative of the Next of Kin with written authorization of Next of Kin to act on his/her behalf
   [ ] Other

3. Authority of the Representative: The REPRESENTATIVE warrants and represents to the FUNERAL HOME that the REPRESENTATIVE is the person or the appointed agent of the Person who by law has the paramount right to arrange and direct the disposition of the remains of the DECEDENT and that no other person(s) has a superior right over the right of the REPRESENTATIVE.

4. IDENTIFICATION: The REPRESENTATIVE certifies to the FUNERAL HOME as follows:

   [ ] The REPRESENTATIVE has viewed the remains and positively identified them as the body of the DECEDENT.

   [ ] The REPRESENTATIVE elects NOT TO IDENTIFY the remains and authorizes the final disposition of the body of the DECEDENT by the FUNERAL HOME without positive identification.

5. INDEMNIFICATION: The REPRESENTATIVE assumes ALL LIABILITY for incorrectly identifying or for failing to identify the body of the DECEDENT and does hereby agree to indemnify and hold harmless the FUNERAL HOME from any claims or causes of action arising in any respect to the REPRESENTATIVE'S act of identification or omission to identify the remains of the DECEDENT.

SIGNATURE OF REPRESENTATIVE: _____

FUNERAL HOME REPRESENTATIVE: _____

Date: _____

**Figure 2–9.** Identification of remains of the decedent.

**Sample Only - TRAUMA**
**Viewing without embalming**

**RELEASE**

I, _____ , hereby release, discharge, and forever hold harmless the _____ Funeral Home and its owners and employees, from any and all claims resulting from my viewing of the body of _____. I explicitly release and discharge the _____ Funeral Home and its owners and employees from any and all claims for loss or damages, including but not limited to personal injury, illness, mental distress or disability of any type, or death, whether or not caused by the _____ Funeral Home, its owners or employees.

Specifically, I have been informed that the body has been damaged by fire. I have been informed that any and all of the remains may be charred and that the superficial layer of skin/tissue is nonexistent due to the fire.

I have been informed that the body is autopsied. I have been informed that the body may give off a pungent odor that may be noticeable as soon as I enter the building.

I have been offered the opportunity to view the body via a photograph and decided to proceed with actual viewing of the body.

I have read this Release and I understand and agree to all of its provisions. If any portion of this Release shall be held invalid, those parts that are not invalid shall continue in full force and effect.

_____

Date: _____

Witness: _____

**Figure 2-10.** Trauma viewing without embalming.

SAMPLE ONLY

**ATTENTION FUNERAL DIRECTOR**

**Name of deceased:** ______________________________

**Date and time of this document:** ______________________________
(DATE) (TIME)

Our embalmer(s) have reviewed the condition of this body immediately prior to transfer to the delivery agent (airport, railroad, private carrier) and have noted any special circumstances below for your convenience. A copy of the EMBALMING CARE REPORT is enclosed.

Occasionally, between the time of departure and arrival, body conditions may change or the transfer may create situations that require additional remedial steps upon arrival. If this body is not satisfactory when received, ***please contact us immediately*** at ______________. We will take all necessary steps to correct any deficiencies.

We appreciate this opportunity to serve one of your client families and trust that everything meets with your satisfaction.

**Special Notes :** ______________________________

**Enclosed Items:**
The following items have been enclosed within the casket:

- ☐ Register Book
- ☐ Thank-You cards
- ☐ Memorial Folders/Prayer Cards
- ☐ Flower cards
- ☐ Personal effects (clothing, etc.)
- ☐ Crucifix/Cross
- ☐ Flag
- ☐ Death Certificates
- ☐ Other

Note: Burial/Transit permit located in head tag envelope.

Thank you for your assistance. If you have concerns about remains, casket or its contents contact us immediately at ______________________.

**Remains reviewed by:**

______________________________
(shipping embalmer )

**Figure 2–11.** Attention funeral director.

# CHAPTER 2 • Fundamentals of Embalming

**DECEDENT CARE REPORT**  **SAMPLE ONLY**

Date: _____  Case Number: _____

## HISTORY & DESCRIPTION

Name of Deceased: _____

Place of Death: _____

Date: _____ Time: _____ Age: _____ Sex: _____ Race: _____ Approx. Height: _____

Approx. Weight: _____ **Identification on body:** _____

Received at Funeral Home: Date: _____ Time: _____ **In House:** _____ **Ship-In:** _____ **Ship-Out:** _____

Permission to Embalm received on the _____ day of _____, 20___ from: _____

Description of personal items **on the body**: itemize on personal effects envelope; place effects in envelope.
Pacemaker _____ Yes _____ No: Permission to remove for cremation _____ Yes _____ No

**CONDITION OF BODY PRIOR TO: ( ) STORAGE: ( ) EMBALMING: ( ) PREPARATION WITHOUT EMBALMING**

| | | | |
|---|---|---|---|
| ___ Abrasions* | ___ Decubitus Ulcers | ___ Gangrene* | ___ Surgical drains* |
| ___ Amputation | ___ Dehydration | ___ Hematoma* | ___ Surgical Incision* |
| ___ Ascites | ___ Dentures (Upper/Lower) | ___ Infectious Disease | ___ Swelling*+ Cause |
| ___ Autopsy | ___ Discoloration (Face/Hands) | ___ IV Leak* | ___ Tattoos* |
| ___ Bruising* | ___ Distention* | ___ Laceration (s) | ___ Tissue Gas* |
| ___ Burns* | ___ Dropsical (anasarca) | ___ Jaundice* | ___ Tracheotomy |
| ___ Catheter, IV | ___ Ecchymosis | ___ Livor Mortis | ___ Trauma* |
| ___ Catheter, Urinary | ___ Edema* (local) | ___ Purge | ___ Tumor* |
| ___ Cast* | ___ Emaciation* | ___ Refrigerated ___ Frozen | |
| ___ Clean Shaven (men) | ___ Facial Hair* (men) | ___ Rigor mortis* | **TREATMENTS** |
| ___ Colostomy | ___ Feeding Tube | ___ Scars* | Topical disinfectant used: |
| ___ Decomposition* | ___ Fractures* | ___ Skin Slip* | _____ |

* Note Location and/or Description on back of form or separate sheet ___ Orifices Packed

**ORGAN / TISSUE DONATION:** _____ Yes _____ No (If Yes, attach paperwork from recovery team.)

## EMBALMING TECHNIQUES

**Primary Injection:** ___ One Point  ___ Split Injection  ___ Six Point  ___ Restricted Cervical

**Other arteries injected:** _____

**Arteries Injected:** ___ Axillary R – L  ___ Brachial R – L  ___ Carotid R – L  ___ Femoral R – L

___ Iliac R – L  ___ Radial R – L  ___ Subclavian R – L  ___ Ulnar R – L

**Drainage:** ___ Femoral R – L  ___ Jugular R – L  ___ Post (Autopsy)

**Drainage Technique:** ___ Concurrent  ___ Intermittent  ___ Alternate

**Mouth Closure:** ___ Mandibular Suture  ___ Muscular Suture  ___ Needle Injector  ___ Dental Tie

___ Cotton  ___ Mouth Former  ___ Dentures (Upper/Lower)  ___ Natural Teeth

**Eye Closure:** ___ Eye Caps  ___ Cotton  ___ Other

**Fluid Dilutions:**
- Pre-injection: _____ oz.  Type: _____
- Humectant: _____ oz.  Type: _____
- Co-injection: _____ oz.  Type: _____
- Dye: _____ oz.  Type: _____
- Arterial: _____ oz.  Type: _____  Index: _____
- Arterial: _____ oz.  Type: _____  Index: _____
- Arterial: _____ oz.  Type: _____  Index: _____
- Total Gallons of Fluid Injected: _____

**Figure 2–12. A and B.** Decedent care report.

**Hypodermic Treatment:** ___Fingers ___Hands ___Face ___Legs ___Torso ___Other:_____

**Surface Treatment** (Manner & Location): _____

**Purge During Injection:** ___Yes ___No (Location & Treatment): _____

**Cavity Treatments:** Cavity Fluid: _____ oz.    Type: _____

**Aspiration:** ___Delayed ___Immediate        **Re-aspiration:** ___Yes ___No

**Autopsy:** ___Cranial ___Thoracic ___Abdominal ___Neck organs ___Tongue  **Viscera Returned:** ___Yes ___No

**Disposition of Viscera:** _____

**Plastic Garments:** ___Coverall ___Pants ___Capri Garment ___Sleeves ___Stockings ___Unionall

**PREPARATION TIME:**    Beginning: _____ AM PM        Ending: _____ AM PM

**Condition & Comments of Body after Embalming    also    Describe ALL Restorative and Cosmetic Treatments**

_____
_____
_____
_____
_____
_____
_____
_____
_____
_____
_____
_____
_____
_____

Embalmers Signature: _____    Date: _____

Hairdresser: _____

Restoration: _____

Cosmetics: _____

Dressing & Casketing: _____

**Figure 2–12. A and B.** Decedent care report. (continued)

**EMBALMING REPORT**
(Confidential)

Embalmer _____ Master No.: _____

Assisted by _____

FUNERAL HOME _____ IN-HOUSE _____ SHIP-IN _____ SHIP-OUT _____

DATE _____ TIME _____ PERMISSION TO EMBALM _____

PROTECTIVE ATTIRE WORN _____ COMMUNICABLE DISEASE _____

NAME _____ DATE OF DEATH _____ TIME OF DEATH _____

CAUSE OF DEATH _____ DOCTOR/MEDICAL-EXAMINER _____

PERSONAL EFFECTS ON BODY _____

AGE _____ SEX _____ RACE _____ HEIGHT _____ WEIGHT _____ FACIAL HAIR _____

NATURAL TEETH _____ DENTURES _____ NO DENTURES _____ OTHER _____

DESCRIBE HAIR _____ DISTINGUISHING MARKS _____

**CONDITIONS PRIOR TO EMBALMING**

<u>GENERAL:</u> CLEAN _____ REFRIGERATED _____ RIGOR MORTIS _____ SURGERY _____

EVIDENCE OF DISEASE _____ EVIDENCE OF TRAUMA _____ TRACHEOTOMY _____ PACEMAKER _____

I.V. PUNCTURE(S) _____ STOMACH FEEDING TUBE _____ COLOSTOMY _____ GAS IN TISSUES _____

SKIN SLIP _____ CATHETER (URINARY) _____ DISCOLORATION(S) _____ PURGE _____

OTHER _____

<u>FACE:</u> NORMAL _____ EMACIATED _____ SWOLLEN _____ TRAUMA _____ EDEMA _____ GAS IN TISSUES _____ LESIONS _____

SKIN-SLIP _____ TUBE MARKS _____ DISCOLORATION(S) _____

OTHER _____

<u>AUTOPSY</u> CRANIAL _____ THORACIC _____ ABDOMINAL _____ PELVIC _____ SPINAL _____

NECK ORGANS REMOVED _____ TONGUE REMOVED _____ PARTIAL AUTOPSY _____ EYES DRAINED _____ EYE(S) REMOVED _____

VISCERA RETURNED WITH BODY _____ PLACEMENT OF VISCERA (AFTER EMBALMING) _____

TISSUES SAMPLES TAKEN (IF NO AUTOPSY PERFORMED) _____

<u>ORGAN DONOR:</u> _____ DESCRIBE _____

ENUCLEATION (WHOLE EYE) _____ CORNEA ONLY _____

**PREPARATION OF THE BODY**

SURFACE DISINFECTION _____ BODY WASHED _____ HAIR WASHED _____ NAILS CLEANED _____

NOSTRILS TRIMMED _____ FACE SHAVED _____ METHOD OF EYE CLOSURE _____

MOUTH SUPPORT IF USED _____ METHOD OF MOUTH CLOSURE _____

ALL ORIFICES DISINFECTED AND PACKED _____

**Figure 2–13. A and B.** Embalming report. **C.** Body outline. *(Used with permission of Darryl G. Shreve.)* **D.** Embalming report.

## PRESERVATIVE TREATMENTS

I. PRIMARY INJECTION PLAN [ARTERY(S)]:

    a. One-point injection _____

    b. Restricted cervical injection _____

    c. Six-point injection _____

    d. Other (describe) _____

    _____

    _____

    TOTAL VOLUME OF SOLUTION INJECTED _____ SOLUTION MIXTURES USED _____
    (indicate Solution Gallon #)

    DRAINAGE SITE _____ DRAINAGE METHOD _____

II. IF THE HEAD IS SEPARATELY EMBALMED (RESTRICTED CERVICAL OR AUTOPSY): _____

    SOLUTION MIXTURE USED _____ VOLUME INJECTED _____

III. AREA(S) RECEIVING AN INADEQUATE AMOUNT OF ARTERIAL SOLUTION: _____

IV. SUPPLEMENTAL ARTERY(S) INJECTED: _____

    TOTAL VOLUME OF SOLUTION INJECTED _____ SOLUTION MIXTURES USED _____
    (indicate Solution Gallon #)

V. SUPPLEMENTAL EMBALMING TREATMENTS (HYPODERMIC, COMPRESSES, GELS, ETC.) _____

VI. CAVITY TREATMENT (UNAUTOPSIED): IMMEDIATE ASPIRATION _____ ; DELAYED ASPIRATION _____

    NAME OF FLUID INJECTED _____ VOLUME INJECTED _____

## ARTERIAL FLUIDS AND SOLUTIONS

**FLUID COMPANY AND NAME:**

    A. WATER

    B. PRE-INJECTION _____

    C. ARTERIAL #1 _____

    D. ARTERIAL #2 _____

    E. CO-INJECTION _____

    F. WATER SOFTENER _____

    G. HUMECTANT _____

    H. DYE _____

    I. OTHER _____

**ARTERIAL SOLUTIONS (MEASURED IN OUNCES PER GALLON; 1 GALLON = 128 FLUID OUNCES)** PLACE THE LETTER OF THE FLUID FROM THE LIST ABOVE IN THE LEFT COLUMN; IN THE RIGHT COLUMN PUT THE NUMBER OF OUNCES USED.

| GALLON #1 | GALLON #2 | GALLON #3 | GALLON #4 | GALLON #5 |
|---|---|---|---|---|
| A ___ (oz) | A ___ (oz) | A ___ (oz) | A ___ (oz) | A ___ (oz) |
| ___ ___ | ___ ___ | ___ ___ | ___ ___ | ___ ___ |
| ___ ___ | ___ ___ | ___ ___ | ___ ___ | ___ ___ |
| ___ ___ | ___ ___ | ___ ___ | ___ ___ | ___ ___ |
| ___ ___ | ___ ___ | ___ ___ | ___ ___ | ___ ___ |

## COMPLETION

AREA(S) OF DISTENSION RESULTING FROM ARTERIAL INJECTION _____

PURGE DURING ARTERIAL INJECTION [DESCRIBE] _____

PURGE TREATMENT _____

EYELIDS GLUED _____ LIPS GLUED _____ INCISION SEAL POWDER _____ INCISIONS GLUED _____

PLASTICS USED: _____ ; EMBALMING POWDER IN PLASTICS _____

**Figure 2–13.** **A and B.** Embalming report. **C.** Body outline. *(Used with permission of Darryl G. Shreve.)* **D.** Embalming report. *(continued)*

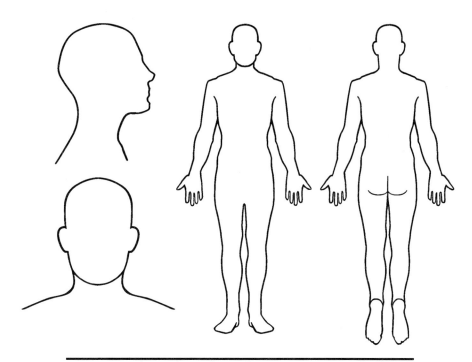

Document conditions observed. Record comments on reverse side of page.

**Figure 2–13. A and B.** Embalming report. **C.** Body outline. *(Used with permission of Darryl G. Shreve.)* **D.** Embalming report. (continued)

**DESCRIPTION OF RESTORATIVE TREATMENTS**

**DESCRIPTION OF COSMETIC TREATMENTS**

**SHIP-IN CONDITIONS AND CORRECTIONS**

Body received from: _____ City/State _____
Describe problem conditions and their correction:

**COMMENTS**

**Figure 2–13. A and B.** Embalming report. **C.** Body outline. *(Used with permission of Darryl G. Shreve.)* **D.** Embalming report. (continued)

## TERMINOLOGY

- **Embalming**—process of chemically treating the dead human body to reduce the presence and growth of microorganisms, retard organic decomposition, and restore an acceptable physical appearance
- **Embalm**—(14c)* (1): to treat (a dead body) so as to protect from decay; (2): to fill with sweet odors: **perfume**; (3): to protect from decay or oblivion: **preserve**; (4): to fix in a static condition—**embalmer** n—embalmment n
- **Decay**—(15c)† (1): to undergo destructive dissolution; (2): implies a slow change from a state of soundness
- **Decay***—decomposition of proteins by enzymes of aerobic bacteria
- **Decompose**—(ca. 1751)† (1): to separate into constituent parts or elements or into simpler compounds; (2): to break up into constituent parts or as if by a chemical process: decay—**decomposition** n
- **Decomposition***—separation of compounds into simpler substances by the action of microbial and/or autolytic enzymes
- **Enzyme**—(1881)† complex proteins that are produced by cells which act as a biological catalyst
- **Preserve**—(14c)† (1): to keep safe from injury, harm, or destruction: **protect**; (2a): to keep intact or free from decay; (2b): **maintain**; (3): to keep or save from decomposition—**preservation** n
- **Preservation***—the science of treating the dead human body chemically so as to temporarily inhibit decomposition
- **Preservative**—(15c)† (1): something that preserves or has the power of preserving; (2): an additive used to protect against decay, discoloration, or spoilage
- **Preservative***—chemicals that inactivate saprophytic bacteria, render unsuitable for nutrition the media upon which such bacteria thrive, and that will arrest decomposition by altering enzymes and lysins of the body as well as converting the decomposable tissue to a formless susceptible to decomposition
- **Protein**—(1844)† one of a class of complex nitrogenous compounds that are synthesized by all living organisms and yield amino acids when hydrolyzed
- **Putrefaction**—(14c)† (1): the decomposition of organic matter; (2): the typically anaerobic splitting of proteins by bacteria and fungi with the formation of foul-smelling incompletely oxidized products
- **Putrefaction***—decomposition of proteins by the action of enzymes from anaerobic bacteria
- **Sanitation**—(1848)† a process to promote and establish conditions that minimize or eliminate biohazards
- **Substrate**—(1807)† a substance acted upon (e.g., protein, fat, carbohydrate), as by an enzyme in the living organism, or embalming chemicals in preserving the dead body
- **Stabilize**—to prevent or retard an unwanted alteration of a physical state. Slowing the onset of the changes of decomposition by the use of refrigeration, dry or wet ice, and the injection of chemicals or nonformaldehyde-containing fluids.

## CONCEPTS FOR STUDY

Define the following terminology:
- Anatomical embalming
- Arterial embalming
- Arterial tube
- Bequeath
- Capillary embalming
- Cavity aspiration
- Cavity embalming
- Cavity fluid injector
- Cavity injection
- Embalming analysis
- Embalming machine
- Hypodermic embalming
- Hypovalve trocar
- Surface embalming
- Trocar

1. Define temporary preservation.
2. Explain the purpose of restoration.
3. Recall the action of enzymes upon body proteins.
4. Summarize the expectations of the embalming process.
5. List the four classifications of embalming.
6. Give another name for arterial embalming; for hypodermic embalming.
7. Describe the function of an arterial tube.
8. Name the two phases of cavity embalming.
9. Give the purpose of embalming analysis.
10. State the action of embalming solution once it reaches the ascending aorta.
11. Explain why arterial embalming might also be called capillary embalming.
12. Name two types of supplemental embalming methods.
13. Describe one surface embalming treatment.
14. Discuss the benefits of anatomical embalming and soft embalming methods.

## FIGURE CREDIT

Figure 2–1A,B is used with permission of Sharon L. Gee-Mascarello.
Figures 2–1C, 2–2 are used with permission of Kevin Drobish.

## BIBLIOGRAPHY

Bass B. *Death's Acre: Inside the Legendary Forensic Lab, the Body Farm, Where the Dead Do Tell Tales.* New York: Putnams, 2003.

Dhonau CO. *Manual of Case Analysis.* The Embalming Book Company Cincinnati, OH, 1924.

Dorn J, Hopkins B. *Thanatochemistry,* 2nd ed. Upper Saddle River, NJ: Prentice Hall, 1998.

*Embalming Course Content Syllabus.* Portland, ME: American Board of Funeral Service Education, 2001.

*Merriam-Webster's Collegiate Dictionary,* 11th ed. Springfield, MA: Merriam Webster, 2003.

Pervier NC. *Textbook of Chemistry for Embalmers.* Minneapolis: University of Minnesota, 1961.

Roach M. *Stiff: The Curious Lives of Human Cadavers.* New York: Norton, 2003.

Spitz WU. *Medicolegal Investigation of Death,* 3rd ed. Springfield, IL: Charles C Thomas, 1993.

Venes D. *Taber's Cyclopedic Medical Dictionary,* 19th ed. Philadelphia: F.A. Davis, 2001.

CHAPTER 3

# Personal Health and Regulatory Standards

## CHAPTER OVERVIEW
- Safe Work Practices
- State and Federal Regulations
- OSHA Bloodborne Pathogens Standard
- OSHA Hazard Communication Rule
- OSHA Formaldehyde Standard
- Safety Data Sheet (SDS)

Embalming has historically encompassed principles and practices that are part of public health. The embalmer, as a sanitarian, grew out of two early twentieth century situations—first, the pandemic flu of 1919; and second, most embalming was performed at the residence of the deceased. The primary role of the embalmer during that time was to clean and sanitize the sick room and tend to the dead. Further understanding of disease transmission and the widespread use of antibiotics occurred later in the century.

Current understanding of the transmission of diseases is coming full circle as researchers study the Covid-19 pandemic caused by the novel coronavirus disease, SARS-CoV-2. Rapid testing and global vaccination programs are being implemented to curb viral spread (**Fig. 3–1**). The sobering impact of the pandemic has so far (August 2021) claimed 4.5 million lives (**Fig. 3–2**). The Delta variant, which appears to be more contagious and more severe than earlier versions of the virus, threatens to claim additional lives. Residual health effects continue to be felt by individuals who have recovered from the virus. Covid-19 has changed ordinary daily living to anything but ordinary for all inhabitants of planet Earth. Health care and death care professionals once again are focused primarily upon public health. In light of the current pandemic, embalming protocols for contagious and infectious diseases have been dramatically affected. As with all emergent diseases, the influx of new information challenges us to stay informed and up-to-date.

The at-risk nature of embalming and decedent care practices, **direct contact** with a dead human, remains until final disposition, is well documented in medical and public health literature. The unembalmed dead human body is a reservoir of potentially harmful agents that pose a pathogenic risk to the living. The process of sanitizing and preserving dead human bodies raises a number of health considerations for individuals engaged in embalming and final care procedures. The embalmer has an ethical responsibility to protect others who come into contact with the deceased, such as family, friends, and members of the community that may attend a funeral or other type of homegoing event.

## SAFE WORK PRACTICES

Human remains must be properly treated with chemicals designed to reduce the risk to pathogenic agents and to stabilize the body from further organic decomposition. Exercise Universal Precautions during any type of contact with unembalmed bodies and when providing care for embalmed remains (**Fig. 3–3**). Wear personal protective equipment appropriate to the task. Safe work practices and engineering controls are reinforced to reduce the exposure levels to formaldehyde and other hazardous chemicals during embalming and final care of the body.

1. Adequate and properly operating air exchange system.
   a. The exhaust ventilation should draw fumes **away** from the embalmer.
   b. Provide an ample supply of incoming clean, fresh air.
2. Prevent spillage of chemicals.
   a. Gently mix embalming solutions and avoid splashing.
   b. Keep the rate-of-flow valve closed on the embalming machine when not in use; close stopcocks on arterial tubes when not in direct use.
3. Keep embalming machines in good repair.
   a. No leakage from within the machine apparatus.
   b. No leakage where hose attachments are made to machine or arterial tube.

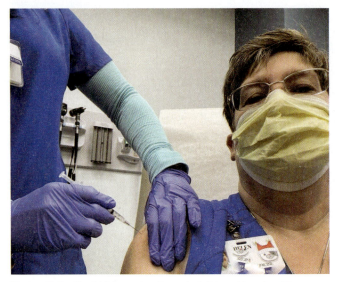

Figure 3–1. Covid-19 vaccination administered to a healthcare worker.

4. Rinse fluid bottles and empty residual chemicals into the arterial solution.
5. Cap all chemical bottles.
6. Keep a lid on the embalming machine tank.
7. Use continuous aspiration of body cavities during the injection of the autopsied body.
8. Clamp all accessible leaking arteries during the injection of the autopsied body.
9. Restrict drainage as much as possible after blood discolorations have cleared
    a. Helps to retain embalming solution within the body.
    b. Lowers the volume of chemicals placed into the waste system.
10. Use closed drainage.
    a. Attach tubing to the drain tube.
    b. Direct heart drainage with a trocar.
11. Cover the waste sink to avoid splashing and aerosolization.
12. Maintain running water to flush drainage from the embalming table.
13. Minimize high water pressure to avoid splashing.

These controls combined with personal protective attire and equipment will greatly reduce exposure to chemicals or their vapors.

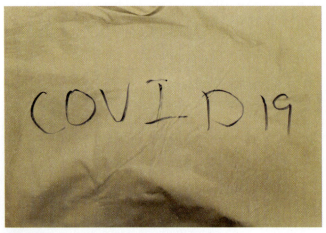

Figure 3–2. Covid-19 warning on body bag.

## OCCUPATIONAL RISKS

### Exposure to Biological Hazards

A 1996 Centers for Disease Control and Prevention (CDC) study reported that there is ample reason for concern about the exposure the embalmers may have to bloodborne and airborne pathogens (McKenna and co-workers, 1996). The CDC analyzed the risk for tuberculosis by determining potential exposure within certain occupational groups, based on historical observation, and the impact that infection within a group could have on public health. The occupational groups were first categorized by their level of risk. The researchers then applied a statistical formula to estimate the number of tuberculosis cases that could be expected within each occupational group. A comparison of the number of cases predicted by the statistical formula for an occupational group and the number of actual cases that were reported for each occupational group showed a strong relationship between the occupation and the risk of contracting tuberculosis.

A notable exception to the association between occupational SES (socioeconomic status) and tuberculosis was the occupation of "Funeral director." Even though this occupation was included in the highest SES category of "Executives, administrative, and managerial occupations," 16 cases were allocated to this occupation where only 4.1 were expected (McKenna et al., 1996, p. 590).

The CDC concluded that funeral directors had an elevated risk of contracting tuberculosis as a result of their contact with dead human bodies.

Gershon and colleagues (1998) reported the results in a Johns Hopkins University study which concluded that funeral home employees who worked as embalmers had a greater exposure to tuberculosis than funeral home employees who did not embalm bodies. The study found that 101 out of 864 (11.7%) funeral home employees who volunteered to be tested reacted to the tuberculin skin test. It was determined that the funeral home employees who engaged in embalming were twice as likely to have a positive tuberculin skin test when compared to the funeral home employees who did not embalm bodies.

Beck-Sague and co-workers (1991) also addressed the potential for occupationally acquired infections among embalmers. In particular, this study suggested that embalmers were at potential risk of acquiring infection as a result of their frequent contact with blood. This study reported that 89 of 539 (17%) morticians who responded to a survey reported contracting infectious diseases attributed to their occupation. Among the most frequently reported diseases in the study were hepatitis, staphylococcal and other skin infections, and pulmonary and skin tuberculosis. The most commonly reported exposure was by skin contact with blood (393 out of 539, or 73%). Needlestick injuries were far more common than cuts. Of the 539 morticians who responded to the survey, 212 (39%) reported a needlestick within 12 months prior to the survey, while 61 (11%) morticians reported having been cut.

Turner and colleagues (1989) reported that embalmers in the Boston area were about two times more likely to test positive for hepatitis B (HBV) infection than a blood donor comparison group. The study also reported that the length of time a person had been working as an embalmer elevated the risk of contracting an HBV infection.

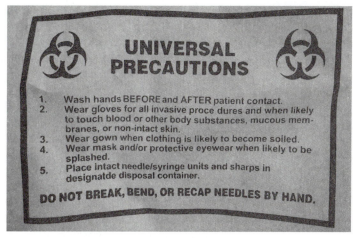

**Figure 3–3.** Universal Precautions label on a body bag.

McDonald (1989) published an editorial which stated that embalmers face much the same risk of exposure to infectious diseases as clinical pathologists. The basis of this finding was the common exposure to blood and body fluids for both pathologists and embalmers. The exposure risk was confirmed when the first documented case of an embalmer being infected with tuberculosis while embalming a dead human body was reported in the *New England Journal of Medicine* on January 27, 2000, by Dr. Timothy Stirling.

Multidrug-resistant pathogens are commonplace. Global travel has created a new environment for the spread of disease-causing organisms and their hosts. Within a period of 24 hours, people, insects, and animal vectors, or foodstuffs can be transported anywhere in the world. This rapid movement makes possible the occurrence and transmission of disease anywhere and at any time. Never before has an embalmer faced such a risk of biological exposure. Outside Magazine in July 1999 stated, "Microbes are still the number three killer in the Western world."

Reported in The Forum December 2009, a publication of the New Jersey Funeral Directors Association: "The incidences of occupationally-contracted infectious, contagious, or communicable disease are low in general and somewhat lower for embalmers than for individuals in other fields, such as health care, the Institute of Occupational Medicine, Edinburgh, Scotland reported in 2004. However, when proper protective measures are not used and given the high probability of percutaneous and mucocutaneous exposures, infectious agent transmission is possible. Therefore, embalmers always should practice universal precautions when handling deceased human bodies, regardless of their known infectious status."

While each body prepared by the embalmer must be considered a potential danger, several more recently diagnosed diseases need to be mentioned, some of which have reference to the previous discussion of antibiotic resistance:

- *Clostridium difficile* produces two toxins and can cause lethal diarrhea often brought on by overuse of antibiotics, found as spores in feces, diapers, and gowns. A new mutation produces 20 times the toxin of the old version.
- *Klebsiella pneumoniae*, a hospital-borne microbe that can infect the urinary tract, gut, and bloodstream.
- *Acinetobacter baumannii*, resistant to almost all antibiotics; found in spinal fluid and between the membranes lining the abdominal wall and the urinary tract. Seen in the very seriously ill and trauma injury wounds. Care with urinary catheters and surgical drainage tubes. Soilborne infects wounds and can penetrate deep into skin, bone, lungs, and blood.
- Methicillin-resistant **Staphylococcus aureus** (MRSA), a pathologic bacterial staph infection. This premier pathogen causes over 102,000 hospital infections a year. MRSA can be found on the skin, in the nose, in blood and urine, and in exudates or fluid from an infected site. Spread by direct physical contact, or contact with contaminated objects.
- Vancomycin-resistant Enterococci (VRE), a pathogenic bacterium, found in open wounds and feces; also associated with invasive devices such as urinary catheters and nasogastric tubes—seen in patients with long-term hospitalization. An especially hardy microbe, it infects blood, urinary tract, and wounds of patients with compromised immune systems.
- Vancomycin-resistant **Staphylococcus aureus** (VRSA), a pathogenic bacterium similar to VRE.
- Vancomycin-intermediate *Staphylococcus aureus* (VISA), a pathogenic bacterium that may be seen in patients with chronic diabetes and kidney disease; found in open wounds.
- *Pseudomonas aeruginosa* causes deadly lower-respiratory infections in sick patients.
- Creutzfeldt-Jakob disease (CJD), a fatal disease caused by a prion (a pathogen smaller than a virus); the causative agent is very difficult, if almost impossible, to destroy. The causative agent appears to be concentrated in cerebrospinal fluid. (See Selected Readings.).
- Human immunodeficiency virus (HIV), a retrovirus that causes acquired immunodeficiency syndrome (AIDS). HIV was identified in 1984. The disease causes a loss of immune functions and the subsequent development of opportunistic infections. HIV is spread through direct contact with contaminated body fluids.
- Hepatitis, an inflammation of the liver brought about by several recognized viruses. HAV, hepatitis A; HBV, hepatitis B; HCV, hepatitis C; HDV, hepatitis D; HEV, hepatitis E; HGV, hepatitis G; GBV, hepatitis GBV. Hepatitis A and E are transmitted by the fecal-oral route; hepatitis B, C, D, G,

and GBV are bloodborne diseases. Embalmers need to be immunized against hepatitis B.

- Tuberculosis, caused by **Mycobacterium tuberculosis**, most commonly affects the respiratory system, but it is capable of affecting almost anybody's system or area. Multidrug-resistant tuberculosis is difficult for physicians to treat. Individuals with lowered immunity can be susceptible to this form of tuberculosis. Worldwide tuberculosis is still a leading cause of death. An embalmer needs to carefully disinfect and dispose of—in a biohazard container—any nasal-oral discharges and sputum when respiratory tuberculosis is present.

## The Female Embalmer and Pregnancy

The choice to continue embalming during pregnancy is a personal decision made by the embalmer. As long as the embalmer feels capable of working in the preparation room and has access to an adequate supply of PPE, she may continue to do so. A pregnant employee can request a change of work assignment when it is determined to be the best course of action by the employee or as the result of the employee's consultation with their health care provider. The health care field offers a comparison; a pregnant worker might not want to change a job assignment until a need arises. According to the Pregnancy Discrimination Act, if a pregnant female is unable to perform her duties, with or without a physician's note, "the employer must treat her the same as any other temporarily disabled employee" (www.eeoc.gov).

## Exposure to Chemical Hazards

The objectives of the embalming process are to preserve, sanitize, and restore the dead human body. These objectives are accomplished by the application of chemicals. Many of the chemicals used in embalming and the related processes contain components that have been categorized as hazardous substances. Dangers associated with using these substances have been well documented in the health and medical literature.

A study conducted by Williams and associates (1984) stated that exposure to formaldehyde, particularly formaldehyde vapor, is probably the most significant of the chemical exposures to which embalmers are subjected. Over the years, a number of other studies have reported on the adverse effects of chronic exposure to formaldehyde (Kerfoot, 1972; Kerfoot and Mooney, 1975; Bender et al., 1983).

Nethercott and Holness (1988) noted that Canadian funeral service workers were more likely to complain about irritations of the nose and eyes than were members of a control group. The study went on to say that those funeral service employees who were in contact with formaldehyde were likely to experience skin and mucous membrane irritation.

Many of the chemicals used in embalming are regulated by state and federal Occupational Safety and Health Administration" (OSHA) standards. Hazardous substance standards adopted in Minnesota, for example, contain a list of nearly 1100 substances controlled because of the hazards that result from their use (State of Minnesota, 1995). Many of the substances on that list are either used in the embalming process or are components of products used in the embalming process. Most notable among the health problems that can result from chemicals in the preparation room are contact dermatitis, eye and nose irritations, and upper respiratory irritations.

Since 1987, the United States Environmental Protection Agency has recognized formaldehyde as a potential carcinogen for tumors in the lung, nasopharynx, and nasal passages. In June 2004, the International Agency for Research on Cancer recognized formaldehyde as a human carcinogen. Presently, the European Union, under its Biocides Directive, is examining the health effects of formaldehyde. The National Cancer Institute released in 2009 the findings of an extensive study of workers with high exposure to formaldehyde—anatomists, pathologists, and funeral personnel. They found these persons to have a statistically increased risk for mortality from lympho-hematopoietic malignancies, in particular, myeloid leukemia.

In 2010, the National Academy of Sciences reviewed the EPA findings that linked formaldehyde and leukemia. NAS disagreed with those findings and determined the EPA document needed revision. A separate study published in Toxicological Sciences in 2011 found no connection between formaldehyde and leukemia in animal studies. The United States Department of Health & Human Services in June 2010 added formaldehyde to the National Toxicology Program list of carcinogenic compounds. Research continues, but a positive link between formaldehyde and leukemia has yet to be established.

## Exposure to Other Hazards of Embalming

In addition to the hazards associated with biological and chemical agents, embalmers are exposed to hazards including heat, ionizing radiation, and nonionizing radiation. Although these hazards may not be as prevalent as chemical or biological hazards, they are worth noting and may necessitate action by a funeral service facility.

### Ventilation and Temperature

Funeral homes must give consideration to the ventilation and temperature in the embalming room. If the temperature of a room is high, an embalmer wearing a full set of PPE may have difficulty regulating core body temperature. PPEs can trap body heat; coupled with inadequate ventilation, and high humidity can cause discomfort.

### Ionizing Radiation

The potential exists for an embalmer to come into contact with a body that has undergone radiation therapy. Institutions that administer radiation treatments monitor radiation levels. Bodies that have undergone radiation treatment are not released until exposure levels are deemed safe. Documentation of the radiation treatment accompanies the body. Contact the radiation officer at the releasing institution for information.

### Nonionizing Radiation

The potential for adverse exposure to nonionizing radiation in the preparation room is remote. Exposure to electromagnetic radiation exists with household products such as microwave ovens or computer monitors.

# REGULATORY AGENCIES

## Legislative Intent

The law is considered the minimum ethic of a community. Members of a society place their trust in funeral service professionals, charging them to discharge their duties in a competent manner. Standards of performance are expected from embalmers and funeral directors.

The issuance of a license to practice mortuary science declares:
1. Embalming is a practice affecting public safety and welfare and is subject to regulation and control in the public interest.
2. The preparation, care, and final disposition of a deceased human body should be attended with appropriate observance and understanding, in addition to having due regard and respect for the reverent care of the human body and for those bereaved and the overall spiritual dignity of humankind.
3. As a matter of public interest, the practice of embalming merits and receives the confidence of the public in that only qualified persons be authorized to embalm in their state of practice.
4. The state codes should be liberally construed to best carry out these subjects and purposes.

## State Regulation

In the United States, the practice of embalming is regulated primarily by the legislative institutions of each individual state to oversee the care and disposition of dead human remains: The Board of Health (or Bureau of Vital Statistics) and the State Board of Examiners (or similar governing body) regulate and license funeral homes, funeral directors, and embalmers. Regulatory agencies promulgate and enforce statutory law as well as rules and regulations governing the disposition of dead human bodies. States regulate a coroner or a medical examiner and the organ and tissue procurement agencies to take actual custody of the dead human body. They also have authority over the disposition of indigent bodies and the procurement of bodies for medical science.

## Federal Regulation

In recent years, federal agencies have come to play an important role in the activities of the funeral establishment and the preparation room. These agencies include the Centers for Disease Control and Prevention (CDC), Environmental Protection Agency (EPA), the Federal Trade Commission (FTC), and the Occupational Safety and Health Administration (OSHA). Four divisions of OSHA directly affect the funeral establishment: (1) General Rule, (2) the Hazard Communication Standard, (3) the Formaldehyde Rule, and (4) the Bloodborne Pathogen Rule. The Transportation Security Administration (TSA) registers providers as *approved shippers* for transportation of human remains by common carriers.

## Federal Trade Commission

In April 1984, the federal government, through the FTC, promulgated a rule governing the activities of funeral directors and embalmers. The rule, which is commonly referred to as the Funeral Rule, was amended by the FTC in 1994. The Funeral Rule applies to **all** states. The following excerpts are reprinted from the Federal Register:

*Misrepresentations*
EMBALMING PROVISIONS—DECEPTIVE ACTS OR PRACTICES. In selling or offering to sell funeral goods or funeral services to the public, it is a deceptive act or practice for a funeral provider to:
1. Represent that state or local law requires that a deceased person be embalmed when such is not the case
2. Fail to disclose that embalming is not required by law, except in certain special cases

PREVENTIVE REQUIREMENTS. To prevent these deceptive acts or practices as well as the unfair or deceptive acts or practices defined in §453.4(b)(1) and §453.5(2) [of the Funeral Rule], funeral providers must:
1. Not represent that a deceased person is required to be embalmed for:
   A. Direct cremation;
   B. Immediate burial; or
   C. A closed casket funeral without viewing or visitation when refrigeration is available and when state or local law does not require embalming.
2. Place the following disclosure on the General Price List, required by §453.2(b)(4) in immediate conjunction with the price shown for embalming: "Except in certain special cases, embalming is not required by law. Embalming may be necessary, however, if you select certain funeral arrangements, such as a funeral with viewing. If you do not want embalming, you usually have the right to choose an arrangement that does not require you to pay for it, such as direct cremation or immediate burial." The phrase "except in certain special cases" need not be included in this disclosure if state or local laws in the area(s) where the provider does business, do not require embalming under any circumstances.

*Services Provided Without Prior Approval*
UNFAIR OR DECEPTIVE ACTS OR PRACTICES. In selling or offering to sell funeral goods or funeral services to the public, it is an unfair or deceptive act or practice for any provider to embalm a deceased body for a fee unless:
1. State or local law or regulation requires embalming in the particular circumstances, regardless of any funeral choice which the family might make; or
2. Prior approval for embalming (expressly so described) from a family member or other authorized person, or
3. The funeral provider is unable to contact a family member or other authorized person after exercising due diligence, has no reason to believe the family does not want embalming performed, and obtains subsequent approval for embalming already performed (expressly so described). In seeking approval, the funeral provider must disclose that a fee will be charged if the family selects a funeral that requires embalming, such as a funeral with viewing, and that no fee will be charged if the family selects a service that does not require embalmings, such as direct cremation or immediate burial.

PREVENTIVE REQUIREMENT. To prevent these unfair or deceptive acts or practices, funeral providers must include on the itemized statement of funeral goods and services selected, required by §453.2(b)(5), the statement: "If you selected a funeral that may require embalming, such as a funeral with viewing, you might have to pay for embalming. You do not have to pay for embalming; you did not approve if you selected arrangements such as direct cremation or immediate burial. If we charge for embalming, we will explain why below."

## Local Regulations

At the local level, various entities such as the zoning board, the local board of health, the waste disposal board, and the water management board also have involvement with the funeral home or the embalming facility.

## EXPOSURE TO EMBALMING HAZARDS: OSHA BLOODBORNE PATHOGENS STANDARD

### Biological Hazards

Health and safety issues associated with embalming are addressed by compliance with **the Bloodborne Pathogens Standard.** The Bloodborne Pathogens Standard is administered by the United States Department of Labor through OSHA. The rule is directly applicable to occupations and professions, including funeral service, where employees are exposed to infectious agents. In addition, many individual states have enacted **Employee Right-To-Know** laws that support or expand the scope of federal OSHA regulations. Embalmers must be aware of the duties and responsibilities that are imposed on them by the laws and rules of the various jurisdictions within which they practice. Compliance with the Bloodborne Pathogens Standard, and any state regulations that support or expand it, are required.

Under the Bloodborne Pathogens Standard, employers are required to conduct an evaluation of their workplace(s) to determine if employees have occupational exposure to infectious agents regulated by OSHA. If such exposure exists, a written **Exposure Control Plan** must be developed to control, minimize, or eliminate employee exposure. Exposure control plans, which by law must be accessible to employees, are to be reviewed and updated at least once per year so that changes in personnel, procedure, and/or work assignments can be documented. The minimum documentation required for an Exposure Control Plan includes exposure determination, methods of compliance, hepatitis B vaccination as well as postexposure evaluation and follow-up, hazard communication, and record-keeping.

### Exposure Determination

Employers are required to examine workplace(s) to determine (1) if occupational exposure to bloodborne pathogens exists and (2) what types of duties are being performed when occupational exposure to bloodborne pathogens occurs. If occupational exposure to bloodborne pathogens is identified, employers must then list all job titles or classifications which have exposure. In a funeral home setting, this might include, but not be limited to, embalmers, intern/ apprentice embalmers, removal personnel, and any other person having **direct contact** with the unembalmed human remains or with any regulated infectious waste materials. Employers must also identify those employees who have "some" occupational exposure to infectious agents. This might include, but not be limited to, hairdressers, housekeepers, maintenance personnel, funeral directors, drivers, and clerical staff. Employers must identify and list duties that involve exposure to infectious agents. Examples of duties that might appear on such a list include removal of human remains, embalming, hairdressing, application of cosmetics, and laundry.

### Methods of Compliance

Compliance with the Bloodborne Pathogens Standard is accomplished by the application of (1) universal precautions, (2) engineering controls, and (3) work practice controls. The basic premise of **universal precautions** is to treat all human remains as if they were potentially infectious. In other words, the embalmer should treat all bodies with the same caution that would be applied for extremely hazardous, potentially fatal infections. By the implementation of this universal caution, the embalmer seeks to prevent "parenteral, mucous membrane, and nonintact skin exposure" (Code of Federal Regulations, 1992). The embalmer avoids needlesticks or cuts that create parenteral exposure by breaking the protective barrier provided by the skin. The embalmer will also avoid other situations that might result in ingestion of contaminated material through the nose or the mouth. The embalmer must take care to avoid allowing infectious agents to invade through the eyes or be absorbed through or otherwise penetrate the skin. Care must also be taken to prevent infectious agents from invading the host by means of an existing break in the skin, such as cuts, scratches, and so on. To seek protection from possible infection, the embalmer will (1) utilize Personal Protective Equipment (PPE); (2) properly decontaminate infected surfaces; (3) properly handle and dispose of infectious wastes; (4) apply appropriate measures to control leaks, drips, and spills of infectious materials; (5) apply proper work practice skills; and (6) properly handle contaminated laundry.

**Engineering controls** are those mechanical systems and devices engineered into the architecture of a building. Engineering controls that are used to provide personal and public health protection should be examined and maintained or replaced on a regular schedule. The examination and maintenance should be documented. Doing so will ensure that the systems and devices are operating at maximum efficiency to reduce exposure. The two primary areas of consideration are **adequate ventilation** and **proper plumbing.**

During embalming, the potential exists for infectious agents to become aerosolized and produce airborne particulates. The purpose of adequate ventilation is to remove contaminated air from the work area for replacement with fresh air. Proper placement of vents for incoming and outgoing air is critical. Outgoing air (discharge) should be at the foot of the embalming table and below the level of the tabletop. The air replacement or incoming air vent should ideally be high on the opposite wall. This configuration provides clean, fresh air in the direction of the embalmer while contaminated air is drawn downward and away from the embalmer's breathing zone.

The number of air exchanges required per hour is determined by numerous factors, primarily the square footage of the room and the nature and scope of room activity. A general requirement for a single-table design might be 15–20 air exchanges per hour. A minimum of 15 air exchanges per hour is currently recommended for the preparation room. (See NFDA Best Formaldehyde Work Practices—2010).

Installation of plumbing devices prevents embalming waste from entering the potable water supply. Examples of engineering controls that reduce water contamination include (1) vacuum breakers on the main water line leading into the building, (2) vacuum breakers on equipment such as hydroaspirators, (3) maintenance of discharge basins and flush sinks in good working order, (4) a suitable water source for the preparation table, (5) eyewash station, (6) drench shower, (7) hand washing station, and (8) adjacent shower facilities for embalmer personal hygiene.

Vacuum breakers installed on aspiration equipment, and water lines leading into the funeral home prevent back-siphonage of water leading from the preparation room to the water lines in the facility. Local and state plumbing codes must be satisfied.

## Work Practice Controls

Work practice controls are common-sense steps taken to avoid unnecessary or excessive exposure to infectious agents. Common work practices that contribute to a hygienic environment include (1) hand washing, (2) proper handling and disposal of contaminated waste and contaminated sharps, (3) avoiding splashing, spraying, or splattering, (4) consistent and proper use of PPE, and (5) housekeeping provisions. Work practice controls must be documented and enforced.

Employees must receive training and instruction on proper hand washing techniques. The sufficient contact time with antiseptic soap and water recommended is 20 seconds. A helpful practice is to wet the hands, apply antiseptic soap, lather generously, and rub hands and fingers together vigorously while singing a song that exceeds the minimum time. The CDC recommends:

1. Using liquid soap and running water at a comfortable temperature, working up a lather and creating friction between the fingers.
2. Rinsing with plenty of running water to remove soap from the hands. Residual soap can cause skin irritation and chapping.
3. Thoroughly drying hands with disposable toweling or air drying. Use the toweling to turn off manual faucets.

Employees must receive training and instruction on the proper use and accessibility of PPE, cleaning and laundering procedures, repair and replacement procedures, disposal procedures for contaminated or damaged PPE, and procedures for proper storage of PPE.

Employers are required to provide a variety of suitable PPE in a range of sizes for all wearers (**Fig. 3-4A-F**). PPE is considered to be appropriate only when it prevents blood and potentially hazardous materials from breaching the protective barrier.

Gloves for embalming use must be of sufficient thickness and provide full protection of the hands and wrists. Heavier mil (13 mil or greater) latex, nitrile, neoprene, rubber, and other high tensile strength materials are more durable and provide greater protection (**Fig. 3-5**). Gloves should be frequently changed throughout the embalming procedure.

The CDC recommends that barrier masks provide protection against inhalation of airborne pathogens and particulates; the mask must cover both mouth and nose and fit the wearer snugly for full efficiency. During embalming, the embalmer should wear a surgical cap, bouffant cap, hood, or other suitable head covering. Hair should be tucked beneath the head covering. The embalmer's forehead, cheeks, and neck should be protected by a face shield. The eyes should be protected by a splash barrier such as safety glasses, goggles, or a combination face-eye shield. The arms, torso, and legs should be protected by a garment or combination of garments that provide full coverage. The feet should be covered by suitable water-resistant, nonslip type of footwear or water-resistant, nonslip shoe coverings. **A rule of thumb for protective garments is that the embalmer should have no exposed skin.** Disposable PPE must be removed after use and properly discarded in an approved biohazard waste container. Launderable PPE must be properly stored for cleaning and disinfection.

Eating, drinking, handling of contact lenses, and application of personal cosmetics are prohibited in work areas. Food items and beverages should never be stored in mortuary refrigeration units.

Employers must ensure that work areas are maintained in clean and sanitary conditions. A written cleaning and disinfection schedule must be implemented. Customarily, terminal room disinfection occurs at the completion of each embalming shift or at the completion of the daily work schedule.

After use, hypodermic needles and other sharps should not be sheared, bent, broken, recapped, or resheathed by hand. Dispose of broken and contaminated sharps in approved biohazard sharps containers. Disposable, retractable scalpels are recommended.

All procedures involving blood or other potentially infectious body fluids should be performed in such a manner as to minimize splashing, spraying, and aerosolization. Blood drainage from the drainage instrument, angular spring forceps, or drain tube must be modified to minimize splashing and reduce aerosolization. Body bridges and various positioning devices lift the decedent and allow blood and waste to freely reach the table drain without splashing. All sinks and basins should be covered to eliminate aerosolization from splashing. All instruments, equipment, and work surfaces must be properly cleaned and disinfected upon contact with blood or other potentially infectious materials. All pails, containers, and receptacles intended for reuse and those that have a potential for becoming contaminated with blood or other potentially infectious materials should be inspected, cleaned, and disinfected on a regular basis or as soon as possible on visible contamination.

## Hepatitis B Vaccination

Hepatitis B vaccination must be made available to all employees who have occupational exposure. The vaccination program must be (1) offered at no cost to the employee; (2) offered at a reasonable time and place; (3) performed by, or under the supervision of, a licensed physician or certified health care professional; and (4) provided according to the recommendations of the U.S. Public Health Service. Employees have the option of accepting or declining the vaccination. If the employee is offered the vaccination and declines, a declination statement must be signed by the employee. If an employee first declines the vaccination and later decides to accept, the declination document is discarded, and the employee must be given the vaccination. Prudent practice is to verify immunity levels with a blood test at regular intervals, annually, or every few years.

## Postexposure Evaluation and Follow-up

In the event that a blood or body fluid exposure incident occurs, employers must immediately implement procedures for postexposure evaluation and follow-up. The postexposure evaluation and follow-up will include (1) a detailed explanation of

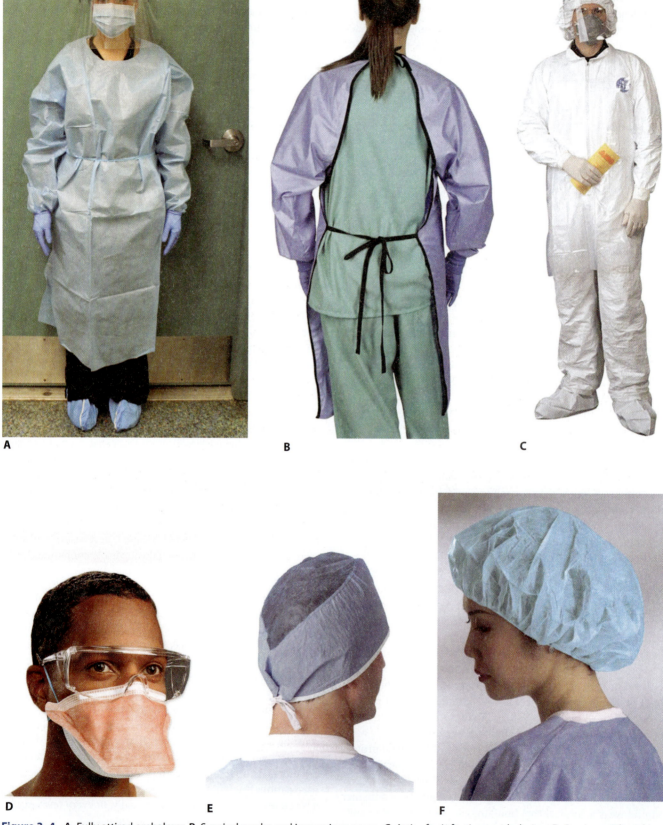

**Figure 3–4. A.** Fully attired embalmer. **B.** Surgical scrubs and impervious gown. **C.** Attire for infectious embalming. **D.** Barrier mask and eyewear. **E.** Surgical cap. **F.** Bouffant head covering.

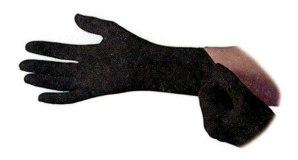

**Figure 3–5.** Nitrile gloves.

the events and circumstances related to the exposure; (2) identification and documentation of the source individual, unless doing so is impossible or prohibited by law; (3) collection and testing of the source blood for HBV and HIV; (4) taking steps necessary to assist in the prevention of infection or disease; (5) offering counseling; and (6) conducting an evaluation of any reported illnesses. It is also prudent to review exposure reduction strategies to limit the potential for future exposure.

### Hazard Communication

The following can be used to label or distinguish containers used to store, transport, or ship blood or other potentially infectious agents: (1) fluorescent orange labels, (2) orange and red labels, (3) predominantly orange and red warning labels, (4) labels with lettering and symbols in contrasting colors, or (5) other suitable substitutes for labels, such as red bags or red containers.

In addition to the labeling provisions required by the Bloodborne Pathogens Standard, employers must also provide information and training to those employees who are exposed to infectious hazards in the workplace. Employers will ensure that all employees with occupational exposure receive training related to bloodborne pathogens and training on methods for dealing with infectious agents. The training must be given at or before the time the employee is assigned a task where exposure exists. Training updates must be repeated at least once per year.

The training program must contain the following components:

1. A copy of the regulatory text must be readily available and accessible to employees at all times.
2. A general explanation of the epidemiology and symptoms of bloodborne diseases must be provided.
3. An explanation of the modes of transmission of bloodborne pathogens must be provided. To satisfy the need for information about epidemiology, symptoms, and modes of transmission, books such as *Control of Communicable Diseases Manual* (Benenson, 1995) have become commonplace in funeral homes as resources that satisfy OSHA compliance standards. This type of reference material provides ready access to information helpful in the identification of infectious agents, as well as information related to the occurrence; reservoir; mode of transmission; incubation period; period of communicability, susceptibility, and resistance; and methods of control.
4. An explanation of the employer's exposure control plan and the means by which the employee can obtain a copy of the written plan must be provided.
5. An explanation of the appropriate methods for recognizing tasks and other activities that may involve exposure to blood and other potentially infectious materials must be provided.
6. An explanation of the use and limitations of methods that will prevent or reduce exposure, including appropriate use of engineering controls, work practice controls, and universal precautions, must be provided.
7. Information on the types, proper use, location, removal, handling, decontamination, and disposal of PPE.
8. An explanation of the basis for selection of PPE. Not all gloves and masks offer equal protection from microorganisms or chemical exposures.
9. Information on the hepatitis B vaccine, including information on its efficacy, safety, method of administration, the benefits of being vaccinated, and that the vaccine and vaccination will be offered free of charge.
10. Information on the appropriate actions to take and persons to contact in an emergency involving blood or other potentially infectious materials.
11. An explanation of the procedure to follow if an exposure incident occurs, including the method of reporting the incident and the medical follow-up that will be made available.
12. Information on the postexposure evaluation and the follow-up required after an exposure incident.
13. An explanation of the signs, labels, and color-coding used to mark biohazardous materials and containers.
14. An opportunity for interactive questions and answers with the person conducting the training session.

### Record Keeping

Employers are responsible for establishing and maintaining accurate records for each employee with occupational exposure to bloodborne pathogens. The employee must receive training on the date of hire or date of being responsible for tasks involving exposure; this date may change as a person's duties change. The record must contain (1) the name and the Social Security number of the employee, (2) a copy of the employee's hepatitis B vaccination, (3) results of any examinations, medical testing, and follow-up procedures that occurred as a result of an exposure incident, (4) employer's copy of any health care professional's written opinion regarding examinations, medical testing, or follow-up in the aftermath of an exposure incident, and (5) a copy of the health care professional's report of any examinations, medical testing, or follow-up in the aftermath of an exposure incident.

Employers must maintain records of each training session. Training records are to be kept for a period of 3 years from the date the training occurred. The record must include (1) the date of each training session, (2) a summary of each training session, (3) the name(s) and qualification(s) of trainer(s), and (4) the names and job titles of all persons attending each training session. Employers are required to make all records available to the employees or their representatives. If either the employment is terminated or the employee transfers to another location or employer, the training records must be made available to the new location or the new employer. If an employer ceases to operate and has no successor, OSHA must be notified so that records can be transferred to an appropriate place and filed for future use.

Embalmers have to make judgments about exposure to potentially infectious agents. Information is vital to the decision-making process, and embalmers should have access to as much information as possible.

The assumption in the embalming process is that all bodies contain infectious agents and, therefore, represent reservoirs in which infectious agents can be found. In as much as the embalming procedure is invasive, it is a given that infectious agents will escape from the body during embalming. The embalmer represents a potential host for the escaped infectious agents because the embalmer will be in direct contact with any infectious agents that are released from the body. In spite of the exposure, infectious agents can be prevented from entering the embalmer with the proper application of work practice controls, engineering controls, and universal precautions. In addition to the controls and physical barriers that can be utilized to protect the embalmer, it is important for the embalmer to maintain good personal health to maintain resistance to infection.

Decontamination of instruments, equipment, the work area, and the body are important weapons in the fight against infectious diseases. In preparation room settings where exposure levels are high, decontamination is accomplished by using physical or chemical means (**Table 3–1**).

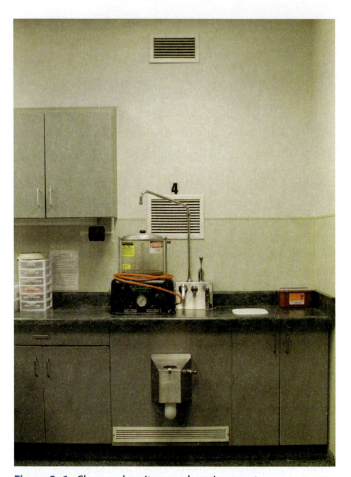

**Figure 3–6.** Clean and sanitary work environment.

Good work practices and universal precautions dictate that the instruments, equipment, counter tops, table tops, walls, floors, light fixtures, sinks, cabinets, and waste receptacles be sanitized and disinfected (**Fig. 3–6**). Disinfection and decontamination activity should occur as necessary during an embalming procedure; concurrent disinfection and decontamination, and then terminal disinfection and decontamination must be done thoroughly at the completion of the embalming process.

A quality topical disinfectant should be applied to the deceased human body followed by bathing of the body during the initial steps of the embalming process. Concurrent cleaning and bathing should occur during the embalming process, followed by thorough final bathing at the conclusion of the embalming process.

Embalmers could consider steam sterilization or **autoclaving,** for contaminated instruments, or immersion of instruments in a suitable cold chemical sterilant. Steam sterilization is seldom used in funeral service because of two considerations. First, autoclaves are very expensive, and second, they are not large enough to hold instruments such as a trocar. Embalmers will find a number of commercially prepared cold chemical sterilants on the market. Cold chemical sterilants have formulations containing acid glutaraldehyde, or alkalinized glutaraldehyde, or formaldehyde in methanol as their active ingredients. Some common microbicides are shown in **Table 3–2**. [Formaldehyde and methanol (formalin) are only sporicidal (a sterilant) at a concentration of 8% or greater.] Selecting disinfectants that

| TABLE 3–1. Breaking the Cycle of Transmission of Infectious Agents in the Preparation Room: Public Health Guidelines for the At-Risk Embalmer "Host" ||
|---|---|
| **Portal of "Host" Entry** | **Infectious Agent** |
| Skin or mucous membrane respiratory tract, alimentary tract, body openings—natural and/or artificial (abrasions, cuts, lacerations, wounds) | Bacteria, fungi (molds and yeasts), viruses, rickettsia, protozoa |
| Proper "barrier" attire<br>Aseptic technique(s)<br>Handwashing, gloves<br>Disinfection and decontamination | Personal health practices<br>Personnel health policies<br>Environmental sanitation<br>Disinfection and decontamination |
| Modes of Transmitting the Infectious Agent | Reservoirs of Infectious Agents in the Preparation Room |
| Direct contact (aerosol or droplet infection) and indirect contact (air, contaminated surfaces) and objects or fomites, body fluids and exudates, insects | Remains, equipment (e.g., hydroaspirators, trocars, razors), instruments, adjacent hard surfaces, air contaminated linens, bandages and dressings, solid and liquid wastes |
| Proper "barrier" attire ||
| Handwashing, gloves ||
| Proper disposition of wastes ||
| Effective air handling system ||
| Concurrent and terminal disinfection ||

**Note:** Proper "barrier" attire may include whole-body covering, head cover, shoe covers, gloves, oral–nasal mask, and eye protection (safety glasses).

## TABLE 3-2. Activity Levels of Selected Microbicides

| Liquid Microbicide[a] | Use Concentration | Activity Level |
|---|---|---|
| Glutaraldehyde, aqueous, e.g., Cidex, Sonacide, Sporicidin | 2.0% | High |
| Formaldehyde + alcohol | 8.0% + 70.0% | High |
| Stabilized hydrogen peroxide | 6.0–10.0% | High |
| Formaldehyde, aqueous | 3.0–8.0% | High to intermediate |
| Iodophors, e.g., Betadine, Wescodyne, HiSine, Losan | 75–200 ppm | Intermediate |
| Iodine + alcohol | 0.5% + 70.0% | Intermediate |
| Chlorine compounds, e.g., sodium hypochlorite as in chlorine bleach | 1000–5000 ppm | Intermediate |
| Phenolic compounds, aqueous, e.g., Amphyl Staphene, O-Syl | 0.5–3.0% | Intermediate to low |
| Quaternary ammonium compounds, e.g., Phemoral, Zepharin Chloride, Diaparine Chloride | 0.1–0.2% aqueous | Low |
| Mercurial compounds, organic and inorganic, e.g., Merthiolate, Mercurochrome, Metaphen | 0.1–0.2% | Low |

[a] Trade names of certain microbicides are given.
From Block SS. *Disinfection, Sterilization, and Preservation*, 3rd ed. Philadelphia: Lea & Febiger; 1983, with permission.

are suited for this application plays an extremely important role. When corrosive disinfectants, such as household bleach, are used, the chrome finish on instruments can be damaged. It may nevertheless be advisable to use household bleach when a known Creutzfeldt-Jakob Disease (CJD) case is being embalmed. Anytime instruments appear to be pitted or the chrome finish is worn away, the instruments should be replaced—because when the surface of an instrument is pitted, it becomes difficult to disinfect. The pitted surfaces are ideal hiding places for microorganisms and also permit air bubbles to build up between the disinfecting solution and the surface of the instrument. When one considers the microscopic appearance of these surface pits, it is plain to see that these instruments pose a greater risk for infection during needlesticks or other sharps injuries. For example, a new suture needle will appear quite smooth under the microscope. When a needlestick occurs, there is a *squeegee effect* when the needle passes through the glove and skin, reducing the number of organisms introduced into the tissues. If the instrument is old or pitted, there is a greatly reduced squeegee effect increasing the number of microorganisms transferred into the embalmer or the body being embalmed. To the embalmer, this translates into an increased risk of infection. For the body being embalmed, this translates into a greater risk of transferring tissue gas bacilli from one body to another.

Following the embalming process, all contaminated surfaces should be decontaminated, cleaned, and disinfected with a suitable disinfectant solution or topical disinfectant (**Table 3–3**).

The following terms in **Table 3–4** are commonly associated with methods of disinfection and sterilization.

**Asepsis**—freedom from infection and from any form of life; sterility

**Bactericidal**—destructive to bacteria

**Bacteriostatic**—inhibiting the growth or multiplication of bacteria (no destruction of viability implied)

**Cleaning**—removal of infectious agents by scrubbing and washing, as with hot water, soap, or a suitable detergent

**Concurrent disinfection**—the cleaning of the body and instruments at the time of embalming the body

**Decontamination**—the use of physical, chemical, or other means to remove, inactivate, or destroy harmful microorganisms or chemicals from a surface

**Disinfectant**—an agent, usually chemical, applied to inanimate objects/surfaces for the purpose of destroying disease-causing microbial agents, but usually not bacterial spores

**Germicide**—an agent, usually chemical, applied either to inanimate objects/surfaces or living tissue for the purpose of destroying disease-causing microbial agents, but usually not bacterial spores

**Primary disinfection**—those disinfection procedures carried out prior to embalming the body. This would include topical disinfection of and washing the deceased human body

**Sanitizer**—an agent, usually chemical, that possesses disinfecting properties when applied to a precleaned object/surface

**Sterilization**—a process that renders a substance-free from all microorganisms

**Terminal disinfection**—the cleaning and disinfection of the body, instruments, and the embalming room following embalming of the body

## Topical Disinfectants in the Preparation Room

Topical disinfectants are used either for the sanitation of the skin and the hair of the dead human body's external orifices or for the sanitation of exposed tissues as a result of trauma, autopsy, organ, and/or tissue donation. These chemicals are also used to disinfect body bags, clothing, medical devices, and protective garments (diapers) removed from the body. Instruments, counter tops and embalming tables, and equipment can also be sanitized with a good topical disinfectant.

The disinfectant needs to be broad-spectrum—meaning bactericidal, fungicidal, virucidal, and ideally tuberculocidal. Read the labels carefully. Instructions for use will be explained. These chemicals are also dated and this needs to be noted. There is a period of time in which the chemical needs to be in contact with the object or the surface being disinfected, and this time element should also be listed.

Areas to be treated ideally need to first be cleaned using a good antiseptic soap. Remove as much contaminated organic matter as possible (blood, sputum, feces, urine, etc.). Apply the chemical as a heavy droplet spray. Give the chemical sufficient time to work. Remove and dry using a disposable towel. Dispose of the towel in a biohazard waste container.

## TABLE 3-3. Acceptable Antimicrobial Procedures/Exposure Intervals

| Objects | Vegetative Bacteria and Fungi and Influenza Viruses<br>*Disinfection* | Tubercle Bacilli, Enteroviruses Except Hepatitis Viruses, Vegetative Bacteria and Fungi, and Influenza Viruses<br>*Disinfection* | Bacterial and Fungal Spores, Hepatitis Viruses, Tubercle Bacilli, Enteroviruses, Vegetative Bacteria and Fungi, and Influenza Viruses<br>*Sterilization* |
|---|---|---|---|
| Smooth, hard surface objects | A—10 min<br>D—5 min<br>E—10 min<br>F—10 min<br>H—10 min<br>L—5 min<br>M—5 min | B—10 min<br>D—10 min<br>G—10 min<br>H—10 min<br>L—10 min | D—18 h<br>J<br>K<br>L—9 h<br>M—10 h<br>M—10 min |
| Rubber tubing, rubber catheters | E—10 min<br>F—10 min<br>H—10 min | G—10 min<br>H—10 min | J[a]<br>K |
| Polyethylene tubing, polyethylene catheters | A—10 min<br>E—10 min<br>F—10 min<br>H—10 min | B—10 min<br>G—10 min<br>H—10 min | D—18 h<br>J[a]<br>K<br>L—9 h<br>M—10 h |
| Lensed instruments | E—10 min<br>F—10 min<br>H—10 min<br>K<br>M—10 min | K<br>M—10 min | K |
| Hypodermic needles | Sterilization only | Sterilization only | J |
| Thermometers[b] | C—10 min<br>K | C—10 min<br>K | D—18 h<br>L—9 h<br>M—10 h |
| Hinged instruments | A—20 min<br>D—10 min<br>E—20 min<br>F—20 min<br>H—20 min<br>L—10 min<br>M—10 min | B—30 min<br>D—20 min<br>G—30 min<br>H—30 min<br>L—20 min<br>M—20 min | J<br>K<br>L—9 h<br>M—10 h |
| Floors, furniture, other appropriate room surfaces | E—5 min<br>F—5 min<br>H—5 min<br>I—5 min | G—5 min<br>H—5 min | Not necessary or practical |

**Key**

A. Isopropyl alcohol (70–90%) plus 0.2% sodium nitrite to prevent corrosion
B. Ethyl alcohol (70–90%)
C. Isopropyl or ethyl alcohol plus 0.2% iodine
D. Formaldehyde (8%)—alcohol solution plus 0.2% sodium nitrite to prevent corrosion
E. Quaternary ammonium solutions (1:500 aq.) plus 0.2% sodium nitrite to prevent corrosion
F. Iodophor—75 ppm available iodine plus 0.2% sodium nitrite to prevent corrosion
G. Iodophor—450 ppm available iodine plus 0.2% sodium nitrite to prevent corrosion
H. Phenolic solutions (2% aq.) plus 0.5% sodium bicarbonate to prevent corrosion
I. Sodium hypochlorite (1:500 aq.—approximately 100 ppm)[a]
J. Heat sterilization, see manufacturers' recommendations
K. Ethylene oxide gas 6 or technical literature
L. Aqueous formalin (40%)
M. Activated glutaraldehyde (2% aq.)
[a]Investigate thermostability when indicated.
[b]Must be thoroughly wiped, preferably with a tincture of soap, before disinfection or sterilization. Alcohol–iodine solution will remove markings on poor-grade thermometers.
**Note:** 1000 ppm of available chlorine is recommended for inactivation of hepatitis B virus and 5000 ppm for inactivation of HIV (AIDS). Thoroughly rinse all inanimate surfaces of any excess formalin prior to application of the hypochlorite disinfectant. Keene (1973) cautions that when formaldehyde reacts with hydrochloric acid, the compound bis(chloromethyl) ether (BCME) may be formed. BCME is a highly toxic, carcinogenic compound.

### TABLE 3-4. Chemical and Physical Methods for Controlling Microbial Contamination

| Method of Decontamination | Temperature Requirement | Minimum Interval of Exposure (min) |
|---|---|---|
| Sterilization: Complete destruction of all forms of microbial life | 285°F (140°C) | —\| (instant) |
| Saturated steam under pressure | 270°F (132°C) | ————\| |
| (autoclaving) | 250°F (121°C) | —————————\| 30 min for hepatitis viruses |
| Ethylene oxide gas | 130°F (54°C) | 2 to 12 h \| |
| Hot air, e.g., oven | 320°F (160°C) | 2 h or more \| |
| Chemical sporicide solution, e.g., | Room temperature | 3 to 12 h or more \| |
| 8.0% formaldehyde plus | | |
| 70% isopropanol, glutaraldehyde[a] | | |
| Disinfection: killing of disease-producing microbial agents, but not resistant spores | | |
| Boiling water or free-flowing steam | 212°F (100°C) | —\| or more, 30 min for hepatitis viruses |
| Chemical germicide solutions, e.g., iodophors, phenylphenols, quarternary ammonium compounds | | Room temperature ————\| or more |
| Sanitization: Chemicals aided by physical methods of soil removal | Maximum of 200°F (93°C) | ——————————\| |

[a]Recommended for high-level disinfection.
Modified from a chart copyrighted in 1967, Research and Development Section, American Sterilizer Co., Erie, PA.

Today, a good topical disinfectant from a mortuary supply company should be effective against tuberculosis, **Staphylococcus aureus**, human immunodeficiency virus (HIV), herpes simplex virus, hepatitis B virus (HBV), methicillin-resistant *S. aureus* (MRSA), and vancomycin-resistant *Enterococcus faecalis* (VRE).

## QUALITIES OF A GOOD TOPICAL DISINFECTANT

1. It is active, not outdated—should have a long shelf life.
2. Will not corrode or stain instruments.
3. It is effective against a wide range of microbes, including viruses and fungi.
4. It destroys microbes and their products quickly.
5. It is a good deodorant for the body.
6. It does not bleach or stains the skin.
7. It is not irritating to the embalmer's skin or respiratory tract.
8. Is not inactivated by the presence of biological debris.

## OSHA: HAZARD COMMUNICATION RULE

### Chemical Hazards

The federal government has mandated that business and industry, including funeral service, comply with regulations related to the safe handling and use of hazardous substances and materials. The Federal **Hazard Communication Rule** requires that employers communicate to employees the dangers that exist in the workplace as a result of hazardous substances or materials, and directs employers to train employees in the safe use and handling of hazardous substances or materials (Code of Federal Regulations, 1988). Under the Hazard Communication Rule, any chemical or a mixture of chemicals that expose employees to a health or physical risk are considered to be hazardous. The symbol used to indicate a biohazard is shown in **Fig. 3-7**.

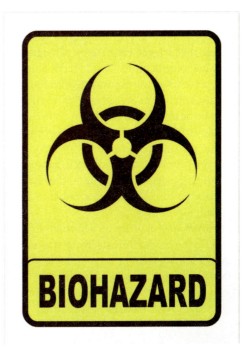

**Figure 3-7.** Biohazard symbol.

Mixtures of chemicals with a composition of 0.1% or more of an ingredient(s) classified as a carcinogen, teratogen, or mutagen are considered to present a physical or a health hazard. Mixtures of chemicals with a composition of 1.0% of an ingredient(s), which, although not being classified as a carcinogen, teratogen, or mutagen, but are classified as hazardous substances, are considered to present a physical or a health hazard. Information about the hazards of using certain materials or substances is provided by **Safety Data Sheets** (SDS), labeling, and training.

### Safety Data Sheets

The Hazard Communication Rule requires manufacturers or suppliers of hazardous materials or substances to include an SDS with each shipment. The SDS contains critical information related to the hazards, exposure levels, and symptoms associated with the material or the substance. An SDS must be kept on file for each hazardous substance or material present in the work area and must be accessible to employees.

### Labeling

Under the Hazard Communication Rule, all containers that hold hazardous substances or materials must be properly marked with the name of the product as it appears on the SDS. To be in compliance, any carton of chemicals containing hazardous materials (hazmats) would be appropriately labeled on the exterior of the box making it clear what the case contained. An SDS would be found in the carton. Because it is likely that each individual bottle of chemical would be removed from the case and stored separately, each bottle would also need to be clearly labeled.

### Training

The Hazard Communication Rule mandates that employers develop a training program that meets the following criteria:

1. The employer must identify hazardous substances found in the workplace by their generic, chemical, trade, and/or common names. This information must then be made known to the employees who may potentially have contact with the identified substances.
2. The employer must identify hazardous substances exposure levels that trigger restrictions. There are standards that mandate certain protective procedures and safeguards be put in place when the exposure to hazardous substances approaches, reaches, or exceeds a level that has been determined to be harmful or injurious.
3. The employer must identify the routes of entry and acute or chronic effects of exposure to hazardous substances. For example, fumes from hazardous substances may be inhaled during normal breathing. Other hazardous substances may be absorbed if they come into direct contact with an employee's skin.
4. The employer must explain the symptoms that accompany exposure. In the case of formaldehyde, the employer might caution the employee to be aware of skin sensitization or irritations of the eyes, nose, and throat.
5. The employer must identify and explain other dangers associated with hazardous substances to which the employee is exposed. Some chemicals, for example, may be flammable or caustic and require special care when being used.
6. The employer must explain emergency treatments that will be employed if there is an exposure incident. If, for example, embalming chemicals get sprayed into the eyes of employees or onto employees' bodies, training should have already been provided on the proper utilization of an eyewash station or a drench shower.
7. The employer must explain to employees the proper use and handling of hazardous substances. Employees, for example, should be taught methods by which they can protect themselves from the dangers of hazardous substances, such as wearing protective equipment and avoiding careless or unsafe use of chemicals.
8. The employer must explain cleanup procedures for leaks and spills. An employer, for example, may require that any spill of embalming chemical on the floor of the preparation room be immediately treated by application of formaldehyde neutralizing spray and wiped up with an absorbent paper towel, which is then placed in a container that is used to handle contaminated materials.
9. The employer must provide information on the name, telephone number, and address of the companies that supply to the workplace those chemicals that are considered hazardous. The employer can easily satisfy this requirement by referring to the manufacturer information section of an SDS included with chemicals.
10. The employer must inform employees of the existence and location of written materials related to hazardous substances that are found in the workplace. In addition, the employer, upon request, must provide access to copies of training materials for employees, representatives of employees, or regulators.

## OSHA: FORMALDEHYDE STANDARD

This standard, which is also part of the federal OSHA requirements, is aimed specifically at addressing hazards associated with exposure to formaldehyde, formaldehyde gas, its solutions, and materials that release formaldehyde. Under the provisions of the Formaldehyde Standard, employers must monitor employees to determine how much exposure exists in the workplace. Studies have shown that exposure to formaldehyde at certain levels will likely cause employees to experience eye, nose, throat, and upper respiratory tract irritation.

Exposure monitoring is accomplished by sampling the air in work spaces where formaldehyde is used. Employers can purchase sampling kits from chemical supply companies and other vendors. Exposure monitoring is intended to determine if the level of exposure to airborne concentrations of formaldehyde in a work area is at or below a specified concentration. The Formaldehyde Standard establishes specific limits on the amount of exposure that is allowed. The specific point at which an 8-hour exposure is unsafe is called the **action level** (0.5 ppm). If sampling reveals that exposure has reached or exceeded the action level, employers are required to take steps to reduce the exposure. The purpose of requiring exposure reduction at the action level is to ensure that exposure does not reach the **permissible exposure limit** (PEL, also called the TWA or time-weighted average). The PEL sets the maximum average exposure over 8 hours that is allowed by OSHA or state governments.

There are two types of tests that must occur in every funeral home where any formaldehyde is used: (1) the **time-weighted average** (over a period of 8 hours) (TWA or PEL), and (2) the **short-term exposure level** (over a period of 15 minutes) (STEL). These tests are to be conducted in a "worst-case" environment. For example, the TWA testing should be done at a time when there is embalming taking place in the preparation room. When test results document worst-case situations that are within the limits specified by OSHA, it is reasonable to conclude that the air quality of the preparation room at all other times is also acceptable.

## Time-Weighted Average

Employers are required to take necessary steps to ensure that no employee is exposed to unsafe concentrations of airborne formaldehyde. If the results of the sampling for formaldehyde indicate that the exposure is below 0.5 ppm over an 8-hour period, the action level has not been reached, no additional TWA testing is needed, **except** if (1) the employer receives a report of an employee's symptoms associated with formaldehyde exposure, or (2) there are any changes in procedure, equipment, chemicals, personnel, or other circumstances that affect the work area.

If TWA sampling reveals an exposure that exceeds the STEL or the PEL, the employer is required to implement steps to reduce the exposure. The employer is then required to (1) place formaldehyde warning signs on areas where the concentration of formaldehyde has exceeded these levels, and (2) begin medical surveillance of employees who work in areas where the concentration of formaldehyde has exceeded the STEL or the PEL. These signs must bear the following information:

**Danger**
**Formaldehyde**
**Irritant and potential cancer hazard**
**Authorized personnel only**

Medical surveillance requires that employers take a series of steps aimed at protecting employees. Those steps include having the employees complete a medical questionnaire, which is then reviewed by a physician who can make recommendations based on the employees' responses. The physician can recommend that the employees are having no ill effects and should return to work or that sufficient cause exists to order that employees be given a medical examination. If the employees are given a medical examination, the physician can recommend that there is no health problem present and employees should return to work, or that a health problem is present and **medical removal** will be ordered.

If medical removal is ordered, the affected employee may not be given preparation duties for up to 6 months. If there is improvement in the physical condition of the employee, the physician may release the employee to return to preparation room duties. If the medical condition of the employee does not improve, (1) the employee may be permanently reassigned to duties other than that in the preparation room, or (2) the employee may be terminated. If employers elect to terminate employees who are medically unable to perform the tasks and duties for which they were hired, there may well be issues related to disability coverage and Worker's Compensation to be addressed.

**Time-Weighted Average Sampling at or Above** 0.75 PPM. In those cases where TWA sampling reveals airborne concentrations of formaldehyde at or above 0.75 ppm, it shows that the permissible exposure limit has been reached. Employers are then required to (1) post formaldehyde warning signs in and around the work area(s), (2) begin medical surveillance, and (3) provide respirators for employees who are assigned to work in the posted area(s).

**Respirators.** There are employers who think that respirators are an easy solution to any problems that arise from formaldehyde concentrations in the preparation area. This is not true! Employers and employees should be aware that OSHA has a respirator standard that must be followed when respirators are put into use in the preparation room. Two of the major provisions of the Respirator Standard are that (1) employees must be fit-tested to see if a respirator is appropriate for them, and (2) a personal respirator must be fitted to each individual employee and refitted regularly.

**The Short-Term Exposure Level.** In addition to the TWA (which is sampled over 8 hours), employers are required to sample for airborne concentrations of formaldehyde over a 15-minute period. If the sampling reveals a concentration of airborne formaldehyde that is **below** 2 ppm, the permissible exposure limit has not been reached, and no further short-term exposure limit testing is required unless (1) the employer receives a report of an employee's symptoms associated with formaldehyde exposure, or (2) there are any changes in procedure, equipment, chemicals, personnel, or other circumstances that affect the work area.

If STEL sampling reveals airborne concentrations of formaldehyde **at or above** 2 ppm, the permissible exposure limit has been reached, and the employer is required to (1) use formaldehyde warning signs, (2) begin medical surveillance, and (3) require employees assigned to duties in the preparation room to wear respirators.

If the initial testing shows airborne concentrations of formaldehyde above either the action level for the TWA or the permissible limit for the STEL, employers must begin periodic testing of the employees. Periodic testing means that employers must retest the work area at least every 6 months if exposure is over the action level and every 12 months if exposure is over the STEL. If employers have two consecutive retests, which are conducted at least 7 days apart, that show concentrations below the action level for the TWA and below the permissible exposure limit for the STEL, the periodic monitoring of employees can be stopped.

See Chapter 7, NFDA Formaldehyde Best Work Practices—2010.

## Methods of Compliance with the Formaldehyde Standard

### Work Practice Controls

Examples of work practice controls for compliance with the formaldehyde standard include:
1. Wearing appropriate protective equipment when handling chemicals to avoid exposure by contact with the skin.
2. Exercising care when handling and pouring chemicals to avoid spills.
3. Handling and pouring chemicals in a way that prevents vapors from escaping into the room.

4. Keeping instruments and equipment in good working condition to prevent spills and vaporization.
5. Keeping the lid on the embalming machine when embalming solution is in the tank.
6. Recapping fluid bottles.
7. Properly rinsing fluid bottles.
8. Continuously aspirating body cavities during autopsy embalming.
9. Controlling drainage and leakage from the body by utilizing a drainage tube with a sufficient length of tubing to reach the bottom of the sink or flush basin reduces chemical splashing.
10. Utilizing a continuous flow of water over the embalming table to rinse and dilute chemicals.
11. Keeping the lid on hazardous waste containers.
12. Maintaining a cover on all sinks and flush basins that the embalming table and aspirator drain into.

### Engineering Controls

Examples of engineering controls for compliance with the Formaldehyde Standard are essentially the same as for biological hazards. They can be considered in terms of proper plumbing and adequate ventilation. Plumbing considerations include the following:

1. Providing vacuum breakers on the main water line leading into the building
2. Providing vacuum breakers on hydroaspirators
3. Maintaining discharge basins/flush sinks in good working order
4. Having a suitable water source for the preparation table

Ventilation considerations include creating multiple vents at varying levels for both incoming and outgoing air. The premise is to introduce fresh air blown toward the embalmer while the contaminated air is being drawn away from the embalmer. As a rule of thumb for a single-table room, the number of air changes ranges from 15 to 20 per hour. This range may vary depending on the contents of the room, the number of bodies that will be embalmed in the room at one time, the shape of the room, weather-related factors, and the preference of the embalmer.

The Formaldehyde Standard also requires employee information and training. Employers must introduce employees, who have occupational exposure, to Safety Data Sheets and identify methods by which employees will have access to the information. Initial training must be provided to employees prior to their being exposed to hazardous substances. In addition, employees must receive additional training if a change in work assignment results in exposure to hazardous substances. Employees must also receive annual updates at intervals of not greater than 1 year. The purpose of the training is to provide employees with information, procedures, and techniques necessary to safely handle substances that contain formaldehyde (see Appendix 1 pages 69–74 for additional hazardous chemicals.)

## ENVIRONMENTAL HEALTH AND SAFETY STANDARDS

The National Funeral Directors Association (NFDA) has drafted a set of Environmental Health and Safety Practices. Permission has been given to reproduce those practices. These practices are not intended to fully meet regulatory compliance or legal standards. Individual state statutory and federal regulatory compliance agencies governing funeral service practices need to be consulted.

If observed conscientiously, the following practices will help funeral directors (and embalmers) meet the highest standards of excellence of the funeral service profession.

- **Secure the preparation room.** Do you have procedures in place ensuring that only trained and authorized personnel enter preparation areas? Never enter preparation areas unless you have received proper training, your vaccinations are up-to-date, and you have selected appropriate PPE, including shoe covers. Do not smoke, eat, drink, apply personal makeup, or handle your contact lenses in preparation areas.

- **Evaluate exposure risks.** Are there special risks or diseases associated with the procedure you are performing? Universal precautions must always be observed, but they may or may not be sufficient to keep you safe.

- **Know the products you are using.** Are you familiar with the labels and the Safety Data Sheets (SDS's) for the products you use? Always retain the current SDS your supplier ships in each new box of chemicals. SDS's for all products you use must be present and readily accessible on the work site. Make sure all containers are labeled properly. Labels and SDS's tell you about the chemicals that the products contain—how to handle and dispose of them, and what to do in the case of an emergency.

- **Prepare for emergencies.** When was the last time your emergency equipment was tested? Know where to find and how to operate drench showers, eyewash stations, fire extinguishers, spill cleanup, and all other emergency equipment. Know exactly where your SDS's are located. Post emergency telephone numbers by all phones.

- **Limit toxicity and waste.** How much of each product are you using and why? Use only the amount of product needed to assure the procedure you are performing is carried out properly. Try to avoid the use of products containing phenol and cresol. Ask your supplier about substitute products that are environmentally friendly. Keep covers on embalming machines. Make sure ventilation systems are clean and running properly. Conduct formaldehyde exposure testing annually. Remember that changes in ventilation, the design of your preparation room, or even the volume of work can change exposure levels. Testing should be performed immediately following such changes.

- **Avoid solvents and chlorinated compounds.** Are you certain that solvents and chlorinated compounds—such as trichloroethylene (TCE) and perchloroethylene (Perc)—are not going down the drain? Found in some cosmetics, adhesives, tissue builders, and cleaning products, these compounds should only be used topically—if used at all. Make sure solvents and chlorinated compounds are never introduced, even in trace amounts, into drains, sinks, embalming tanks, or groundwater. Gauze or cotton containing these compounds and residue in empty containers should never be tossed into a dumpster or commingled with other wastes. Check SDS's to determine whether special handling or disposal is required for products containing these compounds.

- **Know how to manage wastewater.** Do you know the composition of your wastewater and the proper disposal practices? Permits and reports may be required. Your disposal system should be sized properly, operated correctly, and maintained regularly. Think of the drain as the beginning—not the end—of your sanitary and embalming waste stream. Even the smallest disposal system problems should be investigated and corrected immediately by using the services of a trained licensed professional. Remember that funeral home expansion may require wastewater disposal system expansion. Septic tanks must be pumped regularly, no less often than every 3 years.
- **Handle sharps carefully.** Are sharps clean, disinfected, and stored safely? Always use appropriate engineering and safety devices for sharps. Syringe caps and scalpel blade removal/disposal devices that do not require manual handling of the blade are a must. Sharps must be discarded in an approved biohazard sharps container.
- **Think before you flip the switch.** Are you being as careful as you should with power-assisted devices? Always follow manufacturer instructions when using power-assisted equipment.
- **Do not just toss it in the trash.** Do you know where to discard recycled materials, biomedical waste, hazardous waste, contaminated PPE, and potentially contaminated laundry? Be sure to differentiate among the waste you produce, as different rules apply to different wastes. Appropriate, clearly labeled waste containers must be present in the work area. Use licensed and reputable disposal firms. Know where wastes are being taken for disposal and ask about the compliance status of the disposal facility. Keep copies of all waste disposal receipts. Manifests must be maintained and ready for inspection.
- **Recycle.** Do you have a recycling program? Talk to your supplier about recycling the products you are purchasing and find out about community recycling programs. Do not throw away materials that should be recycled.
- **Keep it clean.** Are you keeping the work area clean and disinfected? Decontaminate work surfaces immediately if they are overtly contaminated, after any spill, and after completing preparation procedures. Wash your hands after every procedure and before you leave the area.
- **Document your work.** Do you always complete embalming reports and file them in the business office? Report any and all incidents and/or accidents to your supervisor immediately to initiate appropriate follow-up action.

## CONCLUSION

The dictates of logic, reason, and research all demand that the dead human body be considered a source of pathogenic microorganisms. Embalmers are charged by the same dictates and by law with the responsibility to implement protective and thorough procedures to ensure that the potential for contagion through exposure to the body is minimized.

$$\text{RISK} = \text{Toxicity} \times \text{Exposure}$$

Proper utilization of the PPE and good disinfectants reduces both toxicity and exposure, thus creating a managed risk.

See Selected Readings section of this text for detailed studies dealing with topics of hazards of infection, treatment of CJD cases, and ventilation and disinfectant studies.

# Appendix 1

## HAZARD COMMUNICATION STANDARD: SAFETY DATA SHEETS (SDS)

The Hazard Communication Standard (HCS) (29 CFR 1910.1200(g)), revised in 2012, requires that the chemical manufacturer, distributor, or importer provide Safety Data Sheets (SDSs) (formerly MSDSs or Material Safety Data Sheets) for each hazardous chemical to downstream users to communicate information on these hazards. The information contained in the SDS is largely the same as the MSDS, except now the SDSs are required to be presented in a consistent, user-friendly, 16-section format. This brief provides guidance to help workers who handle hazardous chemicals to become familiar with the format and understand the contents of the SDSs.

The SDS includes information such as the properties of each chemical; the physical, health, and environmental health hazards; protective measures; and safety precautions for handling, storing, and transporting the chemical. The information contained in the SDS must be in English (although it may be in other languages as well). In addition, OSHA requires that SDS preparers provide specific minimum information as detailed in Appendix D of 29 CFR 1910.1200. The SDS preparers may also include additional information in various section(s).

**Sections 1 through 8** contain general information about the chemical, identification, hazards, composition, safe handling practices, and emergency control measures (e.g., fire-fighting). This information should be helpful to those that need to get the information quickly. **Sections 9 through 11 and 16** contain other technical and scientific information, such as physical and chemical properties, stability and reactivity information, toxicological information, exposure control information, and other information, including the date of preparation or last revision. The SDS must also state that no applicable information was found when the preparer does not find relevant information for any required element.

The SDS must also contain Sections 12 through 15 to be consistent with the UN Globally Harmonized System of Classification and Labeling of Chemicals (GHS), but OSHA will not enforce the content of these sections because they concern matters handled by other agencies.

A description of all 16 sections of the SDS, along with their contents, is presented below:

## Section 1: Identification

This section identifies the chemical on the SDS as well as the recommended uses. It also provides the essential contact information of the supplier. The required information consists of the following:
- Product identifier used on the label and any other common names or synonyms by which the substance is known.
- Name, address, phone number of the manufacturer, importer, or other responsible parties, and emergency phone number.
- Recommended use of the chemical (e.g., a brief description of what it actually does, such as flame retardant) and any restrictions on use (including recommendations given by the supplier)[1].

## Section 2: Hazard(s) Identification

This section identifies the hazards of the chemical presented on the SDS and the appropriate warning information associated with those hazards.

The required information consists of the following:
- The hazard classification of the chemical (e.g., flammable liquid, category[1]).
- Signal word.
- Hazard statement(s).
- Pictograms [the pictograms or hazard symbols may be presented as graphical reproductions of the symbols in black and white or be a description of the name of the symbol (e.g., skull and crossbones, flame)].
- Precautionary statement(s).
- Description of any hazards not otherwise classified.
- For a mixture that contains an ingredient(s) with unknown toxicity, a statement describing how much (percentage) of the mixture consists of ingredient(s) with unknown acute toxicity. Please note that this is a total percentage of the mixture and not tied to the individual ingredient(s).

## Section 3: Composition/Information on Ingredients

This section identifies the ingredient(s) contained in the product indicated on the SDS, including impurities and stabilizing additives. This section includes information on substances, mixtures, and all chemicals where a trade secret is claimed. The required information consists of:
- Substances
  - Chemical name.
  - Common name and synonyms.
  - Chemical Abstracts Service (CAS) number and other unique identifiers.
  - Impurities and stabilizing additives, which are themselves classified and which contribute to the classification of the chemical.
- Mixtures*
  - Same information is required for substances.
  - The chemical name and concentration (i.e., exact percentage) of all ingredients which are classified as health hazards and are:
    - Present above their cut-off/concentration limits or

- Present a health risk below the cut-off/concentration limits.
- The concentration (exact percentages) of each ingredient must be specified, except concentration ranges may be used in the following situations:
  - A trade secret claim is made,
  - There is batch-to-batch variation, or
  - The SDS is used for a group of substantially similar mixtures.
- Chemicals where a trade secret is claimed*
- A statement that the specific chemical identity and/or exact percentage (concentration) of composition has been withheld as a trade secret is required.

## Section 4: First-Aid Measures

This section describes the initial care that should be given by untrained responders to an individual who has been exposed to the chemical. The required information consists of:
- Necessary first-aid instructions by relevant routes of exposure (inhalation, skin and eye contact, and ingestion).
- Description of the most important symptoms or effects, and any symptoms that are acute or delayed.
- Recommendations for immediate medical care and special treatment needed, when necessary.

## Section 5: Fire-Fighting Measures

This section provides recommendations for fighting a fire caused by the chemical. The required information consists of:
- Recommendations of suitable extinguishing equipment, and information about extinguishing equipment that is not appropriate for a particular situation.
- Advice on specific hazards that develop from the chemical during the fire, such as any hazardous combustion products created when the chemical burns.
- Recommendations on special protective equipment or precautions for firefighters.

## Section 6: Accidental Release Measures

This section provides recommendations on the appropriate response to spills, leaks, or releases, including containment and cleanup practices to prevent or minimize exposure to people, properties, or the environment. It may also include recommendations distinguishing between responses for large and small spills where the spill volume has a significant impact on the hazard. The required information may consist of recommendations for:
- Use of personal precautions (such as removal of ignition sources or providing sufficient ventilation) and protective equipment to prevent the contamination of skin, eyes, and clothing.
- Emergency procedures, including instructions for evacuations, consulting experts when needed, and appropriate protective clothing.
- Methods and materials used for containment (e.g., covering the drains and capping procedures).
- Cleanup procedures (e.g., appropriate techniques for neutralization, decontamination, cleaning or vacuuming; adsorbent materials; and/or equipment required for containment/ clean up)

## Section 7: Handling and Storage

This section provides guidance on the safe handling practices and conditions for the safe storage of chemicals. The required information consists of:
- Precautions for safe handling, including recommendations for handling incompatible chemicals, minimizing the release of the chemical into the environment and providing advice on general hygiene practices (e.g., eating, drinking, and smoking in work areas is prohibited).
- Recommendations on the conditions for safe storage, including any incompatibilities. Provide advice on specific storage requirements (e.g., ventilation requirements).

## Section 8: Exposure Controls/Personal Protection

This section indicates the exposure limits, engineering controls, and personal protective measures that can be used to minimize worker exposure. The required information consists of:
- OSHA Permissible Exposure Limits (PELs), American Conference of Governmental Industrial Hygienists (ACGIH) Threshold Limit Values (TLVs), and any other exposure limit used or recommended by the chemical manufacturer, importer, or employer preparing the safety data sheet, where available.
- Appropriate engineering controls (e.g., use local exhaust ventilation, or use only in an enclosed system).
- Recommendations for personal protective measures to prevent illness or injury from exposure to chemicals, such as personal protective equipment (PPE) (e.g., appropriate types of eye, face, skin, or respiratory protection needed based on hazards and potential exposure).
- Any special requirements for PPE, protective clothing, or respirators (e.g., type of glove material, such as PVC or nitrile rubber gloves; and breakthrough time of the glove material).

## Section 9: Physical and Chemical Properties

This section identifies physical and chemical properties associated with the substance or mixture. The minimum required information consists of:
- Appearance (physical state, color, etc.);
- Upper/lower flammability or explosive limits;
- Odor;
- Vapor pressure;
- Odor threshold;
- Vapor density;
- pH;
- Relative density;
- Melting point/freezing point;
- Solubility(ies);
- Initial boiling point and boiling range;
- Flash point;
- Evaporation rate;
- Flammability (solid, gas);
- Partition coefficient: n-octanol/water;
- Auto-ignition temperature;
- Decomposition temperature; and
- Viscosity.

The SDS may not contain every item on the above list because information may not be relevant or is not available. When this occurs, a notation to that effect must be made for that chemical property. Manufacturers may also add other relevant properties, such as the dust deflagration index (Kst) for combustible dust, used to evaluate a dust's explosive potential.

## Section 10: Stability and Reactivity

This section describes the reactivity hazards of the chemical and the chemical stability information. This section is broken into three parts: reactivity, chemical stability, and other. The required information consists of:

- Reactivity*
  - Description of the specific test data for the chemical(s). This data can be for a class or family of the chemical if such data adequately represent the anticipated hazard of the chemical(s), where available.
- Chemical stability*
  - Indication of whether the chemical is stable or unstable under normal ambient temperature and conditions while in storage and being handled.
  - Description of any stabilizers that may be needed to maintain chemical stability.
  - Indication of any safety issues that may arise should the product change in physical appearance.
- Other*
  - Indication of the possibility of hazardous reactions, including a statement whether the chemical will react or polymerize, which could release excess pressure or heat, or create other hazardous conditions. Also, a description of the conditions under which hazardous reactions may occur.
  - List of all conditions that should be avoided (e.g., static discharge, shock, vibrations, or environmental conditions that may lead to hazardous conditions).
  - List of all classes of incompatible materials (e.g., classes of chemicals or specific substances) with which the chemical could react to produce a hazardous situation.
  - List of any known or anticipated hazardous decomposition products that could be produced because of use, storage, or heating. [Hazardous combustion products should also be included in Section 5 (Fire-Fighting Measures) of the SDS.]

## Section 11: Toxicological Information

This section identifies toxicological and health effects information or indicates that such data are not available. The required information consists of:

- Information on the likely routes of exposure (inhalation, ingestion, skin, and eye contact). The SDS should indicate if the information is unknown.
- Description of the delayed, immediate, or chronic effects from short- and long-term exposure.
- The numerical measures of toxicity [e.g., acute toxicity estimates such as the LD50 (median lethal dose)]—the estimated amount [of a substance] expected to kill 50% of test animals in a single dose.
- Description of the symptoms. This description includes the symptoms associated with exposure to the chemical, including symptoms from the lowest to the most severe exposure.
- Indication of whether the chemical is listed in the National Toxicology Program (NTP) Report on Carcinogens (latest edition) or has been found to be a potential carcinogen in the International Agency for Research on Cancer (IARC) Monographs (latest editions) or found to be a potential carcinogen by OSHA.

## Section 12: Ecological Information (nonmandatory)

This section provides information to evaluate the environmental impact of the chemical(s) if it were released to the environment. The information may include:

- Data from toxicity tests performed on aquatic and/or terrestrial organisms, where available (e.g., acute or chronic aquatic toxicity data for fish, algae, crustaceans, and other plants; toxicity data on birds, bees, plants).
- Whether there is a potential for the chemical to persist and degrade in the environment either through biodegradation or other processes, such as oxidation or hydrolysis.
- Results of tests of bioaccumulation potential, making reference to the octanol–water partition coefficient ($K_{ow}$) and the bioconcentration factor (BCF), where available.
- The potential for a substance to move from the soil to the groundwater (indicate results from adsorption studies or leaching studies).
- Other adverse effects (e.g., environmental fate, ozone layer depletion potential, photochemical ozone creation potential, endocrine-disrupting potential, and/or global warming potential).

## Section 13: Disposal Considerations (nonmandatory)

This section provides guidance on proper disposal practices, recycling or reclamation of the chemical(s) or its container, and safe handling practices. To minimize exposure, this section should also refer the reader to Section 8 (Exposure Controls/Personal Protection) of the SDS.

The information may include:

- Description of appropriate disposal containers to use.
- Recommendations of appropriate disposal methods to employ.
- Description of the physical and chemical properties that may affect disposal activities.
- Language discouraging sewage disposal.
- Any special precautions for landfills or incineration activities.

## Section 14: Transport Information (nonmandatory)

This section provides guidance on classification information for shipping and transporting of hazardous chemical(s) by road, air, rail, or sea. The information may include:

- UN number (i.e., four-figure identification number of the substance).
- UN proper shipping name[1].
- Transport hazard class(es)[1].
- Packing group number, if applicable, based on the degree of hazard[2] <https://www.osha.gov/Publications/2>.

- Environmental hazards [e.g., identify if it is a marine pollutant according to the International Maritime Dangerous Goods Code (IMDG Code)].
- Guidance on transport in bulk (according to Annex II of MARPOL 73/78[3] <https://www.osha.gov/Publications/3> and the International Code for the Construction and Equipment of Ships Carrying Dangerous Chemicals in Bulk (International Bulk Chemical Code (IBC Code)).
- Any special precautions which an employee should be aware of or needs to comply with in connection with transport or conveyance either within or outside their premises (indicate when information is not available).

### Section 15: Regulatory Information (nonmandatory)

This section identifies the safety, health, and environmental regulations specific for the product that is not indicated anywhere else on the SDS. The information may include:

Any national and/or regional regulatory information of the chemical or mixtures (including any OSHA, Department of Transportation, Environmental Protection Agency, or Consumer Product Safety Commission regulations).

### Section 16: Other Information

This section indicates when the SDS was prepared or when the last known revision was made. The SDS may also state where the changes have been made to the previous version. You may wish to contact the supplier for an explanation of the changes. Other useful information also may be included here.

### Employer Responsibilities

Employers must ensure that the SDSs are readily accessible to employees for all hazardous chemicals in their workplace. This may be done in many ways. For example, employers may keep the SDSs in a binder or on computers as long as the employees have immediate access to the information without leaving their work area when needed and a backup is available for rapid access to the SDS in the case of a power outage or other emergency. Furthermore, employers may want to designate a person(s) responsible for obtaining and maintaining the SDSs. If the employer does not have an SDS, the employer or designated person(s) should contact the manufacturer to obtain one.

## References

OSHA, 29 CFR 1910.1200(g) and Appendix D. United Nations Globally Harmonized System of Classification and Labelling of Chemicals (GHS), third revised edition, United Nations, 2009. These references and other information related to the revised Hazard Communication Standard can be found on OSHA's Hazard Communication Safety and Health Topics page, located at: http://www.osha.gov/dsg/hazcom/index.html

**Disclaimer:** *This brief provides a general overview of the safety data sheet requirements in the Hazard Communication Standard (see 29 CFR 1910.1200(g) and Appendix D of 29 CFR 1910.1200). It does not alter or determine compliance responsibilities in the standard or the Occupational Safety and Health Act of 1970. Since interpretations and enforcement policy may change over time, the reader should consult current OSHA interpretations and decisions by the Occupational Safety and Health Review Commission and the courts for additional guidance on OSHA compliance requirements. Please note that states with OSHA-approved state plans may have additional requirements for chemical safety data sheets outside of those outlined above. For more information on those standards, please visit: http://www.osha.gov/dcsp/osp/statestandards.html*

# Appendix 2
## Hazardous Chemicals

The following three examples represent chemicals commonly used in the preparation room. Synonyms, dilution limits, and health effects come from a safety data sheet (SDS) directory, which is available to the public on the Internet at the University of California, one of many sites that offer SDSs. The term "SDS" or the specific chemical name should be used when doing a search. A complete list of hazardous chemicals may be obtained by contacting the NFDA, 13625 Bishop's Drive, Brookfield, WI 53005, for its publication, *Hazard Communication Program*. It is important to understand that the severity of the health effects listed for the chemicals will depend on the amount of material in the product, the frequency and duration of your exposure, and your individual susceptibility. Some states with their own OSHA programs have replaced the Federal Hazard Communication Rule with an Employee Right-to-Know Rule. For example, the State of Minnesota recognizes 1025 hazardous chemicals and provides a list of these chemicals in its Employee Right-to-Know Rule.

## EXAMPLES OF HAZARDOUS CHEMICALS

**Formaldehyde.** [formic aldehyde; paraform; formol; formalin (methanol-free); fyde; formalith; methanal; methyl aldehyde; methylene glycol; methylene oxide; tetraoxymethalene; oxomethane; oxymethylene; when in aqueous solution, the term formalin is often used.]

| OSHA Action Level: 0.5 ppm | OSHA TWA (PEL) 0.75 ppm | OSHA STEL 2 ppm |
| --- | --- | --- |

**Health Effects: Ingestion.** *Acute Exposure*—Liquids containing 10–40% formaldehyde cause severe irritation and inflammation of the mouth, the throat, and the stomach. Severe stomach pains will follow ingestion with possible loss of consciousness and death. Ingestion of dilute formaldehyde solutions (0.03–0.04%) may cause discomfort in the stomach and the pharynx.

**Health Effects: Eye Contact.** *Acute Exposure*—Formaldehyde solutions splashed in the eye can cause injuries ranging from transient discomfort to severe, permanent corneal clouding and loss of vision. The severity of the effect depends on the concentration of formaldehyde in the solution and whether or not the eyes are flushed with water immediately after exposure.

*Note:* The perception of formaldehyde by odor and eye irritation becomes less sensitive with time as one adapts to its use. This can lead to overexposure if a worker is relying on formaldehyde's warning properties to alert him or her to potential overexposure.

*Chronic Exposure*—permanent corneal clouding and loss of vision.

**Health Effects: Skin Contact.** *Acute Exposure*—Formalin is a severe skin irritant and a sensitizer. Contact with formalin causes white discoloration, smarting, drying, cracking, and scaling. Prolonged and repeated contact can cause numbness and a hardening or tanning of the skin. Previously exposed persons may react to future exposure with allergic eczematous dermatitis or hives.

*Chronic Exposure*—a hardening and tanning of the skin. Sensitive persons can develop allergic eczematous dermatitis and hives.

**Health Effects: Inhalation.** *Acute Exposure*—formaldehyde is highly irritating to the upper respiratory tract and eyes. Concentrations of 0.5–2.0 ppm may irritate the eyes, nose, and throat of some individuals. Concentrations of 3–5 ppm also cause tearing of the eyes and are intolerable to some persons. Concentrations of 10–20 ppm cause difficulty in breathing, burning of the nose and throat, cough, and heavy tearing of the eyes; and concentrations of 25–30 ppm causes severe respiratory tract injury leading to pulmonary edema and pneumonitis. A concentration of 100 ppm is immediately dangerous to life and health. Deaths from accidental exposure to high concentrations of formaldehyde have been reported.

*Chronic Exposure*—Formaldehyde exposure has been associated with cancers of the lung, nasopharynx, and oropharynx, and nasal passages. Prolonged or repeated exposure to formaldehyde may result in respiratory impairment. Rats exposed to formaldehyde at 2 ppm developed benign nasal tumors and changes of the cell structure in the nose as well as inflamed mucous membranes of the nose. Structural changes in the epithelial cells in the human nose have also been observed. Some persons have developed asthma or bronchitis following the exposure to formaldehyde, most often as the result of an accidental spill involving a single exposure to a high concentration of formaldehyde.

**Incompatibilities:** Strong oxidizing agents, caustics, strong alkalies, isocyanates, anhydrides, oxides, and inorganic acids. Formaldehyde reacts with hydrochloric acid to form the potent carcinogen, bis-chloromethyl ether. Formaldehyde reacts with nitrogen dioxide, nitromethane, perchloric acid and aniline, or peroxyformic acid to yield explosive compounds. A violent reaction occurs when formaldehyde is mixed with strong oxidizers. Oxygen from the air can oxidize formaldehyde to formic acid, especially when heated. Formic acid is corrosive.

**Found in:** Embalming adhesive gel, feature builder, embalming spray, sanitizing embalming spray, preservative cream, arterial embalming chemicals, preservative/disinfectant gel, supplemental embalming gel, accessory embalming chemical, incision sealer, preinjection chemicals, bleaching agents, cavity embalming fluid/gel.

**Phenol** (benzenol; carbolic acid; hydroxybenzene; monohydroxybenzene; monophenol; oxybenzene; phenic acid; phenyl alcohol; phenyl hydrate; phenyl hydroxide; phenylic acid; phenylic alcohol)

| | |
|---|---|
| OSHA TWA (PEL) for skin: 5 ppm | ACGIH TWA (PEL) for skin: 5 ppm |
| NIOSH-recommended TWA (PEL): 5 ppm | NIOSH-recommended ceiling: 15.6 ppm |

**Health Effects: Ingestion.** *Acute Exposure*—Inhalation may cause severe irritation of the mucous membranes, profuse sweating, headache, intense thirst, nausea and vomiting, abdominal pain, diarrhea, salivation, cyanosis, tinnitus, twitching, tremors, and convulsions. The central nervous system (CNS) may initially be stimulated followed by severe, profound depression progressing to coma. The heart rate may increase, then become slow and irregular. The blood pressure may increase slightly and then fall markedly with dyspnea and fall in body temperature. Stertorous breathing, mucous rales, and frothing at the mouth and nose may indicate the presence of pulmonary edema that may be followed by pneumonia. Methemoglobinemia and hemolysis have been reported occasionally. Death may occur from respiratory, circulatory, or cardiac failure. If death is not immediate, jaundice and oliguria or anuria may occur. Ingestion of 250 ppm is immediately dangerous to life or health.

*Chronic Exposure*—Symptoms of chronic phenol poisoning may include vomiting, difficulty swallowing, ptyalism, diarrhea, anorexia, headache, vertigo, muscle weakness and pain, mental disturbances, dark or smoky urine, and possibly skin eruptions. Extensive damage to the liver and kidneys may be fatal. Hind limb paralysis has been reported in animals. Pathologic findings, in animals repeatedly exposed to phenol vapors, include extensive necrosis of the myocardium, acute lobular pneumonia, vascular damage, and liver and kidney damage.

**Health Effects: Skin Contact.** *Acute Exposure*—Contact with 0.5% solutions may cause local anesthesia, 1% solutions sometimes cause skin necrosis, and 10% solutions may cause burns. Phenol burns may be severe, but painless due to damage to nerve endings. The skin may turn white, and later yellowish-brown and may be deeply eroded and scarred. Gangrene may occur at the site of contact. Vapors and liquid may be readily absorbed through the skin to cause systemic effects as detailed in acute inhalation exposure. There have been several reports of cardiac arrhythmias associated with application of solutions of phenol, hexachlorophene, and croton oil to the skin. Profound coma and death have been reported to occur within 10 minutes following skin contact. Pathologic findings included congestion of the lungs, liver, spleen, and kidneys.

*Chronic Exposure*—Prolonged exposure may cause a blue or brownish discoloration of the tendons over the knuckles of the hands, dermatitis, vitiligo, and rarely, skin sensitization. Symptoms of chronic phenol poisoning may occur as detailed as under chronic inhalation exposure. Evaluated by Registry of Toxic Effects of Chemical Substances (RTECS) as producing carcinogenic and neoplastic tumors in mice.

**Health Effects: Eye Contact.** *Acute Exposure*—Phenol vapors have caused marked irritation from brief, intermittent industrial exposure to 48 ppm. Concentrated liquid or solid may cause severe irritation with redness, pain, and blurred vision. Concentrated phenol in human eyes has caused chemotic conjunctiva, hypesthetic, white cornea, edematous eyelids, and severe iritis. In some cases, the eyelids have been so severely damaged that they required plastic surgery. The final visual results have varied from complete recovery, to partial recovery, to blindness, and loss of the eye. Crystalline or concentrated aqueous phenol on rabbit eyes causes almost instantaneous white opacification of the corneal epithelium. Eight hours later, the cornea was anesthetic, the surface ulcerated, and the stroma opaque. Five weeks later, entropion, scarring of the conjunctiva, and opacity of the cornea occurred.

*Chronic Exposure*—Repeated or prolonged exposure to phenol vapors may cause conjunctivitis and has caused gray discoloration of the sclera with brown spots near the insertion of the rectus muscle tendon.

**Health Effects: Ingestion.** *Acute Exposure*—Ingestion may cause immediate intense burning of the mouth and the throat, white or brownish stains and areas of necrosis on the lips and in the mouth and esophagus, marked abdominal pain, pale face, and contracted or dilated pupils. Systemic effects may occur as detailed under acute inhalation exposure. The approximate lethal dose in humans is 140 mg/kg.

*Chronic Exposure*—Persons ingesting phenol-contaminated well water experienced diarrhea, dark urine, and sores and burning in the mouth. Other symptoms of chronic phenol poisoning may occur as detailed under chronic inhalation exposure. Administration of phenol in the drinking water in rats for three generations produced stunted growth at 7000 ppm over two generations; offspring of rats given 10,000 ppm died; at 12,000 ppm animals did not reproduce. Other reproductive effects have also been reported in animals.

**Incompatibilities:** *Alkalies:* acetaldehyde, aluminum and alloys, aluminum chloride plus nitrobenzene, 1,3butadiene, boron trifluoride, diethyl etherate, calcium hypochlorite, formaldehyde, lead and alloys, magnesium and alloys, metals and alloys, oxidizers (strong), peroxodisulfuric acid, peroxomonosulfuric acid, plastics, rubber, sodium nitrate, trifluoroacetic acid, sodium nitrite, zinc, and alloys.

**Found in:** Embalming cauterant; embalming chemical disinfectant; cavity embalming fluid/gel, preservative/disinfectant gel; accessory embalming chemical.

**Glutaraldehyde** (1,5-pentanedial)

| | |
|---|---|
| OSHA PEL: 0.2 ppm | ACGIH TLV: 0.2 ppm |

**Health Effects: Inhalation.** *Acute Exposure*—Irritation, headaches, may cause nose and throat irritation and burning, difficulty in breathing.

*Chronic Exposure*—None known.

**Health Effects: Ingestion.** *Acute Exposure*—May cause nausea, vomiting, and systemic illness.

*Chronic Exposure*—None known.

**Health Effects: Skin Contact.** *Acute Exposure*—Sensitization dermatitis.

*Chronic Exposure*—None known.

**Health Effects: Eye Contact.** *Acute Exposure*—Loss of vision. *Chronic Exposure*—None known.
  **Incompatibilities:** Strong oxidizing agent.
  **Found In:** Arterial, cavity, and accessory embalming fluids; humectant; tissue filler; disinfectant and preservative gels.

## OTHER HAZARDOUS CHEMICALS

The following is a sample listing of commonly used chemicals found in the compounding of products used in the preparation room. Each of these toxic chemicals is explained in more detail on the SDS that accompanies the product.

**Acetone** (2-propanone; dimethylformaldehyde; dimethyl ketone; beta-ketopropane; methyl ketone; propanone; pyroacetic ether)—A narcotic in high concentrations which can cause skin irritation. Prolonged inhalation can cause headache, dryness, and throat irritation. A dangerous fire risk when exposed to heat, flame, or oxidizers. Found in: accessory embalming chemicals, external sealing composition, lip tint, solvents, and sealants.

**Alkyl dimethylbenzyl ammonium chloride**—This material belongs to the chemical family called quaternary ammonium compounds. It is a skin and eye irritant has moderate-to-high oral toxicity and is moderately toxic via skin absorption. Found in: cold disinfectant, embalming spray, and embalming cauterants.

**Amaranth** (trisodium salt of 1-[4-sulfo-1naphthylazo]-2-naphthol-3,6-disulfonic acid)—Formerly known as red dye #2, this member of the azo dye family is a suspected human carcinogen. It is no longer acceptable in food, drugs, or cosmetics. Found in: coloring powder for arterial fluids.

**Amitrole** (2-amino-1,2,4-triazole)—Moderate-to-low oral toxicity. Listed by International Agency for Research on Cancer (IARC) and National Toxicology Program (NTP) as a possible carcinogen. Found in: cavity fluid.

**Ammonia**—Causes nose and throat irritation; may cause bronchial spasm, chest pain, pulmonary edema, and skin burns. Incompatible with hypochlorite (household bleach) that is often used to disinfect the preparation area after embalming. Found in: cleaning agents used to neutralize formaldehyde.

**2-Butoxyethanol** (butyl Cellosolve, ethylene glycol monobutyl ether)—Mildly irritating to the skin, and can be absorbed through contact. It is a strong respiratory and eye irritant, and exposure may result in transient corneal clouding; repeated overexposure can cause fatigue, headache, nausea, and tremors. It is a moderate fire risk, which will react with oxidizers. Found in: arterial embalming chemicals.

**Camphor**—High-to-moderate ingestion hazard. Local exposure may cause irritation. Found in: embalming fluid.

**Carbon tetrachloride** (tetrachloromethane)—Can cause depression, nausea, vomiting, and local skin irritation; prolonged exposure and absorption through the skin could produce liver and kidney failure. Found in: organic solvents.

**Chlorine salts** (hypochlorites)—Chlorine salts produce chlorinated vapor causing moderate-to-severe skin and eye irritations, tissue damage, and moderate-to-severe respiratory irritation. They are strong oxidizers and are highly reactive, and can be a serious fire risk when exposed to reducing agents (acids) or petroleum derivatives. Found in: embalming deodorant, bleach, and disinfectants.

**Chloroform** (trichloromethane)—Formerly used as an anesthetic, chloroform causes depression and skin and eye irritation; prolonged exposure can lead to cardiac and respiratory arrest or paralysis; chronic exposure may cause liver damage. Listed in IARC and NTP as a possible carcinogen. Found in: accessory embalming chemical sealant.

**Cresol** (2-hydroxy-4-methylphenol)—The health effects are similar to those of phenol but not as severe. It is corrosive to skin, eyes, and mucous membranes, capable of causing burns at point of contact, and can be absorbed through the skin. Chronic low-level exposure can cause skin rash and discoloration, gastrointestinal disturbances, nervous system disturbances, and kidney and liver damage. It is a moderate fire hazard that can react vigorously with oxidizing materials. Found in: disinfectant and accessory embalming chemicals.

**Diethanolamine**—A severe eye irritant and mild skin irritant which is moderately toxic through ingestion. It can react with oxidizers. Found in: humectant and arterial embalming fluid.

**Diethylene glycol**—A skin and eye irritant which is highly toxic through inhalation. It can react with oxidizers. Found in: arterial and cavity embalming fluids.

**Dimethylformamide**—A strong irritant to skin and other tissues, it is readily absorbed through the skin. Inhalation or skin contact can cause gastrointestinal disturbances, facial flushing, elevated blood pressure, CNS disorders, and liver and kidney damage. It is a moderate fire risk which can be an explosion hazard when exposed to flame. Dimethylformamide is reactive with a variety of halogenated materials and organics. Found in: solvents.

**Ethyl acetate**—Irritates the eyes, gums, skin, and respiratory tract. Repeated overexposure can cause conjunctivitis and corneal clouding; high concentrations can result in congestion of the liver and kidneys. Ethyl acetate is a dangerous fire risk. Found in: embalming cosmetic spray, cavity fluid, sanitizing spray, and sealing lacquer.

**Ethyl alcohol** (denatured ethanol, SD alcohol)—Ethyl alcohol is generally not considered an occupational health hazard, but its flammability makes it a safety hazard. The terms "SDA" or "SD alcohol" mean "specially denatured alcohol." SDA is ethyl alcohol to which another substance, such as *tert*-butyl alcohol, has been added to make it unfit for human consumption. Found in: cavity fluid, cosmetics.

**EDTA** (ethylenediaminetetraacetic acid)—EDTA is found in a variety of products as either tetrasodium or disodium salt. Both react chemically to bind calcium, which inhibits the blood clotting mechanism. EDTA is a skin irritant, causing dryness and cracking. Found in: arterial fluids, preinjection fluids, co-injection fluids, cavity fluids.

**Ethylenedichloride** (1,2-dichloroetheneor1,1-dichloroethene)—A strong irritant to skin and eyes which is toxic via inhalation and skin absorption. Ethylene dichloride is listed in IARC as a possible carcinogen. It is a dangerous fire risk. Found in: embalming fluid and cavity fluid.

**Ethylene glycol** (1,2-ethanediol)—Moderately irritating to skin, eyes, and mucous membranes; very toxic through inhalation, producing depression and damage to blood-forming organs. Ethylene glycol does not readily vaporize at room temperature, and inhalation would be likely only by heating or mechanical action (aerosolization). Ingestion can lead to respiratory, renal, and cardiac failure. Brain damage may also result. Chronic exposure can cause anorexia, decreased urinary output, and involuntary rapid eye movement. Ethylene glycol is combustible and can react violently with certain acids and oxidizers. Found in: arterial and cavity embalming chemicals, external embalming seal, tissue surface embalming seal, anticoagulant/clot remover, and water correctives.

**Ethylene glycol monomethyl ether** (methyl Cellosolve)—Moderately toxic via inhalation, ingestion, and skin absorption. May cause conjunctivitis, transient corneal clouding, and upper respiratory tract irritation. Found in: cosmetics.

**Formic acid** (methanoic acid)—Corrosive to skin, eyes, and mucous membranes. Formic acid has a moderate-to-high oral toxicity, and can be absorbed through the skin. It is a moderate fire risk. Found in: supplemental embalming chemicals and bleaching agents.

**Hexylene glycol** (2,4-hexanediol)—An eye, skin, and mucous membrane irritant which is moderately toxic through inhalation and ingestion. Large oral doses can have a narcotic effect. A low fire risk, hexylene glycol can react with oxidizers. Found in: arterial embalming fluid.

**Isobutane** (2-methylpropane)—While otherwise practically nontoxic, the inhalation of isobutane can cause suffocation. A dangerous fire risk when exposed to heat, flame, or oxidizers. Found in: aerosol propellants, cosmetics, insecticides, and deodorants.

**Isopropyl alcohol** (2-propanol)—An eye, nose, and throat irritant, in high concentration, it causes mild narcotic effects, corneal burn, and eye damage. Drying to the skin, isopropyl alcohol is moderately toxic via ingestion. Ingestion or inhalation of heavy vapor concentrations can cause flushing and CNS depression. As little as 100 mL can be fatal if ingested. It is a dangerous fire risk and a moderate explosion risk when exposed to heat, flame, or oxidizers. Found in: cavity and accessory embalming fluids, feature builder, cosmetics, color concentrate, fungal inhibitors, preinjection chemicals, liquid embalming cosmetics and sprays, tissue filler, supplemental embalming gels, aerosol deodorant, sealing lacquers, and solvent thinners.

**Methyl alcohol** (wood alcohol, methanol)—A skin, eye, and respiratory tract irritant which is moderately toxic via inhalation, and moderately to highly toxic through ingestion. The main target is the CNS, but it also affects the eyes, optic nerve, and possibly the retina. Overexposure can cause depression, sight impairment, weakness, and gastrointestinal disturbances. Severe overexposure can result in cardiac depression. Because methyl alcohol is metabolized slowly, sufficient daily intake can lead to cumulative exposure symptoms. Methyl alcohol is a dangerous fire and explosion risk when exposed to heat, flame, and oxidizers. Found in: arterial, cavity, and accessory embalming fluids and gels; cleaning and disinfecting fluids, gels and solvents; tissue fillers; embalming cauterants; bleaching agents; cosmetics; and color concentrates.

**Methyl ethyl ketone** (2-butanone)—Repeated exposure can cause skin irritation and inflammation; vapors can produce eye, nose, and throat irritation. Methyl ethyl ketone is highly volatile and a narcotic by inhalation, affecting both the CNS and the peripheral nerves. Methyl ethyl ketone can react violently with aldehydes and acids. It is a dangerous fire risk and moderate explosion risk when exposed to heat, spark, or flame. Found in: embalming cosmetic spray, sealing lacquer, and thinners.

**Methylene chloride** (dichloromethane)—High oral toxicity, very dangerous to the eyes, causing corrosion of eye tissue. Because it vaporizes readily, inhalation is an important hazard, resulting in CNS depression, headache, dizziness, nausea, vomiting, and a feeling of intoxication. The material can also irritate the respiratory tract, cause liver damage, and exacerbate coronary artery disease. Chronic exposure can cause skin, CNS, and liver damage. The material is a suspected human carcinogen. The body metabolizes methylene chloride into carbon monoxide, lowering the blood's ability to carry oxygen. The problem is intensified for smokers and those with anemia or related conditions. Found in: external embalming sealants, aerosol insecticides and deodorizers, cosmetic sprays, and solvents.

**Mineral spirits** (naphtha, hexane, and heptane distillates)—Moderately toxic via ingestion and moderately irritating to skin, eyes, and mucous membranes, the mist is highly irritating to the respiratory tract. Symptoms of overexposure often resemble drunkenness. Chronic overexposure can lead to photosensitivity, headache, nausea, dizziness, indigestion, and lack of appetite. Mineral spirits are incompatible with strong oxidizers and are a highly dangerous fire risk when exposed to heat, flame, or spark. Found in: liquid embalming cosmetics and sprays and organic solvents.

**Molding plaster** (calcium sulfate, gypsum, plaster of Paris)—Generally considered a nuisance dust, although prolonged or repeated exposures can induce lung disease. Found in: cavity desiccant and embalming powders.

**Nitrocellulose**—A dangerous fire and explosion hazard when in dry form. Less flammable when wet. Found in: feature builder and sealing lacquer.

**Orthodichlorobenzene** (1,2-dichlorobenzene)—Moderately toxic via inhalation and ingestion; irritating to skin, eyes, and upper respiratory tract. Acute exposure can induce narcotic symptoms. Repeated or prolonged skin contact with liquid can cause burns. Chronic exposure may cause lung, liver, and kidney damage. It is a moderate fire risk when exposed to heat or flame and can react violently with oxidizing materials. Found in: cavity and supplemental embalming chemicals and gels, and bleaching agents.

**Oxalic acid** (ethanedioic acid)—Highly irritating and caustic to skin. Damage is characterized by cracks, fissures, slow-healing ulcerations, blue skin, and yellowish, brittle nails. Highly irritating to tissues via ingestion. It can cause corrosion of mucous membranes, severe gastrointestinal disturbances, and acute poisoning. The major effects of inhalation of dusts and mists are corrosion and ulceration of the nose and the throat, severe eye irritation, nosebleed, headache, and nervousness. Chronic exposure can cause upper respiratory and gastrointestinal disturbances, urinary disorders, gradual weight loss, and nervous system disturbances. Found in: embalming adhesive gels.

**Paradichlorobenzene** (1,4-dichlorobenzene)—Moderately toxic via inhalation; symptoms include irritation of skin, eyes, and upper respiratory tract. Prolonged or chronic skin exposure can cause burns. In liquid form, it can be absorbed through the skin. Chronic exposure can cause liver, kidney, and lung damage. It is a moderate fire risk and incompatible with oxidizers. Found in: deodorizing powders.

**Paraformaldehyde**—Can produce formaldehyde when heated. Paraformaldehyde has moderate oral toxicity and low dermal toxicity. It is a moderate fire risk and can react with oxidizers. Found in: embalming/deodorizing powders, sealing powders, cavity desiccants, and hardening compounds.

**Paratertiary pentyl phenol** (*p*-tert-amyl phenol)—A skin and eye irritant; it is moderately toxic through skin contact and ingestion, and is slightly flammable. Found in: cavity embalming solutions, disinfectant sprays, antiseptic soaps, and bleaching agents.

**Propane**—Propane can cause suffocation and, at very high concentrations, can cause CNS depression. It is a dangerous fire and explosion risk when exposed to heat, flame, or oxidizers. Found in: propellants, aerosol embalming sealants, cosmetic sprays, and insecticide/miticide sprays.

**Propylene glycol** (1,2-propanetriol, 1,3-propanetriol)—A skin and eye irritant. Found in: cavity embalming fluid.

**Quartz** (crystalline silicon dioxide)—Prolonged, repeated exposure to quartz can lead to lung disease characterized by shortness of breath and a troublesome, unproductive cough. Quartz can react violently with certain fluorine-containing compounds. Found in: finishing powder.

**Quaternary ammonium compounds**—Skin and eye irritant; a common cause of skin inflammation; highly toxic via ingestion; symptoms include nausea, vomiting, possible convulsions, and collapse. Found in: disinfectants, cavity, and accessory embalming fluids.

**Sodium hypochlorite**—Strongly irritating and corrosive to tissues. A strong oxidizing agent that will react violently with organic acids and formaldehyde. It is moderately toxic via inhalation and ingestion. Found in: household bleach and other bleaching agents.

**Sodium pentachlorophenate**—Widely used as a fungicide and disinfectant, the material has high toxicity via inhalation and ingestion and is highly irritating to the skin. Found in: arterial embalming chemicals.

**Talc**—Mainly regarded as a nuisance dust, prolonged or repeated exposure may lead to lung disease, although the mechanism of inducement is unclear. Found in: drying powder.

**Toluene** (1,2-dimethylbenzene)—Skin, eye, and respiratory tract irritant. Prolonged or repeated contact can cause drying of skin. Overexposure can produce narcotic effects, depression, headache, dizziness, nausea, fatigue, lack of coordination, and a burning sensation of the skin. Acute poisoning, however, is rare. It is a dangerous fire risk when exposed to heat, spark, or flame. Found in: external embalming sealers, lip cosmetics and cosmetic sprays, sealing lacquer, solvents, and thinners.

**Trichloroethane** (1,1,2-trichloroethane)—A moderate skin and eye irritant causing inflammation and producing CNS depression, dizziness, drowsiness, incoordination, and psychological disturbances. Trichloroethane can also cause gastrointestinal disturbances and irregular heartbeat. High doses can have a narcotic effect and cause heart failure. Found in: cleaning solvents, sanitizing embalming sprays, aerosol lanolin skin creams, and cosmetics.

**Trichloroethylene**—A strong eye and skin irritant which can be absorbed through contact. Overexposure can cause CNS depression, headache, dizziness, tremors, nausea, vomiting, fatigue, and irregular heartbeat. Symptoms may resemble those of alcohol intoxication. Addiction and weakness in the extremities have been reported. Chronic exposure can damage the liver and other organs. Found in: cleaning solvents.

## CONCEPTS FOR STUDY

Define the following terms:

- Action level
- Airborne pathogen
- Aerosolization
- Asepsis
- Bactericidal
- Bacteriostatic
- Biological hazard
- Bloodborne pathogen
- Bloodborne Pathogens Standard
- Cold chemical sterilant
- Concurrent disinfection/decontamination
- Decontamination
- Disinfect
- Employee Right-To-Know laws
- Engineering controls
- Exposure control plan
- Formaldehyde Standard
- Germicide
- Hazard Communication Rule
- Safety Data Sheet (SDS)
- Occupational Safety and Health Administration (OSHA)
- Permissible Exposure Limit (PEL)
- Respirator Standard
- Sanitizer
- Squeegee effect
- Short Term Exposure Level (STEL)
- Sterilization
- Terminal disinfection/decontamination
- Time-weighted Average (TWA)
- Universal precautions
- Work practice controls

1. In addition to biological and chemical hazards, what other occupational hazards do embalmers face?
2. What is the minimum documentation required for a Bloodborne Pathogen Exposure Control Plan?
3. Describe the basic premise of universal precautions.
4. What are the two primary areas of consideration for engineering controls?
5. List a variety of types of personal protective equipment.
6. Describe the provisions of hepatitis B vaccination and postexposure evaluation and follow-up.

## FIGURE CREDIT

Figures 3–1, 3–3 are used with permission of Sharon L. Gee-Mascarello.
Figures 3–2, 3–4A, 3–6, 3–7 are used with permission of Kevin Drobish.

## BIBLIOGRAPHY

An Embalmer's Odds of Contracting Diseases. *The Forum,* December 2009.

Beck-Sague C, Jarvis W, Fruehling J, et al. Universal precautions and mortuary practitioners: Influence on practices and risk of occupationally acquired infection. *J Occup Med* 1991;33:874–878.

Bender JR, Mullin LS, Grapel GJ, et al. Eye irritation response in humans to formaldehyde. *Am Ind Hygiene Assoc J* 1983;44:463–465.

Benenson AS, ed. *Control of Communicable Diseases Manual,* 16th ed. American Public Health Association, 1995.

*The Bloodborne Pathogen Rule.* Code of Federal Regulations. Title 29 CFR Part 1910, Occupational Safety and Health Administration, Department of Labor, Toxic and Hazardous Substances. The Bloodborne Pathogen Rule 1910.1030, 1992.

Burke P, Sheffner A. The anti-microbial effects of embalming chemicals and topical disinfectants on the microbial Flora of human remains. *Health Laboratory Sciences* October 1976.

Code of Federal Regulations. Title 29: Subtitle B—Regulations Relating to Labor: Chapter XVII—Occupational Safety and Health Administration, Department of Labor; Part 1910, Hazard Communication 1910.1200, 1988.

Collison K, Adams J. The CDC advises us not to panic about CJD. *Dodge Mag* September 1999.

Collison K. Hepatitis A to G. *Dodge Mag* January 1999.

Environmental Health and Safety Practices. Brookville, WI: National Funeral Directors Association, 2004.

Gershon R, Vlahov D, Escamilla-Cejudo J, et al. Tuberculosis risk in funeral home employees. *J Occup Environ Med* May 1998;40:497–503.

Kerfoot EJ. Formaldehyde vapor emission study in embalming rooms. *The Director* 1972:42.

Kerfoot EJ, Mooney TF. Formaldehyde and paraformaldehyde study in funeral homes. *Am Ind Hygiene Assoc J* 1975;36:533–537.

McDonald L. Blood exposure and protection in funeral homes. *Am J Infect Control* August 1989;17:193–195.

McKenna MT, Hutton M, Cauthen G, et al. The association between occupation and tuberculosis. *Am J Resp Crit Care Med* 1996;154:587–596.

Nethercott JR, Holness DL. Contact dermatitis in funeral service workers. *Contact Dermatitis* 1988;18:263–267.

State of Minnesota. Minnesota Rule Chapter 5206.0400, Subpart 5. *Employee Right-To-Know Standards.* Minneapolis, MN: Department of Labor and Industry, 1995.

Turner S, Kunches L, Gordon K, et al. Occupational exposure to human immunodeficiency virus (HIV) and hepatitis B virus (HBV) among embalmers: A pilot seroprevalence study. *Am J Pub Health* October 1989;79:1425–1426.

Williams TM, Levine RJ, Blunden PB. Exposure of embalmers to formaldehyde and other chemicals. *Am Ind Hyg Assoc J* 1984;45:172–176.

CHAPTER 4

# The Preparation Room

## CHAPTER OVERVIEW
- Requirements and Regulations
- Design Considerations
- Equipment and Supplies
- Instruments and Devices for Mortuary Use

The primary purpose of a well-designed and organized preparation room is to provide a safe, efficient, and comfortable environment for its workers. Funeral home and decedent care facilities are governed by a variety of laws and regulations from federal, state, and local agencies. Businesses that employ workers must adhere to workplace regulations on all applicable levels. A brief and general review of regulations governing the preparation room environment follows. References apply to generally accepted and standard requirements. Best practice is to consult with experts to assure adherence and observance of requirements.

## GENERAL REQUIREMENTS

1. Admittance to the preparation room is by authorization. The room is kept strictly private during body preparation. Admittance should be limited to:
    a. Licensees, registered funeral service students, and registered trainees.
    b. Those authorized by state statute or rules and regulations, such as coroners, medical examiner personnel, and law enforcement.
2. Limited authorized persons:
    a. Maintenance employees.
    b. Hairstylist, cosmetologist, persons with other responsibilities.
    c. Employees performing business functions.
    d. Individuals performing cultural or religious customs.
3. Room signage must be in compliance with laws and regulations:
    a. Strictly private area.
    b. Required OSHA warnings.
4. Secure the preparation room:
    a. State regulations may require security locks.
    b. Establish a security plan for the handling of the remains of high-profile deceased persons.
    c. Inventory and label personal effects and securely store.
    d. Preparation room should not be located so that it becomes a passage to other building areas.
5. Maintain the dignity of the remains. Be sure that:
    a. The deceased is properly identified.
    b. The deceased is covered; modesty cloth for genital areas.
6. Maintain the highest ethical and moral standards of care and confidentiality:
    a. Guard loose talk and remarks.
    b. Disclose nothing with unauthorized persons; all information relating to the deceased is confidential.
    c. No unauthorized photography.
7. Maintain a clean and healthy environment.
    a. Properly dispose of clothing of the deceased: (1) launder and return to the family; or (2) dispose with proper authorization.
    b. Proper disposition of all waste materials: (3) statutes, rules, and regulations vary for individual states.
    c. Maintain ventilation, heating, and cooling systems in proper working order.
    d. Maintain all mechanical and plumbing devices.
    e. Perform and document regular maintenance and cleaning of the preparation room.
8. Maintain an adequate supply of chemicals and associated sundry items necessary for embalming and decedent care, restorative, and cosmetology treatments.
9. Maintain an adequate number of tables and positioning devices per case volume.
10. Document decedent care activities for every decedent in the care of the facility through the use of embalming decedent care reports and other applicable forms.

## Occupational Safety and Health Administration Requirements

Occupational Safety and Health Administration (OSHA) prescribes in detail the physical and environmental requirements that employers must meet to provide a safe workplace. These requirements are enforced through workplace inspections, warnings, and citations. In the event of failure to correct continual noncompliance or serious violations, substantial fines are levied.

Four areas of OSHA directly impact the funeral service practitioner:

(1) General Rule
(2) Hazard Communication Standard
(3) Formaldehyde Standard
(4) Bloodborne Pathogens Standard

## Right-to-Know Laws

Right-to-know laws provide workers with direct access to information about the health risks of chemicals used in the workplace. Posting requirements for this information is mandatory.

## New Construction

The following floor plans are design examples for new preparation room construction: the station concept (**Fig. 4–1A,B**) and the central embalming and decedent care facility (**Fig. 4–1C**). Note that combination funeral home and crematory operations are not allowed in some states.

## Building Permits

New construction and facility remodeling requires a building permit. The permit application will require detailed site plans and specifications to be submitted. Plumbing, electrical, heating, and cooling systems and other construction requirements require permitting. Best practice is to consult a professional for guidance with building ordinances.

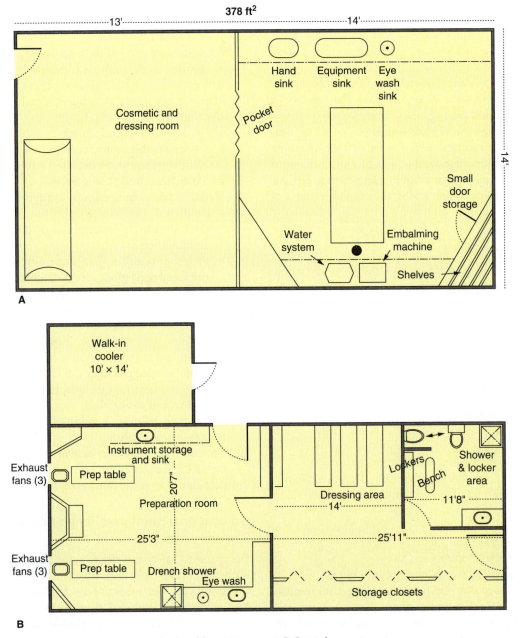

**Figure 4–1.** **A.** Single table arrangement. **B.** Multiple table arrangement. **C.** Central care arrangement.

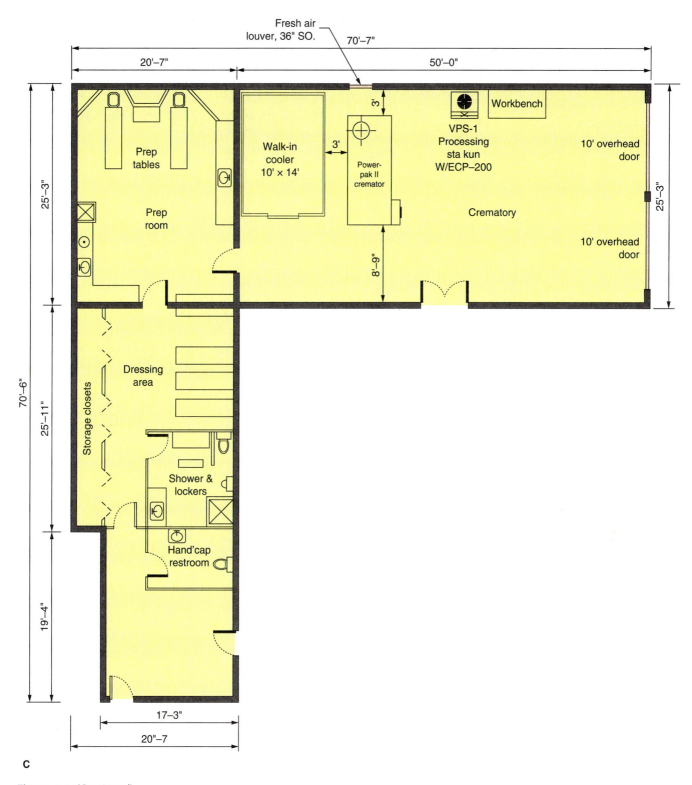

**Figure 4-1** (Continued)

## State Codes and Local Ordinances

Codes and ordinances vary between localities and may change with time. Best practice is to maintain up-to-date compliance with respect to all requirements. Each state may have a Board of Health and a Board of Mortuary Science that enact regulations governing the minimum standards for preparation rooms in that state. As an example, the Board of Embalmers and Funeral Directors of Ohio outline the following rules and regulations requiring minimum facility and equipment standards for the embalming room as it pertains to the preparation of human remains.

**Ohio. Chapter 4717-1-16.** *If embalming will take place at the funeral home, the funeral home shall maintain on the premises a preparation room which shall be:*

- *adequately equipped*
- *maintained in a sanitary manner for the preservation and care of dead human bodies.*

*Such rooms shall:*

- *contain only articles, facilities, and instruments necessary for the preparation of dead human bodies for burial or final disposition*
- *be kept in a clean and sanitary condition*
- *shall be used only for the care and preparation of dead human bodies*

*The minimal requirements for the preparation or embalming room shall be as follows:*

1. *Sanitary floor (cement or tile preferred).*
2. *All instruments and appliances used in the embalming of a dead human body shall be thoroughly cleansed and sterilized using an appropriate disinfectant immediately at the conclusion of each individual case.*
3. *Running hot and cold water with a lavatory sink for personal hygiene.*
4. *Exhaust fan and intake vent, permanently installed and operable with the capacity to change the air in the room a minimum of fifteen times each hour.*
5. *Sanitary plumbing connected with sewer, cesspool, septic tank, or other department of health approved system.*
6. *Porcelain, stainless steel, metal-lined, or fiber-glass operating table.*
7. *All opening windows and outside doors shall be adequately screened and shielded from outside viewing.*
8. *All hydro-aspirators shall be equipped with at least one air breaker.*
9. *Containers for refuse, trash, and soiled linens shall be adequately covered or sealed at all times.*
10. *First-aid kit and eyewash.*
11. *The embalming or preparation room shall be strictly private. A "private" sign shall be posted on the door(s) entering the preparation room. No one shall be allowed therein while the body is being embalmed except the licensed embalmers, licensed funeral directors, apprentices, officials in discharge of their duties, and other authorized persons.*
12. *All waste materials, refuse, used bandages, and cotton shall be destroyed in accordance with all applicable OSHA and EPA regulations.*
13. *Every person, while engaged in actually embalming a dead human body, shall be attired in a clean and sanitary smock or gown covering the person from the neck to below the knees and shall wear impervious rubber gloves, and shall wear any and all items required under any applicable OSHA regulations.*
14. *All bodies in the preparation room should be treated with proper care and dignity and should be properly covered at all times.*
15. *Ingress and egress of the preparation room must be situated so that functions in the funeral home will not impede or interfere with entering or exiting said room.*
16. *Sufficient emergency lighting.*

# DRESSING ROOM

A *dressing room* is used for purposes other than arterial embalming; also called a *holding* or *staging area*. The room is used for decedent care activities such as, but not limited to:

- Temporary storage
- Minimal preparation for identification viewing
- Grooming and hairstyling
- Restorative treatments
- Cosmetic application
- Dressing and casketing
- Religious and cultural practices
- Cavity aspiration or reaspiration

An excerpt from the State of Ohio rule states the use for a holding room:

*If embalming will not take place at the funeral home, the funeral home shall maintain on the premises a holding room which shall be adequately equipped and maintained in a sanitary manner for the holding of dead human bodies. Such holding room shall be kept in a clean and sanitary manner and used only for the holding and storage of dead human bodies. The minimum requirements for the holding room shall be as follows:*

1. *Sanitary floor;*
2. *Running hot and cold water with a lavatory sink for personal hygiene;*
3. *All opening windows and outside doors shall be adequately screened and shielded from outside viewing;*
4. *Containers for refuse, trash, and soiled linens shall be adequately covered or sealed at all times;*
5. *The holding room shall be strictly private. A "Private" sign shall be posted on the door(s) entering the room. No one shall be allowed therein while the body is being held except the licensed embalmers, licensed funeral directors, apprentices, officials in discharge of their duties, and other authorized persons;*
6. *All bodies in the holding room should be treated with proper care and dignity and should be properly covered at all times;*
7. *Ingress and egress of the holding room must be situated so that functions in the funeral home will not impede or interfere with entering or exiting said room.*

# PREPARATION ROOM LOCATION

## Basement

The basement of a facility is often where space is most readily available. Ceiling height can be limited in this area due to overhead plumbing lines and ducts for heating, ventilation, and cooling systems (HVAC). When sewer drains are substantially above floor level, plumbing challenges may be present. Without an elevator or floor lift, stairs can present both an inconvenience and hazard.

## First or Second Floor

The first floor can be the most logical and least costly location of a preparation room when space allows. Natural light is favorable for working conditions. Room access must be secure and not immediately adjacent to public areas.

## PREPARATION ROOM SIZE AND EFFICIENT USE

Frequency of preparation room usage is a determining factor in selecting an optimal size.
- Base room size on case volume.
- Design the space for optimal efficiency.
- Select materials for floors, countertops, cabinets, walls, and all other surfaces that can be efficiently cleaned and disinfected.
- Install an adequate number of embalming tables.
- Include dressing tables; folding or nonfolding styles.
- Include a lifting device; movable floor lift or overhead hoist.
- Reduce the items available in the immediate preparation area to include only those routinely accessed during embalming, such as instruments, fluids, sundry items, and positioning devices.
- Store surplus items and those not routinely used, such as plastic garments, in an adjacent area.

## ROOM DESIGN CONSIDERATIONS

Consult an architect for new construction or remodeling. Consideration of movement and function within the preparation room is paramount to its overall efficiency.

### Storage Cabinets and Countertops

Consider ample storage cabinets. Although space should be provided for working quantities of supplies, the preparation room should not serve as a storage room. Ready-made base cabinets are customarily 24 inches deep; custom cabinets may be necessary.

### Table Arrangements

There are virtually as many table arrangements as there are sizes and shapes of embalming rooms. Table arrangements are limited only by the size and shape of the room. The embalming **station design** creates one or more fully equipped operating areas within a larger area (**Fig. 4–2A–C**).

Adjacent stations accommodate decedent care procedures other than arterial embalming (**Fig. 4–3**). The separate stations are appointed with the specific supplies needed for the functions such as restoration, cosmetic application, hairstyling, dressing, casketing, and temporary staging of the deceased.

## FLOORING

Flooring must be durable and easy to clean. Avoid materials that create a slipping hazard when wet. **Epoxy** coatings provide a seamless and nonslip surface that is easy to clean and

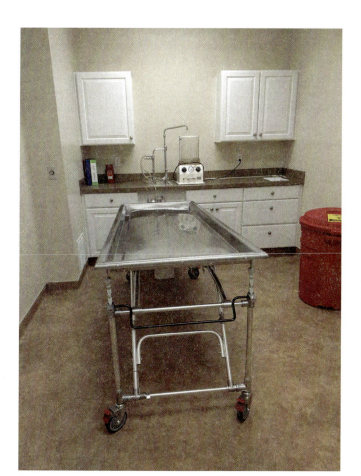

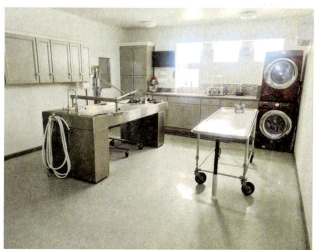

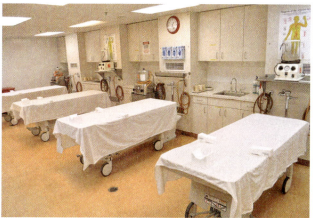

**Figure 4–2.** **A.** Single station design. **B.** Two station design. **C.** Central embalming; multiple station design.

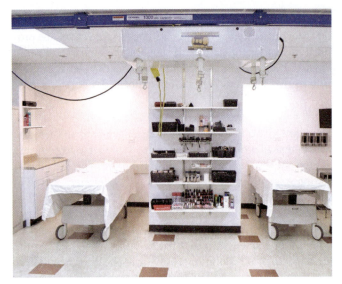

**Figure 4–3.** Decedent care stations.

disinfect. Epoxy coverings can be used over cement, tile, wood, and other types of flooring. **Clay or ceramic tiles** require grouting between the tiles; the grout is porous and must be sealed before use. Avoid glazed ceramic tiles that become slippery when wet. **Vinyl tile** is also seamless, resilient to cleaning products, and comfortable to stand on for hours at a time. **Paint** must be selected for impermeability to spilled materials. Choose a type that will seal the underlying floor surface.

## WINDOWS, DOORS, CEILINGS, AND WALLS

### Windows

Window selection is based on the location of the preparation room within the building. Privacy must always be ensured in the preparation room. Window glass cannot be transparent and allow visibility into a preparation area. Vented glass block installations provide privacy, and like conventional windows, allow incoming fresh air.

### Doors

Preparation room doors must be secured to deny access to unauthorized persons. Conventional locks require keys. Touchpad locking devices require only a code; the code can be readily changed when the need arises. A conventional door opening is 30-inches wide. 36-inch width is mandatory in many localities to accomodate caskets, mortuary equipment, and stretchers.

### Ceilings and Walls

Materials selected should be impervious and able to be kept clean and sanitary. Wall material must be wipeable and readily disinfected upon contamination or soiling. Some materials for walls include glazed masonry block, ceramic tile, and impervious wallboards and paints.

### Sound Insulation

Sound insulation should not be overlooked. Sounds created during embalming, such as the noise of the embalming machine, running or flushing water, instrument handling, and the use of mortuary devices, should not be heard beyond the preparation room. Special density cellulose fiber structural board can be used in ceilings, walls, and floors to lessen sound transmission.

## PLUMBING CONSIDERATIONS

### Eye Wash and Drench Shower Requirement

OSHA regulations address emergency shower and eyewash and eye/face wash station equipment needs. See 29 Code of Federal Regulations (CFR) 1910.151(c). The general requirement is applicable to all facilities that require the installation of emergency shower or eyewash station equipment as a form of first aid.

Sizes of water supply lines leading to and from the preparation room are determined by local ordinance. Sufficient water pressure is necessary for the proper functioning of the hydroaspirator, used during cavity aspiration. Low water pressure reduces suction. Small supply lines and older galvanized pipes are often the cause of low pressure. Wastewater disposal must be in compliance with code to prevent health risks.

### Backflow

Backflow is the reverse flow of liquids within a system caused by siphonage and pressure variables. Siphonage is created by a vacuum or partial vacuum in the water supply system. Siphonage is also caused by ordinary gravity. Water departments enforce codes that require backflow prevention. A device called a *backflow preventor* is a one-way valve installed in the water supply line that services the facility. Because of the serious nature of backflow problems, OSHA has addressed the problem nationally. Subpart J of the Occupational Safety and Health Act pertains to general environmental controls. Paragraph 1910.141(b) (2)(ii) contains the following statement: "Construction of non-potable water systems carrying any other non-potable substance shall be such as to prevent backflow or back-siphonage into a potable water system."*

### Hydroaspirator with Vacuum Breakers

The hydroaspirator (**Fig. 4–4**) is an aspirating device that creates a vacuum when water is run through it. Hydroaspirators are equipped with a vacuum breaker so aspirated material flowing through the device does not enter the water supply if a sudden drop in water pressure occurs. The hydroaspirator is attached to a water faucet over a flush sink. A clear plastic hose connects the aspirator to the trocar. A lever on the aspirator directs the flow of water in the same manner as a shut-off valve on a natural gas or water supply line. When the lever is *in-line,* or vertical with the unit, water flows from the unit into the hose; when the lever is horizontal, suction is created within the hose for aspiration. However, the lever operation is different on a *water control unit*.

Placement of the hydroaspirator is important for proper functioning. The device is attached to the faucet approximately 2 inches above the sink rim and the discharge hose situated below the rim to contain effluent. Large diameter clear tubing is attached so the embalmer can readily see the materials being aspirated. In cases of purge, visual inspection allows the embalmer to determine the source of the purge.

---

*This revision was published in **Federal Register**. 1973;38:10930.

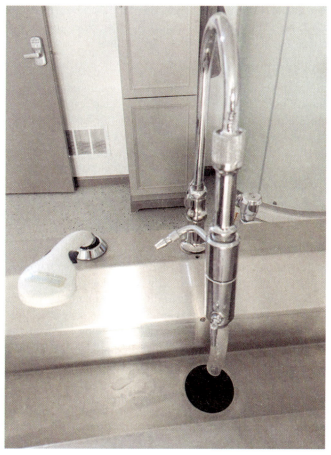

**Figure 4-4.** Hydroaspirator.

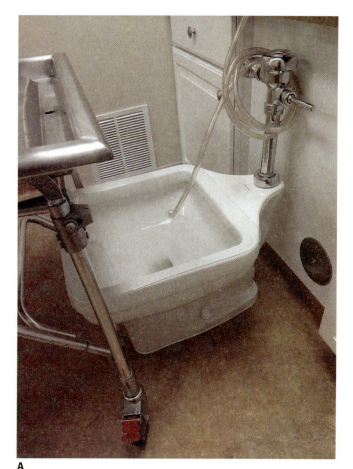

A

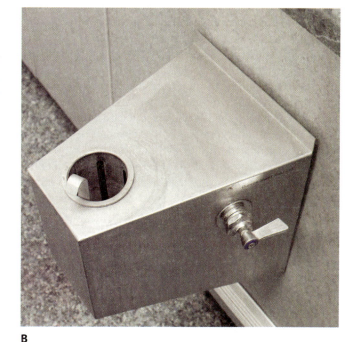

B

**Figure 4-5. A.** Flushable basin design. **B.** Wall-mounted installation.

### Electric Aspirator

The electric aspirating device requires electricity instead of water to operate and create suction. The device is free standing. Electric aspirators are commonly selected when low water pressure is an issue.

### Water Supply

Code compliance may require hot and cold water in the preparation room. A minimum temperature requirement of 130°F or 145°F may also be enforced. OSHA requires that all steam and hot water pipes be insulated when employee contact with the pipes is probable. Convenient water service to the embalming table, the embalming machine, and sinks create efficiency in the work environment. Water can be supplied directly from service sinks or from overhead. When the table is permanently installed, a supply line can be hidden inside the table.

### Sinks

There are many choices for selecting a waste sink for the embalming table; flushable basins and wall-mounted installations are customary (**Fig. 4–5A,B**). The flush valve incorporates a vacuum breaker. Local ordinances may require minimum ratings to be established at the valve for adequate flushing. Hand sinks should be located conveniently for the embalmer to wash hands between glove changes. Touchless faucets may be installed to avoid the handling of faucet controls. Controls for knee and foot operation are also available as well as elbow or forearm operation.

## VENTILATION

Adequate room ventilation is essential (**Fig. 4–6**). Preparation room ventilation requirements are determined by the size of the room. Calculations from a ventilation engineer will determine

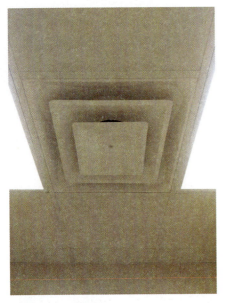

**Figure 4–6.** Ceiling ventilation.

the minimum number of room air changes per hour that are required in a specific setting.

A number of states have adopted 12–20 air exchanges per hour for an average-size embalming room. Formaldehyde is a chemical irritant. Formaldehyde gas may cause severe irritation to the mucous membrane of the respiratory tract and eyes. A study by Morrill reported sensory irritation (itching of eyes, dry and sore throat, increased thirst, and disturbed sleep) in paper-process workers at 0.9–1.6 ppm formaldehyde. Bourne and Seferian reported from another occupational setting intense irritation of eyes, nose, and throat at levels ranging from 0.13 to 0.45 ppm. More recent studies by Kerfoot and Mooney and Moore and Ogrodnik† conducted in funeral homes indicate that concentrations from 0.25 to 1.39 ppm evoke numerous complaints of upper respiratory tract and eye irritation and headache among embalmers. Schoenber and Mitchell report that acute exposure to formaldehyde phenolic resin vapors at levels around 0.4–0.8 ppm causes lacrimation and irritation of the upper as well as the lower respiratory tract. The levels at which serious inflammation of the bronchi and lower respiratory tract would occur in humans are unknown; inhalation of high levels, however, has caused chemical pneumonitis, pulmonary edema, and death.

Emerging technology and thought in the design and construction of preparation rooms reflect the recognition that because formaldehyde is heavier than air, exhaust systems located at or near floor level, when combined with the introduction of uncontaminated air from the ceiling level, are an efficient method of ventilation. In addition, such systems have the added advantage of drawing fumes and contaminants down and away from the operator's face during the embalming procedure. The key to the creation of an embalming environment protective of the embalmer's health and comfort is airflow and adequacy of ventilation. The number and location of windows and doors are components of the total ventilation system. Cross-ventilation requires windows on opposite walls. In choosing the location of the exhaust, care should always be taken so that air flows away from the operator. The grill on the exhaust fan, and on all other grills in the room, should be easily removable for cleaning.

### Air Conditioning

Although there are many different air conditioning units to choose from, the size of the room in cubic feet determines the size of the unit needed. When the entire funeral home is air conditioned by the same unit, independent controls are installed in the preparation room. Separate controls help to compensate for ventilation, which impacts climate more drastically in this location compared to the remainder of the facility.

## PREPARATION ROOM EQUIPMENT

### Mortuary Refrigeration

Refrigeration units are more commonplace in funeral homes. Units vary in size and design. The purpose of cooling units is to slow postmortem changes in the deceased body. Maximum temperature for cooling units is determined by state law; minimum temperature should remain above freezing. Access to the area containing the cooling unit must be locked by key or touch pad. An entry–exit log is kept for decedents stored in the unit. Identification tags or bands are attached to the body and to the body bag. Human remains need to be positioned in a **supine** position, lying face upward, with shoulders and head elevated. A maintenance cleaning schedule is necessary to document sanitation of the cooling unit.

### Body Lifts

Lifting devices are essential for heavy lifting and for use by a single operator. Floor lifts are manually operated; customarily hydraulic. Ceiling hoists require electricity for operation (**Fig. 4–7**). Both devices have safe operation limits for weight.

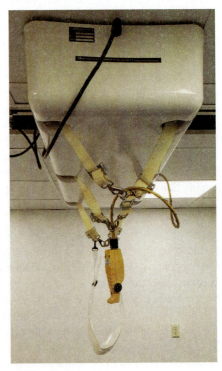

**Figure 4–7.** Ceiling hoist.

---

†See Selected Readings for complete Kerfoot and Mooney Study and Moore and Ogrodnik studies.

Lifts are used for both transferring and elevating a decedent. For example, to move the deceased from the mortuary cot to the embalming table, from the embalming table to a dressing table, or from a shipping container and into a casket.

## Body Transfer Board

Flexible polyethylene body transfer boards are strong, nonabsorbent, and easily cleaned. Placed beneath the body, transfer boards are used to move the remains from the mortuary cot to the preparation room table for embalming and decedent care and between various other surfaces such as dressing tables and mortuary refrigeration trays. Transfer boards can also be used to move the decedent into a casket, alternate container, combination unit, or other receptacle.

## Tables

Numerous types of materials are used in the construction of embalming tables; stainless steel and porcelain are commonly selected because of the stain-resistant finish. Some tables are stationary, others are movable (**Fig. 4–8A–D**). Movable tables

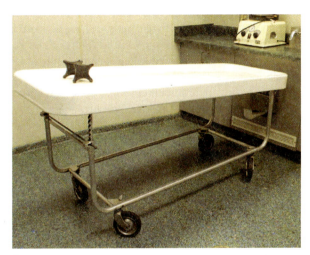

A

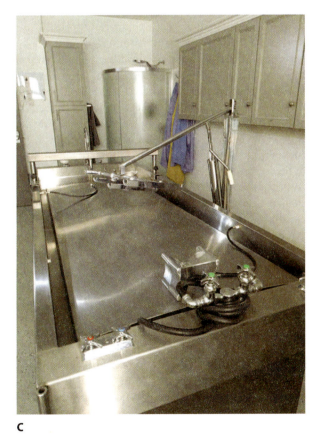

C

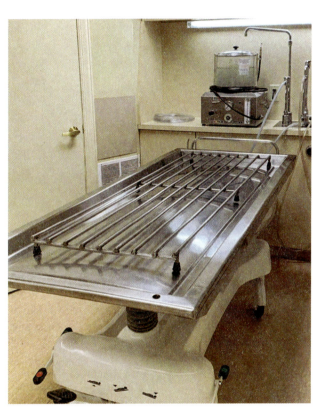

B

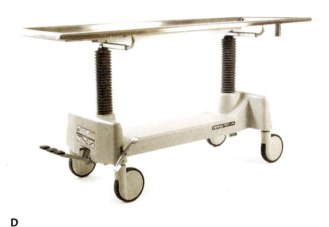

D

**Figure 4–8.** **A.** Porcelain embalming table. **B.** Stainless steel table with custom body positioning device. *(Used with permission of Melissa A. Cyfers.)* **C.** Custom-designed stationary stainless table. Supply line for table water and hoses for embalming solution are installed internally in the base of the table. The foot end incorporates a leg lift. **D.** Hydraulic embalming table.

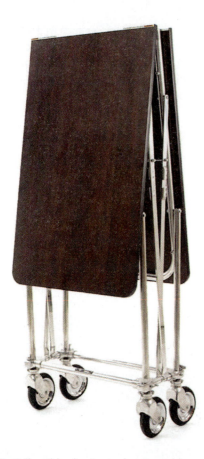

**Figure 4–9.** Collapsible aluminum dressing table.

have locking wheels. Tables are adjustable, manually or by hydraulics. Body bridges can be used to elevate the body above the table. Drainage is easily flushed away from the body and the embalmer.

At the completion of the embalming, the body may be transferred from the embalming table to a dressing table (**Fig. 4–9**). Dressing tables may be entirely stainless or aluminum with a laminated tabletop. The frame has wheels, is adjustable in height, and some are collapsible for storage. Dressing tables are unsuitable for embalming; there is no drain channel or drainage hole in the dressing table.

## Injection Apparatus

Most arterial embalming is done using electric machines for the injection of arterial solution. To be complete, however, several older mechanical methods are considered in this discussion. These devices are generally used today when the electronic machines are not working or when there is an electrical failure. Basically, six devices can be used to inject arterial solution: (1) gravity percolator, (2) bulb syringe, (3) combination of gravity percolator and bulb syringe, (4) hand pump, (5) air pressure machine, and (6) centrifugal pump.

### Gravity Percolator (Historical Injection Method)

The arterial solution is poured into a large glass reservoir, called a *percolator* that has a delivery hose attached to the bottom of the bowl. The percolator is elevated above the body to create the pressure necessary in the delivery hose to allow the embalming solution to flow into the arterial system. Approximately, one-half (0.43) pound of pressure is obtained for each foot of height the device is raised above the injection point (for every 28 inches of height, 1 pound of pressure is created). Because of the ceiling height restrictions in most preparation rooms, pressure is limited with gravity injection. This method of injection is still in use for the injection of anatomical bodies used for dissection. Gravity embalming provides a slow, steady method of injection that allows the body to accept the embalming solution at a slower rate. A greater volume of the arterial solution is retained by the body tissues.

### Bulb Syringe (Historical Injection Method)

This handheld and hand-operated device consists of a rubber bulb with hoses attached to either end. A one-way valve in the device allows for this pump to operate. One hose is placed into a container of embalming solution. Arterial solution flows into the bulb when the device is relaxed. Once the bulb is full, squeezing the bulb forces the arterial solution into the delivery hose and into the body. It is important to remember that the solution actually passes through the bulb syringe. Pressures are unknown and it does require the use of one hand. As pressure builds within the body, the bulb syringe becomes more difficult to squeeze.

### Combination Gravity and Bulb Syringe (Historical Injection Method)

In this method of injection, the delivery hose from the gravity percolator connects to the bulb syringe. The body can be embalmed by the gravity method, but pressures and rate of flow can be increased periodically by squeezing on the bulb syringe. The combination produces a greater pressure and rate of flow of the arterial solution.

### Hand Pump (Historical Injection Method)

This handheld device is a pump with two slip-hubs to which hoses can be attached. One hub delivers air to create pressure; the other hub creates a vacuum. Arterial solution does *not* flow through the hand pump. The arterial solution is placed in a jar and the lid is sealed into position. Air pumped by the hand pump enters through the hose leading from the hand pump to the jar. A delivery hose, which drops to the bottom of the jar, then carries the solution out of the jar and into the body. A careful check is necessary to be certain that air is not injected into the body when all of the arterial solution is injected. By attaching the air hose to the other hub of the hand pump, air can be withdrawn from the jar; thus, a vacuum created within the jar. A trocar can be attached to the free end of a hose which is attached by a gooseneck inserted into the jar lid. The aspirated contents will flow into the jar. No aspirated material passes through the hand pump.

### Embalming Machines

The motorized, centrifugal pump embalming machine is the most widely practiced method of arterial solution injection (**Fig. 4–10A–E**). An extensive variety of machines are available with numerous features. Most of these machines have large volume tanks, holding up to $3\frac{1}{2}$ gallons of solution. With the motorized pump, a constant preset pressure can be maintained in addition to the preset rate of flow of arterial solution into the body. It is always recommended that pressure be adjusted prior to arterial injection. The rate of flow can be determined once the arterial injection begins.

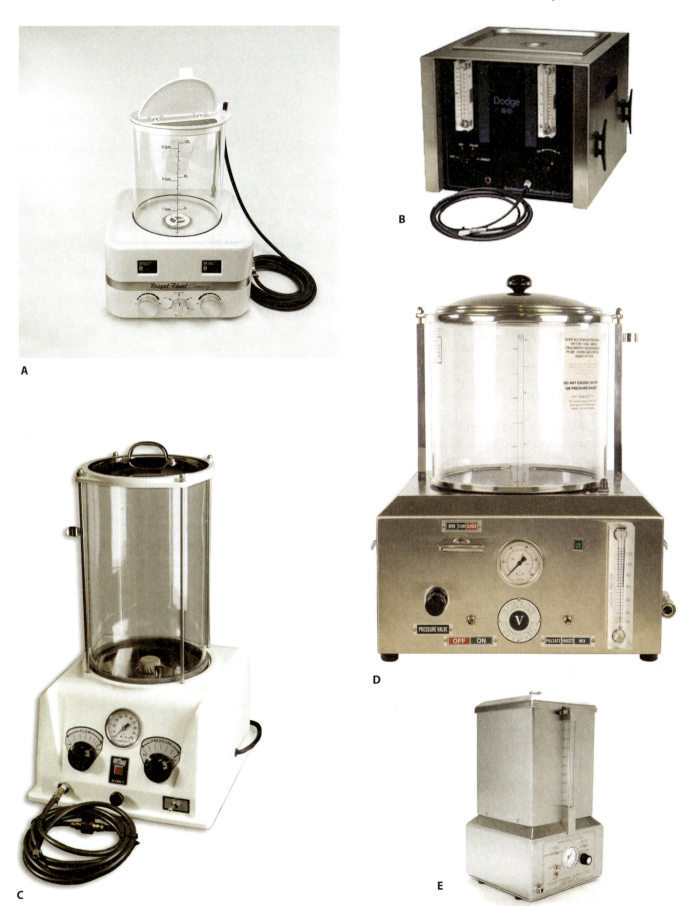

**Figure 4–10.** **A.** Frigid embalming machine. **B.** Dodge Automatic Pressure embalming machine. **C.** ESCO Porti-boy embalming machine. **D.** Pierce Duotronic embalming machine. **E.** NoAyr embalming machine. *(All images used with permission.)*

## Air Pressure Machine (Historical Injection Method)

The air pressure machine operates like the hand pump but is motorized. The motor-assisted air pressure machine relieves the embalmer from manually operating the device. The air pressure machine, like the hand pump, can be adapted to aspiration. Embalming solution and aspirated materials *do not* flow through the machine. The machine provides only air pressure or a vacuum. The delivery hose from the machine is attached to a reinforced plastic jar or metal pressure tank. The jar is the source of arterial solution, and also it will be the container into which aspirated materials will collect. This device can be very dangerous and pressures must be carefully observed. Some will produce pressures and vacuum up to 30 psi.

## Current Air Pressure Machines

Air pressure injection is widely used in Asia, Great Britain, and Europe. The air pressure embalming machine requires electricity only temporarily; when pressure is created within the machine, the power is turned off. The embalming solution, under pressure, will flow through the delivery hose into the artery (**Fig. 4–11**). Unlike historical counterparts, the embalming solution does flow through the machine.

During the embalming, it may become necessary to reset pressure and rate of flow to establish good distribution of the embalming solution. The pressure ranges in the motorized force pump can be very great. Some machines are capable of producing up to 200 pounds of pressure. In some machines, the motorized centrifugal pump runs at a constant speed. In others, the speed can be varied, and in yet other machines, two separate motors operating at different speeds are available. Many of these machines can produce a pulsating injection of solution into the body.

Several terms must be explained at this point. **Pressure** is the force required to distribute the embalming solution throughout the body and is measured in pounds per square inch (psi). The **rate of flow** is the amount of embalming solution that enters the body in a given period and is measured in ounces per minute (opm). **Potential pressure** is the pressure

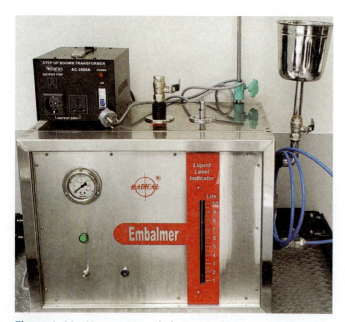

**Figure 4–11.** Air pressure embalming machine.

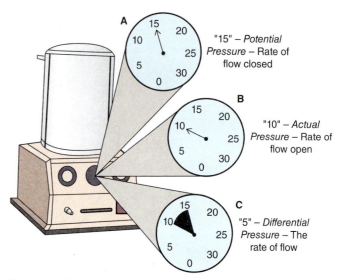

**Figure 4–12.** Centrifugal pump. **A.** Potential pressure (15), rate of flow closed. **B.** Actual pressure (10), rate of flow open. **C.** Differential pressure (5) indicates rate of flow.

reading on the gauge of the centrifugal machine, indicating the pressure in the delivery line of the machine with the rate-of-flow valve closed or the arterial tubing clamped shut.

**Differential pressure** is the difference between the potential pressure reading and the actual pressure reading; this is an indicator of the **rate of flow. Actual pressure** is the reading on the pressure gauge on the centrifugal pump when the rate-of-flow valve is open and the arterial solution is entering the body.

In the example described in **Fig. 4–12**, with the rate-of-flow valve **closed,** the potential pressure is 15 psi. The differential pressure is 5 psi and the actual pressure when the rate of flow valve is open is 10 psi. If the rate-of-flow valve were open until the gauge dropped to 5 psi, the differential would be 10 psi, or it can be said that the flow rate would be twice as fast as the previous setting. The differential pressure reading indicates the amount of resistance in the body, in the arterial tube, and in the delivery hose running from the machine to the arterial tube. The differential is also an important indicator of the rate of flow. Flow rate gauges may be added as an option to the centrifugal embalming machine.

There has been much misunderstanding in regard to the pressure that may exist inside the body as a result of the injection of solution. The fact that a pressure gauge reading on the embalming machine indicates a given pressure at which the fluid is leaving the delivery hose does not necessarily mean that this pressure exists within the body.

## INSTRUMENTATION

An embalming chemical supply catalog lists many instruments, most of which come in a variety of sizes and modifications. Many instruments have multiple uses. Unlike a surgical procedure, embalming is not performed under sterile conditions; instruments can be reused throughout the embalming process. Most instruments are made of stainless steel and plated with nickel or chrome for protection against rust or chemical agents. Instruments are chemically treated to be heat resistant and durable.

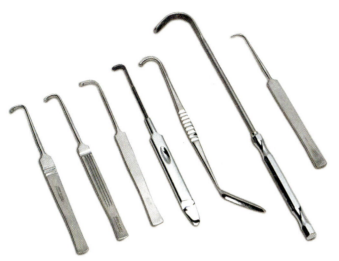

**Figure 4–13.** Various aneurysm hooks and aneurysm needles.

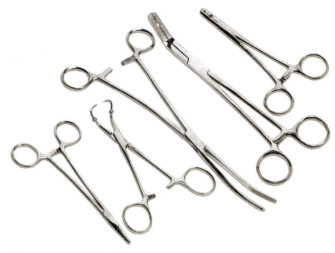

**Figure 4–15.** Various hemostats.

## General Instruments

### Aneurysm Hook and Aneurysm Needle

Aneurysm hooks and needles are curve-tipped instruments chiefly used for the blunt dissection of tissues to locate and raise arteries and veins (**Fig. 4–13**). The hook secures and elevates the vessels for use. A feature of the aneurysm needle is an "eye" in the hook, used to pass suture thread around a vessel. The instrument is useful during feature setting to lift the eyelid for insertion of an eye cap and to separate the lips for placement of dentures or a mouth former. The aneurysm hook has a variety of other uses. A combination instrument, such as the aneurysm hook/grooved director serves two functions (**Fig. 4–14**).

### Bistoury Knife

The bistoury knife is a curved cutting instrument designed for blunt dissection. The bistoury knife is customarily used during embalming to open arteries and veins.

### Hemostat (Locking Forceps)

A wide variety of hemostats are available (**Fig. 4–15**). The hemostat can be used to clamp leaking vessels. A modification is the **arterial hemostat**, which is used to hold the arterial tube securely in an artery (**Fig. 4–16**). The ends of hemostats may be curved or straight, serrated or smooth, or plain or rat-toothed. **Dressing or packing forceps** are very long hemostats used for packing orifices or handling contaminated bandage dressings (**Fig. 4–17**).

### Scalpel

The scalpel is a sharp cutting instrument used for making incisions. Disposable scalpels are best practice to reduce the risk of injury during blade replacement (**Fig. 4–18**). Retractable blade

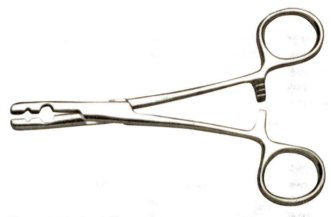

**Figure 4–16.** Arterial hemostat.

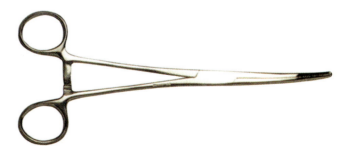

**Figure 4–17.** Dressing forceps.

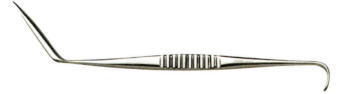

**Figure 4–14.** Grooved director and aneurysm hook combination instrument.

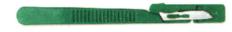

**Figure 4–18.** Disposable scalpel.

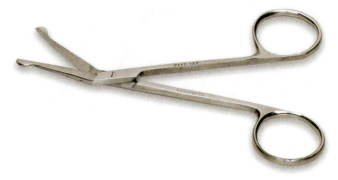

**Figure 4–21.** Bandage scissors.

### Scissors

Surgical scissors are used for cutting. Like the bistoury knife and scalpel, scissors can also be used to open arteries and veins. **Arterial scissors** are designed exclusively for opening vessels. The angled tip and short blades prevent cutting entirely through the vessel. A cutting blade is designed into the crux of the instrument for cutting needle injector wires. Scissors vary in length, and their tips may be straight or curved, pointed or blunt. **Bandage scissors** are designed to cut bandages; one or both blades are flat and paddle-shaped (**Fig. 4–21**). The paddle is placed against the skin to prevent tissue damage while cutting the bandage or dressing.

### Separator

The separator keeps vessels elevated above the incision. This instrument can be made of hard rubber, bone, or metal. In a combination instrument, the separator may have a bistoury knife at the opposite end (**Fig. 4–22**).

### Postmortem Suture Needles

A variety of **postmortem suture needles** are available (**Fig. 4–23**). Postmortem needles are used to close autopsy incisions as well as incisions made to raise vessels for injection. **Half-curved** needles are predominately straight in design with a slightly curved cutting tip. **Double-curved** needles resemble the letter "s." The **circle needle** resembles the letter "c." The half-curved **Loopuypt** needle is designed with an angled grip for secure handling. The patented *spring eye* is designed to make threading a needle easier; the eye is not a completed circle but a split eye. The ligature or thread is pulled between the split eye rather than through a traditional closed eye.

### Spring Forceps

The spring forceps is an instrument used for grasping and holding tissues. The limbs of the forceps may be straight, curved, or angular (**Fig. 4–24**). The tips of forceps may be serrated, smooth, or rat-toothed. **Angular spring forceps** used as a drainage device are sometimes called *drainage forceps*. Most embalmers use several types and lengths of spring forceps. This instrument is available in a large variety of lengths.

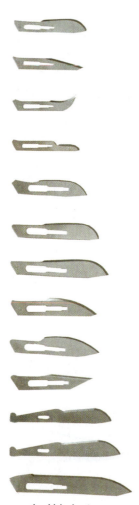

**Figure 4–19.** Various scalpel blade sizes.

scalpels nearly eliminate risk; the blade retracts into the handle after use. Non-disposable scalpels require blade replacement; numerous blade sizes are available (**Fig. 4–19**). OSHA requires a biohazard **sharps container** for the disposal of all sharp and contaminated items, including used scalpel and razor blades. The opening in the container prevents reaching into the container for retrieval of items after disposal. Containers come in a variety of sizes (**Fig. 4–20**).

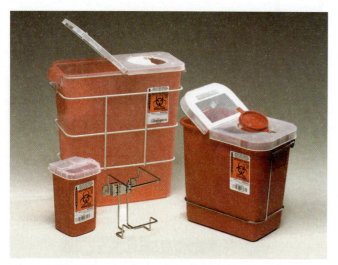

**Figure 4–20.** Biohazard sharps containers.

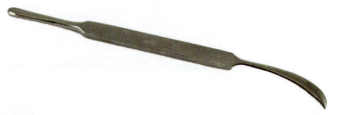

**Figure 4–22.** Separator and bistoury combination.

CHAPTER 4 • The Preparation Room

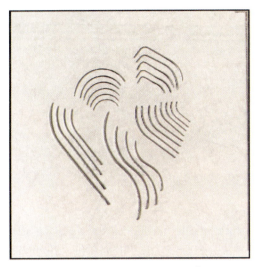

**Figure 4–23.** Various postmortem suture needles.

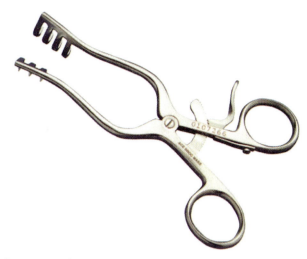

**Figure 4–25.** Retractor.

### Surgical Retractors

Retractors are designed for grasping, retaining, or holding back tissues. Retractors (**Fig. 4–25**) and incision spreaders (**Fig. 4–26**) are used for embalming purposes to hold open an incision during blunt dissection and raising of vessels.

### Ligature or Suture Thread

Ligature or suture thread is used to close incisions as well as the entry sites used for trocar. Ligature is available in various cords or *twists*; three-cord or three-twist combines three thread fibers; five or seven cords have five or seven cords, respectively. Three-cord thread is thinner than ligature of higher numbers. Suture ligature is available in nylon, cotton, and linen; waxed or unwaxed. Dental floss is a light and very strong material used for the restoration suturing of visible areas and is easily concealed with mortuary waxes or cosmetics. A device called a threader or thread passer is used to pass the ligature beneath a vessel (**Fig. 4–27**).

## Injection Instruments

### Arterial Tubes

There are many types, lengths, and sizes of arterial injection tubes (**Fig. 4–28**). Small diameters are used for infants, and distal arteries in adults, such as the radial and ulnar; large diameters are used for femoral and iliac arteries. Carotid tubes are designed short in length and large in diameter. The hub of the arterial tube is the attachment end; the male hub of the arterial tube attaches to the female hub of the stopcock or

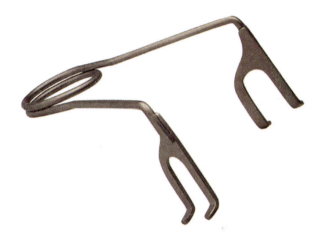

**Figure 4–26.** Incision spreader.

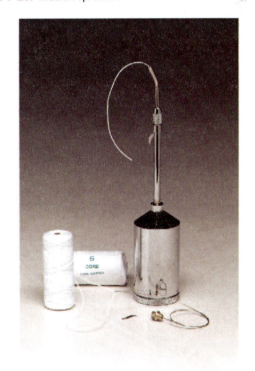

**Figure 4–27.** Threader and 5-cord ligature (suture thread).

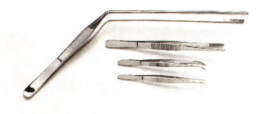

**Figure 4–24.** Angular spring forceps and various spring forceps.

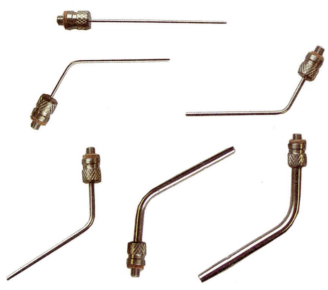

**Figure 4–28.** Various threaded hub arterial tubes.

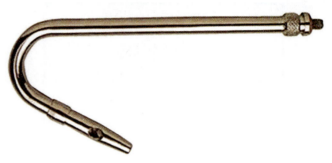

**Figure 4–30.** Hairpin arterial tube.

### Stopcock

The stopcock attaches to the delivery hose; the arterial tube attaches to the stopcock. The stopcock starts and stops the flow of fluid from the arterial tube into the artery. Stopcocks are available in the same hub styles as arterial tubes (**Fig. 4–32**).

### Y-Tube

The Y-tube was developed for the embalming of autopsied bodies to allow arterial injection of both legs simultaneously; also used for injection of both arms or both sides of the head at the same time (**Fig. 4–33**). Double-Y tubes allow injection of four arteries simultaneously (**Fig. 4–34**). Y-tube assemblies are available; assemblies include the Y-tube, stopcocks, hosing, and arterial tubes (**Fig. 4–35**).

### Hypovalve Trocar

The hypovalve trocar is designed for hypodermic injection only (**Fig. 4–36**). The valve is thumb-controlled to start and stop the flow of the solution.

## Drainage Instruments

### Drain Tube

The drain tube is a drainage device inserted into a vein **toward** the heart. Drain tubes keep the vein expanded and can be closed to build circulatory pressure. The stirring rod within the device is activated to fragment large clots. The iliac drain tube is long; insertion at the external iliac vein reaches the heart; the tip is directed into the right atrium. Iliac tubes are made of flexible rubber or curved metal (**Fig. 4–37**). Jugular drain tubes are a straight design, large in diameter and shorter in length (**Fig. 4–38**); axillary drain tubes are slightly curved

other type of instrument. Numerous hub styles are available. Some arterial tubes are threaded at their hub to allow interchangeability with different intermediate instruments, such as stopcocks or other attachments that fix the arterial tube to the delivery hose on the embalming machine. The types of hub connections that affix the arterial tube to the delivery hose include the threaded hub, slip hub (**Fig. 4–29**), quick connect hub, and Luer-lok hub. Other arterial tubes come premanufactured as a single piece with one of these types of connections, lacking the ability to be interchanged. Arterial tubes can be curved or straight. The hairpin arterial tube is designed with a long shaft that places the attachment well below the incision space (**Fig. 4–30**). The Luer-Lok hub was developed exclusively for high-pressure injection (**Fig. 4–31**). The Luer-lok is attached by fitting the arterial tube onto the stopcock and twisting with a quarter turn similar to attaching a hypodermic needle to a syringe.

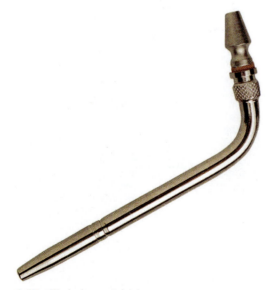

**Figure 4–29.** Slip hub arterial tube.

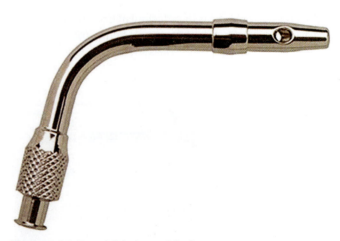

**Figure 4–31.** Luer-lok hub arterial tube.

CHAPTER 4 • The Preparation Room   77

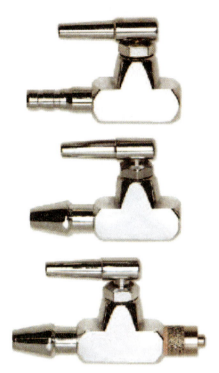

Figure 4–32. Stopcocks.

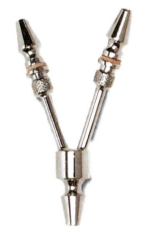

Figure 4–33. Y-tube.

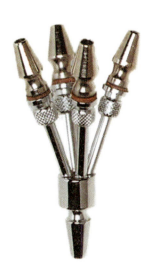

Figure 4–34. Double Y-tube.

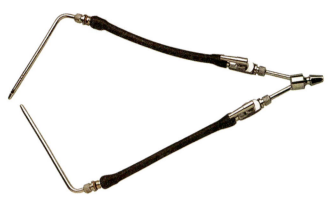

Figure 4–35. Y-Tube assembly.

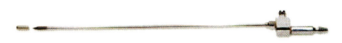

Figure 4–36. Hypovalve trocar.

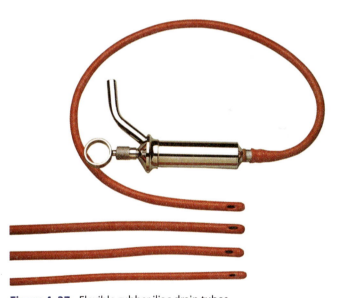

Figure 4–37. Flexible rubber iliac drain tubes.

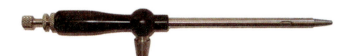

Figure 4–38. Jugular drain tube.

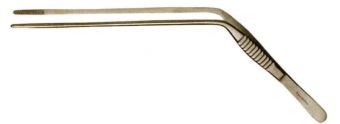

**Figure 4–39.** Angular spring forceps.

and small in diameter. The axillary drain tube is ideal for the small femoral and iliac veins in the infant. Hosing attaches to the outlet on the drain tube; the tubing reaches to the table drain for disposal. Drain tubes are advised for infectious embalming when containing drainage is necessary.

### Angular Spring Forceps
The angular spring forceps is a drainage instrument for use in the internal jugular vein, directed toward the heart (**Fig. 4–39**). Forceps allow clotted materials to be grasped and pulled from within a vein.

### Grooved Director
The grooved director is used to expand the vein and guide a drain tube or drainage device into place (**Fig. 4–40**). The grooved director can also be used to guide an arterial tube into a sclerosed artery.

## Aspirating Instruments
### Autopsy Aspirator
An autopsy or post aspirator is designed with numerous openings, holes, or slots in the head of the instrument to

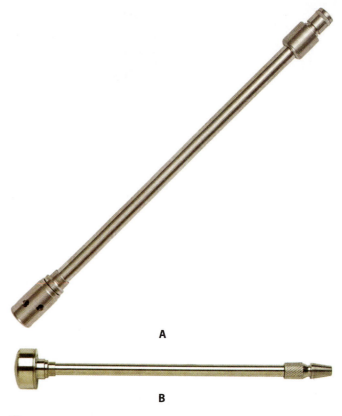

**Figure 4–41.** **A.** Autopsy aspirator with quick connect hub. **B.** Slotted autopsy aspirator with slip hub.

prevent clogging (**Fig. 4–41A,B**). The device is used to aspirate blood and arterial solution that have been collected in the autopsied cavities.

### Nasal Tube Aspirator
The nasal tube aspirator attaches to the aspirating hose and is inserted into the nostril or throat for limited aspiration of the nasal and throat cavities (**Fig. 4–42**).

### Trocar
The trocar is a long hollow needle used for cavity aspiration and injection. Trocar lengths and diameters are variable; collapsible versions are available for compact storage; the pistol grip is designed for single-handed operation (**Fig. 4–43A–C**). Trocar points are actually multisided blades; the points are

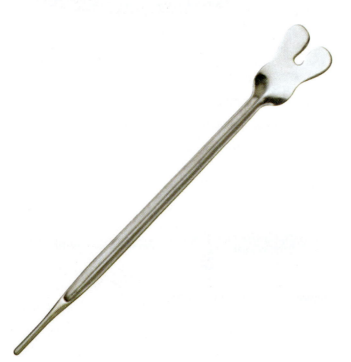

**Figure 4–40.** Grooved director.

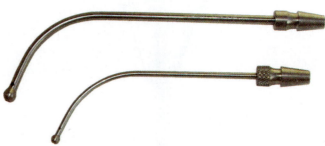

**Figure 4–42.** Nasal tube aspirators.

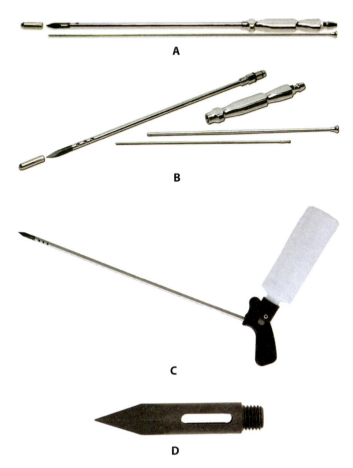

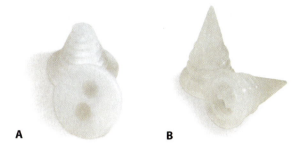

**Figure 4–45.** A. Trocar buttons. B. Multiclosure trocar buttons.

**Figure 4–43.** A. Standard adult trocar. B. Collapsible trocar. C. Evolution injector. D. Trocar point.

threaded for removal and replacement when dull (**Fig. 4–43D**). The handle may have a threaded, slip, or quick connect hub. Infant trocars are shorter in length and smaller in diameter. Infant-size trocars are also used for supplemental hypodermic injection.

### Cavity Fluid Injector
The cavity fluid injector screws onto the cavity fluid bottle. An attached length of tubing secures to the trocar. When the device is inverted, cavity fluid flows through the trocar into the body cavities (**Fig. 4–44**). The cavity fluid bottle attaches directly to a hub on the trocar, without the need for tubing, when using the Evolution injector.

### Trocar Button
A threaded nylon device is available in various sizes and lengths used for closing the trocar insertion site (**Fig. 4–45A,B**). The trocar button may also be used to close small punctures, surgical drain openings, and intravenous line punctures. They are available in several sizes.

### Trocar Button Applicator
The trocar button applicator is the device used to manually insert the trocar button (**Fig. 4–46**).

## Feature Setting Devices
### Eye caps
Eye caps are plastic disks inserted beneath the eyelids to maintain closure and contour the closed eye (**Fig. 4–47A,B**). Eye caps are available in a variety of shapes and sizes; caps may be clear or opaque.

### Mouth Formers
Mouth or expression formers are plastic devices used to maintain closure and contour the mouth. Formers create natural mouth curvature when natural teeth or dentures are missing (**Fig. 4–48**). Mouth formers may also be used overtop teeth or dentures to enhance expression. Mouth formers are available in a variety of shapes and sizes; formers may be clear or opaque.

### Needle Injector
A needle injector is a manual device used to embed a barb attached to the end of a metal wire into the mandible and maxilla for closure of the jaw in a fixed position (**Fig. 4–49**). Several styles of manual needle injector devices are available. An electric version of the injector is also available.

## Positioning Devices
Numerous styles of positioning devices enable the embalmer to properly position the head, arms, hands, and feet of the deceased.

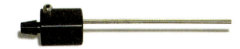

**Figure 4–44.** Cavity fluid injector.

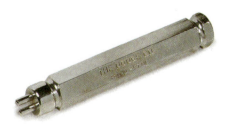

**Figure 4–46.** Trocar button applicator.

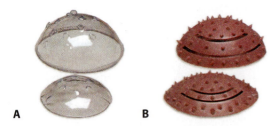

**Figure 4–47.** **A.** Clear perfection eye caps. **B.** Opaque oval eye caps.

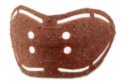

**Figure 4–48.** Mouth former also called an expression former.

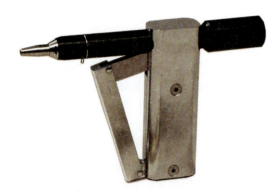

**Figure 4–49.** Needle injector.

Most are constructed of metal, hard rubber, or plastic. Positioning devices vary considerably in design (**Fig. 4–50A,B**). Metal devices secure and elevate the arms or feet using an adjustable platform. Strap devices secure the arms across the abdomen with an adjustable strap.

### Body Rests and Bridges

Numerous styles of body rests and bridges are available to aid in the positioning of the decedent. These devices are made from plastic or metal (**Fig. 4–51A,B**).

### Head or Positioning Blocks

Head and positioning blocks are used to elevate the head and neck, arms, and feet (**Fig. 4–52**). The positioning block has various uses. Blocks may be made from metal, plastic, or styrofoam.

## PLASTIC UNDERGARMENTS

Plastic garments are applied for use beneath clothing. The plastic garment protects clothing from soiling and contains minor leakages and odors. Plastic garments are available in various styles and sizes (**Fig. 4–53**).

- Pants: covers the torso, from the lower abdomen to the upper thigh.
- Coveralls: covers the trunk, from the upper thigh to the axillary space, or armpit.
- Stockings: covers legs to feet.
- Sleeves: covers upper arms to wrists.
- Shirt Jacket: covers the upper torso, from the neck to the waist, including the arms.
- Capri pants: combines pants and stockings.
- Unionall: covers the full body, except the head, neck, and hands.

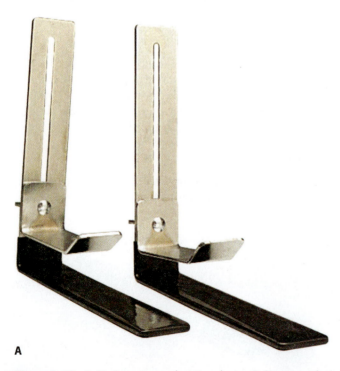

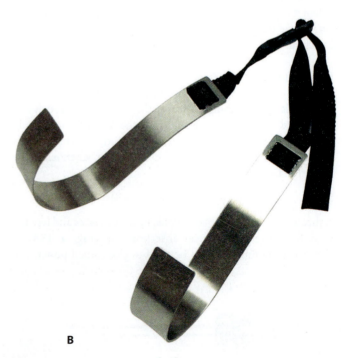

**Figure 4–50.** **A.** Stationary arm elevation device. **B.** Strap positioning device.

# CHAPTER 4 • The Preparation Room

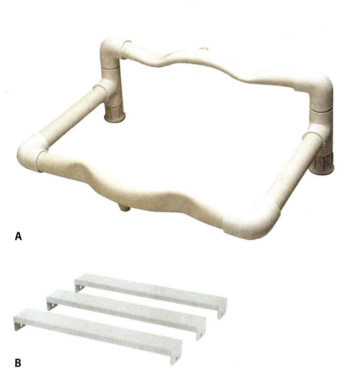

**Figure 4–51.** A. General purpose positioning device. B. Body bridges.

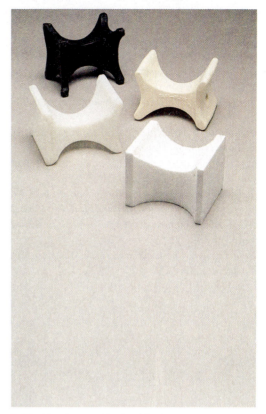

**Figure 4–52.** Head or positioning blocks.

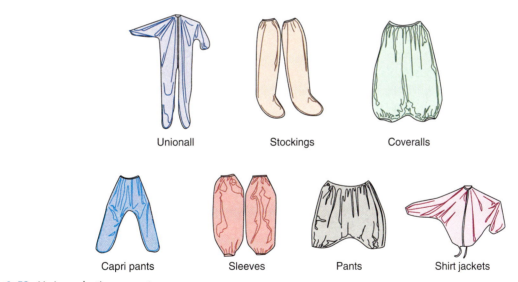

**Figure 4–53.** Various plastic garments.

## FIGURE CREDIT

Figures 4–2C, 4–3 are used with permission of Personal Care Center SCI Colorado Funeral Service-Denver.

Figures 4–5B, 4–8A are used with permission of Kevin Drobish.

Figures 4–8D, 4–9, 4–13, 4–15, 4–16, 4–17, 4–18, 4–19, 4–20, 4–21, 4–22, 4–23, 4–24, 4–26, 4–27, 4–32, 4–33, 4–34, 4–36, 4–42, 4–43 A,B, 4–44, 4–45A,B, 4–46, 4–47A,B, 4–48, 4–49, 4–51B, 4–52 are used with permission of Kelco Supply Company.

Figures 4–14, 4–25, 4–28, 4–29, 4–30, 4–31, 4–35, 4–37, 4–38, 4–39, 4–40, 4–41A,B, 4–43C,D, 4–50A,B, 4–51A are used with permission of The Dodge Company.

A special note of gratitude to the following for allowing the author to photograph their facilities:

Chris Janowiak, Janowiak Funeral Home, Belleville, MI (Figures 4–2A, 4–5A, 4–6)

Dick Kaatz, Kaatz Funeral Directors, William R. Hamilton Chapel, Mt. Clemens, MI (Figures 4–2B, 4–4, 4–8C)

Fred Voran, Jr., Voran Funeral Home, Allen Park, MI (Figure 4–7)

## BIBLIOGRAPHY

Bourne H, Seferian S. Formaldehyde in wrinkle-proof apparel processes: Tears for my lady. *Ind Med Surg* 1959;28:232.

Hendrick DJ, Lane DJ. Occupational formalin asthma. *Br J Ind Med* 1977;34:11.

Johnson P. NIOSH. Health Hazard Evaluation Determination Report HE 79-146-670, March 1980.

Kerfoot E, Mooney T. Formaldehyde and paraformaldehyde study in funeral homes. *Am Ind Hyg Assoc J* 1975;36:533.

Moore LL, Ogrodnik EC. Occupational exposure to formaldehyde in mortuaries. *J Environ Health* 1986;49(1):32–35.

Morrill E. Formaldehyde exposure from paper process solved by air sampling and current studies. *Air Cond Heat Vent* 1961;58:94.

Porter JAH. Acute respiratory distress following formalin inhalation. *Lancet* 1975;2:876.

Proctor NH, Hughes JP. *Chemical Hazards of the Workplace*. Philadelphia, PA: JB Lippincott, 1978:272.

Riccobono PX. *Current Report: Bureau of National Affairs*. October 1979:471.

Sakula A. Formalin asthma in hospital laboratory staff. *Lancet* 1975;2:876.

Schoenber J, Mitchell C. Airway disease caused by phenolic (phenol–formaldehyde) resin exposure. *Arch Environ Health* 1975; 30:575.

U.S. Department of Labor. *Occupational Safety and Health Standards (OSHA) for General Industry*. January 1978.

USDHEW/PHS/HRA. *Minimum Requirements of Construction and Equipment for Hospitals and Medical Facilities*. National Technical Information Service, DHEW Publication No. (HRA) 74-4000, September 1974.

Whitaker L. The preparation room. *Dodge Mag*, The Dodge Company, Cambridge, MA. 1997–1998;89(2)–90(3).

# CHAPTER 5

# Death: Agonal and Postmortem Changes

**CHAPTER OVERVIEW**
- Progression of Somatic Death
- Antemortem Changes
- Postmortem Physical and Chemical Changes
- Intrinsic and Extrinsic Factors
- Signs and Order of Decomposition
- Expert and Inexpert Tests of Death

## PROGRESSION OF SOMATIC DEATH

Death might be thought of as the point when the last breath is drawn. Death is actually a process and not a moment in time. The dying process can be described as an expanding inability of the body to sustain the physiologic and metabolic processes that are necessary for life. In higher biological organisms, like humans, these changes result in a cessation of integrated tissue and organ functions: loss of heartbeat, cessation of spontaneous breathing, and absence of brain activity. The dying process is a series of physical and chemical changes that begin before the legal pronouncement of death and continue for some time afterward. In the sequence of death, there is a point of irreversibility when life can no longer be sustained. When this point is reached, death is final. Yet, physical and chemical changes will continue **postmortem** (after death).

The **antemortem** (before death) interval is known as the **agonal period**. The person is said to be **moribund**, or actively dying during this stage. The length of the agonal period cannot be measured in defined parameters. It could be quick, as in death from sudden fatal injuries. Or linger for an extended time, as in death from chronic illness. When the agonal period is prolonged, signs of imminent death may be noticed: the **death rattle** and **death struggle**. A death rattle is a gurgling, or rattling in the throat caused by the accumulation of mucous and exacerbated by loss of the cough reflex. The death struggle presents as reflexive twitching of the muscles, marking the final efforts to sustain life.

Progression to **somatic death** is realized once the body loses ability to sustain physiologic and metabolic activity. *Soma* means body; somatic death is defined as death of the entire body. Somatic death proceeds in an orderly progression: clinical death, brain death, biological death, and postmortem cellular death.

- **Clinical death** occurs when spontaneous respiration and heartbeat irreversibly cease.
- **Brain death** occurs in a sequence of events that are a function of time without oxygen. The first part of the brain to die, usually in 5 or 6 minutes, is the cerebral cortex. Next the midbrain dies, followed by the brain stem.
- **Biological death** is the irreversible phase of somatic death and represents the cessation of simple body processes. The organs in the body no longer function.
- **Postmortem cellular death** is the process during which individual cells die. It may take a matter of hours depending on numerous variables.

Even after the process of dying has begun, a surplus of oxygen, nutrients, and other vital elements remain at the cellular level. Individual cells sustain metabolic activity by using these stored essential elements. At some point, the surplus is depleted and the cells are overcome by autolytic processes and die. This is **postmortem cellular death**. Cells that are more active and/or specialized have higher demands and will die more quickly. Cellular death continues beyond somatic death. Approximate progression of time for cellular death is shown:

| | |
|---|---|
| Brain and nervous system cells | 5 minutes |
| Muscle cells | 3 hours |
| Cornea cells | 6 hours |
| Blood cells | 6 hours |

> **ANTEMORTEM PERIOD**
> *Cellular death*
> Necrobiosis: the physiologic or natural death of cells as they complete their life cycles.
> Necrosis: the pathologic death of body cells as a result of disease processes. For example, decubitus ulcers and gangrene.
> Agonal period: the period occurring just before death.
>
> **POSTMORTEM PERIOD**
> *Stages of Somatic death*
> Clinical death
> Brain death
> Biological death
> Postmortem cellular death

## SIGNS OF DEATH

1. Cessation of respiration
2. Cessation of circulation
3. Muscular flaccidity
4. Changes in the eye, including:
   a. Clouding of the cornea
   b. Loss of luster of the conjunctiva
   c. Flattening of the eyeball
   d. Dilated and unresponsive pupils
5. Postmortem lividity
6. Rigor mortis
7. Algor mortis
8. Decomposition

## CHANGES DURING THE AGONAL PERIOD

The length of the agonal period influences the postmortem condition of the body. A prolonged agonal period increases the likelihood that the embalmer will encounter cases where (1) disease processes have progressed, (2) secondary infections are present, and (3) drug therapies have altered tissue conditions and chemical balance in the body.

Changes occurring during the agonal period can be related to their effect on (1) temperature of the body, (2) ability of the blood vessels to circulate blood, (3) moisture content of the tissues, and (4) translocation of microorganisms within the body.

### Temperature Changes

There are two agonal temperature changes. **Agonal algor** is a cooling or decrease in body temperature prior to death. This is common when death occurs slowly; metabolism and circulation also slow. **Agonal fever** is an increase in body temperature just prior to death. This is common with infection, toxemia, and certain types of poisoning. Elevated temperatures stimulate microbial growth.

### Circulatory Changes

There are three circulatory changes in the agonal period. **Agonal hypostasis** is the settling of blood into the dependent tissues of the body. Slowing of circulation allows the force of gravity to overcome the force of circulation. **Agonal coagulation** occurs as the circulation of blood slows and the formed elements of the blood begin to clot and congeal. **Agonal capillary expansion** is the dilation of pores within the capillaries in an effort to send more oxygen to the tissues and the cells.

### Moisture Changes

There are two changes in tissue moisture during the agonal period. **Agonal edema** is an increase in the amount of moisture, or fluids, in the tissues and the body cavities. The edema can result from disease processes and from agonal capillary expansion. **Agonal dehydration** is a decrease in the amount of moisture, or fluids, in the tissues and the body cavities.

The relationship between agonal edema and agonal dehydration can consider in terms of shifts in the balance and location of body moisture. Tissue fluids that flow or gravitate to other areas of the body create a shift in the moisture balance. One area may become edematous while another will become dehydrated. In agonal capillary expansion, the increased size of the openings in the capillary walls, while intended to allow more oxygen into the tissues, also allows fluids to flow out of the capillaries and into the intercellular spaces. This movement of fluids constitutes a shift in the moisture balance by which the greater amounts of moisture flow to the intercellular spaces while the moisture within the capillary will be reduced.

### Translocation of Microorganisms

**Translocation** is the movement of microorganisms from one area of the body to another. Organisms normally confined to a specific area of the body by natural body defenses are able to move as the body loses its ability to keep them in check. Most of these microbes naturally reside in the gut. Translocation may be the result of the organism (1) having natural motility, (2) entering the blood stream and circulating to other parts of the body, or (3) gravitating to other parts of the body during hypostasis or shifts in tissue moisture.

## POSTMORTEM CHANGES

Postmortem changes are classified as either physical changes or chemical changes (**Table 5–1**). Postmortem changes are generally more pronounced with the passage of time. The condition of the body continues to change during the interval between death and embalming (**Fig. 5–1**). A main objective of the embalming process is to suspend decomposition changes. When the interval between death and embalming is lengthy, complications are anticipated. For this reason, embalmers prefer to begin the embalming process as soon as possible.

**Physical changes** are produced by the forces of nature. On the molecular level, physical changes rearrange molecules. Natural forces cause changes in the physical state of the body or body tissues. However, natural physical changes do *not* change the chemical composition of the body. For example, the force of gravity can move blood from one area of the body to another. No new products are formed by this movement; blood simply changes physical location.

## CHAPTER 5 • Death: Agonal and Postmortem Changes

### TABLE 5–1. Postmortem Physical and Chemical Changes

| Change | Classification | Description |
|---|---|---|
| Algor mortis | Physical | Cooling of the body to the temperature of the surrounding environment |
| Dehydration | Physical | Loss of moisture from the surface of the body to the surrounding atmosphere |
| Hypostasis | Physical | Gravitation of blood and body fluids to dependent areas of the body |
| Livor mortis | Physical | Postmortem intravascular blood discoloration brought about by the presence of blood in the dependent surface vessels of the body |
| Increase in blood viscosity | Physical | Postmortem thickening of the blood is caused primarily by the loss of the liquid portion of the blood to the tissue spaces |
| Endogenous invasion of microorganisms | Physical | Relocation of microorganisms in the body as a result of the cessation of natural and metabolic activities |
| Postmortem caloricity | Chemical | Temporary rise in body temperature after death |
| Change in body pH | Chemical | Change in body tissues from slightly alkaline in life (pH 7.38–7.40) to acidic (pH 6.0–5.5) during rigor, then a return to alkaline in decomposition |
| Rigor mortis | Chemical | Temporary postmortem stiffening of body muscles by natural body processes |
| Postmortem stain | Chemical | Extravascular color change brought about by hemolysis; liberated hematin seeps through the capillary walls and into the body tissues; cannot be removed by arterial injection and venous drainage |
| Decomposition | Chemical | Separation of compounds into simpler substances by the action of bacterial and/or autolytic enzymes |

**Chemical changes** are generated by chemical activities that result in the formation of new chemical substances. At the molecular level, chemical change involves making or breaking bonds between atoms. Postmortem processes are largely dependent on autolytic enzymes, which stimulate chemical reactions between substances found in the tissues. As existing substances react chemically with one another, new chemical compositions are formed.

### Postmortem Physical Changes

Postmortem physical changes impact embalming and are triggered by cessation of blood circulation, gravity, and surface evaporation (**Table 5–2**). The following are classified as postmortem physical changes:
1. Algor mortis
2. Hypostasis
3. Livor mortis
4. Dehydration
5. Increased viscosity of the blood
6. Endogenous invasion of microorganism

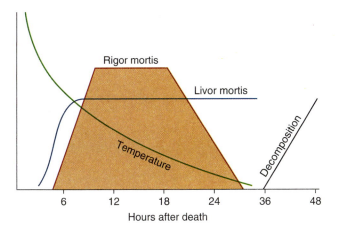

**Figure 5–1.** Principal postmortem changes.

### TABLE 5–2. Embalming Significance of Postmortem Physical Changes

| | |
|---|---|
| Algor mortis | Slows the onset of rigor mortis and decomposition<br>Helps to maintain blood in a liquid state<br>Can increase the degree of livor mortis and postmortem stain |
| Hypostasis | Responsible for livor mortis<br>Hemolysis can cause postmortem stain<br>Increases tissue moisture in dependent tissues |
| Livor mortis | Discoloration can vary from slight reddish hue to almost black, depending on blood volume and viscosity<br>Intravascular; can be cleared during arterial injection<br>Can be "set" as a stain if excessively strong uncoordinated embalming solution is injected<br>Can help capillary expansion<br>Clearing is a sign of fluid distribution |
| Dehydration | May be gravitated or massaged from an area<br>Accompanied by increased blood viscosity<br>Can create postmortem edema in the dependent tissues<br>Darkens skin surface; does not respond to bleaching<br>Causes shrinking and wrinkling of features<br>Extreme condition can retard further decomposition; desiccation<br>Extreme condition can create preservation |
| Increase in blood viscosity | Thickened blood and coagulation<br>Increased vascular resistance during arterial injections<br>Restricts blood drainage |
| Endogenous invasion of microorganisms | Pathologic hazard to embalmer<br>Promotes and aids decomposition |

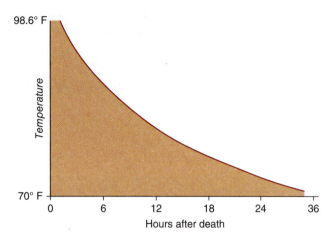

**Figure 5–2.** Algor mortis versus time.

## Algor Mortis

Algor mortis is the postmortem cooling of the body over time (**Fig. 5–2**). For example, when the surrounding environment temperature is cooler than body temperature, the temperature of the deceased body will cool to the temperature of the surrounding environment. The rate at which the body cools is dependent upon a number of variables. Factors within the body are called **intrinsic factors;** factors involving the surrounding environment are called **extrinsic factors**.

Intrinsic factors include (1) the ratio of body surface area to body mass, (2) body temperature at the time of death, and (3) a combination of the effects of the ratio of surface area to body mass and body temperature at the time of death.

During life, body heat is lost to conduction, radiation, and convection as the blood circulates through the superficial vessels of the skin. The blood is warmed again as it circulates back through the body's internal organs. A larger body will have more surface area to lose body heat, but that potential to lose heat can be offset by body mass. A smaller body will have less surface area to lose body heat and would therefore require less body mass to offset the loss of heat. In death, there is no opportunity for the blood to regain the lost heat because there is no circulation. Therefore, if a body has a larger surface area from which heat can be lost, its temperature will decrease more rapidly, unless there is something to offset the potential to lose heat. Here again, heat loss can be offset by body mass. In short, a body with more mass will be better insulated against heat loss and will, therefore, cool at a slower rate. Infants, for example, are more likely to cool faster because, among other factors, they have a higher ratio of surface area as compared with their body mass (Walter, 1989).

If the body temperature is elevated at the time of death, it will take longer for the body to cool to the temperature of the surrounding environment because the temperature will simply have farther to drop. Body temperature can elevate because of increased metabolic activity, the presence of fever, or an inability of the body to regulate its temperature. Likewise, low body temperature at the time of death will influence the length of time for the body to cool to reach a point of equilibrium with the surrounding environment. Body temperature can decrease as a result of exposure to cold or an inability of the body to regulate its temperature.

Rapid cooling of the body by refrigeration or natural means helps to slow the onset of rigor mortis, slow the onset of decomposition, and keep the blood in a liquid state. These are all advantageous for embalming. A body that has been cooled rapidly will, however, be more likely to have discoloration from livor mortis and postmortem staining.

Extrinsic factors that affect postmortem cooling of the body include (1) body coverings and (2) the surrounding environment. Body coverings include clothing or other coverings that protect the skin from direct exposure to the environment. In addition to providing added insulation, an external covering will also retard or prevent heat loss that results from conduction, radiation, and convection.

The surrounding environment itself will affect the rate at which a body loses heat. A body submerged in 70°F water, for example, would lose heat more rapidly than in 70°F air temperature, because water would conduct heat away from the body more quickly than air.

## Hypostasis

Hypostasis is a process by which blood settles, as a result of gravitational movement within the vessels, to the dependent, or lower parts of the body. The designation of dependent changes depending on the position of the body. For example, if a body were lying on its back, the back of the body becomes dependent; blood will settle, or gravitate into the tissues of the back of the body.

Gravitational movement of the blood is affected by constrictions, ligatures, and other factors that impede free movement of the blood within the vessels. **Contact pallor** refers to the areas where blood movement has been inhibited. It is most obvious in areas where the body has been in contact with a surface. The weight of the body pressing against the dependent capillary beds prevents the blood from settling into the dependent area. Although the surrounding area may be discolored, the area in contact with the surface will not discolor (**Fig. 5–3**).

Thinner, or less viscous blood flows with less resistance and will gravitate to dependent parts of the body more readily. Factors that affect the viscosity of the blood influence the speed at which postmortem hypostasis takes place. Some factors include refrigeration, medication, and disease processes.

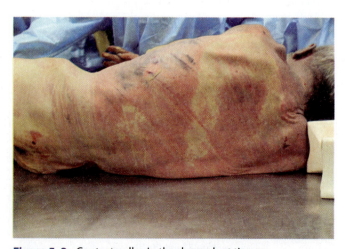

**Figure 5–3.** Contact pallor in the dependent tissues.

Conversely, factors that thicken, or increase viscosity, will slow the rate at which postmortem hypostasis takes place. Possible factors include heat, medication, and disease processes.

The embalming significance of hypostasis lies in the postmortem discolorations that can result from the gravitational movement of blood. In embalming terminology, hypostasis describes the *process* by which blood gravitates to the dependent parts of the body, *not the discoloration*.

### Livor Mortis

Livor mortis is a postmortem intravascular blood discoloration that occurs as a result of hypostasis. Livor mortis is also known as **postmortem lividity** or **cadaveric lividity**. The discoloration may first be noticed as dull reddish patches appearing approximately 30–90 minutes after death. As it becomes more established over time it can take on a deep reddish-blue appearance. Livor mortis can be reduced or removed during the embalming process as embalming solution flushes the pooled blood from the capillary beds of the area (**Fig. 5–4**).

Two factors play an important role in the degree of intensity of livor mortis: blood volume and blood viscosity. In cases where excessive bleeding has taken place, either internally or externally, there will be less blood available to pool. This may reduce the instance or intensity of livor mortis. Likewise,

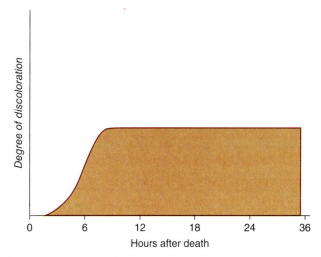

**Figure 5–4.** Livor mortis.

if blood is thicker and not readily subject to gravitation, the appearance of livor mortis may be affected (**Table 5–3**).

### Dehydration

The loss of water and fluids from body tissues is called *dehydration*. There are two basic factors at work in postmortem

| TABLE 5–3. Embalming Considerations and Blood Discolorations | | | | |
|---|---|---|---|---|
| Antemortem Hypostasis (a.m.) | Postmortem Hypostasis (p.m.) | Livor Mortis | Postmortem Stain (p.m.) | Formaldehyde Gray |
| Occurs prior to death or during the agonal period | Begins at death | Seen as soon as blood fills superficial vessels; begins approximately 20 min after death; depends on p.m./a.m. hypostasis | Normally occurs approximately 6 h after death; cause of death and blood chemistry vary rate | Normally occurs approximately 6 h after death; cause of death and blood |
| Intravascular | Intravascular | Intravascular | Extravascular | Intravascular or extravascular |
| Movement of blood to dependent tissues | Movement of blood to dependent tissues | p.m. blood discoloration as a result of p.m./a.m. hypostasis | p.m. blood discoloration as a result of hemolysis | Embalming discoloration |
| a.m. physical change | p.m. physical change | p.m. physical change | p.m. chemical change | — |
| | Speed depends on blood viscosity | Color varies with blood volume and viscosity and the amount of $O_2$ in blood | May occur prior to, during, or after arterial fluid injection | Seen after arterial fluid injection |
| a.m. | p.m. | p.m. | p.m. | p.m. |
| — | — | Pressed on skin clears | Pressed on skin does NOT clear | Seen as a gray stain |
| — | — | Removed by blood drainage | Not removed by blood drainage | Methemoglobin HCHO + blood |
| — | Arterial injection stops progress | Arterial injection (mild) clears/with drainage | Strong solutions bleach and "set" livor as stain | — |
| | Speeded by cooling of body, low blood viscosity | Speeded by cooling, blood "thinners," low blood viscosity, CO deaths | Speeded by cooling, rapid red blood cell hemolysis, CO deaths | Speeded by poor drainage |

loss of body moisture: **surface evaporation** and **gravitation,** or hypostasis of blood and body fluids.

Surface evaporation results from the passage of air over the surface of the body and exposure to direct air currents. Maintaining coverage of the body, the use of moisturizing agents such as massage cream or stone oil, and preventing direct air exposure help to reduce dehydration.

Gravitation, or hypostasis of the blood and body fluids is the physical movement of those fluids to the dependent regions of the body. Elevated, or nondependent areas dehydrate more quickly as fluid is lost. Conversely, fluids settle in the dependent areas; overaccumulation of tissue fluids causes a condition known as **postmortem edema.** Another mechanism leading to postmortem edema is **imbibition.** Imbibition is the ability of the cells to draw moisture from the surrounding area into themselves.

As dehydration occurs, the blood becomes increasingly viscous. Eventually the formed elements of the blood will stick together in clumps, a process that creates what is referred to as **sludge.** Obviously, sludge does not lend itself to establishing good drainage during arterial embalming.

Dehydration causes tissues to darken, shrink, and wrinkle (**Fig. 5–5**). Initially, areas of dehydration were present in yellow and reddish hues. As moisture loss continues, the tissues will progressively darken. Dehydration is discussed here as a postmortem change prior to embalming; note that dehydration can also be exacerbated by excessive moisture loss during embalming and can continue after embalming (**Fig. 5–6**).

### Increase in Blood Viscosity

Viscosity refers to the thickness of a liquid or its resistance to flow. Blood has four components: (1) plasma, (2) red blood cells, (3) white blood cells, and (4) platelets. The liquid component of blood is the plasma; a mixture of water, sugar, fat, protein, and salts. After death, blood can thicken, or increase in viscosity, due to dehydration. As the tissue moisture is lost to the surrounding air, plasma moves through the capillary walls into the tissue spaces. Surface evaporation continues the drying process. Blood remaining in the body thickens and blood cells clump together. Thickened arterial blood clogs the smaller arteries during arterial injection. Thickened venous blood will

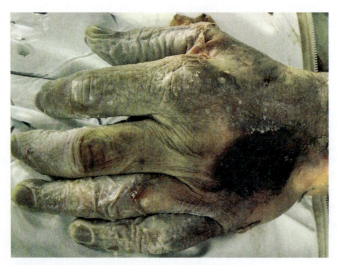

**Figure 5–5.** Severe dehydration of the hand.

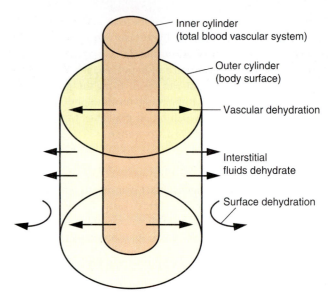

**Figure 5–6.** Total vascular system and the effects of dehydration before and after embalming.

inhibit drainage. Hypostasis favors the liquid blood, leaving behind the more viscous blood. Rapid blood thickening can diminish the degree of livor mortis by slowing the settling of blood into the dependent tissues.

### Endogenous Invasion (Translocation) of Microorganisms

*Following somatic death, the structurally intact epithelial, fascial and other tissue barriers undergo a loss of structural integrity. This permits body-wide translocation, or re-distribution, of systemic microflora; creating alternate body fluid and body tissue reservoirs of host contamination. All body fluids and body tissues can become reservoirs of infectious agents within a relatively short postmortem interval.\**

Endogenous invasion of cerebrospinal fluid by bacterial agents associated with the colon occurs within 4–6 hours of death. *The colon, designated as the postmortem origin of "indicator" organisms recovered from extraintestinal sampling sites, seems to be the primary source of many of the translocated microbial agents.* The isolation of indicator organisms and nonindicator organisms, sampled from the left ventricle of the heart, the lungs, the urinary bladder, and the cisterna cerebellomedullaris, indicates the extent to which microbial agents of low, moderate, and high virulence can translocate within 4–8 hours postmortem. The postmortem multiplication of systemic and translocated recoverable microbial agents may begin within 4 hours of somatic death and reach peak densities of $3.0$–$3.5 \times 10^6$ organisms per milliliter of body fluid or per gram of body tissue within a 24–30 hours postmortem interval.†

Postmortem factors contributing to the translocation of endogenous microflora include (1) chemical and physical

---

*See Selected Readings, "Summary of Guidelines Submitted to OSHA from the National Funeral Directors Association Committee on Infectious Disease," 1989.

†See the Selected Readings section for the complete Rose and Hockett reprint.

changes, (2) movement and positional changes of the body, (3) passive recirculation of blood from contaminated body sites, (4) thrombus fragmentation and relocation, and (5) the inherent true motility of many of the intestinal bacilli. Translocated organisms can exit any type of body opening, contaminate animate and inanimate surfaces, and become aerosolized (droplet infection particles) or dried particles (droplet nuclei), expanding the potential spread of biological hazards.

For the embalmer, the most troublesome organism is **Clostridium perfringens**, an anaerobic, spore-forming bacillus responsible for true tissue gas. Postmortem translocation of *C. perfringens* can produce intense embalming and preservation challenges. Gases that cause tissue distension and accelerate the decomposition cycle can appear within 1 or 2 hours of death. Decomposition changes can be so rapid and severe that viewing of the body may not be recommended.

## Postmortem Chemical Changes

The significance of postmortem chemical changes: rigor mortis, postmortem stain, postmortem caloricity, shifts in pH, and decomposition are outlined in **Table 5-4**.

### Postmortem Caloricity

Metabolism is defined as the *sum of all chemical reactions that occur within a cell.* Metabolism is dependent upon oxygen. There are two phases of metabolism: (1) **anabolism**, the building phase; and (2) **catabolism**, the breakdown phase.

Catabolism releases heat and energy. When death occurs, cells retain a supply of oxygen and metabolism continues for a time. Postmortem metabolism creates heat that can elevate postmortem temperature, also known as *postmortem caloricity*.

### Postmortem Stain

Postmortem stain is the extravascular blood discoloration brought about by the **hemolysis** of blood. Hemolysis is the *rupture or destruction of red blood cells*. After death, blood settles into the vessels of the dependent areas of the body by a process known as **hypostasis**. Blood pooling in the dependent areas caused by hypostasis results in the intravascular discoloration known as **livor mortis**. Approximately 6–10 hours after death, hemolysis of red blood cells begins and leads to the extravascular discoloration called **postmortem stain**. Rapid onset of hemolysis is frequent during mortuary refrigeration and in deaths from carbon monoxide poisoning (**Fig. 5-7**).

Each red blood cell contains several million hemoglobin molecules. The family of hemoproteins, or heme, is the component of hemoglobin responsible for the red pigment in blood. During hemolysis, heme passes through the walls and pores of the capillaries and collects in the tissue spaces causing discoloration. The discoloration is extravascular and is permanently fixed in the tissues as stain.

Tardieu spots result from the rupture of capillaries; appearing approximately 18–24 hours postmortem. Like all extravascular blood discolorations, they do not respond to clearing during arterial injection and blood drainage. They appear as dark pinpoint hemorrhages in the same dependent areas as livor mortis and postmortem stain. In time, they may leave a marbling pattern in the tissues. Tardieu spots are very common in slow deaths and death by asphyxia (DiMaio and DiMaio, 2001, p. 24).

### Shift in Body pH

In the field of chemistry, degrees of acidity or alkalinity of a substance are expressed in pH values. The neutral point, where a solution would be neither acidic nor alkaline, is pH 7. Increasing acidity is expressed as a number less than 7 and increasing alkalinity as a number greater than 7. Maximum acidity is pH 0 and maximum alkalinity is pH 14. Because each unit on the scale represents a logarithm, there is a 10-fold difference between each unit (*Taber's Cyclopedic Medical Dictionary*).

Normal pH for a body is approximately 7.4. After death, blood pH drops and tissue fluid moves into the acid range (approximately 3 hours after death). The body remains acidic during rigor mortis and then gradually, as the decomposition process advances, the body becomes increasingly alkaline.

During life, the carbohydrates (glycogen) stored in the liver and muscles are broken down to pyruvic and lactic acids by the oxygen present. Normally, this pyruvic acid is oxidized to carbon dioxide, water, and energy. The energy, in turn, is used to build up the adenosine triphosphate (ATP) of the body by converting adenosine diphosphate and adenosine monophosphate to ATP. The oxygen present in life prevents the buildup of lactic acid by oxidizing it to carbon dioxide and water. After death occurs, the oxygen is gradually used up, and the lactic acid is no longer inhibited and begins to accumulate in the muscle tissues. This buildup of acid occurs during the first hours after

| TABLE 5-4. Embalming Significance of Postmortem Chemical Changes | |
|---|---|
| Rigor mortis | Creates extravascular resistance<br>Body positioning challenges<br>Feature setting challenges<br>Tissue distention during arterial injection<br>Increases demand for preservative<br>Reduces the absorption of preservative<br>pH changes affect chemical reaction of embalming solution<br>Nonuniform dye coloration<br>False sign of preservation |
| Postmortem stain | Extravascular discoloration; not cleared during arterial injection alone<br>Gray discoloration when reacting with embalming chemicals<br>Sign of delay between death and embalming<br>Indicates an increased demand for preservative |
| Postmortem caloricity | Accelerates the rigor mortis cycle<br>Accelerates decomposition |
| Shifts in pH | Interferes with arterial solution reactions<br>May result in blotchy appearance of dye on the skin surface |
| Decomposition | Poor distribution of embalming solution<br>Tissues easily distend during arterial injection<br>Increased demand for preservatives<br>Manifested by discoloration, odor, skin-slip, gases in cavities and tissues, purge |

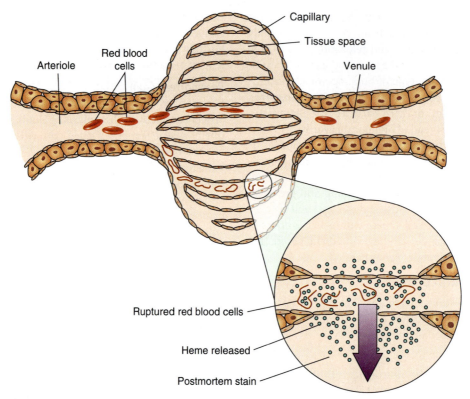

**Figure 5–7.** Postmortem stain.

death (approximately the first 3 hours). This cycle is closely and directly related to the cycle of rigor mortis. The pH will drop to an acid level of approximately 6.0 and has been recorded as low as 5.5.

As a result of the acid buildup in the tissues, conditions become right for the breakdown of the soft proteins of the body. Later, as the protein breaks down, there is a gradual buildup in the tissues of nitrogen products such as ammonia and amines. The ammonia, which is basic, neutralizes the acids present in the tissues from carbohydrate breakdown. As the body contains much more protein than carbohydrates, the ammonia products gradually begin to build to a point where the pH of the tissues becomes basic (or alkaline). During decomposition the tissues are found to have an alkaline pH.

### Rigor Mortis

Rigor mortis is the postmortem stiffening of muscles by natural processes. This condition affects only the muscles, and usually all of the muscles of the body are affected. Once the condition passes, it does not recur. Usually, the muscles are relaxed as death occurs. This is called **primary flaccidity**. If the body is embalmed while the muscles are flaccid, the proteins will react well with the preservative and tissue fixation will occur. If the body is embalmed while rigor is fully developed, the stiffness of the muscles will impede distribution. The proteins of the muscles are tightly bound together so that they are less reactive. Within 36–72 hours, rigor mortis passes naturally from an unembalmed body. This is called **secondary flaccidity**. In this phase, there will be a greater demand for preservative because muscle protein has been broken down to some extent. Rigor results from the body's inability to resynthesize ATP that causes the muscle proteins to lock together and form an insoluble protein. Rigor marks the end of muscle cell life and is generally observed in the average body 2–4 hours after death (**Fig. 5–8**). The minimum temperature at which rigor occurs is 32°F; the ideal temperature for occurrence is 98°F to 100°F. Rigor mortis is halted if the body temperature is elevated above 120°F and if the body is exposed to temperatures below 32°F (American Board of Funeral Service Education, 2016).

"Rigor, when it develops, involves all the muscles at the same time and at the same rate. However, it becomes most evident in the smaller muscles" (DiMaio and DiMaio, 2001, p. 27). Rigor is first demonstrated in the small muscles and moves gradually into the large muscle groups. Rigor appears to begin in the involuntary muscles of the eye, and then moves to the jaw

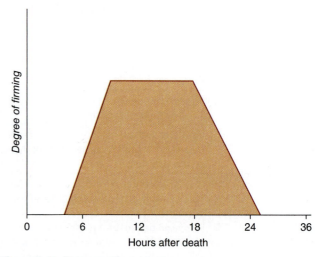

**Figure 5–8.** Rigor mortis.

and face, neck, upper extremities, trunk, and lower extremities. The directional occurrence of rigor mortis from the face to the feet is known as Nysten's law; named for French pediatrician, Pierre Nysten (1774–1817).

Rigor mortis can be relieved by flexing, bending, rotating, and massaging the affected joints and muscles. Once relieved, rigor does not return. Cold stiffening is a condition which may be mistaken for rigor and is caused by solidification of body fats and tissues during exposure to cold temperatures.

*Cadaveric spasm* is associated with rigor mortis. Cadaveric spasms are sudden involuntary movement or convulsion brought about by involuntary muscular contractions. When rigor mortis occurs irregularly in the different muscles, it can cause cadaveric spasms (*Stedman's Medical Dictionary*).

### Decomposition

Decomposition is the process by which dead organic substances are broken down into simpler substances. Decomposition of living organisms begins after death (**Fig. 5–9**). The three major biochemicals in the body are proteins, carbohydrates, and lipids. Of the three, proteins are most important from the standpoint of structure and function. Proteins are the primary component of connective tissue, tendons, cartilage, ligaments, skin, hair, and nails. They are responsible for body movements by the action of contractile proteins found in the muscles. Proteins play a number of other roles in body function and can be described as essential elements to the living body.

Proteins are also essential to embalming; successful embalming is achieved by establishing cross-linkages between proteins of the body and proteins of microorganisms. Proteins are large molecules that contain elements of carbon, hydrogen, oxygen, and nitrogen. The chemical bond that links two proteins together is called a **peptide bond** or **peptide linkage**. It is possible for many proteins to link together. During decomposition, the protein chains break down. If the breakdown is caused by catalytic enzymes, the enzymes are called **proteases**.

**Autolysis.** In human remains, the enzymes of decomposition have two different sources: **saprophytic bacteria** and **lysosomes**. Bacteria maintain the normal microflora of the human digestive tract. After death, they translocate and increase in number by using dead organic matter for their nutrition. Aerobic bacteria may also enter the body through the respiratory tract. They deplete the tissues of oxygen, producing chemical conditions favorable for anaerobic organisms, most of which originate in the intestinal tract.

In addition to bacterially caused decompositions, living cells have their own self-destructing mechanisms. During life, organelles called lysosomes contain the digestive enzymes of a cell. As the pH changes from alkaline to acidic, the membranes surrounding the lysosomes rupture. As the cells' own digestive enzymes are released, they digest the surrounding cellular material. This process is called **autolysis**, which means cellular self-decomposition. The products of autolysis are amino acids, sugars, fatty acids, and glycerol. These substances are sources of food and energy for microorganisms. Therefore, autolysis also favors microbial destructive action on human remains.

*Hydrolysis* has been called the single most important factor in the initiation of decomposition. It is a chemical reaction in which the chemical bonds of a substance are split by the addition, or taking up of water (*Taber's Cyclopedic Medical Dictionary*). The result of this reaction is the formation of simpler compounds which have water's hydrogen ion (H1) and hydroxyl ion (2OH) on either side of the chemical bond (*Stedman's Medical Dictionary*). When hydrolysis occurs, water is broken apart, another compound is broken apart, and new products are formed. The process requires (1) water, (2) catalysts, and (3) compounds with which to react. Hydrolysis is the first chemical reaction in the putrefactive process. During hydrolysis large protein molecules are broken down into smaller fragments called **proteoses**, **peptones**, and **polypeptides**. These intermediates are a good food source for bacteria, which increase dramatically during putrefaction. As degradation continues, the final products are amino acids.

These amino acids undergo further chemical changes. Amines, carbon dioxide, and water are some of the products. **Amines** are organic compounds that are considered to be derivatives of ammonia. **Ptomaines,** or foul amines are a group of malodorous amine compounds formed by the action of putrefactive bacteria. Commonly called corpse odors, indole, skatole, cadaverine, and putrescine are examples of foul-smelling alkaline substances.

Decomposition of the tissues and organs within the body is called **putrefaction**. **Decay** is the decomposition through biological and chemical agents. Some authorities restrict the term putrefaction to the decomposition of proteins by **anaerobic bacteria** (can live without oxygen) and use the term **decay** for the decomposition of proteins by **aerobic bacteria** (require oxygen to live).

Water is abundant in the human body and is therefore present and available for hydrolysis during life and after death. Hydrolysis requires the presence of a **catalyst**, which is a substance that influences the rate of a chemical reaction, without itself becoming part of the products of the reaction. Enzymes found within cells act as catalysts. After death, tissues become slightly acidic. This shift in pH causes the lysosomes within the cells to rupture. Lysosomes are cell inclusions that contain digestive enzymes. In the presence of water, the released enzymes begin to digest the carbohydrates, fats, and proteins of the cell. The end products of the hydrolysis of the proteins are amino acids. As proteins hydrolyze, the resulting products make more and more sites available for union with the preservative. It can be stated then that hydrolytic processes greatly increase the preservative demand of the body tissues. The presence of amino

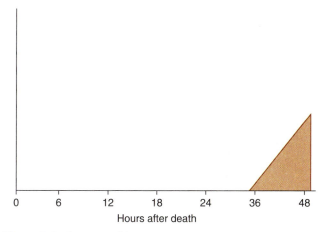

**Figure 5–9.** Decomposition.

acids increases formaldehyde demand because there are more sites available for a union with formaldehyde. Carbohydrates are reduced to monosaccharides (simple sugars), and fats are reduced to fatty acids and glycerine.

The rate at which hydrolysis occurs is speeded by heat and slowed by a cold environment. A mild acid pH can also stimulate hydrolysis. As the process continues, more and more nitrogen end products are produced. This causes the pH to shift to an alkaline condition. The alkaline (or basic) condition now provides an excellent medium for bacterial growth. With this growth of bacteria, the process of putrefaction greatly increases.

**Catalysts.** In the previous discussion of the types of decomposition reactions, it was shown that catalysts were needed for chemical reactions to take place. A **catalyst** is a substance that speeds up the rate of a chemical reaction without itself being permanently altered in the reaction. Inasmuch as decomposition is a chemical change, the presence of catalysts is needed in addition to the reactants. In every chemical reaction there is a **transition state,** where chemical bonds of reactants are broken and new chemical bonds are formed. At this point in a reaction, there is a higher level of energy needed. That boost of energy is provided by the catalyst. Enzymes serve as catalysts. Enzymes are also proteins and are therefore influenced by temperature and pH.

It is known that there are temperature fluctuations related to the agonal period and to the period between cellular death and embalming. It is also known that after death, the pH of the body changes from its normal 7.4 to a more acidic pH. As the body becomes somewhat acidic, it also becomes a favorable environment for microorganisms to multiply and contribute to decomposition. As the process continues, the pH of the body shifts back to alkaline, which is an excellent environment for enzymes to accelerate decomposition.

**Decomposition of Carbohydrates.** The breakdown of carbohydrates does not have any significant effect on embalming. Carbohydrates are stored in the body as glycogen (a polymer of glucose). The process by which glucose breaks down is called **fermentation.** We say, therefore, that fermentation is the bacterial decomposition of carbohydrates under aerobic conditions. The products of this breakdown of carbohydrates are organic acids, but they are not produced in sufficient quantity or strength to alter the overall alkaline environment that exists in a decomposing body and do not produce any foul odors. The final products of the breakdown are carbon dioxide and water.

**Decomposition of Lipids.** Body fats are broken down by hydrolysis that occurs in the presence of enzymes called *lipase*. The products of this breakdown are glycerol and fatty acids. These by-products do not significantly affect embalming because they do not change the alkaline environment, nor do they give off any foul odors. The final product of fat decomposition is **adipocere,** commonly known as "grave wax." Adipocere is a grayish-white waxy substance caused during hydrolysis and hydrogenation of lipids (fatty cells). Adipocere formation favors warm, moist environments with anaerobic conditions. The presence of adipocere has been noted after disinterment and disentombment of bodies interred or entombed for extended periods of time. Adipocere is resistant to bacterial action and remains stable for long periods. Forensic exhumation studies illustrate the ability of adipocere to slow decomposition, even after a century.

**Decomposition Order.** Decomposition proceeds at different rates in various body areas. Cells, tissues, and organs that contain high levels of moisture and autolytic and bacterial enzymes break down before similar structures that contain less water and autolytic and bacterial enzymes. The optimum temperature for decomposition is 98°F. The process is greatly slowed or stopped at temperatures below 32°F or above 120°F (American Board of Funeral Service Education, 2016).

Order of decomposition of the body compounds:
1. Carbohydrates
2. Soft proteins
3. Fats
4. Hard proteins
5. Bones

The vascular system is one of the last organ systems to decompose. Even in advanced decomposition it would be possible to inject some preservative chemicals in an attempt to slow decomposition and control odor. However, blood coagulation and sludge may make drainage difficult to establish.

**Signs of Decomposition.** There are five classic signs of decomposition: *color, odor, skin slip, gases,* and *purge* (**Fig. 5–10**). Decomposition in the dead human body is not a uniform process. It may be present in one location and absent in another. Decomposition can also be present without all five "signs" being present at the same time. For example, a body may evidence decomposition by skin slip and color changes but exhibit no abdominal gases or purge.

**Color Change.** The first external color change that occurs in the unembalmed body is a greenish discoloration over the right lower quadrant of the abdomen. This discoloration is caused by the combination of hydrogen sulfide (a product of putrefaction) with hemoglobin from the blood. In many bodies this discoloration follows the surface outline of the large intestine, which is located just beneath the abdominal wall. The abdomen as a whole gradually discolors and the chest, neck, and upper thighs are affected in time.

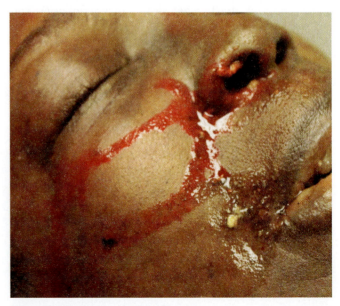

**Figure 5–10.** Lung and stomach purge.

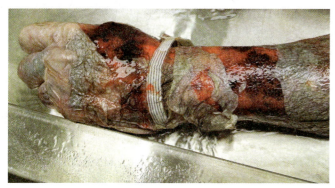

**Figure 5–11.** Desquamation or "skin slip" evident in advanced stage of decomposition.

The blood trapped in the superficial vessels gradually breaks down, staining the surrounding tissues. The outline of the veins on the surface of the skin is easily detected. This purplish brown discoloration of the superficial veins is most pronounced in the veins of the shoulder, upper chest, lower abdomen, and groin. Sometimes this type of discoloration is referred to as **marbling**. An early discoloration that occurs as a result of the hemolysis or breakdown of red blood cells is postmortem stain.

**Odor.** As the proteins of the body decompose, putrefactive odors become apparent. This odor is caused by foul-smelling amines, mercaptans, and hydrogen sulfide.

**Desquamation (Skin Slip).** The superficial skin layer weakens as deeper layers undergo autolysis. Hydrolysis of collagen and elastin causes the superficial skin to slough or "slip" (**Fig. 5–11**). As decomposition progresses, accumulations of gases and liquids form blisters between the layers of skin. When a blister is ruptured, the skin will easily slough. As the superficial skin desquamates, the exposed surface is moist and appears shiny. Exposed tissue rapidly dehydrates, firms, and darkens.

**Gases.** As decomposition progresses, gases begin to form in the viscera. This formation of gas generally starts in the stomach and intestines. Later, gases form in the body tissues. Gas accumulation causes the abdominal cavity to swell, and later the body tissues become distended. Gases in the tissues can actually be moved by the application of pressure. As the gas moves through the tissues, it can be palpated as a crackling sensation. This movement is called **crepitation**. Weakened areas, such as the eyelids, scrotum, and breasts easily distend with gases. In time, eyelids, cheeks, and lips distend and the tongue protrudes.

**Purge.** Purge is defined as the evacuation of gases, liquids, and semisolids from a natural body orifice. In decomposition, purge is generally caused by the buildup of gas pressure in the abdomen. The pressure forces gases, liquids, and semisolids along the path of least resistance, usually a body orifice. Purge originating from the stomach is generally acidic and can be foul-smelling. Stomach purge resembles undigested food material, sometimes similar to coffee grounds. Purge originating in the lungs is frothy in appearance due to the presence of air bubbles. If blood is also present in the lungs, the purge is a frothy-red color. Stomach and lung purge usually exit from the oral and nasal orifices. Anal purge consists of fecal material and exits the anal orifice.

**Taphonomy.** Taphonomy is the scientific study of decomposition; the study of processes (such as burial, decay, and

| Category Title and Time | Stage | Changes |
|---|---|---|
| Category 1. Fresh: 1–6 days | 1 | putrid odor, lividity, rigor mild |
|  | 2 | abdominal green, hemolysis, intense rigor → rigor passed, desquamation, dehydration of features and fingers |
|  | 3 | hemolysis, tissues soften, desquamation |
| Category 2. Bloat: 7–23 days | 4 | body swelling begins, head and face discolored, marbling of superficial veins, bullae or blebbing on the skin surface |
|  | 5 | moderate swelling, head and trunk discolored |
|  | 6 | maximum body swelling |
| Category 3. Destruction/Active Decay 24–50 | 7 | gases released, soft tissues putrefied, total breakdown of the blood |
|  | 8 | partially skeletonized, adipocere, mummification |
| Category 4. Dry/Skeleton 51–64 | 9 | skeleton with ligaments |
|  | 10 | skeleton with no soft tissues |

**Figure 5–12.** Categories of decomposition.

preservation) that affect remains. In 1981, Dr. William Bass established the first Forensic Anthropology Center at the University of Tennessee, Knoxville. Also known as the "body farm," a purpose of the facility is to study decomposition rates of human remains for crime scene investigation. Environmental factors play a major role in influencing the rate of decomposition. For example, bodies that receive full exposure to sunlight decompose faster than bodies submerged in cool water, or buried beneath the soil. Scientists established categories to describe rates of decomposition based upon time intervals (**Fig. 5–12**).

## TESTS OF DEATH

### Expert Tests

The legal pronouncement of death is a medical function. Expert tests of death are performed by trained and legally certified medical personnel.

- **Stethoscope**—an instrument used to mediate sounds produced in the body. This instrument would be used to listen for sounds of respiration or cardiac activity (*Taber's Cyclopedic Medical Dictionary*, 2001, p. 2055).
- **Ophthalmoscope**—an instrument used to examine the interior of the eye, especially the retina. This instrument would be used to examine the blood vessels in the retina for signs of circulating blood. Because it is a light source, it could also be used to detect responses in the pupils of the eyes (*Taber's Cyclopedic Medical Dictionary*, 2001, p. 1510).
- **Electroencephalogram (EEG)**—a record of the electrical activity of the brain (*Taber's Cyclopedic Medical Dictionary*, 2001, p. 675).

- **Electrocardiogram (ECG, EKG)**—a record of the electrical activity of the heart (*Taber's Cyclopedic Medical Dictionary*, 2001, pp. 672, 748).
- **Evoked response**—method of testing the function of certain sense organs, even if the subject is unconscious or uncooperative. For example, in a living patient, an **auditory evoked response** will appear on an electroencephalograph if sound reaches the brain. If there is no evoked response, the technician may conclude that sound did not reach the brain (*The Merck Manual of Diagnosis and Therapy*, 1982). Brain death would be one reason for the absence of an evoked response.

### Inexpert Tests

An **inexpert test** of death does not legally confirm a death. Inexpert tests are carried out when the equipment and expertise required to perform an expert test is unavailable.

- **Fogging a mirror**—a mirror is placed beneath the nose. Fogging of the mirror can indicate breathing and presence of life.
- **Ligature test**—a finger is ligated with string or a rubber band. Blood circulation can be indicated when the ligation causes swelling or discoloration in the finger.
- **Ammonia injection test**—a small amount of ammonia is injected subcutaneously. A localized, reddish skin reaction can indicate presence of life.
- **Pulse**—digital pressure is applied to a pulse point. A beating pulse can indicate heartbeat.
- **Listening for respiration or heart beat**—place an ear over the chest of the individual. The sound of breathing or heartbeat can indicate presence of life.

## CONCEPTS FOR STUDY

Define the following terminology:

- Adipocere
- Agonal algor
- Agonal capillary expansion
- Agonal dehydration
- Agonal edema
- Agonal fever
- Agonal hypostasis
- Agonal period
- Anabolism
- Autolysis
- Biological death
- Brain death
- Cadaveric spasm
- Catabolism
- Clinical death
- Contact pallor
- Death rattle
- Death struggle
- Decay
- Desquamation
- Extrinsic factors
- Fermentation
- Hemolysis
- Imbibition
- Intrinsic factors
- Moribund
- Postmortem cellular death
- Postmortem chemical changes: Rigor mortis, Postmortem stain, Postmortem caloricity, Shifts in pH, Decomposition
- Postmortem physical changes: Algor mortis, Hypostasis, Livor mortis, Dehydration, Increase in blood viscosity, Endogenous invasion of microorganisms
- Primary flaccidity
- Ptomaine
- Putrefaction
- Secondary flaccidity
- Sludge
- Somatic death
- Taphonomy
- Translocation

1. Recall environmental conditions that could speed the decomposition of a dead human body and those that could slow decomposition.
2. Discuss how agonal changes can affect the postmortem condition of the body.
3. State the order of decomposition of body compounds.
4. List the five classic signs of decomposition.
5. Discuss the process of hypostasis and explain how the progression of events leads to livor mortis and postmortem stain.
6. Discuss the pH changes that occur in the dead human body after death.
7. Evaluate inexpert tests of death and offer thoughts on why this might be beneficial for the embalmer to know.

## FIGURE CREDIT

Figures 5–3, 5–5 are used with permission of Sharon L. Gee-Mascarello.
Figures 5–10, 5–11 are used with permission of Kevin Drobish.

## BIBLIOGRAPHY

American Board of Funeral Service, *Course Content Syllabus,* 2016.
DiMaio DJ, DiMaio VJ. *Forensic Pathology,* 2nd ed. Boca Raton, FL: CRC Press, 2001.
*The Merck Manual of Diagnosis and Therapy.* Rahway, NJ: Merck, Sharp & Dohme, 1982:1941.
*Stedman's Medical Dictionary,* 26th ed. Baltimore: Williams & Wilkins, 1995.
*Taber's Cyclopedic Medical Dictionary,* 19th ed. Philadelphia: Davis, 2001.
Walter JB. *Pathology of Human Disease.* Philadelphia: Lea & Febiger, 1989:327.

CHAPTER 6

# Embalming Chemicals

## CHAPTER OVERVIEW
- Types of Embalming Chemicals
- Chemical Components of Embalming Fluids
- Preservative Action Upon Cellular Proteins
- Natural or "Green" Options

## PRECAUTIONS

Preservative and supplemental embalming chemicals are packaged in concentrated form and not diluted until time of use. Cavity fluids, accessory chemicals, bleaching agents, gels, powders, and solvents are used in concentrated form. Most chemicals are irritating to living tissue. Personal protective equipment (PPE) must be worn to prevent injury from direct skin contact with chemicals. Preparation room ventilation must create adequate air exchange to reduce exposure to chemical fumes.

Product containers should be tightly sealed and safely stored when not in use. Chemical spills must be addressed and exposure incidents immediately reported. Safety data sheets (SDSs) are available for all hazardous chemicals used during embalming. The SDS contains specific product information, including instructions for safe use, spill-handling procedures, and potential hazards associated with a particular material or product.

## BASIC COMPONENTS AND PURPOSES

Six general chemical groups provide the basic components of the various embalming formulations (**Fig. 6-1**):
1. Preservatives
2. Disinfectants (germicides)
3. Modifying agents
    a. Buffers
    b. Anticoagulants (water conditioning agents)
    c. Surfactants (wetting agents, surface tension reducers, penetrating agents, or surface-active agents)
    d. Humectants
4. Dyes (coloring agents)
    a. Cosmetic (active)
    b. Noncosmetic (inactive)
5. Vehicles
6. Perfuming agents

These chemicals are combined in various concentrations to produce vascular (preservative) embalming fluids, cavity fluids, supplemental embalming fluids, and some accessory chemicals used in the preparation of the dead human body. The listed groups of chemicals are added to the concentrated embalming fluid to control the adverse effects of the main preservative chemical (commonly formaldehyde), to maintain stability of the fluid, and to lengthen its shelf life. The functions of these various chemicals can be understood by looking at the following terms that are associated with embalming chemicals and fluids:

- **Arterial fluid (embalming, vascular, or preservative fluid)**—the concentrated, preservative embalming chemical.
- **Arterial solution (embalming solution, primary dilution)**—the in-use solution composed of the concentrated embalming fluid diluted with water and/or other additive (supplemental) chemicals for injection into the body.
- **Cavity fluid**—the concentrated chemicals injected into the body cavities following aspiration during cavity embalming. Cavity fluid can also be used for surface and hypodermic embalming treatments.
- **Supplemental fluid**—fluid injected for purposes other than preservation and disinfection. Supplemental fluids enhance the effectiveness of the preservative fluid. They may be injected prior to the main preservative solution, or mixed into the preservative solution (preinjection, coinjection, water conditioning fluids).
- **Accessory chemicals**—a group of chemicals used in addition to vascular and cavity embalming fluids; most are applied to the body surface (embalming gels and powders).
- **Special purpose fluids**—fluids designed for use with specific body conditions that require a high preservative (not limited to: burns, edema, decomposition, jaundice, and renal failure).

## HISTORICAL: ESTABLISHMENT OF MINIMUM STANDARDS

To understand the significance of the preservative chemical in an embalming fluid, it is helpful to review the historical establishment of minimum standards for disinfection of remains. After the turn of the twentieth century (about 1906), formaldehyde became a widely used component of embalming fluids. Various state health departments required that for embalmed

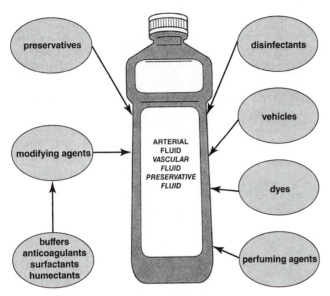

Figure 6–1. Components of arterial fluid.

bodies to be considered disinfected, a minimum amount of formaldehyde must be used. This established the standard amount of formaldehyde to be incorporated into all embalming formulations. At that time, the minimum amount was used without distinction, for both bodies dead from noninfectious diseases, and those dead from infectious and contagious diseases. The minimum standard established was not less than the following: 1 gallon of 14% of a 40% solution of formaldehyde (5.6%) for every 100 pounds of body weight for "normal" cases and 1 gallon of this same strength for every 75 pounds of body weight for infectious and contagious disease cases.

In these early years, the manufacturers of embalming fluid sold their product, prediluted with water. Embalming fluid was sold in half gallon glass bottles, ready for injection. Later, due to the high cost of bottling, packing, and shipping, much of the water was omitted, and the concentrated solutions were sold in smaller, pint bottles. To uphold state-required minimum standards, each pint bottle had to contain at least 8.96 oz of 40% formaldehyde and the same proportion of other added chemicals. These strong formaldehyde-based fluids acted harshly on body tissues, causing dehydration, darkening, and graying of body tissues. They also did not distribute or diffuse well. The use of strong embalming solutions (approximately 5.75%) was enforced in the years immediately following the influenza pandemic of 1918–1919 (H1N1 virus with genes of avian origin). To overcome the adverse effects of formaldehyde on the body, a variety of supplemental fluids, such as blood solvents (later known as preinjection solutions), were developed. Coinjection and jaundice fluids were developed for use as early as 1910. The development of penetrating agents and motorized injection in the mid-to-late 1930s, brought milder arterial solutions. The recommended use of the milder solutions continued until the early 1970s. One gallon of a 1–1.5% arterial solution injected for every 50 pounds of body weight was considered adequate. Further research demonstrated that a minimum 2% formaldehyde-based arterial solution was necessary to effectively disinfect body tissues. Today, general application of the "50-pound rule" may be inadequate. Analysis of the body conditions present, the length of time between death and final disposition, and numerous other factors determine the proper selection of arterial fluids, solution strengths, and volume necessary to produce optimal results.

## FORMALDEHYDE-FREE ALTERNATIVES

The assurance of safe work environments, coupled with concern for our natural environment drives manufacturers of embalming chemicals to seek alternatives to harmful chemicals. Some are revisiting ingredients used in formulations for preservation prior to the discovery of formaldehyde. Less toxic formulations may reduce adverse impact to air, soil, and water quality. Formaldehyde-free embalming and cavity fluids are available. These products offer effective sanitation for short-term, temporary preservation.

Natural products are antiseptic in nature and can precipitate and coagulate proteins. Most do not produce tissue firmness. Composition includes oil ingredients derived from gums and resins of plants, including a variety of spices. Certain alcohols, capable of adding and retaining moisture serve as vehicles for temporary preservatives.

Since the period of the Egyptians, and throughout embalming history, various ingredients have been used to preserve the dead human body. In the eighteenth and nineteenth century, redistilled wine or brandy was a popular preservative, better known as "rectified spirits." Reference for their use is found in the Bible.

## "GREEN" OR NATURAL BURIAL

Eco-friendly death care, also referred to as "green" or natural burial provides the simplest preparation of the human body followed by interment in a largely untouched landscape (**Fig. 6–2**). Traditional embalming and grave liners are not permitted. Green burial requires the use of nontoxic products that do not generate a SDS. The Green Burial Council was founded in 2005 to establish standards for green burial and to certify green burial sites. In North America, 200 green burial sites and eight conservation burial sites have been certified. Funeral homes offering green burial options that meet the Council's standards also receive this certification.

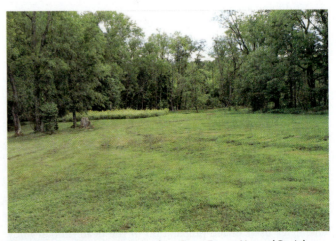

Figure 6–2. Green burial meadow, Penn Forest Natural Burial Park. *(With permission of Kevin Drobish.)*

## NATURAL ORGANIC REDUCTION OR HUMAN COMPOSTING

Natural organic reduction (NOR), or human composting, is an alternative method of final disposition. NOR is defined as the contained, accelerated conversion of human remains to soil. In 2019, Washington-based Recompose led the efforts to legalize the NOR process, which can be performed in Washington state as of May 2020. Recompose opened its first facility in December 2020. In 2021, Colorado and Oregon became the second and third states to legalize human composting.

The "laying in" process at Recompose involves placing the unembalmed decedent into a cradle and surrounding them with plant materials (**Fig. 6–3**). The cradle is placed into a vessel where microbes break everything down on the molecular level, resulting in the formation of nutrient-dense soil. Following a two-month process, the soil created can be used to enrich conservation land, forests, or gardens.

## ALKALINE HYDROLYSIS OR WATER CREMATION

Alkaline hydrolysis is a method of final disposition that uses one-quarter the energy of flame-based cremation. Since the mid-1990s, alkaline hydrolysis has been used in the disposal of cadavers donated for research. The process involves the use of lye (potassium hydroxide) and heat to reduce the body to soft, porous bone and residual liquid. Further reduction of the remaining bones produces cremated remains. Alkaline hydrolysis is legal in 18 states. Hawaii lawmakers are considering two bills that would allow the process. According to traditional Hawaiian burial practices, bones are preserved and protected in the belief that they carry a person's spiritual essence. Alkaline hydrolysis is also practiced in parts of Australia, Canada, and Mexico (Baja California). *Also called: aquamation, biocremation, resomation, flameless cremation, or water cremation.*

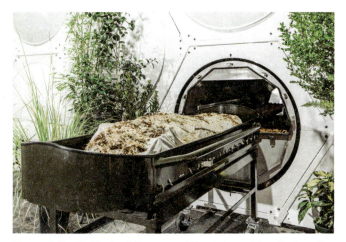

**Figure 6–3.** The "laying in" process at Recompose. Decedent-replica in cradle, covered with plant materials. *(Photo taken by Sabel Roizen. Used with permission of Recompose.)*

## GENERAL CHEMICAL PRINCIPLES OF EMBALMING FLUIDS

Formaldehyde and methyl alcohol are the main chemicals common to almost all embalming preservative solutions. The remaining ingredients used to produce embalming fluids vary immensely. There is no general agreement on what constitutes a "standard" embalming fluid. Embalmers have varying preferences for the results they desire. Some prefer strong, fast-acting fluids that produce a high degree of firmness; others prefer milder, slower-acting fluids that leave tissues flexible. The "20-index" embalming fluid made by one company can produce different results than a fluid from another company. Fluids may differ by grade of formalin; types of alcohol; surfactants (anionic, nonionic, or cationic); anticoagulants; modifiers; pH of the solution; buffers used to maintain pH; and physical features, such as specific gravity and surface tension.

## CHEMICAL COMPONENTS OF EMBALMING FLUIDS

### Preservatives

Chemical compounds classified under "preservative or fixative chemicals" are the agents in the chemical preservative solution which react with proteins. Such compounds change a protein from a state in which it is easily decomposed to a state in which it will endure and not undergo putrefaction, for a temporary period of time. Reaction of a preservative and a protein changes the nature of the protein molecule. Aldehydes, for example, react with various forms of nitrogen found in proteins. Such reactions produce an altered protein structure and water.

Formalin (37% formaldehyde by mass, 40% by volume), as the commercial source of formaldehyde, is still the most commonly used chemical for this purpose. Other examples of preservative and/or fixative chemicals are paraformaldehyde, formaldehyde polymerization products or formaldehyde "donors," light aldehydes, glyoxal, glutaraldehyde, phenol, phenolic derivatives, and some alcohols.

### Formaldehyde and Formaldehyde-Type Preservatives

#### Formaldehyde

Formaldehyde is a colorless gas at ambient temperature. It has a strong, irritating odor and is very soluble in water. The commercial source of formaldehyde is an aqueous solution of formaldehyde gas, called formalin.

Formaldehyde was discovered in 1859 by the Russian scientist Alexander Butlerov (1828–1886). Nine years later, German scientist Wilhelm Von Hofmann conclusively identified formaldehyde and found a reliable way to make it through the oxidation of menthol with air using a metal catalyst. This basic process is still used today in the manufacture of formaldehyde.

Formaldehyde is a naturally occurring substance; produced by every living organism and is essential to the functioning of the human body. Formaldehyde is produced in the atmosphere by lightning and is off-gassed when cooking certain vegetables, such as cabbage and Brussels sprouts. A study published in the May 2010 issue of The Director, a publication of the National Funeral Directors Association states that *formaldehyde is readily biodegradable and does not accumulate in the body or in the environment.*

Formaldehyde is readily used in industry to produce
- resins used to manufacture buttons, composite wood products (i.e., hardwood plywood, particleboard, and medium-density fiberboard), insulation;
- household products such as glues, permanent press fabrics, paints and coatings, lacquers and finishes, and paper products;
- decaffeinated coffee;
- preservatives used in some medicines, vaccine production, cosmetics, dishwashing liquids and fabric softeners; and
- fertilizers and pesticides.

Formaldehyde is also a by-product of
- emissions from unvented, fuel burning appliances, such as gas stoves and kerosene space heaters;
- cigarette smoke.

Formaldehyde is also a known toxin. Acute exposure can cause irritation of the eyes, nose, and throat. Skin irritation is common with direct contact. In 1987, the Formaldehyde Rule was established (OSHA 29CFR1910.1048). Since the 1980s, various organizations including the National Cancer Institute (NCI) have investigated the long-term exposure effects of formaldehyde upon workers in higher risk occupations: anatomists, pathologists, embalmers, and laboratory workers. NCI has suspected formaldehyde to be a causative agent of leukemia and to yield a definite increase in the risk of various types of cancers. In 1987, the Environmental Protection Agency (EPA) classified formaldehyde as a probable carcinogen. In 2004, the International Agency for Research on Cancer (IARC) classified formaldehyde as a known carcinogen.

A 2009 NCI study revealed, "the number of years of embalming practice and related formaldehyde exposures in the funeral industry associated with statistically significantly increased mortality from myeloid leukemia and associations with brain cancer, is unclear." The agency concluded that the biological mechanism of formaldehyde as a leukemogenic is lacking and that a considerable amount of missing data and further studies were warranted.

Occupational exposure to formaldehyde is influenced by a host of variable factors: ventilation system efficiency in preparation rooms, PPE choices, types and strengths of embalming chemicals selected, short- and long-term exposure times, and accuracy of reporting. Furthermore, embalming frequency is declining while direct cremation and other available final disposition options are increasing. Fewer embalming procedures lead to reduced formaldehyde exposure for embalmers.

**Formalin.** Formalin is an aqueous solution containing 37% formaldehyde gas by mass in water, or in water and methyl alcohol. The solution has a density slightly greater than water and corresponds to a solution that is 40% formaldehyde by volume. The National Formulary (NF) grade of formalin contains an average of 7% methyl alcohol, 37.0% minimum—37.3% maximum formaldehyde, and the remainder water. The alcohol present in the solution stabilizes formaldehyde so it will not precipitate.

The 37% by mass (40% by volume) solution is the regular product of commerce. There are also solutions available containing 40, 55, and even 70% by mass formaldehyde in alcohol. The higher concentrations are subject to precipitation. The precipitate is **paraformaldehyde**, a solid form of formaldehyde. The formaldehyde that drops out of solution to the bottom of the container is not available for chemical reaction. This results in a weaker concentration of formaldehyde in the top layers of the solution and a nonuniform overall concentration.

The definition of index: *an embalming fluid will be said to have formaldehyde index, N, when 100 mL of fluid, at normal room temperature, contain N grams of formaldehyde gas.* For example, a 20-index embalming fluid contains 20 grams of formaldehyde gas per 100 mL of concentrated fluid. Index identifies only the absolute formaldehyde gas present in any given product. Index is not a measure of the total aldehyde concentration present. Historically, index referred to the percentage strength of concentrated embalming fluid (the amount of absolute formaldehyde gas by volume, not to the amount of formalin).

The chemistry of formaldehyde is a highly specialized field of study. The disinfectant properties of formaldehyde, which depend on its concentration, have been extensively studied. Formaldehyde is classified as a high-level disinfectant (8% formaldehyde plus 70% alcohol) or an intermediate-to-high level disinfectant (4–8% formaldehyde in water). Formaldehyde exerts broad-spectrum action upon microorganisms. When carried by a vehicle that increases cellular diffusion, formaldehyde effectively destroys putrefactive organisms. Formaldehyde preserves tissues by forming new chemical compounds. The new compounds are stable and unfit as nutrition for the organisms that drive the cycle of decomposition.

Consider an example that illustrates the action of formaldehyde on albuminous materials; **albumin** is a simple form of protein that is soluble in water and coagulable by heat. New resins are formed that are neither formaldehyde nor albumin. These resins may be hard resins, soft resins, or semihard resins, depending on the control chemicals used in combination with the formaldehyde (modifying or plasticizing materials). Now consider the button on your clothing. The button is an example of a resin. Formaldehyde was used to manufacture that button. Injury would result from direct contact with formaldehyde. Yet the button, produced with formaldehyde could be placed in your mouth without harm. This is because the new compound (the button) differs from its original component (formaldehyde).

During embalming, formaldehyde acts quickly upon direct contact with tissues. The more formaldehyde that reaches a body area, the greater the action upon the tissues in that area. A greater amount of preservative is also absorbed by the tissues closest to the site of injection.

Compare the action of formaldehyde upon tissue with the action of a sponge placed into water. The sponge absorbs or *takes up* water. How much water it absorbs, depends upon how much water is available and how long the sponge remains in the water. If an embalming solution is hurried through the circulatory system as the result of high pressure and excessive drainage, remote tissue areas will receive little to no formaldehyde.

There are both advantages and disadvantages to the use of formaldehyde in embalming. The advantages, or effectiveness of formaldehyde outweighs its disadvantages.

### Formaldehyde Disadvantages
- Rapidly coagulates blood
- Constricts capillaries
- Fixes discolorations
- Converts tissues to a gray hue (when it mixes with residual blood)
- Dehydrates tissues
- Deteriorates with age
  - Oxidizes to formic acid
  - Decomposes to an alcohol and organic salt in a strongly alkaline pH
- Unpleasant odor
- Eye, nose, skin, and throat irritant

### Formaldehyde Advantages
- 100% organic (quickly broken down in the air by sunlight or by bacteria in soil or water)
- Inexpensive
- Bactericidal
- Inhibits yeast and mold growth
- Rapidly destroys autolytic enzymes
- Converts body proteins to insoluble resins
- Inhibits tissue decomposition
- Small percentage of formaldehyde needed to act upon a large amount of protein
- Produces rapid tissue fixation
- Deodorizes *ptomaines*, the foul amines formed during putrefaction
- Sublimates or undergoes sublimation when changing forms of matter, going directly from a solid to gas without becoming liquid first

**Paraformaldehyde.** Paraformaldehyde is a polymer of formaldehyde. It is a white, powdery solid containing from 85% to 99% formaldehyde. The NF grade of paraformaldehyde contains 95% formaldehyde. Paraformaldehyde is generally prepared from water solutions of formaldehyde by processes involving evaporation and distillation until concentration to a point at which solidification or precipitation takes place. Paraformaldehyde is used in powdered preparations, such as embalming and hardening compounds.

**Trioxane.** Another polymer of formaldehyde is trioxane (trioxymethylene), a colorless crystalline material with an odor resembling chloroform. This material is incorporated into formulations to act as an accessory preservative. Trioxane is costly in comparison to other forms of formaldehyde.

**Other Aldehydes.** Examples of lower or "light" aldehydes include acetaldehyde, propionaldehyde, and pyruvic aldehyde (methylglyoxal); higher aldehydes include furfural and benzaldehyde. The main requirement of an aldehyde is that it possesses denaturing and cross-linking properties that enable it to produce a firm tissue.

**Condensation Products (Formaldehyde "Donor" Compounds, Formaldehyde Reaction Products).** Aliphatic nitrohydroxy compounds are formed as the result of a condensation reaction between nitroparaffins (nitromethane, nitroethane, etc.) and certain aldehydes. Compounds of this type, in the presence of the proper catalyst, such as potassium carbonate, give off formaldehyde at a slow rate. When in solution, formaldehyde condensation products exhibit an acidic pH and need the alkaline catalyst to release the formaldehyde.

Other types of formaldehyde "donor" compounds are the methylol derivatives of hydantoin. These also liberate formaldehyde at a slow rate. Both types are used in low-odor or "fumeless" products. These complex organic substances make it possible to formulate fluids that do not produce irritating fumes. The formaldehyde is released after being distributed to all soft tissue areas where the usual preservative action is exerted. Disadvantages include slow reaction rate and high cost.

### Dialdehydes
Chemical compounds that contain two aldehyde functional groups in the same molecule are called *dialdehydes*. As far back as 1941, several firms in this industry investigated the possibility of using the then-known dialdehyde compounds available on a commercial scale. The principal dialdehyde and probably the only one available at that time in large commercial quantities and at an economical price, that made its use in embalming formulations feasible was glyoxal, the lowest member of the dialdehydes. On November 2, 1943, a patent (US Patent 2333182) was granted relating to the use of glyoxal in embalming fluid formulations.

**Glyoxal.** Glyoxal is available commercially as a 30% yellowish, aqueous solution containing small amounts of ethylene glycol, glycolic acid, formic acid, and formaldehyde. It is also available as a special 40% clear solution. Because it contains a chromophore group, glyoxal solution tends to stain tissue yellow. This feature limits the use of glyoxal mainly to cavity fluid formulations, especially because its optimal pH range of activity is about 9 to 10.

**Glutaraldehyde.** In the early 1950s, a method was developed that made it possible to manufacture the five-carbon, straight-chain dialdehyde glutaraldehyde in commercial quantities. Glutaraldehyde was first employed as an embalming and fixative agent in early 1955 and was subsequently patented for use in embalming preparations. When used for such purposes, it is commercially supplied as a stable 2.5% aqueous solution that has a mild odor and a light color. Glutaraldehyde reacts through cross-linking to insolubilize both protein and polyhydroxy compounds. The pH of the commercial solution is 3.0 to 4.0, and the specific gravity is 1.058 to 1.068. While still used in the United States, glutaraldehyde is not currently permitted for use in embalming formulations in Europe and Great Britain.

An interesting feature of glutaraldehyde is that, unlike other aldehydes, it is capable of reacting with protein structures over a wide pH range. This is an important advantage for an aldehyde in embalming, because after death, tissue pH varies in different parts of the body and as time elapses between death and embalming. In their pure forms both glyoxal and glutaraldehyde are liquids at ambient temperature, whereas formaldehyde is a gas.

In combining with proteins and tissue, glutaraldehyde changes the nature of the proteins, makes them unsuitable as food for bacteria, and makes them resistant to decomposition changes. At the same time, less moisture is removed from the tissues as the result of the chemical reaction between glutaraldehyde and proteins, compared with formaldehyde. In addition, glutaraldehyde used as a disinfecting agent is effective against most microorganisms, including viruses and spores making it many times more effective as a disinfectant than formaldehyde.

### Phenol

Phenol ($C_6H_5OH$), also known as *carbolic acid*, is classified as both preservative and germicide. Phenol is a coal-tar derivative that is a colorless crystalline solid. Upon exposure to strong light or metallic contamination, it darkens and assumes an amber or reddish-brown appearance in solution. The color change does not impact the potency of phenol to any great extent. Phenol readily penetrates the skin and is rapidly absorbed by protein structures. Phenol and phenolic derivatives assist formaldehyde in forming insoluble resins with albumins.

### Properties of Phenol

- Preservative
- Germicide
- Fungicide (mold inhibitor)
- Bleaching agent
- Cautery agent
- Reducing agent
- Drying agent

Historically, phenol was one of the most commonly found components of both arterial and cavity fluids. Phenol causes a "putty gray" discoloration of the tissues. For this reason, phenol is primarily used in cavity fluids; less commonly in arterial formulations. Phenol is a strong mold inhibitor (fungicide), making it an ideal ingredient in fluids used for the anatomical embalming of medical cadavers. Formulations containing phenol are often used as bleaching agents to lighten surface discolorations on the skin. Injected subcutaneously with a hypodermic syringe, phenol is an ideal drying and reducing agent. Applied as an external pack, phenol is a powerful cautery agent.

Phenol is a strong irritant to the living skin, eyes, and mucous membranes. PPE must be worn to protect the embalmer during use. Acute skin contact can produce second-degree burns (**Fig. 6–4A**). Due to the local anesthetizing properties of phenol, burns may be painless. Scarring is likely to remain after tissues have healed (**Fig. 6–4B**).

The most powerful germicides among the phenols are not water soluble. Halogenated phenols found in embalming formulations include **ortho**-phenylphenol, **para**-chloro-**meta**-cresol, dichloro-**ortho**-phenylphenol, tribromothymol, and sodium salts of these and other phenol-related chemicals. A fluid containing three main ingredients, such as phenol, methyl alcohol, and formaldehyde, is called a *triple-base fluid*. Double-base fluids contain two main ingredients such as formaldehyde and methyl alcohol, formaldehyde and phenol, or methyl alcohol and phenol.

### How Preservatives Work

Biochemistry is a complex subject and beyond the scope of this textbook. The intent of this section on preservation is to give a brief explanation of how the main types of chemicals used in embalming preserve tissue. The makeup of amino acids and proteins is briefly described in the following paragraph.

The embalming process is primarily focused on the proteins of the body. Disinfection and preservation are achieved through the cross-linking of proteins, both those of the body and those of microorganisms. An amino acid is an organic

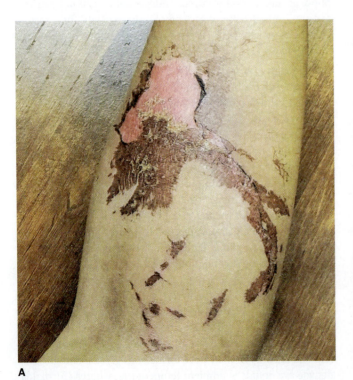

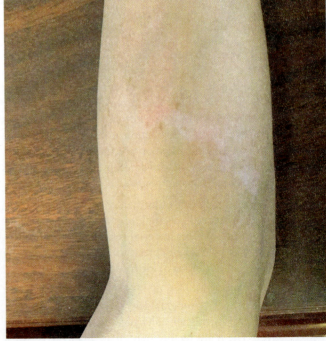

**Figure 6–4.** **A.** Phenol burn to living tissue. **B.** Evidence of scarring to healed tissue.

compound that contains both an amino ($NH_2$) group and a carboxyl (COOH) group. Twenty amino acids are necessary for the growth and metabolism of the human body. When two or more amino acids are joined together, a polypeptide is formed. These compounds are the building blocks of proteins. The site that joins the amine group of one peptide and the carboxylic acid of another peptide is called the *peptide bond*, or *peptide linkage*. The twenty different amino acids are linked in a specific sequence, in chains up to thousands of units, to form proteins. Since amino acids are the building blocks of proteins, they are also found as end products of protein breakdown (decomposition). The fact that amino acids contain $NH_2$ allows them to be preserved or cross-linked.

### Action of Preservative Compounds, or Mechanisms

Chemical mechanisms refer to the manner in which electrons and atoms transfer or move in chemical reactions. There are several compounds that affect preservation of proteins. These compounds or chemicals include **aldehydes, phenol** and its derivatives, **alcohols, acids,** and **salts**.

**Formaldehyde.** Also known as methanal, methyl aldehyde, methylene oxide, formic aldehyde, and oxymethylene. The line formula for formaldehyde is HCHO; the molecular formula is $CH_2O$; represented structurally as $H_2C=O$. Formaldehyde achieves preservation by cross-linking proteins at the peptide linkage. Other terms used for this action include fixating, denaturing, and coagulating protein. This concept is easily demonstrated by an example: the cooking of an egg. The albuminous portion of the egg (the egg white) is a clear fluid prior to cooking; the application of heat changes the egg white to a semisolid. The protein of the egg has been denatured, or coagulated, or fixated. The denaturing of protein happens during the embalming process by inserting a methylene bridge ($—CH_2—$) between the nitrogens in the amino groups of adjacent proteins. One of the properties of formaldehyde is that it combines with water to form methylene glycol, the source for the methylene bridge. The oxygen atom in formaldehyde links to a hydrogen atom from each of the two amino groups to form water. Proteins, by nature, attract and hold water molecules between the various amine, $RNH_2$, and carboxylic acid, COOH, groups found throughout their structure. Proteins in living tissue are coiled and folded in order to perform a specific function. Embalming denatures protein by causing these folds and coils to become undone, or cross-linked (**Fig. 6–5**). When the preservative reacts with the amine and acid portions of these folds, it releases the water molecules that were attracted by the partial polarity of the amino acids, hence the dehydrating effect of formaldehyde on tissue. In addition to the dehydration of tissue, the loss of water normally found in and around the proteins causes a gelling, or coagulation of the protein. This produces the firming effect upon embalmed tissue.

Disinfection and inactivation of proteolytic enzymes is achieved by the same mechanism, as most bacteria/enzymes have protein, or are protein in nature.

**Phenol.** Also known as carbolic acid or hydroxybenzene. The line formula is $C_6H_5OH$. Phenol is a crystalline solid at room temperature, very soluble in water, and is weakly acidic.

Phenol does not preserve by cross-linking the protein as formaldehyde does. It preserves by penetrating the phospholipid bilayer of the cell and dissociating in the cytoplasm of the cell. The dissociation of the acidic hydrogen causes the negative charge that is left on the benzene ring to become delocalized. In this delocalized form, phenol inhibits further decomposition of proteins and inactivates proteolytic enzymes as well as destroying bacteria.

**Alcohols.** One-carbon methyl alcohol or methanol, wood alcohol, two-carbon ethyl alcohol or ethanol, and three-carbon propyl alcohol or propanol and its isomer isopropyl alcohol preserve tissue and disinfect in a manner similar to phenol. However, the hydroxyl groups, OH, in these alcohols do not dissociate or produce an acidic hydrogen. The destruction of proteolytic enzymes and proteins is achieved by removing the water in the cell, which is necessary for normal metabolism to take place.

**Salts.** Various salts have been used in embalming products since the early days of embalming. Among the more commonly used compounds are potassium acetate, sodium nitrate, and some salts of aluminum. After 1906, many states prohibited the use of the salts of the heavy metals in embalming compositions. Salts preserve by desiccation. Salts pull the water from the cells, depriving them of the water needed for normal metabolism. This type of preservation does not produce the results desired for acceptable appearance. Egyptian mummification relied on salt (natron) for tissue desiccation.

One of the main forces that allow tissue to be preserved and bacteria to be disinfected, is the formation of water or removal of water, from the substance that is being preserved. The mechanisms affecting this change in the proteins differ. The end result is similar; the proteins are rendered unsuitable as food for bacteria and/or resistant to both putrefactive and saprophytic decomposition.

### Germicides

An important purpose of embalming is to sanitize the tissues of the body. Germicides are incorporated into arterial, cavity, and coinjection fluids, and surface disinfectants. The embalmer uses surface sanitizing agents when topically treating the

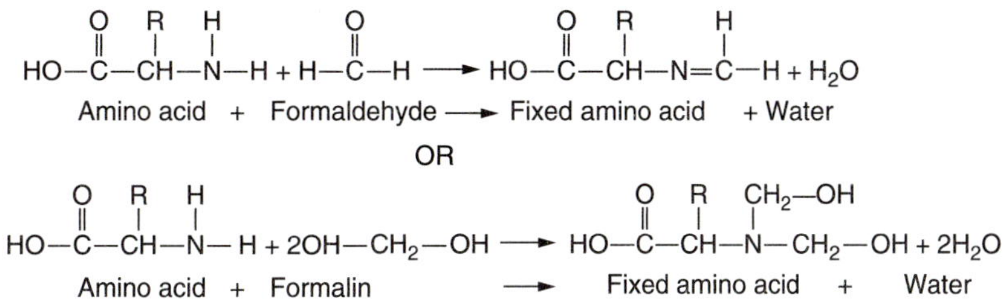

$$HO-\overset{\overset{O}{\|}}{C}-\overset{\overset{R}{|}}{CH}-\overset{\overset{H}{|}}{N}-H + H-\overset{\overset{O}{\|}}{C}-H \longrightarrow HO-\overset{\overset{O}{\|}}{C}-\overset{\overset{R}{|}}{CH}-\overset{\overset{H}{|}}{N}=\overset{}{C}-H + H_2O$$

Amino acid + Formaldehyde ⟶ Fixed amino acid + Water

OR

$$HO-\overset{\overset{O}{\|}}{C}-\overset{\overset{R}{|}}{CH}-\overset{\overset{H}{|}}{N}-H + 2OH-CH_2-OH \longrightarrow HO-\overset{\overset{O}{\|}}{C}-\overset{\overset{R}{|}}{CH}-\overset{\overset{CH_2-OH}{|}}{N}-CH_2-OH + 2H_2O$$

Amino acid + Formalin ⟶ Fixed amino acid + Water

**Figure 6–5.** Cross-linking of proteins by formaldehyde produces tissue firming.

surfaces of the body as well as the nasal and oral cavities. The autopsied cavities such as abdominal, thoracic, pelvic, and cranial are treated with sanitizing agents.

Germicides kill, or render disease-causing microorganisms incapable of reproduction. As microbes are made of proteins and the enzymes they make are also protein in nature, most of the preservative chemicals act as germicides. Formaldehyde, phenol, and phenolic derivatives are germicidal. Glutaraldehyde in an alkaline pH is particularly effective. Quaternary ammonium compounds such as Roccal and zephiran chloride are good examples of germicides incorporated into cavity fluids.

### Quaternary Ammonium Compounds

These materials are used chiefly for their germicidal and deodorizing qualities. They consist of mixtures of alkyl radicals from $C_8H_{17}$ to $C_{18}H_{37}$, that is, high–molecular-weight alkyl dimethyl benzyl ammonium chlorides. Aqueous solutions are usually neutral (pH 7). These compounds are compatible neither with the wetting agents used in arterial fluids, nor with many of the coloring materials incorporated into such fluids. Consequently, their use is restricted to cavity fluids and specialty formulations used for cold sterilization of instruments, linens, gowns, clothing, and other items; cleaning agents for mold proofing remains; and deodorant sprays.

## Modifying Agents

Modifying agents control the rate of action of the main preservative chemicals of embalming formulations. Many preservatives, when used alone, exert adverse effects that interfere with good embalming results. For example, when used alone, formaldehyde is so harsh and astringent that it sears the walls of the small capillaries and prevents diffusion of the preservation solution to remote soft tissue areas. It is necessary to control the rate of fixation so that the firming action is delayed long enough to permit thorough saturation of tissue cells. When the hardening effect of the aldehyde is delayed, the more uniform the distribution of the coloring or staining agent. Buffers, humectants, water conditioners, and inorganic salts control the rate of chemical action, modify the adverse color reaction produced by the preservative chemical in the tissues, and control capillary restriction or other undesirable results produced by the preservative materials.

1. **Buffers.** Agents that serve to control the acid–base balance of fluid and tissues.
2. **Humectants.** Agents that help to control tissue moisture balance.
3. **Anticoagulants (water conditioning agents).**
4. **Surfactants (wetting agents, surface tension reducers, penetrating agents, or surface- active agents).**

It should be pointed out that many chemicals in the preceding list serve similar functions. Many buffers can also act as water conditioners and anticoagulants. In addition, some of these chemicals are also inorganic salts and contribute to the osmotic qualities of the embalming solution. Even humectants can play a role in influencing osmotic quality. Because certain chemicals have multiple uses in embalming solutions, specific chemicals appear under different headings. For example, in a discussion of the anticoagulants, buffers are also reviewed.

### Buffers

Buffers stabilize the acid–base balance of the embalming fluid and assist in stabilizing the pH of the tissues where the embalming fluid reacts with the cellular proteins. The tissues of the body after death contain varying levels of acids or bases. Normal body pH is about 7.38 to 7.4 after death. During the rigor mortis cycle, the tissues have an acid pH resulting from carbohydrate breakdown. Postrigor, the tissues become basic as a result of protein breakdown. These reactions are not uniform throughout the body; tissues will vary in pH depending on rigor mortis and decomposition cycles. In addition, the cause of death can influence tissue pH. Buffers play a very important role in providing a good pH medium for the reaction of preservative with body proteins. Many of the compounds used as anticoagulants serve as buffer pairs. Examples are borates, carbonates, phosphates, and salts of ethylenediaminetetraacetic acid (EDTA).

**Borates.** In a report released by the Public Health Service in 1915, it was found that borax (sodium borate) was a good, efficient stabilizer of formalin, providing a desired degree of alkalinity that rendered formalin stable for long periods. It has been found to reduce the hardening and graying actions of formaldehyde. Depending on the specific type of formulation and other compounds present, in addition to borax, boric acid may also be added to certain embalming formulations. Formulations containing a well-balanced mixture of borates have been found to keep formaldehyde stable beyond 2 years. The loss in formaldehyde strength in such instances is insignificant.

**Carbonates.** Sodium carbonate is used alone or in combination with borates to modify the action of formaldehyde on tissue. Magnesium carbonate is also used sometimes and may be added to the formalin prior to combination with the other chemicals in a formulation. From all indications, it would appear that carbonates are not as efficient as borates in preventing the deterioration of formalin over long periods.

In a **Report and Review of Research in Embalming and Embalming Fluids** by the Minnesota State Department of Health, N.C. Pervier and F. Lloyd Hansen of the University of Minnesota studied the tissue reaction to injections of formaldehyde at various pH values. These investigators found that addition of a strong base, such as sodium hydroxide, improved tissue coloring; however, the high concentration of sodium hydroxide used caused deterioration of the preservative. When they injected formaldehyde solutions containing 1%, 2%, and 3% acid (HCl), the tissue tended to assume a putty-gray coloration. Since pH extremes are detrimental to formaldehyde, today, most arterial fluids are found to be slightly alkaline (with a pH of 7.2–7.4).

### Humectants

Humectants are described as having a coating action; they wrap the formaldehyde molecule and prevent formaldehyde from making direct contact with albuminous material until the tissues are thoroughly saturated and bathed with the preservative solution. The formaldehyde is "under shackles" for a time, and as it travels through the capillaries and to the tissue cells, it gradually sheds its shackles and, on release, acts on the albuminous material. Humectants bring about cellular hydration. The addition of humectant compounds to embalming fluids assists in making the tissue more flexible. In some instances, such materials are also called plasticizing agents because of their pliable effects. These compounds include glycerine, sorbitol, glycols, and other polyhydroxy alcohols. Cosmetic oils, lanolin, and its derivatives are also used for their emollient properties.

**Glycerine.** A by-product of the manufacture of soap, glycerine can be classified as an alcohol. It has also been produced synthetically from petroleum products. Although glycerine is not itself a germicide and has no preservative qualities, it does increase the germ-killing power of other chemicals, probably because it is an excellent solvent for disinfecting chemicals; its good solvent ability makes it an efficient carrier for the chemicals. Glycerine is also a good lubricator and is hygroscopic, which means it has affinity for moisture. If retained in the tissues, it helps to prevent dehydration.

**Sorbitol and the Glycols.** Sorbitol is probably used more extensively today in embalming fluids than is glycerine. Chemically, it has a straight chain of six carbon atoms and six hydroxyl groups, whereas glycerine has three carbon atoms and three hydroxyl groups in its structure. Commercially, sorbitol is generally available as a 70% aqueous solution. An important characteristic of sorbitol is that it loses water at a slower rate than glycerine, and consequently, for controlling the rate of moisture loss, it is more efficient than glycerine. One disadvantage of sorbitol solutions is that at very low temperatures, sorbitol precipitates from solution. Different types of glycols (mainly propylene, ethylene, and diethylene) are also found in embalming preparations. Sometimes, these materials are used alone with formaldehyde; in other instances, they may be incorporated into a formulation already containing either glycerine, sorbitol, or both.

Ethylene glycol is a colorless, syrupy liquid with very little odor. It is readily soluble in water. Because of its hygroscopic properties it is used as a moisture-retaining and softening material.

Propylene glycol is reported to be superior to glycerine as a general solvent and inhibitor of mold growth. Like ethylene glycol, it is colorless, odorless, and completely soluble in water.

**Emulsified Oils.** Materials such as lanolin and silicon are not in themselves water soluble, but certain fractions or derivatives are used that can easily be dispersed in aqueous solutions. It is the purpose of these materials in embalming fluid to mitigate the drying effect of the preservative agents. Highly penetrative oils of the oleate and palmitate types are also employed to help reduce the drying effect of aldehydes. Use of such materials requires an emulsion system that is able to maintain the formulation in a stable and uniform state over a long period.

**Gums—Vegetable and Synthetic.** The use of vegetable and synthetic gums is generally prompted by the need to restore moisture to tissue or to maintain the normal appearance of tissue when the subject is to be held for a period of time prior to burial. These materials, when added to water, swell and retain moisture as the gum molecule is distributed to the soft tissue areas. Because of their molecular size, the gums, on taking up moisture, are actually trapped in the capillary bed and aid both in restoring moisture to the area and in filling out the tissues to overcome the emaciated appearance.

As these materials are large molecular entities they are generally added to the arterial embalming solution after the initial injection has been made and all surface discolorations have been cleared. Use of such compounds prior to complete removal of blood from the tissues may interfere with proper distribution of the injected preservative solution. Examples of vegetable gums include **karaya** and **tragacanth.** The synthetic gums are generally formed from cellulose and have varying composition.

### Inorganic Salts
The inorganic salts used in embalming fluids serve a variety of functions. They can act as buffers, anticoagulants, preservatives, germicides, and water conditioners. Their use is quite simple in that they can be dissolved in the limited space of the 16-oz standard bottle of concentrated embalming fluid. By controlling the amount of inorganic salts used, the fluid remains balanced, as some of the salts do not "settle out" of the concentrated fluid. A role for salts in any solution is their ability to control the osmotic qualities. This is true in embalming fluid. Once the embalming solution reaches the capillary beds, it is very important that the solution be able to pass through the microscopic pores of the capillaries and enter the tissue spaces. Inorganic salts maintain an osmotic quality of the embalming solution that helps to draw fluid from the capillaries into the tissue spaces. Likewise, special fluids are used on bodies whose tissues are saturated with edema. Special-purpose fluids draw excess tissue moisture (edema) from the tissues and back into the capillaries, where it is removed as drainage. It is the osmotic qualities of special-purpose fluids that cause the dehydration (see Chapter 21).

### Anticoagulants (Water Conditioners or Softeners)
Anticoagulants are an important component of embalming fluids for numerous reasons:

First, to improve drainage by keeping blood in a liquid state and soften clotted material.

Second, to reduce water hardness. Calcium, magnesium, and iron found in hard water hinder preservative chemicals from penetrating soft tissues and achieving preservation.

Third, the dyes in the arterial fluid work best under slightly alkaline conditions. Arterial fluids cannot be compounded to remain alkaline over long periods of time. Aldehydes, especially formaldehyde, break down and lose strength under alkaline conditions. The alkaline condition is created at the time of use by the addition of water softeners. Dye intensity and uniformity is also enhanced by the addition of a water conditioner.

Fourth, formaldehyde also functions better as a fixative agent under slightly alkaline conditions. As previously mentioned, the alkaline solution is created at time of use to maintain effectiveness.

**Borates.** In addition to its function as a stabilizer of formaldehyde, sodium borate also serves to prevent or reduce coagulation. Sodium borate (borax, sodium tetraborate, or pyroborate) is a white crystalline powder that is readily soluble in a mixture of water and glycerine. Boric acid is a white powder that is often used in combination with borax.

**EDTA.** The sodium salts of EDTA are very effective sequestering or chelating agents, which means that they very readily combine with calcium ions to prevent blood coagulation and also to remove hardness chemicals from the water supply. Generally, these materials are not found in arterial fluids. These agents are alkaline and are not compatible with the other compounds in embalming fluids over a long shelf life. Such materials are used most advantageously as separate formulations; that is, in the form of supplemental or accessory chemicals that are added to the embalming solution at the time of use.

**Other Materials.** Among the other compounds often used as anticlotting materials are magnesium sulfate (Epsom salts), sodium chloride, sodium sulfate, and sodium phosphates. At one time or another, these compounds have been recommended for use in capillary wash solutions, and some are still used in arterial fluid formulations. This class of chemicals also contains some of the materials employed in buffer systems to maintain a constant pH in a fluid formulation. These are used in combination with those mentioned earlier.

### Surfactants (Wetting Agents)

Probably one of the greatest developments that has occurred in the chemistry and physics of embalming since the discovery of formaldehyde is the principle of removing body liquids by lowering their surface tension. It is necessary, before complete circulation may take place in the body, to remove the liquid that is held in the capillaries. Capillary attraction, or the force that attracts and holds liquid in the capillary tubes, is the result of surface tension. If the surface tension of the liquid in these tiny tubes is lowered, the liquid easily loosens and flows out.

Much has been said and written about the important role and use of surfactants (**surface-active agents, tension breakers, tension reducers**) in embalming formulations. Actually, there is no industry that has not investigated these compounds and found them adaptable for a variety of uses. The chemical structure of surfactants is rather complex: one part of the molecule has a strong attraction or affinity for water, whereas the other part of the molecule dislikes water. This latter part of the molecule has an affinity for nonaqueous liquids. Such a complicated molecular makeup functions to lower or reduce the surface tension of the solution to which the surfactant is added. In a water-and-oil mixture the surfactant destroys the surface tension of the components so that the oily mixture is more easily dispersible in water. Other materials are made "water soluble" in a similar manner.

It should also be remembered that each cell in the soft tissues of the body is surrounded by a film of body liquid mostly water in composition. For easy, rapid penetration of the cell, this surface film must be dispersed. Such chemical substances, then, are used in embalming fluids for three reasons.

First, by lowering the surface tension of the preservative solution (the embalming solution), surfactants aid or cause the embalming solution to flow more readily and rapidly through the capillaries. Second, **all** of the millions of tissue cells are literally bathed by the embalming solution and become thoroughly preserved. Naturally, the technique of injecting the solution and draining employed by the embalmer can assist or handicap the function of the surfactant. The process of moving the solution through the body being embalmed is a technique that should be planned and controlled by the embalmer to ensure that a sufficient amount of preservative chemicals is uniformly distributed throughout the body. It is also important that some of the normal moisture lost during embalming be replaced to safeguard against dehydration.

Second, by reducing the capillary attraction (which is a phenomenon of surface tension) of blood and body liquids, surfactants cause the almost immediate clearing of blood from the capillaries. Surface tension is reduced, and the liquid more readily moves and flows out of the capillary bed and through the venous drainage system. Since two things cannot occupy the same space at the same time, the capillaries must be emptied of blood before injected solution can flow through them to reach the tissues of the body. Only the solutions that pass by osmosis through the capillary walls into the intercellular spaces have any chance of being absorbed by the tissue cells. The embalmer must help the solution reach the tissues by employing the necessary physical manipulation such as massage and intermittent or restricted type of drainage.

Third, by increasing the ability of the solution to filter through the semipermeable capillary walls in a uniform manner, it is possible to incorporate coloring agents into the solution and obtain a normal appearance internally.

### Surface Tension and Embalming Solutions

Solids, liquids, and gases are all made up of molecules arranged in characteristic patterns depending on the material being studied. These molecules have an affinity or attraction for one another. Again, depending on the materials under study, this degree of molecular attraction differs. For example, the attractive force is greater between water molecules than it is between alcohol molecules. At 20°C, the surface tension of water is 72.75 dynes per centimeter, and for methyl alcohol it is 22.61 dynes per centimeter. (Note: a dyne is the force required to accelerate a 1gram mass 1 centimeter per second.) Water has a surface tension value more than three times that of methyl alcohol and penetrates much more slowly. In other words, the lower the surface tension value, the faster the rate of penetration by the liquid substance.

The surface tension of water is lowered by the addition of surfactants. Wetting or penetrating chemicals tend to destroy the bonds or attractive forces that normally exist between water molecules so that they seemingly break away from each other. The net effect of such physiochemical action is to cause liquids to diffuse and penetrate more readily through cellular tissue.

Surface tension is also defined as the contractive forces that cause liquids to assume the shape in which they have the least surface, that is, a sphere. Wetting agents reduce this contractive force.

In embalming solutions, the addition of surfactants in proper concentrations produces better penetration of the preservative chemicals in a more uniform manner. This enables the preservative solution to more readily displace the body fluids from all cellular tissue and replace them to achieve the embalming function. Also, coloring agents are uniformly distributed through the use of surfactants. The even diffusion of such agents throughout the soft tissues results in a more natural color and appearance.

Surface tension changes with the variations in temperature. As the temperature rises, the surface tension value of a solution decreases. In embalming, this means that if lukewarm water, also called *tepid water*, is used to prepare the solutions for injection, the resultant solution may be expected to penetrate more rapidly because of the lowered surface tension value. Also, keep in mind that the chemical reaction between preservative chemicals and the tissues will take place more rapidly as a result of using tepid water. The fixative or firming action will also occur faster than usual. Cool water is routinely used when mixing embalming solutions.

Surfactants also increase the germicidal activity of chemical solutions. It is believed that this is due to an increased speed of penetration into the bacterial cells as a result of the lowering the surface tension of the solution.

### Surfactants and Surface Tension

From the preceding discussion it might appear that the embalmer could easily make their embalming technique more efficient by simply adding an extra surfactant to the embalming solution. This is not true. Surfactants function best in very low concentrations and must be carefully selected by experienced chemists with respect to the other substances present in the formulation. It is necessary to determine compatibilities among all the components of an embalming fluid and the surfactant, and the amount of surfactant to use to produce a properly well-balanced chemical formulation. Addition of extra surfactant to an embalming solution may result in excessive drainage as well as oversaturation of tissue.

The following considerations, which must be thoroughly explored by the chemist in evaluating specific applications for any given surfactant, serve to illustrate the complex nature of such chemicals. The discussion is by no means complete.

Surface-active agents are generally classified into three groups: anionic, cationic, and nonionic. In brief, if the surfactant molecule tends to ionize, then it is either anionic or cationic. If it does not ionize in solution, it is nonionic.

Surfactants such as soap, alkyl sulfonates, alkyl aryl sulfonates, salts of thioalcohols, and oils are **anionic**. These compounds are compatible with other anionic and nonionic agents. They are not normally compatible with and are frequently precipitated from solutions by cationic materials and by certain inorganic cations such as aluminum, calcium, and magnesium.

An example of **cationic** surfactants is the quaternary ammonia compounds. The principal disadvantage of these compounds is that they are inactivated by anionic substances such as soap which is routinely applied to the external surface of the body.

**Nonionic** surfactants do not ionize in solution but owe their surface activity and water solubility or dispersibility to nonionized polar groups within the molecule, such as hydroxyl or ether linkages. Ethylene oxide condensation products with amides and fatty acids belong to this group (specific examples are the Atlas "Tweens" and "Spans").

In actual chemical formulating practice, the result to be achieved by the end product must be kept in mind in deciding the type of surfactant to employ. Most generally, a blend of such materials is incorporated into embalming fluids to achieve the results mentioned at the beginning of this discussion.

### Dyes (Coloring Agents)

Coloring agents added to embalming fluids to produce an internal cosmetic effect within the tissues of the decedent are called **active dyes** (**Fig. 6–6A**). Active dyes are available in a variety of shades to simulate natural tissue complexion. These dyes have high staining qualities. As they diffuse from the circulatory system, they impart color to the superficial tissues. **Inactive dyes** merely lend color to the fluid in the bottle (**Fig. 6–6B**).

Active dyes are usually a blend of dyes, mainly coal–tar derivatives. Red dyes of various shades and degrees of intensity are usually blended in an attempt to restore a natural color to the tissues. The coloring materials selected for use in any given embalming fluid formulation depend to a great extent on the pH of the solution. Examples include eosin, erythrosine, ponceau, fluorescein, amaranth, and carmine.

### Types of Coloring Agents

Coloring materials may be placed into two classes: natural and synthetic. **Natural coloring agents** are vegetable colors such as cudbear, carmine, and cochineal. **Cudbear** is a purplish red powder prepared from lichens by maceration in dilute ammonia and caustic soda and fermentation. **Carmine** is an aluminum and calcium salt of carminic acid. **Cochineal** is a red-coloring matter consisting of the dried bodies of the female insects of *Coccus cacti*. The coloring principle is carminic acid, $C_{22}H_{20}O_{13}$. This class of dyes is not generally incorporated into modern solutions.

**Synthetic coloring agents** are the coloring materials used in modern fluids and are mainly coal–tar derivatives. They are economical to use and are the most permanent if they are chemically compatible with the other substances in the fluid. Many different types and shades are available under rather confusing diversified commercial names and chemical nomenclature. For better solubility, most of the coal–tar dyes are supplied as sodium or potassium salts of the synthetic coloring matter. These materials then may be said to be dyes of alkali metal salts that have been reacted with coal–tar compounds. Several dyes are available.

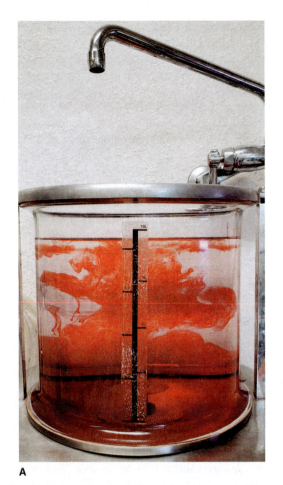 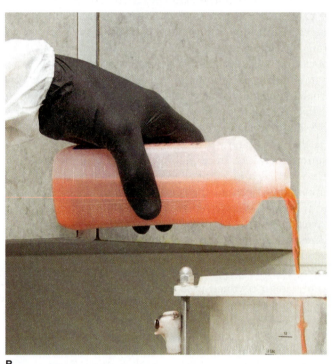

Figure 6–6. **A.** Active dyes impart color to the tissues. **B.** Inactive dyes lend color to the fluid in the bottle.

| | |
|---|---|
| • Eosin | Known as tetrabromofluorescein, $C_{20}H_8Br_4O_5$; red crystalline powder |
| • Erythrosine | Brown powder that forms cherry red solutions in water; known chemically as the sodium salt of iodeosin, $C_{20}H_6I_4Na_2O_5$, FD&C No.3 |
| • Ponceau | Dark red powder that is soluble in water and acid solutions; forms a cherry red solution and is a naphthol disulfonate compound |
| • Amaranth | Coal–tar azo dye, $C_{20}H_{11}N_2Na_3O_{10}S_3$, that forms a dark red-brown color in water but is only slightly soluble in alcohol. FD&C No. 2 |
| Other synthetic dyes include croceine scarlet, rhodamine, rose bengal, acid fuchsin, and toluidine red. | |

**Coloring Materials in Embalming Fluids.** Coloring materials belong to a group known as *biological stains*, as such materials are used in clinical laboratories to stain different types of tissue for study under the microscope. The coloring agents used in fluids must be stable in the presence of formaldehyde, must be water soluble, should impart a natural flesh color to the tissues, and should have high tinctorial or staining qualities so that small amounts can produce the desired color. This last requirement is important because arterial fluids are diluted before use.

The coal–tar dyes possess the requirements of a coloring agent for use in embalming fluids. Molecularly they are fine enough to diffuse evenly and uniformly through tissue cells. As soon as surfactants (wetting agents) began to be used in embalming solutions, it was found possible to add staining materials to the formulations because wetting agents diffused the dye very effectively. The specific material that is to be used in any given formulation must be carefully selected, as some dyes produce different coloring effects at different pH values and different extents of dilution.

Natural color materials such as the vegetable dyes are considered too unstable for use in embalming fluids. Some have good color-fast features but do not diffuse evenly because of their large molecular structures.

Newer environmentally friendly nontoxic formaldehyde-free embalming fluids contain such dyes as erythrosine (FD&C Red 3) because it is biodegradable. This type of dye is compatible with natural or "green burial."

### Perfuming Materials (Masking Agents, Re-odorants)

Reodorants or perfuming agents are selected not only for their power in covering harsh chemical odors but also for the pleasant odor they impart to the embalming solution. Perfuming agents do not eliminate odors from the body. By blending special synthetic essential oils with the harsh preservative chemicals in a formulation, the harshness or "raw" odor of the solution is reduced and replaced by a more pleasing scent.

Floral compounds such as wisteria, rose, and lilac types, along with nondescript essential oils and aromatic esters, are used quite extensively in embalming formulations because of their strong aroma. This property makes it possible to cover objectionable fumes during brief exposures. Such materials are made water soluble through the medium of nonionic surfactants.

If the formulation does not contain a high concentration of formaldehyde or other irritating chemicals, it is possible to use synthetic compounds that give off odors resembling spices (clove, cinnamon), fruit (strawberry, peach, etc.), mint (spearmint, peppermint, menthol), and many other aromas designed by the essential oil chemist. Sassafras, oil of wintergreen (methyl salicylate), and benzaldehyde have been among some of the more commonly used materials for this purpose.

Low odor products presented as "fumeless" or "odorless" are based on the use of "donor" compounds that release the aldehyde upon contact with the tissues. The embalmer notices only the perfuming agent.

The essential oils used in embalming fluids are selected on the basis of their stability in the presence of preservative chemicals and their ability to remain in solution when water is added. Some essential oils possess antiseptic properties.

### Vehicles (Diluents or Carriers)

The active preservatives and other compounds in the formulation must be dissolved in a common solvent. As water is an essential part of tissue, its use in embalming solutions facilitates the diffusion and penetration of the active preservative components of fluids. The vehicle or carrier must be a solvent or mixture of solvents that keeps the active substances in a stable and uniform state during transport through the circulatory system to all parts of the body.

To maintain the proper density and osmotic activity, or in other words the proper chemical and physical balance of the formulation, the vehicle or diluent may include glycerine, sorbitol, glycols, or alcohols in addition to water.

> **CONCEPTS FOR STUDY**
>
> Define the following terminology:
> - Active dyes
> - Anticoagulants
> - Buffers
> - Disinfectants
> - Formaldehyde
> - Formalin
> - Glutaraldehyde
> - Humectants
> - Inactive dyes
> - Modifying agents
> - Paraformaldehyde
> - Perfuming agents
> - Phenol
> - Preservatives
> - Surfactants
> - Vehicles (diluents)
>
> 1. List the advantages and disadvantages of formaldehyde and glutaraldehyde.
> 2. Recall the purpose of modifying agents.
> 3. Paraphrase the function of anticoagulants in dissolving blood clots.
> 4. Anticoagulants are sometimes referred to as water conditioners. How do they condition the water?
> 5. What is the role of surface tension in the embalming process?
> 6. Differentiate among cationic, anionic, and nonionic surfactants.
> 7. What is the difference between active and inactive dyes?
> 8. What is meant by a vehicle in embalming fluids and what is its purpose?

## FIGURE CREDIT

Figures 6–2, 6–6 are used with permission of Kevin Drobish.
Figures 6–4A,B, 6–6 are used with permission of Sharon L. Gee-Mascarello.

## BIBLIOGRAPHY

American Board of Funeral Service, *Course Content Syllabus*, 2016.

Block SM, ed. *Disinfection, Sterilization, and Preservation*, 5th ed. Philadelphia: Lippincott Williams & Williams, 2001.

Dorn JM, Hopkins BM. *Thanatochemistry: A Survey of General, Organic, and Biochemistry for Funeral Service Professionals*, 3rd ed. Upper Saddle River, NJ: Prentice Hall, 2010.

Eckles College of Mortuary Science, Inc. *Modern Mortuary Science*, 4th ed. Philadelphia: Westbrook, 1958:206.

*Encyclopedia of Industrial Chemical Analysis*, Vol. 12. *Embalming Chemicals*. New York, NY: Wiley, 1971.

Champion Co. Enigma: Champion's fourth generation chemostasis infusion chemicals: Embalming redefined for the 21st century. In: *Champion Expanding Encyclopedia of Mortuary Practices*, No. 657. Springfield, OH: Champion Co., 2009.

Formaldehyde Council Inc., www.formaldehyde.org. Champion Co. General chemical principles of embalming fluids. In *Expanding Encyclopedia of Mortuary Practice*, Nos. 365–371. Springfield, OH: Champion Co., 1966.

Dodge Co. Green embalming: A paradigm shift. In *Dodge Magazine*, Vol. 103, No. 1, Cambridge, MA: Dodge Co., Winter 2011.

Dodge Co. In Search of the Perfect Embalming Chemical. In *Dodge Magazine,* Vol. 102, No. 4, Cambridge, MA: Dodge Co., 2010.

New Jersey State Funeral Directors Assn. Putting Alternative Preservatives to the Test. In *The Forum*, Vol. 76, No. 3, Wall, NJ: New Jersey State Funeral Directors Assn., January 2010.

New Jersey State Funeral Directors Assn. The Future of Formaldehyde. In *The Forum*, Vol. 75, No. 3, Wall, NJ: New Jersey State Funeral Directors Assn., January 2009.

National Funeral Directors Association. *Memorial Business Journal*, Vol. 12, No. 9, March 4, 2021.

Penn Forest National Burial Park- general info from the web page.

Walker J. *Formaldehyde*, 3rd ed. ACS Monograph No. 159, New York, NY: Reinhold, 1964.

CHAPTER 7

# Use of Embalming Chemicals

**CHAPTER OVERVIEW**
- Work Practice Controls
- Arterial Preservative Fluids
- Supplemental Vascular Fluids
- Cavity Fluids
- Accessory Embalming Chemicals

## WORK PRACTICE CONTROLS IN THE USE OF CHEMICALS

During the course of embalming and decedent care, the embalmer handles a variety of chemicals. Safe work practices are created and adopted to reduce exposure to all chemicals classified as hazardous. Hazardous chemicals require a safety data sheet (SDS). The SDS is instrumental in identifying chemical classifications. Personal protective equipment (PPE) is selected according to the nature and scope of the exposure to hazardous chemicals (**Fig. 7-1**). Use of PPE is the best practice during all facets of decedent care. The following work practice controls serve as a guide for safe handling and use of embalming chemicals.

1. *Wear eye protection.* Face shields, safety glasses, and other types of eyewear protect from chemical splashes.
2. *Wear protective and/or impervious garments.* Aprons, lab coats, and other coverings serve as a barrier to prevent skin contact with chemicals. Protective garments also prevent soiling of the embalmer's clothing. Surgical scrubs are recommended as best practice.
3. *Wear gloves.* Surgical gloves are produced from different types of material. Nitrile has a high chemical resistance to formaldehyde. Tests that measure *breakthrough duration* indicate higher longevity before glove failure in nitrile compared to latex. Latex allergies are also a consideration.
4. *Activate room ventilation systems* (**Fig. 7-2**). Adequate room air exchanges provide fresh air and reduce airborne populations.
5. *Keep a binder of chemical SDSs.* SDSs for all in-stock chemicals are required. Maintain an updated collection in a location immediately accessible to the preparation room. A second binder is kept in a general work area. SDSs are also available online.
6. *Pour embalming fluid into the embalming machine after it is filled* (**Fig. 7-3**). Adding the chemical first, followed by water or another diluent, creates excess fuming.
7. *Rinse chemical bottles after use.* Use water to flush remaining chemicals from bottles prior to disposal.
8. *Replace the cap or lid on bottles and containers after use.*
9. *Keep the lid on the embalming machine.*
10. *Flush formaldehyde from work surfaces regularly.* Disinfectants containing strong oxidizers, like household bleach (sodium hypochlorite), can react negatively with formaldehyde.

Never use embalming chemicals as an antiseptic for first aid. Embalming chemicals are not for use on living tissue and may cause injury. If chemical splashes occur, flush the area immediately with cold running water. Use the emergency drench shower or eyewash station. Report all exposure incidents and seek medical attention as needed. Dilute chemical spillage immediately before cleaning the area. Irrigate the spill with running water; neutralize the spill with household ammonia. Evacuate the room after large spills until fumes subside.

## FORMALDEHYDE BEST MANAGEMENT PRACTICES

The following recommendations from the National Funeral Directors Association suggest practices for handling formaldehyde-based products. The same practices can be applied to all hazardous chemicals used in the preparation room.

**1.0 Ensure adequate and effective ventilation in the preparation room.**

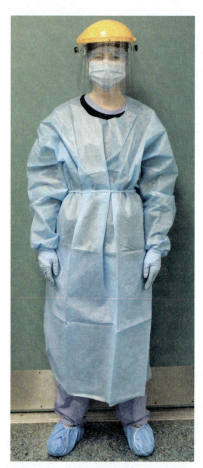

**Figure 7-1.** Embalmer in personal protective equipment (PPE).

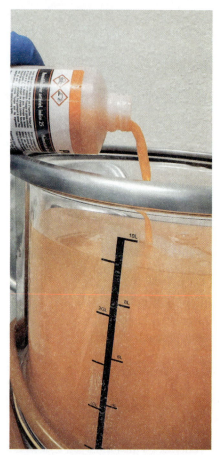

**Figure 7-3.** Pouring fluid into an already filled tank to reduce fumes.

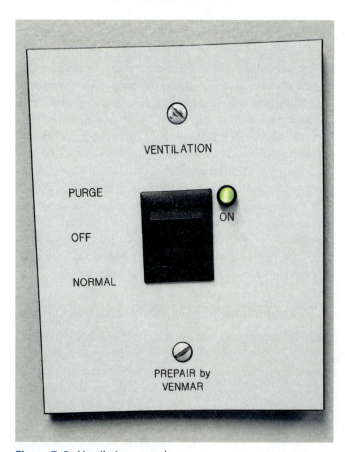

**Figure 7-2.** Ventilation controls.

1.1 Have no fewer than 15 air changes per hour in the preparation room.

1.2 Employ a local exhaust ventilation (LEV) system for added capture of formaldehyde emissions.

1.3 Provide a source of fresh, clean air that prevents excessive negative pressure and improves quality in the preparation room.

1.4 Establish a standard operating procedure (SOP) for ventilation system activation whenever an individual is in the preparation room.

1.5 Vent waste air from the preparation room HVAC system to the outdoors.

1.6 Monitor the effectiveness of the preparation room HVAC system no less than annually.

1.7 Do not use ozone generators.

2.0 Select and use the proper embalming product in considering the environmental, health, and safety characteristics of the product and the condition of the remains.

2.1 Make a practice of using the least concentrated solution and reserving the most highly concentrated solution for the most difficult cases.

2.2 Substitute environmentally friendly products for traditional embalming products.

2.3 When mixing embalming solutions, always add arterial fluids to water.

3.0 Take precautions in the preparation room to limit formaldehyde exposure and emissions during routine embalming.

3.1 Institute work practices to avoid formaldehyde spills, and if spills occur, clean spills of formaldehyde immediately.

3.2 Always keep the lid on the embalming machine.

3.3 If embalming wastewater is discharged into a sink, always use a sink cover to limit splashing and exposure.

3.4 Use all appropriate personal protective equipment to avoid skin and eye contact with formaldehyde-containing products (and any chemical products of any type).

3.5 Limit exposure to formaldehyde and bloodborne pathogens through the use of a drain tube.

3.6 Follow the funeral home's written 30-day cleaning, decontamination, and inspection schedule to ensure proper functioning of eyewash stations and emergency showers.

4.0 Observe special precautions to limit formaldehyde exposure and emissions when embalming organ procurement cases and autopsied remains, as such embalming may increase the embalmer's formaldehyde exposure risk.

4.1 Employees may elect to use a properly fitted respirator, even when measured exposure limits do not exceed OSHA standards.

4.2 Carefully monitor and restrict the use, to the greatest extent possible, of the most highly concentrated formaldehyde products, such as osmotic gels, hardening compounds, and disinfecting sprays.

5.0 Be familiar with and follow all federal, state and local environmental, OSHA, and health requirements that apply when embalming is performed.

## ARTERIAL FLUIDS

An **arterial fluid** (embalming, vascular, or preservative fluid) is the concentrated embalming fluid that contains the following types of chemicals—preservatives, germicides, vehicles, dyes, perfuming, and modifying agents. This concentrated **arterial fluid** is added to water to form the **arterial solution** called the **primary dilution**.

## ARTERIAL SOLUTION STRENGTH

Solution strengths using formaldehyde-based arterial fluids are as follows:
- **Mild** solution strength: 1.0–1.99%
- **Moderate** solution strength: 2.0–3.99%
- **Strong** solution strength: 4.0% and above

A **pre-injection fluid** is a **supplemental fluid** that is injected **before** the injection of the preservative arterial solution. Its purpose is to expand the vascular system, promote drainage, and prepare the tissues for reception of the preservative arterial solution. A **co-injection fluid** is a **supplemental fluid** that is mixed and injected along with the arterial solution. The co-injection fluid is designed to enhance the distribution and effectiveness of the arterial solution.

Arterial and cavity fluids are packaged in concentrated form, commonly in 16-ounce (pint) plastic bottles. Fluids may also be packaged in 32-ounce bottles, 1-gallon, and multi-gallon cubes. Preservative arterial fluids are diluted at the time of use. Supplemental fluids are also added to the solution at time of use. Cavity fluids are not diluted; cavity fluid is used full strength.

Product catalogs, company websites, and product labels provide useful information for the embalmer. Technical advice and recommendations may also be available online. Ultimately, the embalmer determines the type, strength, and volume of fluid to be used during the pre-embalming analysis.

**Table 7–1** lists various arterial embalming chemicals.

### Preservative Formaldehyde Arterial Fluids

1. Index
    a. *High-index:* 26–38 and above
    b. *Medium-index:* 16–25
    c. *Low-index:* 5–15

**TABLE 7–1. Various Arterial Chemicals Used in Embalming**

| Aldehyde-Based Vascular Fluid (Preservative) | Supplemental Fluid |
|---|---|
| Index | Pre-injection |
| High | Co-injection (standard) |
| Medium | Internal bleach |
| Low | Tissue gas |
| Nonformaldehyde | Edema corrective |
| Color | Germicide booster |
| Noncosmetic | Humectant (restorative) |
| Cosmetic | Water corrective |
| Reds | Dyes |
| Suntan | Pink tints |
| Firming speed | Suntan tints |
| Fast | |
| Slow | |
| Firmness | |
| Soft | |
| Mild | |
| Hard | |
| Antidehydrant | |
| Humectant | |
| Nonhumectant | |
| Special purpose | |
| Jaundice | |
| High-index | |
| Dehydrating | |
| Nondehydrating | |
| Tissue gas | |
| Infants | |

2. Color
   a. *Noncosmetic:* fluids that contain little or no active dye and do not color the tissues
   b. *Cosmetic:* fluids that contain an active dye that colors the tissues
3. Firming speed
   a. *Fast-firming:* fluids buffered to firm tissues rapidly
   b. *Slow-firming:* fluids buffered to firm body tissues slowly
4. Degree of firmness
   a. *Soft:* fluids that are buffered and contain chemicals to control the preservative reaction to produce very little firming of the tissues.
   b. *Mild:* fluids that are buffered and contain chemicals to control the preservative reaction to produce medium firming of the tissues.
   c. *Hard:* fluids that are buffered and contain chemicals to control the preservative reaction to produce very definite firming of the tissues.
5. Moisturizing qualities
   a. *Humectants:* fluids that contain large amounts of chemicals that act to add and retain tissue moisture.
   b. *Nonhumectants:* fluids that do not contain chemicals that add or retain moisture.

## Special-Purpose Arterial Fluids

1. *Jaundice fluids:* fluids compounded to lessen or remove the discoloration of jaundice.
2. *High-index special-purpose fluids:* a group of chemicals used in the preparation of extreme cases, such as edema, renal failure, and decomposition.
   a. *Dehydrating:* fluids compounded to accelerate dehydration of the tissues.
   b. *Nondehydrating:* fluids compounded with large amounts of controlled preservatives to prevent tissue dehydration.
3. *Tissue gas fluids:* fluids designed to arrest and control the causative agent of tissue gas (*Clostridium perfringens*).

## Eco-friendly Arterial Fluids

1. Biodegradable and environmentally friendly products only
2. Do not contain formaldehyde
3. Produce minimal to no firming of tissues
4. Provide temporary stabilization only
5. May be approved for green and natural burial

## ARTERIAL FLUID DILUTION

The mixture of arterial fluid with water and/or supplemental fluids (arterial solution) is called the **primary dilution.** Upon injection, the arterial solution becomes further diluted when it makes contact with tissue fluids; this is called the **secondary dilution.** To obtain optimum results, the types of arterial chemicals, strength and volume of the arterial solutions, and the techniques of arterial injection and drainage will vary with each body. **Each deceased human body has a preservative demand specific to that individual.** Preservative demand is determined during pre-embalming analysis: (1) physical conditions of the body, (2) amount of body protein, (3) antemortem pathological conditions, (4) antemortem effects of therapeutic drugs and chemotherapy, (5) postmortem conditions, (6) postmortem interval, and (7) interval between preparation and disposition. As arterial injection proceeds, the embalmer adjusts the strength and volume of subsequent solutions to support ongoing analysis: adequate distribution of the solution to all body areas, clearing discolorations, and meeting the preservative demands of the body. The conditions present, interval between embalming and final disposition, and preferences of the embalmer determine the degree of tissue firmness necessary.

At the onset of embalming, when body conditions are unremarkable, milder solutions can be used to clear intravascular blood discolorations. Subsequent injections are increased in strength to achieve desired firmness and preservation. Mild solutions are not recommended for advanced conditions such as renal failure, generalized edema, and early signs of decomposition; stronger initial solutions are indicated.

A number or value, called an **index** measures the percentage of aldehyde in the concentrate. The index is shown on the label of formaldehyde-based arterial fluids (**Table 7–2**). Index is defined as *the amount of formaldehyde gas, measured in grams, dissolved in 100 mL of solution.* Index is a measure of formaldehyde only. Glutaraldehyde-based fluids and other nonformaldehyde fluids do not use the term index. Instead, preservative strength may be expressed as a *factor.* When formaldehyde is used in combination with other preservatives in the formulation, index is not used.

A simple mathematical equation uses index to determine the strength of an arterial solution.

$$c \times v = c' \times v'$$

Index × volume of arterial fluid
= strength of solution × volume of solution

$c$ is the index, or concentration.
$v$ is the volume of arterial fluid.
$c'$ is the solution strength, or total concentration.
$v'$ is the volume of solution.

Note that the index of the arterial fluid ($c$) and the volume of arterial fluid ($v$) reference the bottle of arterial fluid. The strength of the solution ($c'$) and the volume of the solution ($v'$) reference the arterial solution contained in the embalming machine tank.

*Example 1:* To prepare a 2% arterial solution using a 25-index fluid, it is necessary to know how much fluid is needed to make a 1-gallon solution of 2% strength. 1 gallon is 128 ounces.

$$c \times v = c' \times v'$$
$$25 \times x = 2\% \times 128 \text{ oz of total solution}$$
$$25x = 256$$
$$x = \frac{256}{25}$$
$$x = 10.2 \text{ ounces of arterial fluid is needed}$$

Approximately 10 ounces of arterial fluid and 118 ounces of water are needed to make 1 gallon of 2% strength arterial solution.

# CHAPTER 7 • Use of Embalming Chemicals

| TABLE 7-2. Preparation of Various Percentage Aldehyde "In Use" Solutions[a] | | | | | |
|---|---|---|---|---|---|
| Concentration Rate per Gallon (oz) | % Aldehyde in Concentrate (Index) | | | | |
| | 15 | 20 | 25 | 30 | 35 |
| 4 | 0.47 | 0.625 | 0.78 | 0.94 | 1.10 |
| 5 | 0.59 | 0.18 | 0.98 | 1.17 | 1.38 |
| 6 | 0.70 | 0.94 | 1.17 | 1.41 | 1.64 |
| 7 | 0.82 | 1.10 | 1.37 | 1.64 | 1.91 |
| 8 | 0.93 | 1.25 | 1.56 | 1.88 | 2.19 |
| 9 | 1.05 | 1.41 | 1.76 | 2.11 | 2.46 |
| 10 | 1.17 | 1.56 | 1.95 | 2.34 | 2.73 |
| 11 | 1.29 | 1.72 | 2.15 | 2.59 | 3.01 |
| 12 | 1.41 | 1.86 | 2.34 | 2.81 | 3.28 |
| 13 | 1.52 | 2.03 | 2.54 | 3.05 | 3.55 |
| 14 | 1.64 | 2.19 | 2.73 | 3.28 | 3.83 |
| 15 | 1.76 | 2.34 | 2.93 | 3.52 | 4.10 |
| 16 | 1.88 | 2.50 | 3.13 | 3.75 | 4.38 |
| 17 | 1.99 | 2.66 | 3.32 | 3.98 | 4.65 |
| 18 | 2.11 | 2.81 | 3.52 | 4.22 | 4.92 |
| 19 | 2.23 | 2.97 | 3.71 | 4.45 | 5.20 |
| 20 | 2.34 | 3.13 | 3.91 | 4.69 | 5.47 |
| 21 | 2.46 | 3.18 | 4.10 | 4.92 | 5.74 |
| 22 | 2.58 | 3.44 | 4.30 | 5.16 | 6.02 |
| 23 | 2.70 | 3.59 | 4.49 | 5.39 | 6.29 |
| 24 | 2.81 | 3.15 | 4.69 | 5.63 | 6.56 |
| 25 | 2.93 | 3.91 | 4.88 | 5.86 | 6.84 |
| 26 | 3.05 | 4.06 | 5.01 | 6.09 | 7.11 |
| 27 | 3.16 | 4.22 | 5.27 | 6.33 | 7.38 |
| 28 | 3.28 | 4.38 | 5.47 | 6.56 | 7.66 |
| 29 | 3.40 | 4.53 | 5.66 | 6.80 | 7.92 |
| 30 | 3.52 | 4.69 | 5.86 | 7.03 | 8.20 |

[a]Fluid ounces × index ÷ by 128 (oz/gal) = % aldehyde in solution.

Source: Used with permission of The Champion Company, Springfield, Ohio.

*Example 2:* Determine the strength of the arterial solution when 7 ounces of arterial fluid is added to one *full* gallon of water (128 ounces).

$$25 \times 7 = x \times 135 \text{ (add 128 ounces of water}$$
$$\text{and 7 ounces of fluid together)}$$
$$175 = 135x$$
$$x = \frac{175}{135} \text{ or } x = 1.29\% \text{ solution strength}$$

## Quantity of Arterial Solution

A 160-pound body contains approximately 10 pints (one and one-half gallons) of blood. During the embalming of the body, this blood is replaced with the arterial solution; a portion of the arterial solution will remain in the vascular system and a necessary portion is needed to move into the tissue spaces to preserve the body cells and tissues. Drainage taken during arterial injection contains blood, tissue fluid, and arterial solution. It is estimated that 50% of the arterial solution can be lost in the drainage (see, **Selected Readings: The Measurement of Formaldehyde Retention in the Tissues of Embalmed Bodies**). It is the arterial solution that is retained by the body tissues that preserves and sanitizes. A review of a number of embalming care reports shows that 3–4 gallons of the proper strength of arterial solution is generally sufficient for the embalming of a 160-pound deceased body. These are bodies without edema, renal failure, or signs of decomposition.

The "50-pound rule" is an outdated guideline concerned primarily with body weight. The premise was to inject a minimum of 1 gallon of arterial solution for each 50 pounds of body weight. This guideline was observed for many years. Presently, individual conditions observed during pre-embalming analysis are considered the guiding factors used to determine solution strength and volume.

## PRESERVATIVE DEMAND

A sufficient quantity of arterial solution at the proper strength must be injected to meet preservative demand following long-term usage of medications. Over a long period of time, medications may increase the demand for preservative. Examples include

- the effect of the drug on the preservative solution;
- the damage the drug has done to the body proteins;
- the damage done to specific organs such as the liver and the kidneys, causing retention of wastes such as ammonia and urea in the tissues; and
- the damage done to the cell membrane—a possible condition in which it is difficult for fluids to pass through the cell membranes.

Consider these points in determining the strength and amount of fluid to inject:

- time interval between death and preparation
- time interval between preparation and disposition
- moisture content in the tissues and body cavities
- renal failure and the buildup of nitrogenous **wastes** in the body
- liver failure and the buildup of toxic wastes in the body tissues
- weight of the body
- amount of adipose tissue compared to muscle tissue
- protein levels of the body
- progress of the postmortem physical and chemical changes, especially the stages of decomposition and rigor mortis
- nature of death—sudden heart attack versus wasting disease; use of life-support systems for many weeks
- chemotherapy and medications given to the individual

## GENERAL GUIDELINES FOR ARTERIAL SOLUTION STRENGTH AND VOLUME

> Embalming the unautopsied body: Inject a sufficient volume (quantity), of arterial solution at a strength (quality) necessary to meet the preservative demands of the body; using a pressure and rate of flow so as to distribute the solution to all body regions causing the solution to diffuse to the tissues and cells without noticeable distension or dehydration. Body regions can vary: some regions may receive insufficient solution while other areas may receive too much. Some body regions may have a higher preservative demand because of disease processes. This may necessitate a separate injection (multi-point) possibly using a different strength of arterial solution.

### General Guidelines

1. General guidelines
   a. The arterial solution must be strong enough to meet the preservative (formaldehyde) demands of the body.
   b. Begin with a mild solution and then increase strength once distribution is established.
   c. If you dilute a high-index fluid to make a mild solution, you will not only dilute the formaldehyde but also dilute the modifying agents.
2. Preferences of the embalmer: embalming is an art and a science. Some embalmers or funeral homes want the bodies to have a natural feel; others prefer that the bodies be very firm to the touch.
3. The 160-pound body contains about 10 pints of blood. By injecting 3–4 gallons of solution, this more than displaces the blood and fills the vascular system and tissue spaces. It is estimated that 50% of injected arterial solution can be lost through drainage.
4. Manufacturer's recommendations: Some fluid companies will offer dilution suggestions.
   a. The minimum injection of 1 gallon per each 50-pounds of body weight rule is outdated.
   b. Body moisture conditions; dilutions for no edema; mild and intense edema.
   c. Specific fluids for specific body conditions, for example, jaundice, decomposition, renal failure, trauma, mortuary refrigeration, edema, and frozen bodies.
   d. Strength is based on the clearing of the blood discolorations; the rule is to inject mild solutions first, followed by stronger solutions.
   e. Manufacturers state that sufficient fluid and solution must be used to achieve the embalmer's desired results.
5. Dr. Jerome F. Frederick—1968: Average body = 160 pounds; contains 10,700 g of protein; needs 470 g of formaldehyde which equals three bottles of a 30-index fluid (see **Selected Readings: The Mathematics of Embalming Chemistry**). *In 2021, the average body weight for males was 200 pounds; females 171 pounds.*
6. Rendon/Rose Hockett guidelines: minimum of 2% strength arterial solution; minimum volume of 3–4 gallons or use the 50-pound rule (see **Selected Readings**).
7. Mortuary Care of Armed Forces Service Members. Minimum of 5% arterial solution strength (see **Selected Readings**).
8. Waterless embalming: No added water. Solution is comprised only of arterial fluid, water conditioner, co-injection, and humectant. Dye can also be added.

## WATERLESS EMBALMING

Waterless embalming is based on the theory that *water does not preserve*. "Waterless" is a misnomer because embalming fluid contains some water in the formulation, primarily as a carrier. The term "waterless" simply means that no water is added by the embalmer. Waterless solutions are composed entirely of a mixture of arterial and supplemental fluids. Co-injection, humectant, and water-conditioner replace water in the solution.

> **WATERLESS SOLUTION EXAMPLE:**
> 16 ounces of a preservative arterial fluid is mixed with 48 ounces of a co-injection, 48 ounces of water corrective, and 16 ounces of humectant to make 1 gallon of solution. Subsequent solutions can be mixed in the same proportions or modified to support the embalming analysis.
> 16 ounces = 1 bottle
> 48 ounces = 3 bottles

Waterless embalming provides maximum tissue preservation using a minimum volume of arterial solution. Restricted cervical injection of a waterless solution is recommended for the following:

- Facial trauma
- Moderate-to-severe decomposition
- Sepsis
- Lengthy mortuary refrigeration
- Frozen tissues
- Tissue gas
- Contagious or infectious conditions
- Poor circulation
- Difficult cases
- Cases requiring reembalming

Sectional injection is recommended for conditions that affect a localized area, such as an extremity:

- Gangrene
- Edema

### Arterial Solution pH

The pH of the arterial fluid is determined by the fluid manufacturer. This is not an element of the fluid that the embalmer determines. Most arterial fluids are buffered to be slightly alkaline in pH, approximately 7.2–7.4. At this pH, the fluid reaction is stable, dyes in the fluid work well, and the tissues do not exhibit a tendency to turn gray. Some fluids are buffered to rapidly react. When using these fluids, the embalmer must be certain that a sufficient volume of fluid has been injected. Because these fluids cause rapid firming of the body, there is a tendency to use an insufficient amount of solution.

With all embalming, after surface blood discolorations have been cleared, intermittent drainage can be employed. Inject a sufficient quantity of solution, making every effort to retain as much solution as possible within the body.

### Arterial Fluid Temperature

Arterial fluids are diluted with cool or room temperature water, sometimes slightly warm or tepid water. In special cases, such as tissue gas or decomposition, arterial fluids are diluted with warmer water; the warmer the water, the faster the chemical reaction of the fluid.

### Density/Specific Gravity

Certain solid chemical substances known as *salts* play an important role in determining the characteristics of the different embalming fluids and in controlling, to a large extent, the reactions between the cellular tissues and the chemical solution. When salt is dissolved in water, it is possible to form solutions of different concentrations depending on the amount of salt added to the water. The more salt (solute) added to the water (solvent), the more concentrated the solution becomes. In other words, the strength of the solution actually indicates how much solute is present. The amount of solute in a solution has a direct effect on the density of the solution.

**Density** is defined as mass per unit volume and is expressed in such units as grams per cubic centimeter. Thus, it can be seen how density relates to the concentration of the solute in the solution. Often, it is desirable to compare the density of a given substance with the density of water. This ratio is called **specific gravity**. If a substance has a specific gravity of 1.5, it means that compared with the density of water, the substance is 1.5 times as dense. Again, as with density, the specific gravity of a solution varies with concentration.

In solutions used in medicine, either the density or the salt concentration of a solution is frequently compared with that of blood. If a solution contains less of a dissolved substance than is found in blood, it is said to be **hypotonic**. If it contains a greater quantity of a dissolved substance than is found in the blood, it is said to be **hypertonic**.

During embalming, blood and other body liquids are eventually replaced with the chemical preservative solution, which changes the nature of tissue. Such change resists decomposition. The penetration of such solution into all soft tissue areas should be thorough to achieve complete preservation and produce the best results. It has been found that a solution that is slightly hypotonic to blood and body fluids produces the best embalming results. In part A of the following illustration, a membranous bag, such as from a section of animal intestine that is "semipermeable," that is, permeable to some materials but not to others, is placed in a container of distilled water. The bag contains a 10% salt solution. In part B of the same illustration, it is observed to increase in volume. This demonstrates that water has passed into the bag (**Fig. 7–4**).

The distilled water, being "hypotonic" (less density), passes to the inside of the bag, which contains the more highly concentrated solution (higher density). The solution in the bag in diagram **A**, then, is hypertonic to the distilled water. What is the importance of all this to the embalming operation and to embalming fluids?

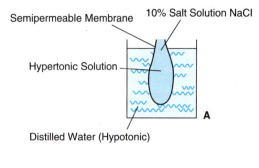
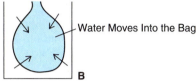

**Figure 7–4.** Semipermeable membrane.

It is known that a solution will penetrate to the side or region containing the higher density solution; this fact is used in compounding fluids and in establishing the proper concentrations to use in embalming. When diluted according to the recommended usage, the resultant solution is slightly hypotonic to blood and body liquids. If less of the concentrated fluid is used, then the resultant solution may be more hypotonic than desired for proper embalming results. The tissues tend to become "waterlogged," which eventually results in skin slip (desquamation) because of the lack of sufficient preservative material.

On the other hand, if too much-concentrated fluid is used, according to the preceding principle, a hypertonic solution results, and it will have the effect of removing too much moisture. This, of course, causes excessive dehydration. In some instances, the embalmer may want to make use of this principle to remove excess moisture from tissue areas, such as in dropsical or edematous cases. The "special" fluids designed for such purposes incorporate this principle.

Briefly, then, an embalming solution that is less dense (i.e., hypotonic) than the tissue liquids will flow rapidly through the capillary walls into the soft tissue areas. If the solution is designed so that it has a greater density (i.e., hypertonic) than the tissue liquids, it will draw tissue liquid through the capillary wall into the circulatory system and away from the soft tissue areas.

### Osmotic Qualities

For the body in which there is no edema or dehydration, the arterial solution should be hypotonic in its osmotic composition. When the solution is hypotonic to the body tissues, the fluid moves from the capillary vessels into the tissue spaces. If these solutions were hypertonic, tissue fluids would move from the tissue space into the capillary vessels causing dehydration and lack of arterial fluid in the tissues. There are instances when hypertonic solutions are desired. Hypertonic solutions are beneficial in reducing skeletal edema (edema of the limbs). These solutions help to move the excess water from the tissue into the capillary vessels by increasing the osmotic permeability of the cell membranes. From there, the water can be removed through drainage. High-index special-purpose fluids are used to create dehydrating hypertonic solutions.

## SPECIAL-PURPOSE ARTERIAL FLUIDS

### High-Index Fluids

High-index arterial fluids have a formaldehyde index ranging from 26 to 38. These fluids are designed for difficult cases, although they may be used for other types of preparations. High-index fluids are also used to fortify the strength of milder or weaker arterial solutions.

*Example.* An embalmer mixes a solution using a 22-index arterial fluid and uses 12 ounces to 1 gallon. If tissue firming is not evident, the second and subsequent gallons are mixed using several ounces of a high-index fluid (26–38) to increase the preservative strength of the solution. Mix solutions from mild to strong, not the reverse.

The Dodge Chemical Company explains the use of a special-purpose high-index fluid: *The more severe the conditions of the body, the stronger the primary solution should be. When little drainage is anticipated, stronger concentrations and less total volume of solution should be used. When normal drainage is achieved, the volume of solution to be used will be governed by the size, weight, and conditions of the body. In general, in treating bodies of "difficult" types, a good rule to follow is: more rather than less chemical—and less rather than more water. Water will not preserve nor will it arrest putrefaction—but it will create swelling and distension.*

The use of high-index fluid is advised for bodies:

- dead for extended periods of time
- that have been frozen or extended refrigeration
- that have undergone extensive treatments with drugs
- that have been institutionalized
- with traumatic injuries for which restorative treatments will be needed
- with evidence of decomposition
- with gangrenous limbs
- that are difficult to firm
- with skeletal edema
- dead from renal failure
- with bloodstream infections
- with tissue gas present
- obese bodies

Some companies produce two types of high-index fluids: **dehydrating** and **nondehydrating.** The nondehydrating fluid is designed to deliver a strong formaldehyde and preservative action with a minimum of dehydration. As with other arterial fluids, it is best to follow the dilutions recommended by the manufacturer. Most of the high-index fluids, when used as a "booster" fluid, work well with standard arterial fluids of other companies. Because of the problems encountered with delayed embalming and the wide use of drug therapy today, *this arterial fluid should always be kept on hand in the preparation room.*

### Jaundice Fluids

Jaundice fluids are special-purpose preservative arterial fluids designed for treating the condition of jaundice. Jaundice fluids are formulated to flush mild jaundice discolorations and prevent the discoloration from intensifying. These fluids may or may not contain formaldehyde. When formaldehyde is used in formulation, the index of the fluid is typically low. Buffers may also be added to prevent pH changes that can cause the conversion of bilirubin to biliverdin.

### *Bleaching Fluids*

Bleaching fluids oxidize the discoloration. The chemicals employed in the formulations include peroxides, citric acid, and phenols. These chemicals are usually employed in an alcohol medium.

### *Coupling Compound System*

The coupling compound system combines a chemical with the bile pigment to decolorize the pigment. A pre-injection coupling compound (e.g., a diazo agent in a nonacidic medium) is injected first. The aldehyde arterial injection follows. The system is complex, time consuming, and not always reliable.

### *Chemical Adduct System*

In the chemical adduct system, a chemical is combined with formaldehyde; later, the formaldehyde is slowly released.

### Tissue Gas Fluid

A variety of fluids have been manufactured by chemical companies to treat the condition known as *tissue gas*. This condition is caused by *C. perfringens*, an anaerobic spore-forming bacterium. Directions for use, if provided, should be strictly followed.

### Nonformaldehyde Preservative Arterial Fluids

Environmental issues and the probable carcinogenic qualities of formaldehyde have been leading to a development of arterial fluids using preservatives other than formaldehyde. Some of these fluids contain preservatives, modifying agents, and dyes that are nontoxic, nonhazardous, and biodegradable. Such fluids can be used for the temporary preservation of bodies being buried in "Green" or "Natural" cemeteries.

Other formaldehyde-free fluids contain chemicals that are not biodegradable and can be considered hazardous to the embalmer or the environment. They do provide a temporary preservation of the body but they cannot be used for bodies that are to be buried in strict Green Cemeteries.

These fluids may produce little or no firming of the body tissues. As indicated, the preservation of the body is very temporary. **Manufacturer's directions for use should be strictly followed.**

## SUPPLEMENTAL FLUIDS

### Pre-Injection Fluid

Pre-injection fluids, also called *primary injection fluids* and *capillary washes*, are designed to prepare the circulatory system for injection of the preservative solution. Pre-injection clears blood discolorations, adjusts the pH of the tissues to prevent graying, reduces blood coagulation, improves distribution and drainage, and minimizes the harsh effects of formaldehyde. Pre-injection fluids are diluted with water for use and contain little or no preservative. Injection of too large of a quantity can waterlog the tissues; one-half to three-quarters of a gallon is usually sufficient. Restricting drainage during the first several minutes of injection promotes vascular expansion and creates intravascular pressure. Best results are obtained when time is allowed for the chemical to work within the vascular system before allowing drainage to continue. Historically, pre-injection fluids were absolutely necessary because the early arterial fluids were so harsh that good drainage and blood clearing did not happen without them.

### Co-Injection Fluid

Co-injection fluids are combined with the arterial fluid and injected at the same time. Use of co-injection enhances the properties of the arterial fluid and improves overall arterial solution distribution and diffusion. Co-injection creates a synergistic relationship with arterial fluid: the two fluids combined are more effective than if the arterial fluid was used alone. Like pre-injection fluid, a co-injection will minimize the harsh effects of formaldehyde.

Co-injection fluids are commonly used in equal amounts to arterial fluid. For methods such as waterless embalming and instant tissue fixation (see Chapter 12), co-injection fluid is used as a diluent in place of water in the solution.

### Water Corrective Fluid

Water corrective fluids remove particulates in tap water and adjust the pH of the solution. A water conditioner is added to any solution that uses water as a carrier, or vehicle. A few ounces added to each gallon of solution is usually sufficient. Overuse can cause uneven diffusion of fluid dyes, resulting in a blotchy appearance. Water corrective chemicals are used as vehicles for waterless embalming solutions. After embalming, a mixture of warm water and several ounces of water conditioner can be used to flush and clean the embalming machine; removing salts and residual chemicals that can clog internal hoses and structures.

### Dyes

Dyes are coloring agents. Inactive dyes merely color the arterial fluid. Active dyes serve several functions:
- Are visible in tissues reached by arterial solution; indication of distribution effectiveness.
- Restores color to the skin; blood drainage pales the tissues.
- Minimizes graying discolorations caused by incomplete blood drainage; *formaldehyde gray*.
- Discolorations caused by jaundice can be counterstained.

Dye can be added at the onset of injection or added toward the end. The amount needed varies. Dyes also vary between suppliers; one brand may require a few drops, another brand may require an ounce or more. Best practice suggests using dyes sparingly to avoid overstaining the tissues. The use of too much dye at the onset may give the false appearance of embalmed tissues and result in under embalming.

### Humectant (Restorative) Fluid

The separately purchased humectant is really a co-injection fluid. The reason for this is quite simple. The humectant is added and injected along with the arterial fluid. Some embalmers use humectants only when the body is dehydrated. Others add extra humectant to all arterial solutions when embalming a body with normal moisture to prevent dehydration. The amount of humectant added to each gallon of solution should follow the manufacturer's directions. Humectants hydrate and add moisture to the tissues and they also prevent tissue dehydration.

Some humectants are colloids, and these viscous colloid mixtures, when injected into the arterial system, have a tendency to draw moisture **out of the tissues** and into the capillaries. If additional humectants are used and solutions are injected into the body with continuous drainage, evidence of dehydration can be seen in such areas as the lips, fingers, and backs of the hands. Most embalmers, when adding humectants to the arterial solution, use intermittent drainage. In this manner, the humectant is held in the capillaries and tissue spaces and does not draw moisture from the tissues.

For a severely emaciated body, add humectant to the final gallon of solution and halt drainage during injection. Closed drainage allows the facial tissues to receive the solution necessary to recontour features. Monitor the facial features closely during injection to produce a natural appearance and avoid distending tissues.

### Edema Reducing Fluid

Edema corrective co-injection fluids are designed to reduce edematous or waterlogged tissues. The edema corrective fluid changes the osmotic qualities of the embalming solution, making it hypertonic to the body fluids, which draws the edema from the tissue spaces back into the venous drainage. The volume of corrective co-injection is dependent upon the severity of the edema.

Edema reducing fluids are very effective in reducing swollen facial tissues, often resulting from vascular or heart surgery. Best results are obtained when the head is separately injected using the restricted cervical injection method along with the corrective treatment. Massage and elevation of the affected area also helps to reduce distension. Excessive volumes of edema reducing fluid may cause tissue dehydration, discoloration, and wrinkling.

### Tissue Gas Co-Injection Fluid

Tissue gas co-injection fluids are germicidal and act on the microbe responsible for tissues gas formation, *C. perfringens*. This co-injection fluid is usually added to an arterial solution. Strictly follow the manufacturer's directions for use.

### Internal Bleach and Stain Remover

This supplemental chemical is added to the arterial solution to lighten blood or decomposition discolorations when they are present on the face or hands.

### Other Supplemental Embalming Products

Supplemental embalming products also include germicidal soaps and detergents, contact embalming liquids and sprays, orifice and topical disinfectants, and formaldehyde absorbent chemicals.

## CAVITY FLUID

Cavity fluid is injected directly into the unautopsied thoracic, abdominal, and pelvic cavities using a trocar. In certain cases, the cranial cavity can be injected using a long needle or hypo-valve trocar. The instrument is directed through the nostril and through the cribriform plate of the ethmoid bone to reach the cranial cavity. Pre-embalming analysis, including body size and weight, indicates the volume of cavity fluid necessary for injection. Routinely, a total of 32–48 ounces of cavity fluid is introduced into the three cavities; more as needed to meet preservative demand. The principal component of cavity fluid is preservative; cosmetic dyes, anticoagulants, and humectants are unnecessary.

Cavity fluid *preserves*, *disinfects*, and *deodorizes* the organs within the cavities, contents of the hollow viscera, and walls of the cavities. There are additional uses for cavity fluids:

- Preservation of viscera removed during autopsy.
- As a surface compress to treat tissues not reached by arterial profusion.
- Injection via hypodermic needle or hypovalve trocar into tissues that lack sufficient arterial preservation.
- As a surface compress to dry and deodorize lesions, gangrenous or edematous tissues, and other pathologic conditions.
- As an arterial fluid in the preparation of difficult cases such as advanced decomposition, tissue gas, and jaundice. Caution: some manufacturers void the warranty on the embalming machine when phenol is placed into the machine.
- To bleach blood discolorations.
- To dry tissues when excisions have been performed.
- For surface preservation of fetal remains.

## Fumeless Cavity Fluids

Fumeless fluids, particularly cavity fluids, are produced by many manufacturers. There are three ways in which fumeless fluids can be produced: (1) covering the formaldehyde odor with a perfuming agent or reodorant, (2) substituting other preservatives for formaldehyde (such as phenol), or (3) using formaldehyde donor compounds (donor compounds do not release formaldehyde until contact is made with the tissues). A concern with masking formaldehyde odor is that the embalmer may not realize that formaldehyde is present and become overexposed. The substitution method is used by many manufacturers; however, other preservatives lack the penetrating qualities of formaldehyde. Formaldehyde donor compounds are used mainly in the production of arterial fluids.

## ACCESSORY EMBALMING CHEMICALS

Accessory chemicals are those used to treat the dead human body for purposes other than arterial embalming or unautopsied cavity treatment. They include autopsy gels, concentrated cautery chemicals, hardening compounds, concentrated preservative powder, concentrated deodorant powder, concentrated disinfectant powder, mold inhibitors, powdered sealing agents, cream or "putty" sealing agents, and surface sealing agents.

## Autopsy (Surface) Gels

These surface preservative gels are available in two viscosities: a gel that is thin and can be poured and a more viscous gel that can easily be applied by brush to surfaces. Preservative gels are used in several ways. They may be

- poured over the viscera returned from an autopsy in the plastic bag in which the viscera have been placed.
- applied to the surface of viscera in partial autopsies.
- used as a preservative in the orbital area after enucleation.
- applied to the walls of cavities and surfaces, such as the cranial cavity and calvarium in autopsied bodies.
- applied as a surface preservative to pathologic conditions such as decubitus ulcerations and gangrenous or necrotic areas.
- applied as a disinfectant and as an odor reducer.
- applied to surface areas of the body that the embalmer feels have received insufficient arterial fluid.
- used to bleach discolored areas such as ecchymoses and postmortem stains.
- used to preserve, cauterize, and deodorize burned tissues.
- used to pack the anal orifice and colostomy opening.

Preservative gels are designed as surface or osmotic preservatives. These adhering and penetrating gels not only preserve tissues but also bleach blood and decomposition discolorations. In addition, they eliminate odors when applied to pathologic conditions such as gangrene and decubitus ulcerations.

As with all preservative chemicals, care should be taken to use gels in a well-ventilated embalming room while wearing proper protective equipment. When the gels are applied to an external surface, they should be covered with cotton or plastic to improve the effectiveness of the gel and to reduce chemical fumes.

Each manufacturer recommends the length of time the gels should remain on a surface to be most effective. Several hours would be a good rule. The embalmer can check from time to time on the working action of the gel. When the gels are applied to necrotic areas (as on the legs), plastic stockings should be placed on the body and the gel should not be removed. The same is true for application over decubitus ulcerations. The compresses should be left in place and plastic garments such as pants or coveralls should be placed on the body.

## Cautery Chemicals

Cauterizing chemicals are liquids that are basically phenol (carbolic acid). Those sold through embalming manufacturers contain about 2–5% of phenol. It should be emphasized that whenever these chemicals are used, the embalmer must wear eye protection. Unlike most embalming chemicals that irritate the eyes, carbolic acid can actually burn and scar eye tissue. Gloves must be worn when handling phenol.

A cautery chemical can be applied to the areas where the skin has been removed, for example, abrasions, skin slip, blisters that have been opened, and burned areas. Phenol is a rapid-acting cautery agent and dries these areas in minutes. Phenol can be used as a surface bleach (applied as a pack) or injected by hypodermic needle subcutaneously. Phenol is a reducing and constricting agent. It can be injected into swollen areas such as black eyes or hematomas and allowed to remain for a time. When external pressure is placed on the swollen area, some of the phenol is forced from the area along with some of the liquids responsible for the swelling. In addition to the above, cautery chemicals are good germicides.

## Tissue Builder (or filler)

A tissue builder is a chemical injected by hypodermic syringe and needle **traditionally after** arterial embalming. It is injected into sunken areas of the face and hands to help restore their natural contour when the body exhibits a great loss of weight to absorb moisture and odor. Common ingredients of hardening compounds:

- Plaster of Paris (dehydrating agent)
- Paraformaldehyde (preservative, disinfectant)
- Aluminum chloride and alum (dehydrating agent, disinfectant, preservative)
- Wood powder (cellulose, very fine sawdust), whiting (calcium carbonate), and clays (moisture absorbing chemicals)

"Dustless" hardening compounds contain Bentonite, an absorbent, heavier particulate clay that creates little dust. When embalming powders are used, the room should be well-ventilated and appropriate PPE worn to protect the embalmer's eyes and airway. Judicious use of powders will reduce airborne particulates that can easily be inhaled.

## Autopsy Compounds

**Autopsy compounds** are used similarly to hardening compounds. Autopsy compounds are specifically formulated for use on the exposed tissues within the cavities of autopsied bodies. They absorb excess moisture, preserve, firm, and sanitize tissues. Autopsy compounds are effective for treatment of full- and split-thickness tissue donors. "Dustless" products replace the paraformaldehyde with formaldehyde-releasing preservative chemicals such as hydroxymethyl-5,5-dimethylhydantoin.

> Autopsy and hardening compounds are not reduced by the cremation process and cannot be separated from the cremated remains. A larger volume of cremated remains may necessitate a larger urn. Use of a minimal amount of these products is recommended when the final disposition is cremation.

## Embalming Preservative Powder

Embalming powders are designed to preserve tissues, but lack the absorbent and drying qualities of a hardening compound. Paraformaldehyde is the primary ingredient of embalming powders. *Para*-dichlorobenzene crystals are added to arrest mildew and mold. Some embalming powders also serve as deodorants and disinfectants. Embalming powders supplement preservation of bedsores, burns, cancerous tumors, necrotic, and traumatized tissues. They can be applied directly to autopsied cavity walls.

Embalming powder can also be placed into the plastic garments used to cover edematous limbs. When bodies are shipped to a distant point for interment, embalming powder can be placed in the casket to control mildews, molds, and odors. Maggots and vermin can be controlled with embalming powder. Consult the product label before using embalming powders; some are preservatives, some are only disinfectants and deodorants. An embalming powder that serves all three purposes is the most beneficial.

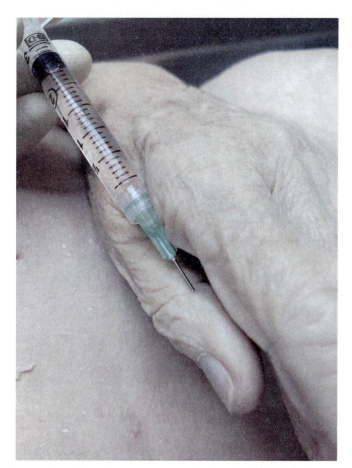

**Figure 7–5.** Hypodermic treatment of fingertips after embalming.

(**Fig. 7–5**). Individual features such as the lips or the fingers can also be treated with this chemical. Once injected beneath the skin, it can be spread through the tissues by digital pressure. It is important to not overfill an area; it is almost impossible to remove the tissue builder once it is injected. Tissue builder contains nitrocellulose and several types of alcohols.

## Solvents

The embalmer uses three solvents in various embalming treatments. A **general solvent** is used for cleansing of the skin surface, usually the face and the hands. Most of these solvents can also be used for cleansing the scalp and hair. They are useful in removing cosmetics from the hair, eyelashes, and eyebrows. Older formulations contained chemicals such as trichloroethylene or acetone. Newer products are free of these chemicals and less toxic to the embalmer. A **tissue builder solvent** (methyl alcohol) is used to clean hypodermic syringes and needles that have been used for the injection of tissue builder. Some embalmers like to store syringes with a few milliliters of solvent in them. Anytime a syringe is used, it should be flushed with this solvent before another chemical is used. A third solvent found in the preparation room is finger nail polish remover, primarily **acetone.**

## Hardening Compounds

Hardening compounds are blends of powdered chemicals designed to dry moist tissues and may contain powdered preservatives, disinfectants, and deodorants. The primary use is the treatment of the cavities and viscera of the autopsied body. Hardening compound is often placed inside of plastic garments

## Mold Inhibitors

Mold inhibitors are applied topically as a gel or spray. The primary ingredient is phenol or thymol. Short-term mortuary refrigeration will retard most mold growth but not stop it entirely. To avoid inhalation, wear PPE and apply a mold inhibiting product before attempting to remove mold growth.

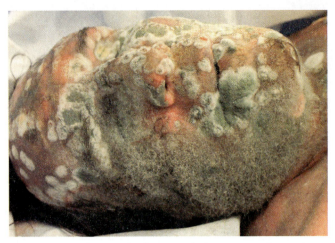

**Figure 7–6.** Mold growth after extended mortuary refrigeration.

Anatomical embalming solutions contain mold inhibitors because long-term refrigerated storage of cadavers is customary; some mold spores have an affinity for cool temperatures (**Fig. 7–6**).

### Incision Sealing Agents

Sealing agents can be applied in two ways: internally or externally. Both applications are designed to prevent leakage from the sutured incision. Internal products are placed into the incision site prior to suturing. Examples are powders and mastic compounds, also called *mortuary putty*. Powders swell as they absorb moisture; excess powders create a bulge beneath the incision. Excessive use also dehydrates the tissue surrounding the incision. Mastic compounds are not water soluble. They can be introduced into the incision site manually with a restorative art spatula or by an injector designed for the purpose. Mastic compounds are used as a substitute for tissue builder and have a variety of restorative uses, including restoration of the eye orbit of donors, as a base for deep wound restorations, and as a barrier in the autopsied cranium.

Externally applied sealing agents are adhesives or glues. Surface glues are available in brush-on or spray applicators. Super adhesives (cyanoacrylics) are widely used for surface sealing applications. Mortuary cosmetics are compatible with most sealing agents. A best practice is to dry tissue surfaces thoroughly before applying surface sealing agents.

## FIGURE CREDIT

Figure 7–1 is used with permission of Kevin Drobish.
Figures 7–2, 7–3, 7–5, 7–6 are used with permission of Sharon L. Gee-Mascarello.

## BIBLIOGRAPHY

American Board of Funeral Service, *Course Content Syllabus*, 2016.
Adams J. Waterless embalming—a valuable technique. In: *Dodge Magazine*, Vol. 102, No. 2. Cambridge, MA: Dodge Co., 2010.
Bedino J. Waterless embalming—an investigation. In: *The Champion Expanding Encyclopedia*, Nos. 619–620. Springfield, OH: Champion Co., 1993:2490–2497.

### CONCEPTS FOR STUDY

Define the following terminology:
- Cavity fluid
- Co-injection fluid
- Hypertonic solution
- Hypotonic solution
- Pre-embalming analysis
- Pre-injection fluid
- Preservative vascular fluid
- Primary dilution
- Secondary dilution

1. List ten work practice controls for the safe handling and use of embalming fluid.
2. Define waterless embalming solution and give several examples for its use.
3. Recall the benefits of pre-injection and co-injection fluids.
4. Discuss five factors that influence preservative demand.
5. List several purposes for addition of an active dye to arterial fluid.
6. Give several uses for mortuary putty (mastic compound).
7. State why the amount of autopsy and hardening compounds reduced when final disposition is cremation.
8. Review the results of excessive use of incision sealing powder.
9. How many ounces of a 25-index arterial fluid are used to prepare 1 gallon of a 2.0% strength arterial solution?
10. How many ounces of a 36-index arterial fluid are used to prepare 1 gallon of a 2.0% strength arterial solution?

Bedino JH. Enigma: Champion's fourth generation chemostasis infusion chemicals: Embalming redefined for the 21st century. In: *The Champion Expanding Encyclopedia of Mortuary Practices*, No. 657. Springfield, OH: Champion Co., 2009.
Dorn JM, Hopkins BM. *Thanatochemistry, a Survey of General, Organic, and Biochemistry for Funeral Service Professionals*, 3rd ed. Upper Saddle River, NJ: Prentice Hall, 2010.
Frigid Fluid Co, Funeral Home Catalog, www.frigidfluidco.com, Northlake, IL. 2004.
Mathews MC. *Embalming Chemistry Note Outline*. Minneapolis, MN: University of Minnesota, 1998.
New Jersey State Funeral Directors Association. Wall, NJ. January 2010.
Pervier NC. *Textbook of Chemistry for Embalmers*. Minneapolis, MN: University of Minnesota, 1961.
Pierce Chemicals; Royal Bond. www.piercechemical.com. Dallas, TX. 2009.
Putting alternative preservatives to the test. In: *The Forum*, Vol. 76, No. 3.
Rendon L. General chemical principles of embalming fluids. In: *The Champion Expanding Encyclopedia*, Nos. 365–371. Springfield, OH: Champion Co., 1966:1478–1504.

CHAPTER 8

# Anatomical Considerations

**CHAPTER OVERVIEW**
- Vessels Identified for Embalming
- Anatomical Features and Surface Landmarks
- Linear and Anatomical Guides
- Anatomical Limits, Origins and Branches

Basic knowledge of human anatomy is fundamental to the embalmer. This enables an efficient approach to solving embalming challenges and ensures successful outcomes. Recognition of anatomical features and the manner in which they relate to underlying structures assists the embalmer in making appropriately placed incisions.

To maintain reliable consistency in references to orientation, standard **anatomical position** is adopted as the *position of reference* for all anatomical nomenclature: the body is erect, feet together, arms at the sides, palms facing forward, and thumbs point away from the body. Consider that a reference to the right side of the deceased always means the deceased's right side, regardless of the viewer's perspective.

Familiarity with the main vessels in the blood vascular system supports the selection of the appropriate arteries and veins for thorough embalming of each body region (**Fig. 8–1A,B**).

In addition to identifying the main vessels used for embalming, the linear and anatomical guides, anatomical limits and origins, and applicable branches are also presented.

The **anatomical guide** is a descriptive reference for locating arteries and veins by means of identifying anatomical structures that are known. A **linear guide** is a line drawn or visualized on the surface of the skin to represent the approximate location of a deeper-lying structure. The **anatomical limit** designates the boundaries of arteries; the point of origin and the point of termination of the artery are given in relation to adjacent structures.

The anatomical guides for the arteries and the veins are the same. However, because venous blood flows in the *direction opposite* that of arterial blood, the anatomical limits and linear guides for veins are *opposite* those of the respective arteries.

## ARTERIES AND VEINS OF THE HEAD AND NECK

The importance of creating an acceptable appearance cannot be understated. The facial features are the most viewable aspect of the deceased body. An illustration of the vascular anatomy of the head and neck emphasizes the areas reached by the numerous branches of the external carotid arteries (**Fig. 8–2**).

## COMMON CAROTID ARTERY AND INTERNAL JUGULAR VEIN

### Anatomical Features

Prominent anatomical features of the chest and neck regions serve as landmarks to visualize the location of the common carotid artery and internal jugular vein:

- clavicle
- mandible
- angle of the jaw
- mastoid process of the temporal bone
- earlobe
- hyoid bone
- sternum
- sternoclavicular articulation
- suprasternal notch
- thyroid cartilage of the larynx

  Three prominent muscles of the neck:
- Sternocleidomastoid muscle (SCM)
- Platysma
- Omohyoid

### Anterior Triangle of the Neck (Anterior Cervical Triangle)

Three lines and their anatomical parallels serve as linear guides to describe the **anterior triangle** of the neck. The linear guide is expressed by drawing or visualizing a line along the midline of the neck between the tip of the mandible and the sternum. Extend this line superiorly along the anterior border of the SCM and then anteriorly along the lower margin of the body of the mandible. High in the neck, the hyoid bone, thyroid, and

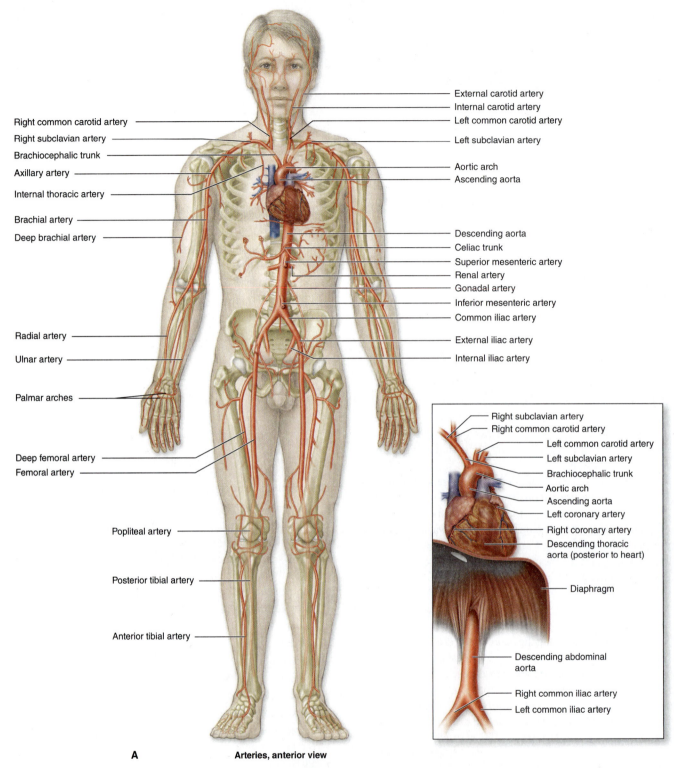

**Figure 8-1. A.** Arteries of the body, anterior view. **B.** Veins of the body, anterior view. (Used with permission from McKinley M et al. *Human Anatomy*. 5th ed. New York, McGraw Hill, 2017, Fig. 23.9AB.)

cricoid cartilages can be palpated along the midline. Located within the anterior triangle is the external carotid artery and several of its branches (Fig. 8-3).

The skin and subcutaneous tissue covering the vessels are thin and underlaid by the thin, cutaneous **platysma** muscle. The platysma is a muscle of facial expression, indicated by the shallow, transverse wrinkles of the neck. The platysma alters skin contour of the neck in a manner similar to the way muscles of facial expression modify the appearance of the face. Significant to the embalmer is that both the common carotid artery and internal jugular vein lie beneath the plane of this muscle.

The **sternocleidomastoid muscle (SCM)** is another useful landmark. Attached to the mastoid process of the temporal bone and the manubrium of the sternum, the SCM courses obliquely

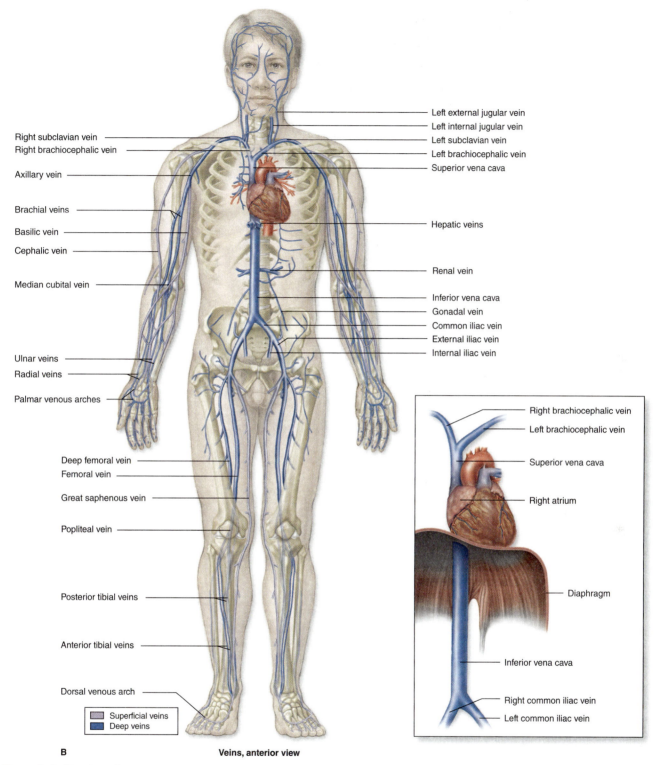

**Figure 8–1** (Continued)

along the side of the neck. The external jugular vein and some of its tributaries lie on the surface of the muscle and could be mistaken for the internal jugular vein. The internal jugular vein is located within the carotid sheath, not on the muscle surface.

The carotid sheath lies posterior and nearly parallel with the SCM. The sheath is an investment of fascia that extends up into the neck and contains the common carotid artery, the internal jugular vein, and the vagus nerve. The nerve is situated between the two vessels. The lower portion of the sheath is crossed anteriorly by the intermediate tendon of the **omohyoid muscle**. The omohyoid is located in the front of the neck, and consists of paired muscle bellies joined by an intermediate tendon. Locating the intermediate tendon guides the embalmer to the carotid sheath.

Once the carotid sheath is dissected, the internal jugular vein and the common carotid artery become visible. The vein lies

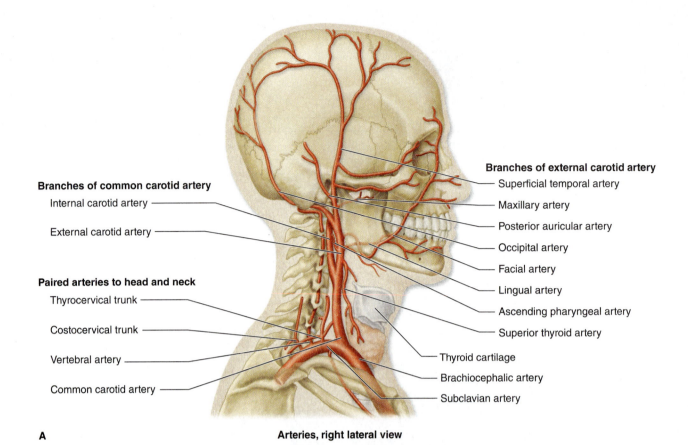

**Figure 8–2.** Arteries and veins of the head and neck, right lateral view. (Used with permission from McKinley M et al. *Human Anatomy*. 5th ed. New York, McGraw Hill, 2017, Fig. 23.10.)

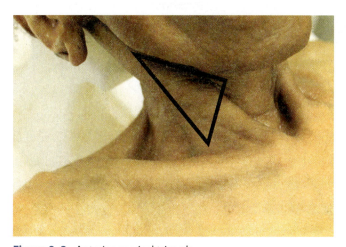

**Figure 8-3.** Anterior cervical triangle.

lateral to, and partially overlaps, the artery. A few variable tributaries of the internal jugular vein may be seen crossing the carotid artery in this area. The artery lies medial, somewhat underneath the vein. The vagus nerve, also called *cranial nerve X*, can be identified between and posterior to the two vessels within the sheath.

In the upper portion of the anterior triangle, the common carotid artery bifurcates to become the internal and external carotid arteries. The external carotid has eight branches, including the facial artery. The internal carotid artery does not have any branches until it enters the cranium.

## Common Carotid Artery

### Linear Guide
Draw or visualize a line on the surface of the skin from a point over the respective sternoclavicular articulation to a point over the anterior surface of the base of the respective earlobes (**Fig. 8–4**).

### Anatomical Guide
The right and the left common carotid arteries are located posterior to the medial border of the SCM, on their respective sides of the neck.

### Anatomical Limit
The right common carotid begins at the level of the right sternoclavicular articulation and extends to the superior border of the thyroid cartilage. The left common carotid begins at the level of the second costal cartilage and extends to the superior border of the thyroid cartilage.

### Origins
The right common carotid is a terminal branch of the brachiocephalic artery. The left common carotid is a branch of the arch of the aorta.

### Branches
There are no branches of the right common carotid, except the terminal bifurcation into the right internal and external carotid arteries. The left common carotid also has no branches, except the terminal bifurcation into the left internal and external carotid arteries.

### Branches of the Right and Left External Carotid Arteries
Ascending pharyngeal, superior thyroid, lingual, facial, occipital, posterior auricular, maxillary, superficial temporal.

### Branches of the Right and Left Internal Carotid Arteries
Branches arising within the carotid canal, in addition to ophthalmic, anterior cerebral, middle cerebral, posterior communicating, and choroidal branches.

### Relationship of the Common Carotid to the Internal Jugular Vein
The internal jugular vein lies lateral and superficial to the common carotid artery; it can also be said that the common carotid artery lies medial and deep to the internal jugular vein.

### Contents of the Carotid Sheath
Internal jugular vein (lateral to artery), vagus nerve (between and posterior to artery and vein), common carotid artery (medial to vein).

## Facial Artery

Sclerotic conditions that occlude the common carotid artery can drastically limit the arterial solution that reaches facial tissues. Other pathological conditions and traumatic injury may cause this artery to be unsuitable for injection. The facial artery may be selected as an alternative to reach the frontal structures of the face, especially the lips and superficial tissues. To raise the facial artery, an incision is made along the inferior border of the mandible, just anterior to the angle of the jaw (**Fig. 8–5**). The artery itself is superficial and requires only a small incision and reduced diameter arterial tube. Following injection,

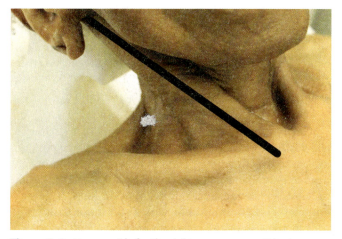

**Figure 8–4.** Linear guide for the right common carotid artery.

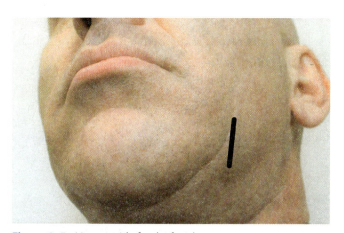

**Figure 8–5.** Linear guide for the facial artery.

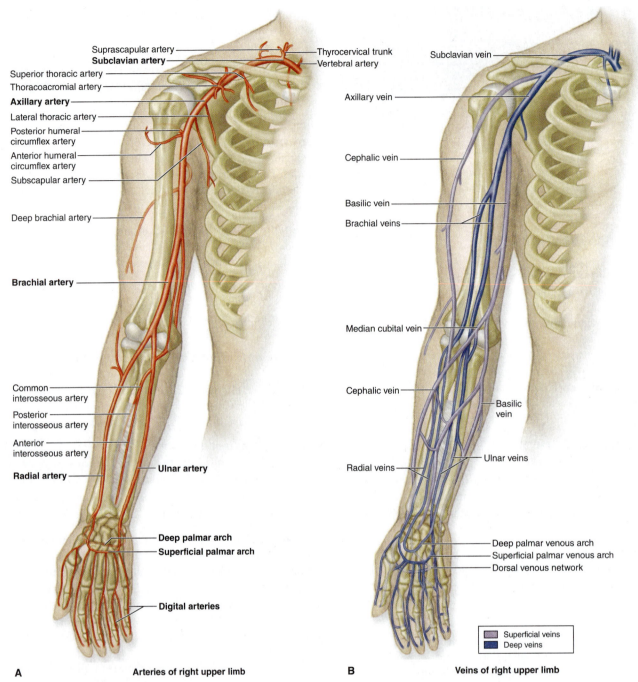

**Figure 8-6.** Arteries and veins of the right upper limb. (Used with permission from McKinley M et al. *Human Anatomy*. 5th ed. New York, McGraw Hill, 2017, Fig. 23.19.)

the incision may be sealed with an adhesive rather than a suture for ideal concealment.

## ARTERIES AND VEINS OF THE UPPER LIMBS

An illustration of the vascular anatomy of the upper limb shows the arteries and veins found in the arm and hand (**Fig. 8-6**).

## THE AXILLA (ARMPIT)

### Anatomical Features

The axilla is the concave area of soft tissue underlying the shoulder joint, known as the *armpit* or *underarm*. When the arm is fully extended (abducted), the axilla is viewed in its entirety. Surface landmarks of the axillary region include the

- ribs,
- intercostal muscles, and
- anterior and posterior axillary folds.

The most obvious boundaries of the axilla are its anterior and posterior walls, which comprise the anterior and posterior axillary folds. The anterior fold can be identified by using one hand to grasp the mass of tissue on the anterior surface of the axilla on the contralateral side of the body. Most of the substance of this fold consists of the pectoralis major muscle with contributions from the pectoralis minor and the subclavius muscles.

The posterior axillary fold can be identified by using one hand to grasp the tissue mass on the posterior side of the axilla on the contralateral side of the body. This fold consists of the latissimus dorsi, subscapularis, and teres major muscles. The medial axillary wall consists of ribs two through six and their intercostal muscles, covered externally by the serratus anterior muscle. The ribs can usually be palpated even if they are not visible on the chest surface. **Palpation** is a method of feeling with the fingers or hands during a physical examination.

The serratus anterior muscle also contributes to the medial wall but is visible as a surface feature only in lean, muscular subjects. The shaft of the humerus makes up a portion of the lateral wall, and although it cannot be seen, is easily palpated. The biceps brachii and coracobrachialis muscles also contribute to the lateral wall. The former is discernible in virtually all subjects, whereas the latter is clearly defined only in lean, muscular subjects.

The apex of the axilla is an opening called the **cervicoaxillary canal**, which transmits structures from the neck into the arm and is bounded by three bony structures: the clavicle, the scapula, and the first rib (**Fig. 8-7**). Of the three landmarks that demarcate this canal, only the first rib is difficult to palpate. The base of the axilla is closed with dome-shaped fascia and skin on which the axillary hair is found.

Familiarity with the surface features of the axilla guides one to the important axillary contents, including the axillary artery and its six branches, the axillary vein, and the many elements of the brachial plexus. The axillary sheath invests the major structures that leave the neck and pass through the cervicoaxillary canal to enter the axilla. Upon incising the axillary sheath, the first structure encountered is the superficial axillary vein. If the arm is fully abducted, the vein lies overtop and partially obscures the axillary artery. Identification of the artery within the sheath may be complicated by the many nerves of the brachial plexus that surround and partially obscure the artery. There are three large nerve cords of the brachial plexus. These nerves are grouped around the middle portion of the axillary artery in positions corresponding to their names: medial, lateral, and posterior.

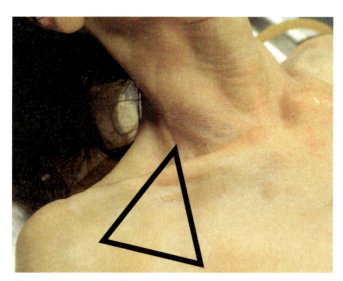

**Figure 8-7.** Cervicoaxillary canal.

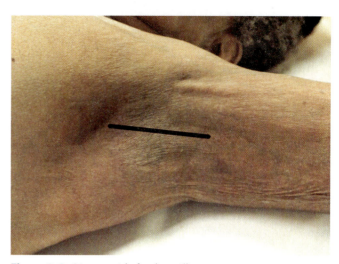

**Figure 8-8.** Linear guide for the axillary artery.

## Axillary Artery

### Linear Guide
Draw or visualize a line on the surface of the skin from a point over or through the center of the base of the axillary space to a point over or through the center of the lateral border of the base of the axillary space. This line is parallel to the long axis of the abducted arm (**Fig. 8-8**).

### Anatomical Guide
The axillary artery is located just behind the medial border of the coracobrachialis muscle.

### Anatomical Limit
The axillary artery extends from a point beginning at the lateral border of the first rib to the inferior border of the tendon of the teres major muscle.

### Origin
The axillary artery is a continuation of the subclavian artery.

### Branches
Highest (supreme) thoracic artery, thoracoacromial artery, lateral thoracic artery, subscapular artery, anterior humeral circumflex artery, posterior humeral circumflex artery.

### Relationship of the Axillary Artery to the Axillary Vein
The axillary artery is located lateral and deep to the axillary vein.

### Incision for Raising the Axillary Vessels
A midaxillary incision is made along the anterior margin of the hairline of the axilla with the arm abducted.

## Brachial Artery

### Linear Guide
Draw or visualize a line on the surface of the skin from a point over the center of the lateral border of the base of the axillary space to a point approximately 1 inch below and in front of the elbow joint (**Fig. 8-9**).

### Anatomical Guide
The brachial artery lies in the bicipital groove at the posterior margin of the medial border of the belly of the biceps brachii muscle.

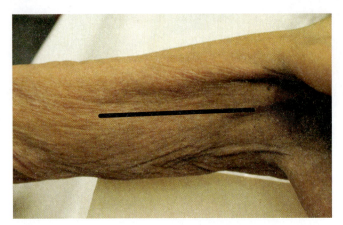

**Figure 8–9.** Linear guide for the brachial artery.

### Anatomical Limit
The brachial artery extends from a point beginning at the inferior border of the tendon of the teres major muscle to a point inferior to the antecubital fossa (the triangular depression in the anterior elbow; also called the elbow pit).

### Origin
The brachial artery is a continuation of the axillary artery.

### Relationship of the Brachial Artery and the Basilic Vein
The accompanying basilic vein is located medial and superficial to the brachial artery. Note the different names for the artery and vein.

### Location of the Incision
The incision is made along with the upper one-third of the linear guide, furthest from the elbow joint.

## DISTAL FOREARM

The distal forearm includes the radial and ulnar arteries for injection of the hands. The radial artery lies on the lateral side of the forearm and the ulnar artery on the medial side. The distal forearm permits easy access to the radial artery. Surface features of importance here are the styloid process of the radius and the tendon of the flexor carpi radialis muscle. In the interval between these two structures lies the radial artery on the anterior surface of the styloid.

A pulse may be obtained here easily in the living subject. The styloid is the most distal and lateral bony structure in the forearm, and just medial to this, one can palpate the tendon of flexor carpi radialis. In the distal region, the fleshy bellies of the muscles tend to yield to long, usually well-defined tendons. Here, a layering of the musculature is evident. In the most superficial layer are four muscles, including the pronator teres, flexor carpi radialis, flexor carpi ulnaris, and palmaris longus. Only the tendon of the pronator teres does not reach the distal forearm.

The second layer consists of one muscle with four tendons, one each leading to digits two through five. This muscle is the flexor digitorum superficialis. The three muscles in the deep group are the flexor digitorum profundus, the flexor pollicis longus, and the pronator quadratus. Of these three, only the pronator has no long tendon. Some of these tendons are useful guides to the radial and ulnar arteries.

Consider first the identification of the radial artery. An additional muscle, the brachioradialis, must be introduced here. This muscle is seen partially in the flexor compartment of the forearm. It is, nevertheless, an extensor muscle. In the proximal forearm, the radial artery is overlaid by the brachioradialis muscle but at no point is the artery crossed by this or any other muscle. **Proximal** indicates proximity; proximal means nearer to the center (trunk of the body) or to the point of attachment to the body. This situation keeps the radial artery superficial and permits easy access to it at any point along its course in the forearm. In the middle and distal forearms, the radial artery lies medial to the brachioradialis and lateral to the flexor carpi radialis. **Distal** refers to distance; distal refers to sites located away from the center (trunk of the body). Its course is described by a line drawn from the middle of the cubital fossa to the medial side of the radial styloid process. It is easiest to approach the artery with an incision in the distal two-thirds of the forearm along this line.

The ulnar artery is located on the medial side of the distal forearm. It lies between the tendon of the flexor carpi ulnaris muscle and the tendons of the flexor digitorum superficialis muscle. Here, it will always be found traveling with the ulnar nerve, with which it should not be confused. Together with the venae comitantes, the nerve and artery will be found in a connective tissue sheath from which the vessels must be freed before beginning injection.

The course of the ulnar artery is indicated by a line curving medially from the midpoint of the cubital fossa to the pisiform bone in the wrist. An incision along the distal one-third of this line permits access to the flexor carpi ulnaris muscle, which is then reflected medially to expose the ulnar artery.

### Radial Artery

#### Linear Guide
Draw or visualize a line on the surface of the skin of the forearm from the center of the antecubital fossa to the center of the base of the index finger (**Fig. 8–10**).

#### Anatomical Guide
The radial artery lies just lateral to the tendon of the flexor carpiradialis muscle and just medial to the tendon of the brachioradialis muscle.

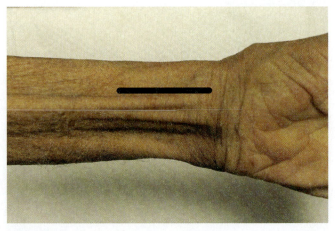

**Figure 8–10.** Linear guide for the radial artery.

## Anatomical Limit
The radial artery extends from a point approximately 1 inch below and in front of the bend of the elbow to a point over the base of the thumb (thenar eminence).

## Origin
The radial artery originates at the bifurcation of the brachial artery.

## Relationship of the Radial Artery and the Venae Comitantes
Two small veins (venae comitantes) lie on either side of the artery. They may be helpful in locating the artery, for they generally contain some blood. The corresponding venae comitantes go by the same name as the artery.

# Ulnar Artery
## Linear Guide
Draw or visualize a line on the surface of the skin from the center of the antecubital fossa on the forearm to a point between the fourth and fifth fingers (**Fig. 8–11**).

## Anatomical Guide
The ulnar artery lies just lateral to the tendon of the flexor carpi ulnaris muscle. (It lies between the tendons of the flexor carpi ulnaris and flexor digitorum superficialis.)

## Anatomical Limit
The ulnar artery extends from a point approximately 1 inch below and in front of the bend of the elbow to a point over the pisiform bone (hypothenar eminence).

## Origin
The ulnar artery originates at the bifurcation of the brachial artery.

## Relationship of the Ulnar Artery to the Venae Comitantes
Two small veins (venae comitantes) lie on either side of the artery. They can be useful in locating the artery, for they generally contain some blood.

# ARTERIES AND VEINS OF THE TRUNK

The arteries and veins of the trunk (**Table 8-1**) are shown in the illustration of the vascular anatomy of the trunk (**Fig. 8–12A,B**).

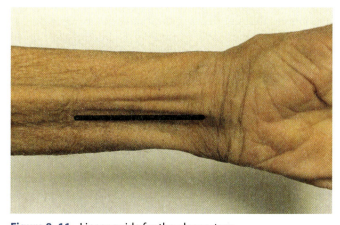

**Figure 8–11.** Linear guide for the ulnar artery.

**TABLE 8–1. Arteries of the Body Trunk**

| Artery | Description | Branches |
|---|---|---|
| Ascending aorta | Originates at the left ventricle; at its beginning, the aortic semilunar valve should close, thus creating the pathway for arterial solution distribution | Right coronary artery<br>Left coronary artery |
| Arch of the aorta | Center of arterial solution distribution | Brachiocephalic artery<br>Left common carotid artery<br>Left subclavian artery |
| Right subclavian | Begins at the right sternoclavicular articulation and extends to the lateral border of the first rib; in the complete autopsy (with neck organs removed), the branches need to be clamped | Vertebral artery<br>Internal thoracic artery<br>Inferior thyroid |
| Left subclavian | Begins at the level of the left second costal cartilage and extends to the lateral border of the first rib | |
| Descending thoracic aorta | Begins at the end of the aortic arch | Its branches include nine pairs of thoracic intercostal arteries |
| Descending abdominal aorta | Extends from the diaphragm to the lower border of the fourth lumbar vertebra | • Parietal<br>• Inferior phrenic<br>• Superior suprarenals<br>• Lumbar<br>• Middle sacral<br>• Visceral (unpaired)<br>• Celiac axis<br>• Superior mesenteric<br>• Inferior mesenteric<br>• Visceral (paired)<br>• Middle suprarenals<br>• Renals<br>• Internal spermatic (male), ovarian (female)<br>• Common iliacs (terminal) |

The aorta is the largest and main artery in the body. When available, the thoracic and abdominal aorta may be used for injection of partial autopsy and organ donation cases. The scope of the autopsy or recovery will determine which area of the aortic vessel is accessible. When the superior portion of the aortic arch remains intact, the ascending aorta may be injected to supply the head, neck, and arms.

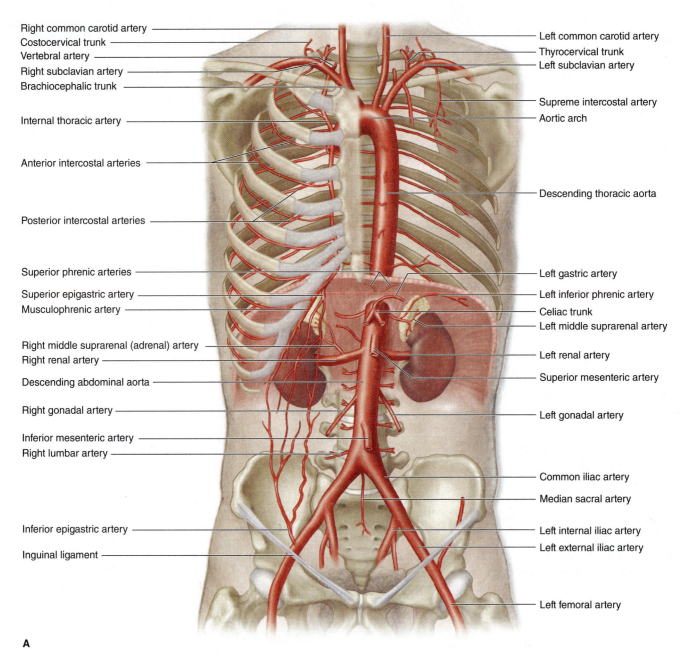

**Figure 8–12.** **A.** Arteries of the trunk. **B.** Veins of the trunk. (Used with permission from McKinley M et al. *Human Anatomy*. 5th ed. New York, McGraw Hill, 2017, Figs. 23.12 and 23.13.)

## ARTERIES AND VEINS OF THE LOWER LIMBS

An illustration of the vascular anatomy of the lower limb shows the arteries and veins found in the leg and foot (**Fig. 8–13A,B**).

### External Iliac Artery and Vein

The common iliac arteries are the terminal branches of the abdominal aorta. The external and internal iliac arteries are the continuations of the common iliac arteries. The external iliac artery lies lateral to the external iliac vein (**Fig. 8–14**).

The external iliac artery extends to a point under the center of the inguinal ligament and becomes the femoral artery as it continues below the inguinal ligament. The term *iliofemoral* is used to describe this area of the inguinal ligament where the same vessel changes names.

The external iliac is the main supply to the lower extremity. The internal iliac supplies the gluteal and pelvic tissues as well as the external genitalia. When available, the internal iliac should also be injected.

## INGUINAL REGION

The area below the inguinal ligament is known as the inguinal region. To locate the femoral artery, two bony prominences serve as landmarks. The anterior superior spine of the ilium and the pubic tubercle serve as attachments for the inguinal ligament and are readily identified. The position of the underlying femoral vessels can be estimated with a manual approach. For the right femoral artery, the embalmer places their left thumb upon the right anterior superior iliac spine and their

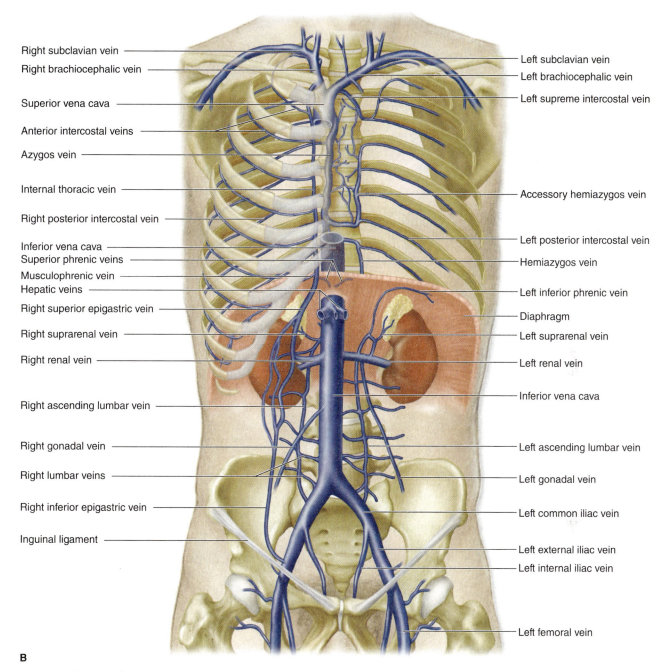

**B**

**Figure 8–12** (Continued)

left middle finger upon the right pubic tubercle. The position of the embalmer's left index finger approximates the location of the right femoral artery. This approach can be reversed for the left artery using the embalmer's right hand.

## FEMORAL TRIANGLE (SCARPA'S TRIANGLE)

The femoral triangle in the upper thigh appears as a triangular depression in the subfascial space. The Italian anatomist, Antonio Scarpa is credited with identifying the anatomical area on the thigh. The contents of the triangle include, from lateral to medial, the femoral nerve, femoral artery, and femoral vein. The anatomical borders of the femoral triangle include the inguinal ligament superiorly, the adductor longus muscle medially, and the sartorius muscle laterally.

Of high importance is the recognition that the femoral vessels are located *within* these boundaries. The femoral vessels are found inferior to the inguinal ligament, along the medial margin of the sartorius muscle and along the lateral margin of the adductor longus muscle (**Fig. 8–15**).

In addition to skin and subcutaneous tissue, the roof of the triangle consists of a thin casing of innervated connective tissue called *superficial fascia*. The deep fascia, or fascia lata, encloses the muscles of the thigh. On the surface of the fascia lata lies the great saphenous vein, which is often mistaken for the femoral vein.

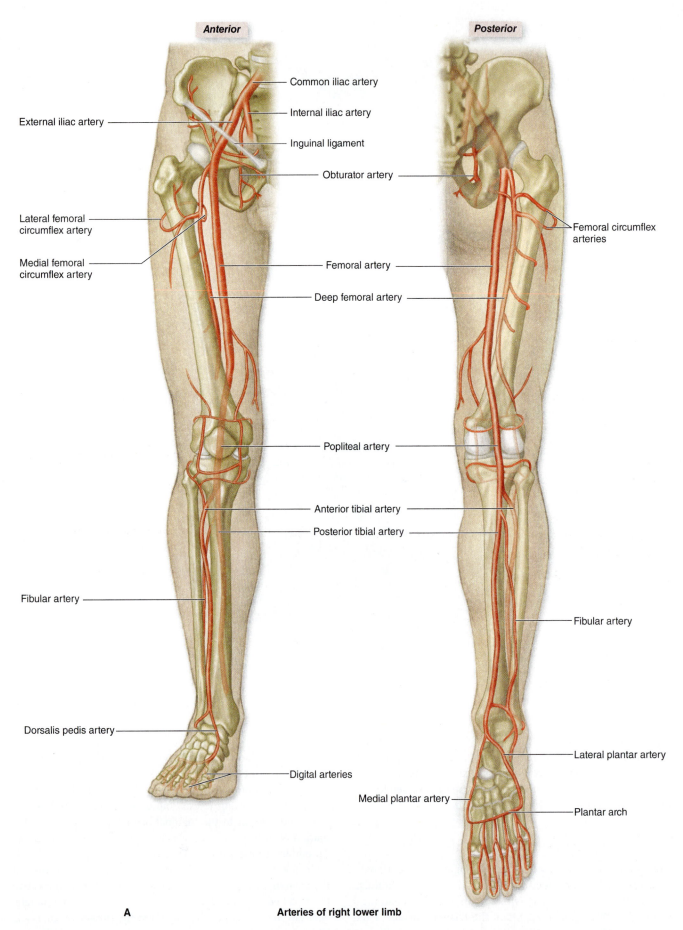

**Figure 8–13.** **A.** Arteries of the right lower limb. **B.** Veins of the right lower limb. (Used with permission from McKinley M et al. *Human Anatomy*. 5th ed. New York, McGraw Hill, 2017, Fig. 23.20AB.)

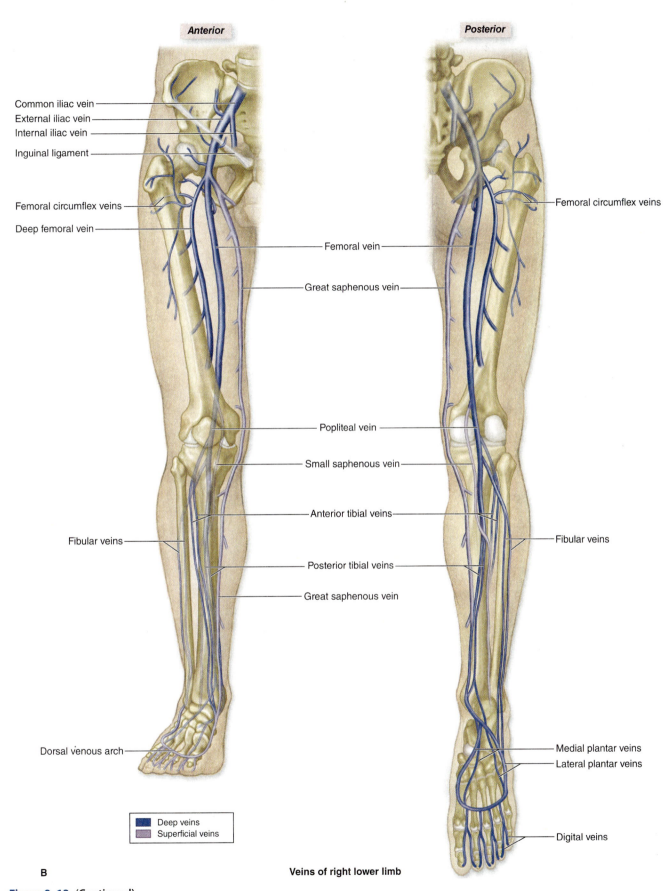

**Figure 8–13** (Continued)

Veins of right lower limb

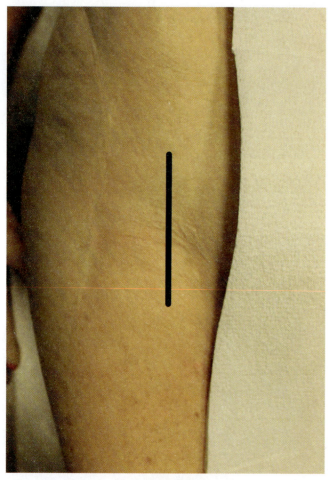

**Figure 8–14.** Linear guide for the external iliac artery.

The roof of the triangle must be incised and reflected to expose the contents. The femoral artery and vein are contained within the femoral sheath. The femoral nerve lies lateral and is not contained in the sheath.

The floor of the triangle is entirely muscular, comprised of the iliopsoas, the pectineus, and the adductor longus.

## Femoral Artery

### Linear Guide
Draw or visualize a line on the surface of the skin of the thigh from the center of the inguinal ligament to the center of the medial prominence of the knee; the medial condyle of the femur (**Fig. 8–16**). The incision is made along with the upper one-third of the linear guide, furthest from the knee.

### Anatomical Guide
The femoral artery passes through the center of the femoral triangle and is bounded laterally by the sartorius muscle (its medial border) and medially by the adductor longus muscle.

### Anatomical Limit
The femoral artery extends from a point behind the center of the inguinal ligament to the opening in the adductor magnus muscle.

### Origin
The femoral artery is a continuation of the external iliac artery.

### Branches
Superficial epigastric, superficial circumflex iliac, external pudendal, profunda femoris.

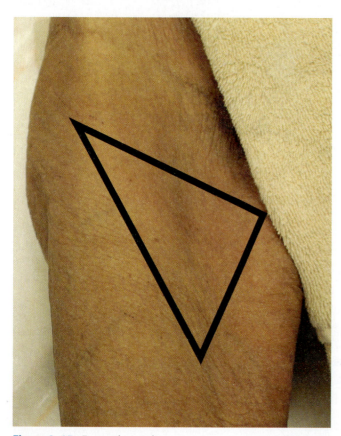

**Figure 8–15.** Femoral triangle.

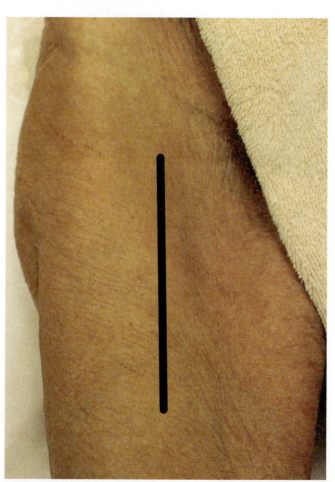

**Figure 8–16.** Linear guide for the femoral artery.

## Relationship of the Femoral Artery and Vein

The femoral artery lies lateral and superficial to the femoral vein.

## Popliteal Fossa

On the posterior aspect of the knee, two sets of tendons and two fleshy muscle heads can be identified. This describes the popliteal fossa as a trapezoid and can be subdivided into an upper femoral and a lower tibial triangle. The upper femoral triangle (not to be confused with the femoral triangle in the inguinal region) is bounded laterally by the long and short heads of the biceps femoris and medially by the tendons of the semimembranosus and semitendinosus muscles. The tibial triangle is limited medially and laterally by the diverging medial and lateral fleshy heads of the gastrocnemius muscle and, to a lesser extent, by the plantaris muscle laterally. The base of each triangle is an imaginary line drawn through the middle of the joint. These surface landmarks serve as guides to the underlying popliteal vessels within the boundaries of the space.

The muscular boundaries of this fossa are overlaid by a roof of deep fascia, subcutaneous tissue, and skin. Intrusion into this space provides access to the popliteal vessels for injection and drainage. After recognizing and dispatching minor vascular and nervous branches external to the deep fascia, the fascia is incised to gain access to the vessels. The major contents of the space include the tibial and peroneal nerves (from the sciatic) and their branches, the popliteal vein and its tributaries, the popliteal artery and its branches, and a generous amount of fat and lymphatic tissue.

As space is approached posteriorly, the first structures to be encountered are the tibial and peroneal nerves. The tibial nerve is the larger of the two and is located directly in the midline. The common peroneal nerve, on the other hand, leaves the sciatic nerve at about midthigh and courses down the lateral aspect of the popliteal space.

With the tibial nerve retracted, the popliteal vein comes into view, lying superficial (posterior) to the popliteal artery, which is the deepest (most anterior) structure in the fossa. The vessels are bound together by connective tissue, which must be loosened and reflected to gain access to the vessels.

Deep (anterior) to the popliteal artery, the floor of the fossa is formed by the lower end of the femur and a portion of the capsule surrounding the knee joint.

### Linear Guide

Draw or visualize a line on the surface of the skin from the center of the superior border of the popliteal space parallel to the long axis of the lower extremity to the center of the inferior border of the popliteal space (**Fig. 8–17**).

### Anatomical Guide

The popliteal vessels are located between the popliteal surface of the femur and the oblique popliteal ligament.

### Anatomical Limit

The popliteal artery extends from a point beginning at the opening of the adductor magnus muscle to the lower border of the popliteus muscle.

### Origin

The popliteal artery is a continuation of the femoral artery.

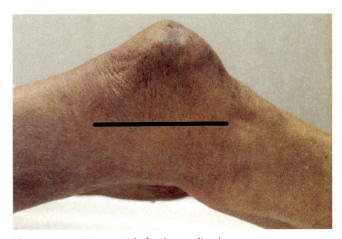

**Figure 8–17.** Linear guide for the popliteal artery.

### Branches

There are five pairs of genicular arteries and five muscular branches.

### Relationship of the Popliteal Artery and Vein

The vein lies posterior and medial to the artery. Because of the location of these vessels, the vein can also be described as lying superficial to the artery.

## DISTAL LEG

In the distal leg, the superficiality of the anterior tibial artery makes it easily accessible as an injection site. The popliteal artery ends by dividing into two terminal branches: the anterior tibial artery and the posterior tibial artery. The branches begin at the lower border of the popliteus muscle. In the distal portion of the leg, the arteries become superficial and can be used as points of injection for the foot. Injection could also be made toward the head to embalm the distal leg and thigh.

The anterior tibial artery is the smaller of the terminal branches of the popliteal artery. As it approaches the distal portion of the leg, it becomes very superficial. It can be raised by making an incision just above the ankle, just lateral to the crest of the tibia. In front of the ankle joint, the anterior tibial artery now becomes the dorsalis pedis artery.

The posterior tibial artery is also one of the terminal branches of the popliteal artery and passes posteriorly and medially down the leg. In the area between the medial malleolus and the calcaneus bone, the artery can be raised by the embalmer for injection of the foot. The artery terminates by dividing into the medial and lateral plantar arteries.

### Anterior and Posterior Tibial Arteries

#### Linear Guide

*Anterior Tibial Artery:* Draw or visualize a line from the lateral border of the patella to the anterior surface of the ankle joint.
*Posterior Tibial Artery:* Draw or visualize a line on the surface of the skin from the center of the popliteal space to a point midway between the medial malleolus and the calcaneus bone (**Fig. 8–18**).

#### Anatomical Guide

*Anterior Tibial Artery:* The anterior tibial vessels are located in a groove between the tibialis anterior muscle and the tendon

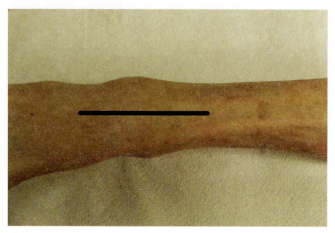

**Figure 8–18.** Linear guide for the anterior tibial artery.

of the extensor hallucis longus muscle. *Posterior Tibial Artery:* The posterior tibial vessels are located between the posterior border of the tibia and the calcaneus tendon.

### Anatomical Limit
*Anterior Tibial Artery:* The anterior tibial artery extends from a point beginning at the inferior border of the popliteus muscle to a point in front of the middle of the ankle joint on the respective sides. *Posterior Tibial Artery:* The posterior tibial artery extends from a point beginning at the inferior border of the popliteus muscle to a point over and between the medial malleolus and the calcaneus of the respective foot.

### Branches and Tributaries of the Vessels
*Anterior Tibial Vessels, Posterior Tibial Vessels:* right and left peroneal branches, right and left dorsalis pedis arteries.

## FOOT
Tendons passing onto the dorsum of the foot from the leg pass posterior to and are restrained by two thickenings of fascia, the superior and inferior extensor retinacula, which lie anterior to the ankle. In addition, the anterior tibial artery and the deep peroneal nerve also pass deep to these retinacula. Only inconsequential superficial nerves and veins lie superficial to these retinacula.

Skin on the dorsum of the foot is thin and loosely applied. The subcutaneous tissue permits easy visualization of the venous network, which is so prominent here. Tendons of two extrinsic muscles of the foot, the extensor hallucis longus, and the extensor digitorum longus, are easily identified as they pass to the great toe and digits two through five, respectively. The dorsalis pedis artery is situated in the interosseous spaces between the tendon of extensor hallucis longus and the first tendon of extensor digitorum longus as it passes to the second digit.

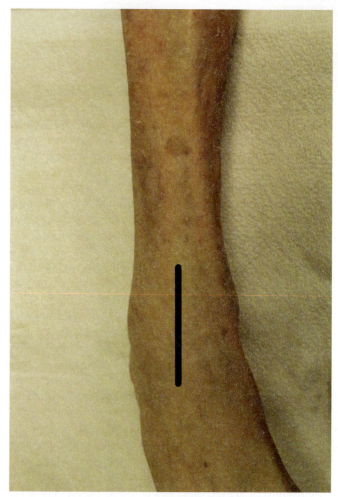

**Figure 8–19.** Linear guide for the dorsalis pedis.

### Dorsalis Pedis Artery
#### Linear Guide
Draw or visualize a line from the center of the anterior surface of the ankle joint to a point between the first and second toes (**Fig. 8–19**).

An incision made from a point midway between the medial and lateral malleoli to the interosseous space will provide access to the dorsalis pedis artery. Supplemental hypodermic embalming of the foot is commonly practiced and is also an effective alternative to arterial injection.

## CONCEPTS FOR STUDY

Define the following terminology:
- Anatomical guide
- Anatomical limit
- Anterior triangle
- Cervicoaxillary canal
- Fascia lata
- Linear Guide
- Omohyoid
- Platysma
- Sternocleidomastoid muscle

1. Define and illustrate the importance of anatomical position.
2. Explain anatomical guide, linear guide, and anatomical limit.
3. Describe the anterior triangle and identify the vessels contained within the triangle.
4. Recall the linear guide and the anatomical guide for the common carotid artery.
5. Explain the relationship of the internal jugular vein to the common carotid artery.
6. Summarize the features supplied by the facial artery.
7. List the three bony structures bordering the cervicoaxillary canal.
8. Describe the axilla and identify the artery found in this space.
9. Recall the linear and anatomical guides and anatomical limits for the brachial artery.
10. Give the origin of the radial and ulnar arteries.
11. Discuss the location of the nerve, artery, and vein within the femoral triangle.
12. Use the term iliofemoral in a sentence.
13. Recognize which areas are supplied when injecting the ascending aorta.
14. List two types of cases that could be embalmed using the abdominal aorta.

## FIGURE CREDIT

Figures 8–3, 8–4, 8–5, 8–7, 8–8, 8–9, 8–10, 8–11, 8–14, 8–15, 8–16, 8–17, 8–18, 8–19 are used with permission of Kevin Drobish.

# CHAPTER 9

# Embalming Vessel Sites and Selections

## CHAPTER OVERVIEW

- Selection of Vessels for Injection and Drainage
- Comparison of Arteries, Veins, and Nerves
- Types of Incisions for the Common Carotid Artery
- Techniques for Raising Vessels
- Types of Incisions for Preparing Vessels

There are numerous sites throughout the human anatomy to raise arteries and veins for arterial embalming. One major objective of the pre-embalming analysis is to determine which sites are most suitable given the conditions present. The vessels selected for injection and drainage should produce the most satisfactory results. Evaluation during embalming often necessitates injection at secondary sites to achieve an optimal outcome. Post-embalming evaluation indicates when supplemental embalming treatments, such as hypodermic and topical treatments, are necessary. The stable condition of the decedent is maintained through periodic monitoring and providing additional care as needed.

## SELECTION OF VESSELS

The arteries most frequently utilized for embalming are
- common carotid,
- femoral (or external iliac if raised at the inguinal ligament), and
- axillary (or brachial).

With respect to comparison in size and diameter, the common carotid artery is usually the largest, followed by the femoral (or, the external iliac). This does occur in the reverse. The axillary artery is the smaller of these vessels. While any artery could be used as an injection site to reach the entire body, the smallest vessels may not be ideal. Sufficient pressures and rates of flow needed to adequately distribute and diffuse the arterial solution could be difficult to achieve and the process could become time intensive. Smaller arteries are usually reserved for secondary injection sites to reach specific areas. The larger, more elastic arteries, like the common carotid and femoral, accept the higher pressures and faster rates of flow necessary to achieve uniform distribution and diffusion of the arterial solution.

The accessibility and condition of the artery are factors for consideration. Vessels with greater flexibility and with few branches are more easily lifted from the incision (**Fig. 9-1**). The common carotid arteries have no branches (except their terminal bifurcation). The femoral arteries and the external iliac arteries (at the inguinal ligament) are not held tightly in position by large numbers of branches. Any vessel presenting with moderate arteriosclerosis will be less flexible. Severe sclerosis can completely occlude the vessel lumen rendering it unusable for injection.

Selection of the vein that will be used for blood drainage is equally as important as the artery used for injection. Each vein that accompanies an artery may be used for blood drainage. The internal jugular vein is companion to the common carotid artery. The femoral vein is companion to the femoral artery. The axillary vein accompanies the axillary artery. And the basilic vein is companion to the brachial artery. The internal jugular vein is the most frequently selected vein for blood drainage. Its close proximity to the right atrium of the heart (the center of venous drainage) makes it an ideal pairing with any selected artery.

## COMPARISON OF ARTERIES, VEINS, AND NERVES

Identification of the many structures found within the incision site guides the embalmer to locate and raise various vessels. To the untrained eye, the external surface of an artery, nerve, and vein look alike. Comparison of the characteristics of arteries, veins, and nerves serves to differentiate between them and ensure correct identification (**Table 9-1**).

**Nerves** are solid structures lacking the lumen present in both arteries and veins. They have a silvery white appearance. Visible surface striations are indicative of the composition of a nerve; bundles of nerve fibers surrounded by connective tissue. When a nerve is incised, the edges fray similar to the ends of a cut rope.

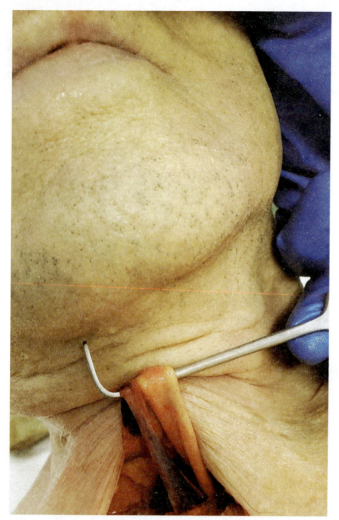

**Figure 9-1.** Elasticity in common carotid artery and internal jugular vein.

**Veins** are thin-walled vessels that contain a lumen. The **lumen** is the opening or inside space of the vessel or other tubular structure. They have a bluish appearance when filled with blood; opaque when not blood-filled. Veins have internal valves to prevent the backflow of circulating blood. Upon mistakenly injecting a vein, the telltale sign is that fluid will not distribute and instead flow back out from the vessel. A vein will collapse upon itself when cut; making the lumen of the vessel difficult to access. The grooved director is helpful to locate and expand the opening for insertion of a drainage device. Postmortem, veins usually contain blood.

**Arteries** are thick-walled vessels. Their off-white color allows the **vasa vasorum** to be seen over the surface of the artery. Vasa vasorum (vv), or "vessels on vessels" are tiny blood vessels that supply the large vessel walls with nutrients. The lumen stands open and pronounced when cut. Arteries may be differentiated from veins and nerves by rolling the vessel gently between a thumb and forefinger. The thick walls will move in opposition. Arteries do not have valves which makes them suitable for injection in either direction of the vessel.

## SELECTING AN ARTERY AS AN INJECTION POINT

The selection of an artery, or arteries for embalming is based on numerous factors. Asking the following questions assists the embalmer in making the best choice:
1. How superficial or deep is the artery?
2. What other structures surround the artery?
3. How close is the artery to the aorta?
4. What is the diametric size of the artery?
5. Will selection of the artery interfere with body positioning?
6. Can the incision be easily concealed when clothing does not cover the incision?
7. Can drainage be taken from the companion vein?
8. In which direction will arterial clots move during injection?
9. Is arteriosclerosis present in the artery?

## TYPES OF INCISIONS FOR THE COMMON CAROTID ARTERY

Several types of incisions are available to raise the common carotid artery and internal jugular vein (**Fig. 9-2A-F**).

**Supraclavicular (anterior lateral):** The incision is made along the clavicle (collar bone) from a point near the sternoclavicular articulation and is directed laterally. Making the incision on the upper surface of the bone prevents the cutting instrument from continuing too deeply and inadvertently damaging the underlying vessels.

**Anterior vertical (parallel):** The incision is made from a point near the sternoclavicular articulation and is directed superiorly along the sternocleidomastoid muscle. The muscle serves as a structural guide for the cutting instrument.

**Posterior vertical (parallel):** The incision is made posterior to the sternocleidomastoid muscle, 2 inches below the lobe of the ear, and is directed inferiorly toward the base of the neck.

**Anterior horizontal:** The incision is made at the base of the neck from a point on the sternocleidomastoid muscle and is directed posteriorly. The anterior horizontal can be visible with collarless shirts or low necklines.

**Semilunar (flap incision):** The incision extends from a point lateral and slightly superior to the sternoclavicular articulation and is directed inferiorly, crosses the upper chest in an arc, and

| TABLE 9-1. Comparison of Arteries, Veins, and Nerves |||
|---|---|---|
| **Artery** | **Vein** | **Nerve** |
| Has a lumen | Has a lumen | Solid structure; no lumen |
| Off-white | Bluish when blood-filled | Silvery white |
| Vasa vasorum visible | Vasa vasorum not visible | Vasa vasorum not visible |
| Thick vessel wall | Thin vessel wall | Solid structure |
| Vessel walls roll between two fingers | Vessel walls do not roll between two fingers | Nerve does not roll |
| Stands open when cut | Collapses when cut | Nerve fibers fray when cut |
| Have no valves | Have valves | Have no valves |
| Not usually blood-filled | Usually blood-filled | Not blood-filled |

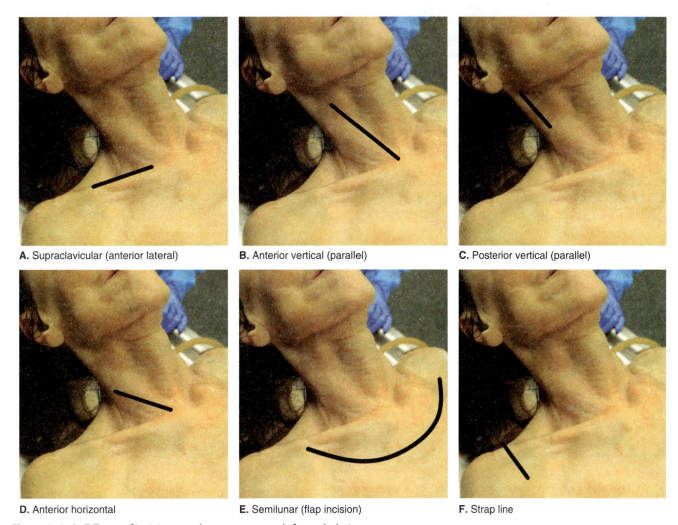

**A.** Supraclavicular (anterior lateral)  **B.** Anterior vertical (parallel)  **C.** Posterior vertical (parallel)

**D.** Anterior horizontal  **E.** Semilunar (flap incision)  **F.** Strap line

**Figure 9–2 A–F.** Types of incisions made to access vessels for embalming.

is directed superiorly to the opposite articulation. Contingent upon which direction the skin flap is to be reflected, the incision resembles either the letter "U" or an inverted "C." The semilunar incision is ideal when both right and left common carotids are raised, as in restricted cervical injection. The semilunar (flap incision) is also a treatment option to assist in the release of gases associated with tissue gas cases.

**Strap line:** The incision is made approximately 2 inches lateral to the base of the neck on the line where the shoulder strap of a sleeveless garment crosses the shoulder. The strap line is deliberately selected to conceal the incision beneath clothing; especially when the clothing style is known in advance and would have exposed an incision made in the neck area.

## LOCATING AND PREPARING VESSELS

After making an incision at the injection site, the embalmer performs blunt dissection to locate the vessels. The identification of adjacent anatomical structures guides the embalmer to finding vessels. Once the vessel is located, its tightly bound fascial covering is removed using an aneurysm hook or blunt-tipped hemostat. Removal of the fascia increases elasticity in the vessel. Ligature is placed around the vessel, and it is elevated for use. Vessels are incised to create an opening for insertion of the respective instruments; an arterial tube into the artery and a drainage device into the vein. To secure the arterial tube in place, an arterial hemostat can be used. The existing ligature can also be tightened around the arterial tube to prevent leakage of embalming solution during injection (**Fig. 9–3**).

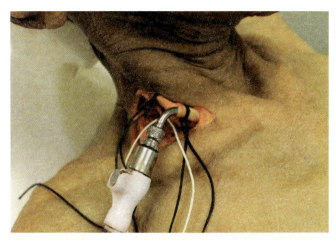

**Figure 9–3.** Ligature secures arterial tube in place.

Following injection, the ligature around both the artery and vein is tied securely to maintain intravascular pressure for thorough diffusion of solution and to prevent any residual leakage.

1. Select instruments.
2. Prepare ligatures.
3. Follow the linear guide to properly position the incision.
4. Make the incision; choose an area where the vessel is most superficial.
5. Perform blunt dissection. Muscle tissue usually can remain intact; vessels lie between the muscles.
6. Observe anatomical guides to locate the vessels.
7. Lift and clean each vessel.
8. Place two ligatures loosely around each vessel; place the first ligature superior and the second inferior.
9. Incise each vessel between the two ligatures.
10. Insert the appropriate instrument into each vessel. Secure arterial tubes in place.
11. Proceed with embalming.

The order in which vessels are raised varies, depending on the depth relationship of the artery to the vein. When both artery and vein are raised in the same location, this sequence minimizes damage to either vessel.

- Raise the superficial vessel first.
- Insert instruments into the deepest vessel first.

*Example.* When raising the internal jugular vein and the common carotid artery, the vein is the superficial vessel. After a ligature is placed around the vein, it is pulled laterally to expose the deeper artery. The artery is described as medial and deep in relation to the vein. Incise the artery, insert and secure the arterial tube. Incise the vein and insert the drainage instrument. Select an arterial tube slightly smaller than the lumen of the artery to avoid damage to the intimal lining. In cases of mild arteriosclerosis, the grooved director can be inserted prior to the arterial tube to verify that the lumen is unrestricted (**Fig. 9–4**).

## MAKING THE INCISION INTO THE ARTERY AND VEIN

An arterial scissors or a scalpel is commonly used to incise the artery for insertion of an arterial tube, and the vein for insertion of a drainage device. Several incision methods are practiced (**Fig. 9–5**).

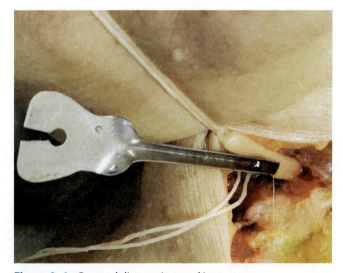

**Figure 9–4.** Grooved director inserted into artery.

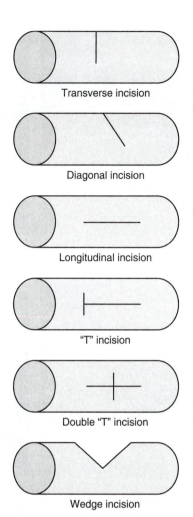

**Figure 9–5.** Types of incisions for opening vessels.

The most common methods are the transverse and diagonal incisions (**Fig. 9–6**). Both incisions are made by cutting from the edge of the vessel to its center or slightly beyond center. The variant for the diagonal incision is to angle the cut toward the center. Incising too far can damage and break the vessel in two. The presence of sclerosis in an artery makes the vessel more fragile and less elastic. As soon as the lumen is observed in a sclerotic artery, discontinue the cut and manipulate the artery as little as possible. Too much tension used to raise the artery can also cause it to rupture.

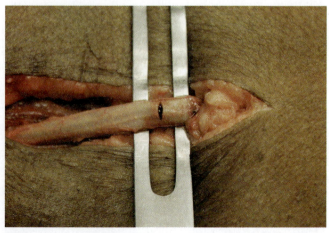

**Figure 9–6.** Transverse incision.

A longitudinal incision begins at the center and runs parallel with the vessel. This method is favored for creating a large opening without compromising the vessel. The larger opening in the vein accommodates greater manipulation of the drainage instrument. In an artery, two opposing arterial tubes can be inserted simultaneously. The longitudinal incision is not recommended for sclerotic arteries. A combination of longitudinal and transverse incision, such as the "T" and double "T" also create a large opening. Two arterial tubes can be placed in opposite directions, and venous drainage can occur from both directions.

The wedge incision removes a wedge-shaped portion from the side of the vessel. The wedge is cut with arterial scissors, double-point scissors, or a scalpel. This method allows the insertion of large diameter instruments. The wedge is not recommended for sclerotic arteries.

## INSTRUMENTS

Commonly used instruments to raise an artery for injection and a vein for drainage.

| Instrument | Use |
| --- | --- |
| Scalpel | Make incisions; superficial dissection; incise the artery or vein |
| Surgical scissors | Make incisions; cut ligatures; incise the artery or vein |
| Arterial scissors | Incise a vessel; some styles cut needle injector wires |
| Aneurysm hook | Dissects fat and fascia; elevates and secures vessels |
| Separator | Elevates and secures vessels |
| Arterial tube | Inserted into artery for injection of embalming solution |
| Drain tube or Angular spring forceps | Inserted into vein for drainage of blood and body fluids |
| Arterial hemostat | Secures arterial tube in artery |
| Spring forceps | Passes ligatures around vessels |
| Grooved director | Expands vein for insertion of the drainage device or guides an arterial tube into an artery |

## VESSELS USED FOR ARTERIAL EMBALMING

The vessels most commonly used for arterial embalming are the right common carotid artery and the right jugular vein. The right common carotid is a terminal branch of the brachiocephalic artery. The left is a branch of the arch of the aorta. The acronym ANV is helpful to describe the relationship of the common carotid artery, vagus nerve, and internal jugular vein. From medial to lateral: artery, nerve, vein.

### Common Carotid Artery

1. Regions supplied
   a. When the injection is directed superiorly, the face and head are embalmed.
   b. When the injection is directed inferiorly, the opposite side of the face and head as well as the remainder of the body receives solution.
2. Considerations
   a. Large in diameter.
   b. No branches (except the terminal bifurcations).
   c. Flexible; rarely sclerotic.
   d. Close to the arch of the aorta, center of circulation in the dead human body.
   e. Supplies fluid directly to the head and the face.
   f. Accompanied by a large vein (internal jugular), which can be used for drainage.
   g. Injection inferiorly will direct arterial coagula away from the head.
3. Precautions
   a. The facial features can distend; solution concentrates in the area nearest injection, and a rapid rate of flow and high pressure can cause immediate swelling.
   b. Instruments improperly positioned can indent the facial tissues.
   c. Clothing may not conceal the incision.
   d. Leakage must be controlled to prevent the visible soiling of clothing.
4. Raising the artery
   a. Take a position at the head of the embalming table.
   b. Turn the head of the body in the direction opposite that of the vessels being raised (i.e., to raise the right common carotid, turn the head to the left).
   c. Place a positioning block beneath the shoulders and lower the head onto the head block.
   d. Make the incision.
   e. Dissect superficial fat, fascia, and divide muscle tissues to expose the artery.
   f. Raise the internal jugular vein first; ligate and pull the vein laterally.
   g. Locate the common carotid artery medial and deep; raise and ligate.

### Internal Jugular Vein

The right internal jugular vein leads directly into the right atrium of the heart through the right brachiocephalic and superior vena cava. The right atrium is considered the center of venous drainage in the dead human body (**Fig. 9-7**). For this reason, the right internal jugular vein is the preferred drainage site. The left internal jugular, also large in size, does not lead directly into the right atrium. Instead, it joins with the left subclavian vein to form the left brachiocephalic vein. The left brachiocephalic vein crosses to the right side of the chest, joins with the opposite brachiocephalic vein, and forms the superior vena cava.

1. Considerations
   a. Large in diameter.
   b. Direct access to the right atrium; easy removal of blood and coagula.
   c. Direct drainage of the face and head.
   d. Accompanied by a large artery (common carotid), which can be used for injection.
2. Precautions
   a. The facial features can distend if clotted material blocks blood drainage.

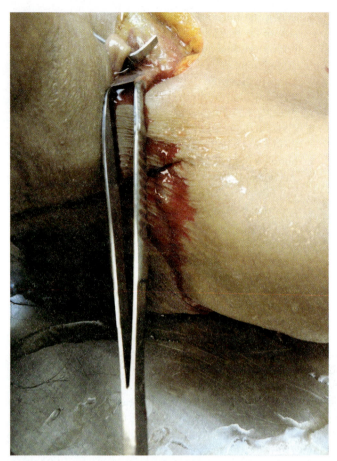

**Figure 9–7.** Angular spring forceps inserted into the right atrium of the heart.

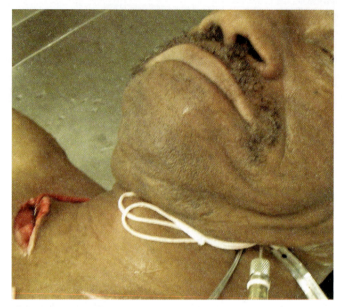

**Figure 9–8.** Facial artery.

   b. Instruments improperly positioned can indent the facial tissues.
   c. Clothing may not conceal the incision.
   d. Leakage must be controlled to prevent the visible soiling of clothing.
3. Raising the vein
   a. Take a position at the head of the embalming table.
   b. Turn the head of the body in the direction opposite that of the vessels being raised (i.e., to raise the right internal jugular, turn the head to the left).
   c. Place a positioning block beneath the shoulders and lower the head onto the head block.
   d. Make the incision.
   e. Dissect superficial fat, fascia, and divide muscle tissues to expose the vein.
   f. Raise the internal jugular vein, gently remove the fascial covering, raise and ligate and pull laterally to expose the artery.

## Facial Artery

The facial artery is one of eight branches of the external carotid artery. The facial artery is usually reserved for injection of the facial tissues when the common carotid artery is either damaged or unavailable. Portions of the common and external carotid may be missing after autopsy, donation, or trauma. Severe coagula or sclerosis can prevent its use entirely. The facial artery may be used to supplement preservation in the event the common carotid did not provide sufficient solution to the facial tissues (**Fig. 9–8**).

The facial artery supplies the medial and soft tissues of the face; the upper and lower lips, the area around the mouth, the sides of the nose, and portions of the lower eyelid. The facial artery is similar in size to the radial and requires use of a small diameter arterial tube.

In life, a pulse can be felt by resting a finger on the inferior margin of the mandible just in front of the angle of the jaw. In this same location, a small incision is made to raise the artery. The platysma muscle is divided by blunt dissection as the aneurysm hook is guided along the inferior margin of the mandible to locate the artery. This small incision is easily sealed after use with a super adhesive.

## Axillary Artery

The axillary artery is a continuation of the subclavian artery. The artery begins at the lateral border of the first rib after passing through the **cervicoaxillary canal**.

In the early years of embalming at the residence, the axillary artery was the preferred site to inject the entire body. Axillary injection was considered very clean. Blood drainage was generally taken directly by trocar from the right side of the heart (*see Direct Heart Drainage method in the section on the Right Atrium*). Early arterial solutions were strong, so large volumes were not injected. Facial discolorations quickly cleared, and the incision was easily concealed.

Today, the axillary artery is used principally as a secondary point of injection when arterial solution reaching the arm or hand is insufficient (**Fig. 9–9**).

The right internal jugular vein is often used for blood drainage as the axillary vein is relatively small and may not evacuate clotted materials.
1. Regions supplied
   a. When the arterial tube is directed toward the hand, the axillary supplies solution directly to the arm and hand.
   b. When the tube is directed toward the trunk, the entire body receives solution.

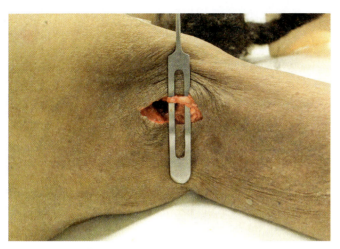

**Figure 9–9.** Axillary artery.

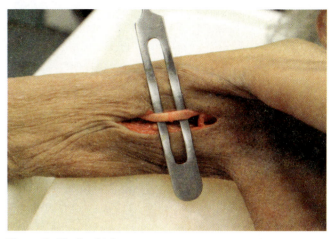

**Figure 9–10.** Brachial artery.

2. Considerations
   a. Arterial solution flows directly into the arm and hand.
   b. The artery is close to the face.
   c. The vessels are superficial.
   d. The artery is close to the center of arterial solution distribution (arch of the aorta).
3. Precautions
   a. The arm must be extended (abducted) to effectively use the vein for drainage.
   b. The artery is small for injection of the entire body.
   c. The companion vein is small for drainage, especially viscous blood.
   d. Facial tissues may distend.
   e. Numerous branches exist.
   f. Vascular anomalies are common.
4. Raising the axillary artery and vein
   a. The arm is abducted slightly less than 90 degrees from the trunk. The incision is made parallel to the linear guide, along the anterior margin of the hairline of the axilla.
   b. The artery is found just anterior and deep to the vein and the brachial plexus. The location of the axillary vein is described as medial and superficial to the axillary artery.

## Brachial Artery

The brachial artery is a continuation of the axillary artery. The brachial artery is used principally as a secondary point of injection to reach the forearm and hand. The right internal jugular vein is often preferred for blood drainage as the accompanying basilic vein is very small. When the arterial tube is directed toward the trunk, the artery can embalm the entire body. However, its small size limits the arterial pressure required to deliver effective overall distribution.

The incision for the brachial artery may be made anywhere along the upper half of the linear guide. The proximal third is preferred; approximately 1 inch above and parallel to the linear guide (**Fig. 9–10**).

Alternatively, the brachial artery can be raised in the area of the antecubital fossa, where the artery divides into the radial and ulnar arteries. The arterial tube can be directed into each of these arteries from this point, avoiding a distal incision in the wrist.

## Radial Artery

The radial artery originates at the bifurcation of the brachial artery and supplies solution directly to the lateral side of the hand (thumb). The arterial tube may be reversed to supplement solution to the arm. The artery is superficial and easily palpated in the wrist. In the living subject, this is a pulse point. The incision is made parallel to the vessel directly on the linear guide, approximately 1 inch above the base of the thumb (**Fig. 9–11**).

## Ulnar Artery

The ulnar artery also originates at the bifurcation of the brachial artery and supplies solution directly to the medial side of the hand (little finger). The arterial tube may be reversed to supplement solution to the arm. The incision is made parallel to the vessel directly over the linear guide (**Fig. 9–12**).

If blood discolorations in the hand do not clear, digital pressure can be applied to one vessel while the other is injected. The application of pressure prevents short-circuiting so that solution can reach both sides of the hand.

Potential for leakage exists from anterior incisions on the wrist. When the hands are positioned at the sides or upon the abdomen, the incision becomes dependent. Post-embalming treatment of the incision must prevent soiling of clothing or fabric.

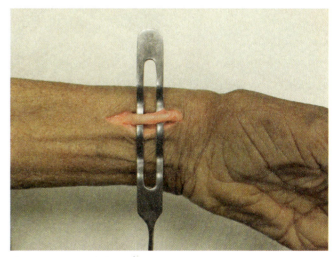

**Figure 9–11.** Radial artery.

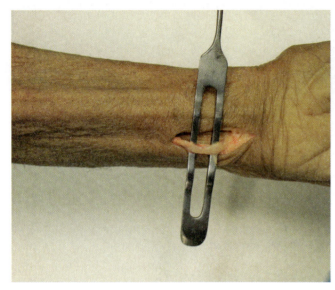

**Figure 9–12.** Ulnar artery.

## Femoral Artery

The second most frequently selected vessels for arterial embalming are the femoral artery and the femoral vein. The femoral artery is a continuation of the external iliac artery and is located superficial and lateral to the femoral vein (**Fig. 9–13**).

Nearest the inguinal ligament, the region is called **iliofemoral** because determination of the exact point where the external iliac artery ends and the femoral artery begins is imprecise.

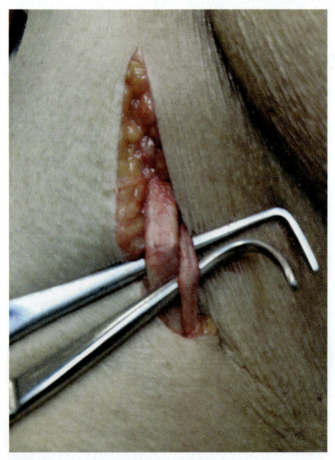

**Figure 9–13.** Femoral artery and femoral vein.

1. Regions supplied
    a. When the injection is directed toward the foot, the leg and the foot are embalmed.
    b. When the injection is directed toward the head, the opposite leg as well as the remainder of the body receives solution.
2. Considerations
    a. Large in diameter.
    b. The incision is not visible.
    c. Both sides of the head and face receive solution simultaneously (important when dye is added to the arterial solution).
    d. The artery is accompanied by a large vein (femoral vein), which can be used for drainage.
3. Precautions
    a. Arteriosclerosis commonly affects this artery.
    b. Vessels may be very deep in obese cases.
    c. Solution reaches the head uncontrolled, especially when large volumes or strong solutions are used.
    d. Arterial coagula can be pushed toward vessels that supply viewable areas.
    e. Large branches can be mistaken for the femoral artery.
4. Incision for the femoral artery and vein
    a. Draw a line centered between the anterior superior iliac spine and the pubic symphysis. The incision is made along the medial edge of this linear guide. The femoral artery lies lateral and slightly superficial to the femoral vein. The acronym VAN is helpful to describe the relationship of the femoral vein, femoral artery, and femoral nerve. From medial to lateral: vein, artery, nerve.
5. Raising the femoral artery and vein
    a. Stand at the right or the left side of the table.
    b. Make the incision parallel to the vessels, on the linear guide through the skin and the superficial fascia.
    c. Dissect superficial fat and fascia bluntly. Observe the great saphenous vein, which is quite superficial.
    d. Locate the sartorius muscle. The vessels are found along the medial side of this muscle.
    e. Locate the femoral artery. Remove the fascial covering. Raise and pass ligature around the superior and the inferior portions of the artery.
    f. Pull the artery laterally; dissect medially and deep to locate the femoral vein.
    g. Remove the fascial covering gently. Raise and pass ligature around the superior and the inferior portions of the vein.
    h. Make an incision into the vein and insert the drainage device toward the heart. Secure the device in place.
    i. Lift and incise the artery. Insert one arterial tube directed toward the head and a second tube directed down the leg. Inject the leg first.

## Femoral Vein

1. Considerations
    a. The vein is large.
    b. Use of a drain tube with attached length of hosing provides a clean method of drainage as well as containment for infectious drainage.

2. Precautions
   Blood drainage from the head, face, and upper body can be severely restricted by
   a. coagula and viscous blood;
   b. edema: ascites and hydrothorax; and
   c. visceral weight.

   The internal jugular vein(s) can be raised to supplement drainage to clear or prevent facial discolorations.

### Popliteal Artery

The popliteal artery is a continuation of the femoral artery and can be used as a secondary injection site when solution has not distributed below the knee. Its location behind the knee makes the popliteal artery less accessible than the tibial arteries. However, in the event that arthritic conditions have caused the legs to draw and the pelvis to twist, the popliteal may become accessible. The location and small size of the popliteal vein makes it unsuitable as drainage site.

To raise the popliteal artery the embalmer should perform either or both of the following:

(1) Roll the decedent to one side and make an incision down the center of the popliteal space, parallel to the artery.

(2) Flex the knee slightly and a make a longitudinal incision along the posterior–medial aspect of the lower third of the thigh, just superior to the popliteal space.

### Anterior and Posterior Tibial Arteries

The anterior and posterior tibial arteries supply arterial solution directly to the portion of the leg below the knee and into the foot. The anterior tibial artery is superficial and easily accessible as an injection site. The incision for raising the anterior tibial artery is made along the lateral margin of the inferior third of the crest of the tibia. In the distal portion of the leg, the artery lies at the superficial margin of the tibia (**Fig. 9–14**).

The aneurysm hook is used to dissect along the tibia to locate the artery. The incision for the posterior tibial artery is made midway between the medial malleolus and the large calcaneous tendon.

### Abdominal Aorta and Thoracic Aorta

The aorta is the largest artery in the body, travelling the length of the torso along its midline. The abdominal aorta and thoracic aorta are found within their respective cavities on the anterior surface of the spinal column. Either can be used for injection following partial autopsy or organ donation. Drainage may be taken directly from the inferior or superior vena cava. The aorta may also be selected for infant embalming when commonly used arteries are too small for injection.

### External Iliac Artery

The external iliac artery passes beneath the inguinal ligament and lies on the lateral side of the external iliac vein. The external iliac is more superficial than the femoral and can be selected as an alternate. The incision is made at the level of the inguinal ligament; an inch inferior or superior (**Fig. 9–15**).

Following a complete trunk autopsy, the external iliac is accessible from within the pelvic cavity. The artery supplies solution to the lower extremity and the anterior abdominal wall.

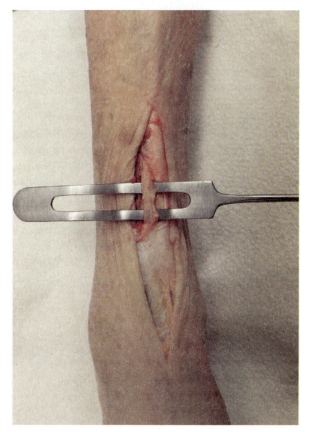

**Figure 9–14.** Anterior tibial artery.

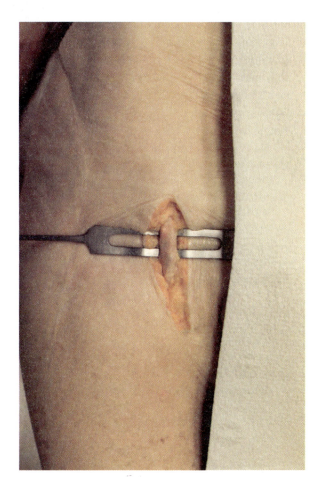

**Figure 9–15.** External iliac artery.

## Internal Iliac Artery

The internal iliac artery supplies embalming solution to the external genitalia, gluteal muscles, and the peroneal regions. Following a complete trunk autopsy, the internal iliac is accessible from within the pelvic cavity.

## Inferior Vena Cava

The inferior vena cava is the largest vein in the body. It is located to the right of the aorta at the posterior abdominal wall. The inferior vena cava is primarily used for blood drainage in cases of partial autopsy or organ donation. A mixture of blood and embalming solution drainage flow directly in the open cavities. The autopsy (or post) aspirator removes the collected drainage to reduce exposure and fumes, and to maintain visibility within the cavities. To build intravascular pressure, intermittent drainage can be created by clamping the inferior vena cava with a hemostat. Alternatively, a cotton compress can be pressed against the vena cava to stop and start drainage.

## Right Atrium of the Heart

The right atrium of the heart is the center for venous drainage in the dead human body. Routinely, during embalming of a nonautopsied body, a drainage device is inserted into the right internal jugular vein and guided into the right atrium. A different method involves piercing the right side of the heart with a trocar and guiding the tip of the instrument directly into the right atrium. **Direct heart drainage** is an historic method first practiced when embalming was done at the residence of the deceased. (*See Chapter 12 Injection and Drainage Techniques.*)

Today, direct drainage from the right atrium is recommended for infectious cases to eliminate contact with blood and bodily fluids. The drainage is contained within the tubing leading to the aspirator instead of freely flowing along the sides of the embalming table. The direct method is also beneficial when drainage is difficult to establish from a vein and to clear stubborn facial discolorations.

## CONCEPTS FOR STUDY

Define the following terminology:
- Diagonal incision
- Double T-incision
- Longitudinal incision
- Multipoint injection
- One-point injection
- Restricted Cervical injection
- Sectional embalming
- Six-point injection
- Split injection
- T-incision
- Transverse incision
- Wedge incision

1. Describe the characteristics of arteries, veins, and nerves.
2. Identify the two arteries most commonly used for arterial embalming.
3. Relate the advantages of using the largest vein for blood drainage.
4. Recall six incisions that can be used to raise the common carotid artery.
5. Analyze nine questions asked in considering an artery as an injection point.
6. Explain the location of the common carotid artery compared to the internal jugular vein.
7. Explain the location of the femoral artery compared to the femoral vein.
8. Describe the function of each instrument used in raising and preparing vessels for injection and drainage.
9. Evaluate the use of a small artery for injection of the entire body.
10. Describe where the incisions are made for raising the radial and ulnar arteries.
11. Critique each type of incision used to open vessels.
12. Review which incisions are not recommended to open sclerotic arteries.
13. Express the function of the grooved director.
14. Defend the use of multiple injection sites to achieve optimal embalming.

## FIGURE CREDIT

Figures 9-1, 9-4, 9-7, 9-8, 9-13 are used with permission of Sharon L. Gee-Mascarello.
Figures 9-2A-F, 9-3, 9-6, 9-9, 9-10, 9-11, 9-12, 9-14, 9-15 are used with permission of Kevin Drobish.
Figure 9-5 is used with permission of Cherie Mascarello.

## BIBLIOGRAPHY

American Board of Funeral Service Education, *Course Content Syllabus*, 2016.

CHAPTER 10

# Embalming Analysis

## CHAPTER OVERVIEW
- Pre-embalming Considerations
- Considerations During Embalming
- Post-embalming Considerations

The **embalming analysis** includes all analytical observations of the deceased human body before, during, and after embalming. Analysis incorporates the disciplines of anatomy, pathology, microbiology, chemistry, and restorative art. Observation, analysis, and corrective treatments continue until the time of final disposition. Periodic monitoring of the body for adverse conditions is the professional duty of the embalmer. Postmortem body conditions, embalming treatments, and any post-embalming corrective treatments are documented on the **Embalming and Decedent Care Report.**

## HISTORICAL METHODS OF ANALYSIS

Vintage embalming textbooks described hundreds of diseases, poisons, and traumatic modes of death. Treatments were concerned only with the specific pathology, specific poison, or specific trauma. No consideration was given to the various intrinsic and extrinsic factors, such as the time interval between death and preparation and evaluation of all other observable postmortem changes. A specific embalming treatment was outlined for each condition.

In the mid-1950s, the method of *body typing* was introduced. Dead bodies were classified by the conditions exhibited rather than by the specific cause of death. Professor Ray E. Slocum of The Dodge Company published a detailed system of body types based primarily on the time between death and preparation, and the degree of postmortem advancement. For instance, separate categories were established for bodies with jaundice and for infants. Six categories described specific chemical formulations necessary for the preparation of the body. Body typing was based on a *recipe method*. The embalmer followed a different recipe for treatment of each different classification. Variations of the *Slocum Method of Body Typing*, now called **pre-embalming analysis,** continue today. Most importantly, without the specific recipes.

The practice of medicine underwent radical change in the 1960s with the extensive development and use of new medications. The embalmer had to consider the influence of therapeutic medications upon postmortem conditions, in addition to consideration of all other postmortem factors.

## PRESENT-DAY METHODOLOGY

Embalmers consider the aggregate, or sum total of factors that are specific to each decedent. Every dead body is treated with respect to individual embalming requirements. Embalming analysis is applied during each phase of embalming, divided into three time periods: *before, during,* and *after* embalming. Embalming analysis is outlined by four steps:
1. Observation and evaluation of postmortem conditions.
2. Proposed methods of treatment.
3. Implementation of treatments.
4. Observation and evaluation of treatment results.

## COMMUNICATION OF POSTMORTEM AND POST-EMBALMING CONDITIONS

Decedent confidentiality must be strictly observed beyond the workplace. Shared information within the workplace is conducted on a need-to-know basis. Communications between various funeral service professionals, primarily the embalmer and the arranging funeral director, and between the professional and the deceased's family are encouraged.

For example, the arranging funeral director should be apprised of any concerns relating to the condition of the body or if additional time is needed for treatments. The height and weight of the deceased are important for selection of a casket and clothing. The expectations by the family related to the viewing of the deceased are important to communicate to the embalmer. For example, the family may assume that a tumor on the forehead will be removed.

## FACTORS CONSIDERED DURING EMBALMING ANALYSIS

The following factors are considered during embalming analysis. Observation and evaluation of these factors help the embalmer to formulate embalming treatments.
- Body conditions, including age, weight, musculature, body build

- Immediate cause and manner of death
- Effects of disease and/or trauma
- Effects of drugs and medical treatments
- Postmortem physical and chemical changes
- Postmortem procedures: refrigeration, autopsy, organ and tissue recovery
- Postmortem interval between death and embalming
- Post-embalming interval between preparation and disposition
- The embalmer also considers the following
- positioning of the body,
- method of mouth and eye closure,
- treatments for visible antemortem swellings that need to be reduced,
- treatments for removing or altering visible antemortem discolorations,
- techniques to use to raise sunken or emaciated facial tissues,
- vessels for injection and drainage,
- strength of the embalming solution,
- volume of the embalming solution,
- injection pressure and rate of flow,
- necessary supplemental embalming treatments, and
- delayed or immediate cavity treatment following arterial injection.

The correct embalming treatment is dictated by the conditions present in the body, not solely by the cause of death. Very few causes of death determine the embalming technique. Three examples could include: death from a contagious or infectious disease, death from a ruptured aortic aneurysm, and death from renal failure.

In making an embalming analysis, three important guidelines should always be considered:
1. *The body must be continually observed and evaluated during all phases of embalming.*
2. *Prepare each body as if an infectious or contagious disease is present. Observe Universal Precautions and Terminal Disinfection Protocols.*
3. *Prepare each body as if viewing and final disposition will be delayed.*

### Extrinsic and Intrinsic Factors

The American Board of Funeral Service Education outlines the following variable factors for consideration during embalming analysis:
I. Preparation of the body
  A. Embalming analysis
    1. Purpose
      a. Pre-embalming considerations
      b. Embalming considerations
      c. Post-embalming considerations
    2. Variable factors encountered
      a. Intrinsic factors
        (1) Cause and manner of death
        (2) Body conditions
          (a) Pathological conditions
          (b) Microbial influence
          (c) Moisture
          (d) Thermal influences
          (e) Nitrogenous waste products
          (f) Weight
          (g) Gas in tissues or cavity
        (3) Presence or absence of discolorations
        (4) Postmortem physical and chemical changes
        (5) Effects of pharmaceutical agents
        (6) Illegal drugs
      b. Extrinsic factors
        (1) Environmental
          (a) Atmospheric conditions
          (b) Thermal influences
          (c) Microbial influences
          (d) Vermin
          (e) Other
        (2) Time intervals
          (a) Time between death and preparation
          (b) Time between preparation and disposition
        (3) Embalmer preferences

## EMBALMING ANALYSIS, PART I: PRE-EMBALMING ANALYSIS

Embalmers consider four major factors in making a pre-embalming analysis: (1) general conditions of the body, (2) effects produced by disease processes, (3) effects produced by drugs or surgical procedures, and (4) effects of the postmortem period between death and embalming.

Sensory mechanisms such as sight, touch, and smell allow the embalmer to observe and evaluate postmortem conditions. Most often, the embalmer does not know, at the time of the embalming, the cause of death or the medications which have been administered. It is also in this phase that treatments must be considered for antemortem conditions produced by trauma or surgery; postmortem events such as refrigeration, autopsy, organ and tissue recovery; and the postmortem changes that have occurred in the body.

> **MOST COMMON EMBALMING VARIABLES**
> Selection of arterial injection sites
> Selection of venous drainage sites
> Selection of arterial and supplemental fluids
> Selection of embalming solution strength and volume
> Selection of injection and drainage techniques
> Selection of injection pressure and rate of flow
> Selection of mouth closure methods
> Selection of suturing methods

## ADDITIONAL PRE-EMBALMING INFORMATION

Additional information may be obtained from the following sources. This information along with the conditions presented by the body will contribute to the pre-embalming analysis and the treatments necessary for the care of the deceased.
1. Certificate of death.

2. Infectious or contagious conditions of the deceased provided by the medical facility.
3. Information concerning the timing of the memorial event and final disposition.
4. Shipping information to another funeral establishment in the same or foreign country. Locations outside of the native country may require specific embalming treatments and the preparation of specific documents.
5. Specific requests from the next-of-kin or authorizing party: such as grooming of facial hair and cosmetic treatments.

## General Intrinsic Body Conditions

The general intrinsic conditions of the body include age, body weight and build, musculature, protein level, and general skin condition.

### Age Considerations

**Child or Infant.** Arteries and veins will be much smaller than in the adult; specially sized instruments are needed for injection and drainage. Solution volumes will also be lessened. Embalming solutions cannot be assumed to be milder; infants and children often require stronger solution strengths. Higher body moisture and additional complications related to disease processes, medications, and the accumulation of toxic wastes as a result of organ failure require stronger solution strengths. Preservative demands are determined during pre-embalming analysis. A needle injector may not be suitable for mouth closure. Positioning will vary from that for an adult.

**Advanced Age.** Conditions such as arteriosclerosis and arthritic legs may eliminate the use of the femoral artery as an injection point. Absence of teeth and dentures may create feature setting challenges. Suturing may be needed for mouth closure when the bones of the jaw are porous and prevent use of the needle injector.

### Weight Considerations

**Emaciated.** Solution strengths may need to be reduced and humectant co-injection fluids added to create natural moisture in the tissues. Dehydration may create challenges with eye closure and mouth closure.

**Obese.** Femoral vessels may be too deep to use for injection. Very large quantities of arterial solution will be needed. The internal jugular vein will afford the best drainage site. Restricted cervical injection will best control arterial solution entering facial tissues. There will be positioning challenges.

### Musculature Considerations

Well-developed musculature usually assimilates preservative well. Protein in muscle tissues readily absorbs preservative, except during the stage of active rigor. The embalmer can anticipate good firming of the body tissues. Intense rigor mortis will prevent good distribution and diffusion of the solution. When wasting diseases, poor musculature, senile (or atrophied) tissues are present, the embalmer can expect incomplete firming of the limbs. Swelling may also be expected if large volumes of mild solutions are injected. Senile, loose tissue does not assimilate the arterial solution as well as healthy, firm tissues.

### Disease Processes and the Cause of Death

The cause of death may not be known at the time of embalming; however, the embalmer can observe the effects that diseases have had on the body. For example, **jaundice** may be caused by the effect of drugs on the liver or red blood cells, obstruction of the bile duct, hepatitis, cancer of the liver, and hemolysis of red blood cells. It is the condition of jaundice that concerns the embalmer, not the disease that caused this condition.

The following excerpts, from an article written by Murray Shor (1972) of the American Academy of Funeral Service, illustrate how the same disease can produce different conditions in different persons.

*Let us begin by examining a very common disease and cause of death today—cancer. This pathological condition may attack and be confined to the stomach. In such an event, the patient would not be able to retain foods, either liquid or solid, for weeks just prior to death. He actually might die of starvation although the primary cause of death would be cancer of the stomach.*

### Primary Condition Unimportant

*Consider that the embalmer is presented with a thin, emaciated, dehydrated subject. The primary cancer of the stomach is less significant. Consider a different patient with cancer. In this subject, the malignancy is of the liver or right suprarenal gland. The attendant enlargement of these structures bears down upon and obstructs the cisterna chyli, the lymph collecting station of the abdomen and lower extremities. This prevents the lymph from returning to the venous system from these areas. All of the parts drained by this system will become edematous and ascites will develop. The primary cause of death in both examples is cancer. In one case, we have a subject with edema, ascites, and anasarca; in the other, an emaciated, dehydrated subject. We should also note here that many other diseases can cause the above-described conditions. When we learn to treat the postmortem conditions, we will treat them successfully, regardless of the cause of death.*

*Let me illustrate this further. In incompetence of the right atrioventricular valve of the heart, the valve fails to close efficiently. During the diastole, blood will regurgitate from the right ventricle to the right atrium. This, of course, reduces the amount of blood the right atrium can receive from the inferior vena cava. In turn, the amount of blood the vena cava receives from its tributaries is minimized. The resulting venous congestion in the lower venous system increases transudation of plasma and results again in edema and ascites. Whether the excess fluid is a result of cancer of the viscera or damage to the heart valves, the embalming treatment is the same.*

### Same Basic Treatment

*By the same token, emaciation, whether caused by cancer of the stomach, actual starvation, or pulmonary tuberculosis, requires the same basic embalming treatment. Further inquiry into cancer shows that obstruction to the passage of bile into the intestinal tract can lead to the very common embalming challenge—jaundice. This condition also can be caused by obstruction of the common bile duct—a disease not usually related to cancer. Here again, it is the symptoms and not the disease that pose an embalming challenge. A disease that is as common as cancer and can produce as varied a group of postmortem conditions is arteriosclerosis.*

*Depending on the vessel or vessels involved, we can get a wide range of different embalming challenges.*

*For example, let us consider renal arteriosclerosis. Here, the blood vessels carrying blood to the kidneys are impaired. As a result, the kidneys diminish in size and efficiency. Nitrogenous wastes and urea instead of passing out of the body via kidney and other excretory organs will remain in the bloodstream and tissue spaces. The result will be uremia, cachexia, and possibly edema and ascites, as in some cancers. Arteriosclerosis can affect the vessels of the brain, causing a* **stroke** *which, in turn, can lead to other abnormalities. One of these is long-term* **paralysis** *of the extremities with the attendant atrophied vasoconstriction. Another is long periods of confinement to bed, with the attendant* **decubitus ulcers***. A third is* **immediate death** *with* **no special embalming challenges***.*

*Again, the decubitus ulcers and the atrophied parts can stem from any other disease that confines the patient to bed for extended periods of time. In all these situations, the resulting conditions cause much greater embalming challenges than the disease that led to them. The embalmer must not overlook the fact that any two or three of the diseases discussed here can and do coexist. So can each disease exist in two or more forms. Therefore, a patient can die with stomach and liver cancer. A patient can have liver cancer and renal or cerebral arteriosclerosis. In reality, then,* **an embalmer should ask, "What conditions exist?"** *rather than "Of what did the subject die?"*

The reader should not construe this article to mean that the author discourages the study of pathology. It is intended, rather, to encourage the student to correlate studies of pathology with embalming. It is incumbent upon the embalmer to learn the embalming treatments for the basic postmortem conditions that create challenges. If the conditions are identified and properly treated, the embalming procedure will succeed regardless of the disease that caused the condition.

## Drug Treatments and Surgical Procedures

Since the 1960s, there has been an increase in the therapeutic use of drugs. Like the hundreds of diseases and their effects on the body, it would be impossible for the embalmer to embalm a body using chemical formulations designed to combat the effects of a specific drug. Most often, a patient is given combinations of drugs, often over a long period. A drug does not always produce the same effects in each person. Here again, it is important that the embalmer have an understanding of the possible effects of drugs and of the fact that embalming challenges often stem from long-term drug therapy.

Some effects of the long-term use of medications, which can affect the embalming of the body, include (1) jaundice, (2) discolorations such as purpura and ecchymosis, (3) edema, (4) difficulty in establishing tissue firmness, (5) loss of hair (alopecia), (6) internal bleeding, (7) renal failure causing an increase in nitrogenous wastes in the tissues, (8) changes in the walls of cells making it more difficult for preservatives to act on body proteins, and (9) swelling of facial tissues (steroids).

### Chemotherapeutic Agents Are Toxic

The one axiom that can be universally applied to all chemotherapeutic agents is that they are toxic. Cellular changes occur when they are used and no matter which drug is administered. Even the relatively innocuous aspirin pill has its effects. Drugs have an effect on the skin, circulatory system, liver, and kidneys. Such changes may be comparatively minor in nature, limited to slight discolorations that respond readily to cosmetic treatment. However, when changes are major, such as acute jaundice or saturation of the body tissues with uremic toxins, the fixative action of the preservatives in the arterial solution is seriously impaired. **Table 10–1** lists some common embalming complications created by the extensive use of drug therapies.

### Blood Thinners

Drugs that thin the blood in life will often reduce postmortem blood clotting in the vascular system. Reduced postmortem clotting will improve distribution and subsequent diffusion of the arterial solution.

Bodies that exhibit a midline scar over the sternum may have underwent open heart surgery, valve repair, or vascular bypass. In the medical setting, anticoagulant or blood thinning medications are administered during surgical procedures. Keeping the blood thin will increase postmortem hypostasis of the blood and intense livor mortis in the dependent tissues. Expansion of the veins in the distal arm will be noted when the arms are lowered to the sides of the body. Vessel expansion and distension is an indicator that good distribution of the embalming solution can be expected.

### Surgery

In making a pre-embalming analysis, choice of embalming technique may be greatly influenced by whether death occurred during or immediately after surgery. Surgery could be the primary factor in an analysis, as illustrated in the following examples.

**Heart Surgery or Aortic Repair.** During these procedures, the heart may be stopped for a period during which an artificial means of life support is used. Frequently, if death occurs during or shortly after this type of surgery, the face and neck are grossly distended with edema. Repair of an abdominal aneurysm may not always be successful, and the interruption in circulation will necessitate sectional arterial injection.

**Abdominal Surgery.** Abdominal surgery on the bowel can result in peritonitis, intense distension of the abdomen, and bloodstream infections (septicemia). These conditions require the use of a strong, well-coordinated arterial solution.

Whenever death follows surgery, there exists the potential for leakage from arteries and veins involved in the surgical procedure. The embalmer should use dyes to indicate the distribution of arterial solution. It may be necessary to inject a greater volume of arterial solution to compensate for solution that may be lost to the abdominal or thoracic cavities.

All surgical bodies should undergo thorough cavity treatment. The formation of tissue gas is always a possibility. Be certain a liberal amount of undiluted cavity fluid is injected into the area where the surgery was performed. Best practice is to inject additional cavity fluid into the tissues surrounding the surgical incision. Re-aspiration and re-injection of the cavities are anticipated.

## Postmortem Interval Between Death and Embalming

Pre-embalming analysis includes observation and evaluation of changes that occur during the postmortem interval

| TABLE 10-1. Embalming Complications Created by Extensive Drug Therapies ||
|---|---|
| Complication | Result |
| Immediate allergic reaction to the drug | Tissues appear swollen |
| | Discolored skin surface |
| | Possible skin eruptions |
| Liver failure | Edema (ascites); edema of lower extremities |
| | Increase in ammonia in the tissues (neutralizes formaldehyde) |
| | Purges caused by rupture of esophageal veins |
| | Gastrointestinal bleeding; fluid loss; possible purge |
| | Hair loss |
| | Jaundice |
| Renal failure | Increase in ammonia in the tissues |
| | Edema of tissues |
| | Gastrointestinal bleeding |
| | Pulmonary edema |
| | Congestive heart failure |
| | Discoloration of the skin (sallow color) |
| | Uremic pruritus of the skin |
| Damage to blood vessels | Skin hemorrhage (ecchymosis, purpura hemorrhages) |
| Damage to the walls | Breakdown of the skin; skin-slip often present |
| Clot formation (poor circulation of embalming fluids) | Breakage during arterial injection (causes discolorations) |
| Loss of cranial hair | Hair restoration may be necessary |
| Growth of facial hair and hair on the forehead on women and children | Hair removal may be necessary |
| Creation of resistant strains of microbes | Disinfection treatment more difficult |
| | Exposure of embalmer to drug-resistant microbes |
| Cell membranes become less permeable | Creates "solid" edema that cannot be removed |
| | Makes passage of arterial solution into cell very difficult |
| Killing one type of microbe can stimulate growth of other types | Antibiotics used to kill bacteria give fungal organisms a chance to multiply |
| | Breakdown of the red blood cell |
| | Liver failure |
| Jaundice | Edema |
| | Drainage difficulties |
| Congestive heart failure | Facial discolorations |
| | Death of the superficial cells |
| | Protein degeneration |
| Scaling of skin (seen on facial tissues and between fingers) | Ammonia buildup in the tissues which neutralizes formaldehyde |
| Difficult tissue firming | Presence of edema |

between death and embalming. The types of body conditions will determine the embalming treatment (**Table 10-2**). Accelerated changes can take precedence over less advanced postmortem factors. Consider that a person who dies of cancer is emaciated and jaundiced, and the body is not discovered in for several days. If the environmental temperature is very high, postmortem changes will be accelerated. Advanced decomposition conditions will determine the strength of the embalming solution despite consideration of other postmortem conditions.

As a general rule, best results are obtained when embalming is done as soon as possible following the death. Three postmortem conditions that interfere most with good distribution of the arterial solution are blood coagulation, rigor mortis, and decomposition. Embalming the body before these changes are established helps to produce better results.

If there is to be a delay between death and preparation, mortuary refrigeration will help to slow the onset of some postmortem changes. Cooling of the body helps to slow postmortem blood coagulation, the onset of rigor mortis, and decomposition. Overextended periods of time, refrigeration can create disadvantages such as dehydration, increased blood viscosity, postmortem edema, intense livor mortis, and postmortem stain. Refrigeration can also create false signs of preserved tissue. Tissue firming is caused by the solidification of fats in the subcutaneous tissues; hemolysis produces discolorations that resemble dyes used in the embalming fluids. **Table 10-3** summarizes the embalming significance of postmortem physical and chemical changes.

# EMBALMING ANALYSIS, PART II: DURING ARTERIAL INJECTION OF THE BODY

The second part of the analysis is an evaluation of the treatments during embalming. When a challenge is encountered, the embalmer must decide what new approach to take to solve the challenge. During this phase of analysis, after the injection of each gallon of arterial solution, the embalmer reevaluates distribution, diffusion, and the results produced. The following are some concerns:

1. What areas of the body are receiving arterial solution? This can be noted by the presence of fluid dyes in the tissues and the clearing of intravascular discolorations such as livor mortis.
2. What areas are not receiving arterial solution? Dyes will not be present and livor mortis, if present, will not be cleared; no firmness will be present.
3. What can be done to stimulate the flow of arterial solution into areas not receiving solution?
    a. Massage along the arterial route that supplies fluid to the area.
    b. Increase the pressure of the solution being injected.
    c. Increase the rate of flow of the solution being injected.
    d. Lower, raise, or manipulate the body area.
    e. Close off the drainage to increase the intravascular pressure.
4. What areas must receive sectional arterial injection? Areas that did not receive solution even after massage and changes in injection protocol must be injected separately.

| TABLE 10-2. Body Conditions and Embalming Treatments ||
|---|---|
| Condition | Treatment |
| Normal body; some livor; dead less than 6 h; no edema; no chemotherapy | Any vessel for injection and drainage, pre-injection; mild to moderate solutions (3–5 gallons, will vary with body size); set tissues to the desired firmness |
| Extensive livor of facial areas; dead less than 6 h; no extreme pathology | Clear discolorations with a mild to moderate solution; jugular and common carotid recommended; step-up strength to set to desired firmness |
| Postmortem stain present; body in or out of rigor; dead more than 6 h | Begin with strong coordinated arterial solutions; continue to increase after circulation is established; restricted cervical injection; slow injection; dye for tracer; sectional injection where needed; hypodermic and surface treatments where needed |
| Decomposition evident | Restricted cervical injection; strong coordinated solutions; dye for tracer; sectional/hypodermic and surface treatments where needed |
| Bodies refrigerated more than 12 h; some rigor; livor | Solution stronger than average; avoid pre-injection; dye tracer; circulation problems expected; restricted cervical injection |
| Jaundice; no edema; yellow | Jaundice fluid; mild solutions (however, must meet preservative demands); femoral vessels if possible, may respond to pre-injection; dye for counterstain |
| Jaundice green | Cannot be cleared; solution strength based on preservative demands; plenty of dye to counterstain |
| Generalized edema of body | Start with solution a little above normal strength; continue to increase; if circulation is poor increase to very strong solutions |
| Localized edema | Treat general embalming based on condition of the tissues; separate sectional embalming of area with edema; hypodermic and surface treatments |
| Extravascular discolorations from chemotherapy or pathology | Use solutions based on size of body, length of time dead, etc.; treat the discoloration when on hands and face with hypodermic and surface treatments |
| Autopsied; dead less than 12 h | Moderate solutions; increase if needed to achieve desired firmness |
| Autopsied; dead more than 12 h; refrigerated | Solutions stronger than normal; dyes for tracing; restricted drainage to help achieve circulation; higher pressure may be needed |
| Death from second-degree burns | Begin with strong solutions; use dye for tracer; death will be related to uremia; may need 100% fluid (waterless solution); do the same if autopsied |
| Localized gangrene/ischemia/possible diabetic | Strong solutions when circulation problems are anticipated; bacterial complications can exist in these bodies; hypodermic/sectional and surface treatments to areas affected; dye for arterial tracing |
| Frozen bodies | Strong solutions; dye for tracer; restricted cervical injection |
| Emaciated with edema | Sectional embalming to separately treat affected areas; reduce edema with strong solutions; enhance emaciated tissues with moderate solutions and added humectant |
| Emaciated | Mild solutions in large volume; add humectants to last injection; restricted drainage |
| Generalized edema with jaundice | Always treat for preservation first; moderate to strong solutions; dye for tracer; inject until edema is treated |
| Trauma of face/black eyes/lacerations/restorative work needed infants/children with no pathological complications | Restricted cervical injection if not autopsied; strong solutions; dye for tracer vessels (iliac/carotid/aorta) if not autopsied; standard arterial fluid; inject strength and volume as needed; based on weight and body conditions; dye for tracing |
| Dehydrated bodies not dead very long | Mild solutions; restricted drainage; humectants in last injection |
| Bodies with chemotherapy, some edema; skin hemorrhage; expect fixation problems | Use restricted cervical injection; strong solutions into trunk areas; dye for tracing; may help force fluid into tissue spaces |
| Eye enucleation/no other remarks | To control solution entering head, use restricted cervical injection when body not autopsied; use a stronger than normal solution; avoid pre-injection |
| Contagious disease | Use solutions a little stronger than normal (2–3%); run plenty of volume; avoid personal contact with "first" drainage; run volume and increased strengths depending on other body conditions (i.e., weight/edema) |
| Obese | Begin with a slightly stronger than normal solution; after blood discolorations clear, strength may continue to be increased; first, vessel choice common carotid/jugular; second, choice external iliac |
| Arteriosclerosis in common carotid | Stronger solution; higher and/or pulsating pressure; dye for tracer; sectional injection; hypodermic (subcuticular) injection and surface (topical) treatment |
| Severe arteriosclerosis in femoral when used as first point of injection | Select common carotid and jugular for primary site as above; hypodermic (subcuticular) injection and surface (topical) treatment of distal legs |

## TABLE 10-3. Postmortem Physical and Chemical Changes

| Change | Embalming Significance |
|---|---|
| **Physical** | |
| Algor mortis | Slows onset of rigor and decomposition |
| | Keeps blood in a liquid state; aids drainage |
| Dehydration | Increases the viscosity of the blood; sludge forms |
| | Partly responsible for postmortem edema; increasing preservative demands |
| | Darkens surface areas; cannot be bleached |
| | Eyelids and lips separate; lips and fingers wrinkle |
| | When severe, may retard further decomposition, i.e., desiccation |
| Hypostasis | Responsible for livor mortis and eventual postmortem stain |
| | Increases tissue moisture in dependent tissue areas |
| Livor mortis | Varies in intensity from slight redness to black depending on volume and viscosity of the blood |
| | Intravascular discoloration; can be cleared |
| | Can be set as a stain if too strong an uncoordinated arterial solution is used |
| | Keeps capillaries expanded; can work as an aid to distribution |
| Increase in blood viscosity | Clearing serves as a sign of arterial solution distribution |
| | Sludge is created; intravascular resistance |
| | Postmortem edema can accompany problem |
| | Blood removal becomes difficult; distribution can be poor |
| Translocation of microbes | Speeds decomposition in various body regions |
| **Chemical** | |
| Rigor mortis | Extravascular resistance |
| | Positioning difficult; features may be hard to pose pH not conducive for good fluid reactions |
| | Tissues swell easily |
| | False sign of preservation (fixation) |
| | After passage, firming is difficult |
| | Decomposition is usually minimal when present |
| | Increases preservative demand |
| Decomposition | Color changes; odor present; purges; skin-slip; gases |
| | Poor distribution of solutions |
| | Increased preservative demand |
| | Rapid swelling in affected tissue areas |

## TABLE 10-3. (Continued)

| | |
|---|---|
| Postmortem stain | Extravascular; cannot be removed; may be bleached or concealed |
| | Generally noticeable six hours postmortem |
| | Increased preservative demand due to delay interval |
| | Reddish tissues falsely indicate the presence of embalming fluid dyes |
| | Tissues turn gray after embalming; cosmetics correct Embalmers Grey |
| Postmortem caloricity | Triggers the rigor and decomposition cycles |
| Shift in the body pH | Interferes with embalming fluid-protein reactions |
| | Dyes can appear blotchy |

5. Has the body as a whole received sufficient arterial solution and has the solution been of sufficient strength?
   a. A high-index arterial fluid can be injected or added to the remaining arterial solution to boost the preservative qualities of the solution.
   b. If there is doubt as to the amount of solution, inject additional amounts as long as there is no distension of the neck or facial tissues; inject until preservation is well established.
6. Has sufficient arterial solution been retained by the body? Retention of embalming solution is necessary to continue the preservation process. After blood and surface discolorations clear; intermittent drainage can be used to help the tissues retain more embalming solution. It has been estimated that more than 50% of the drainage is arterial solution. (**See Selected Readings:** The Measurement of Formaldehyde Retention in the Tissues of Embalmed Bodies.)
7. Is the arterial solution having too much of a dehydrating effect on the tissues? A humectant co-injection fluid can be added.
8. Should additional fluid dye be added for internal coloring of the tissues? Additional dyes may be added throughout the embalming procedure.
9. If purge begins from the mouth or nose, what are its origin and cause? Let the purge continue during the arterial injection unless the purge is arterial solution. If the purge is arterial solution and drainage continues, inject an additional arterial solution to make up for the preservative lost in the purge. If the purge is arterial solution and there is no drainage, it can be assumed there is a major rupture in the vascular system. Consider multisite or sectional injections.
10. Are the tissues firming? This will depend on several factors. In conditions such as renal failure, emaciation, edema, and wasting degenerative diseases, firming may be very difficult to establish. Poor firming can also be a result of the type of arterial fluid being used. (Some fluids have a slow firming action, and others produce less firming of body tissues.) If there is doubt as to the preservative needs

of the tissues, the arterial solution can be increased in strength either by preparing a new solution using a higher-index fluid or by using more concentrated fluid per gallon. A high-index fluid can be added to boost the strength of the solution being injected.

11. Does another site need to be selected for drainage? For example, when injecting and draining from the right femoral artery and vein, there is little drainage, and the face and neck begin to discolor and veins of the neck become prominent. These changes indicate that drainage should be taken from a location above the heart, such as the internal jugular vein.

> **TO INCREASE ARTERIAL SOLUTION STRENGTH**
> 1. Prepare a solution using a higher-index arterial fluid.
> 2. Add a higher-index arterial fluid to the present solution.
> 3. Add more concentrated arterial fluid to the present solution.

## EMBALMING ANALYSIS, PART III: EVALUATION OF THE BODY AFTER ARTERIAL EMBALMING

### Post-embalming Monitoring and Treatments

Embalming analysis is an ongoing process from the time of receiving the decedent into the embalmer's care until the final disposition of the body. During the process of **post-embalming monitoring,** the embalmer continues to check for adverse changes on a periodic basis. Adverse changes could include the presence of gas in the tissues or cavities, odor, purge, color changes in visible areas, and skin slip.

When an embalmed body has been received from another funeral establishment, an evaluation must be made of all body areas. Some of the following treatments may be necessary: (1) re-injection of a particular body area, (2) supplemental preservative treatments, (3) cavity re-aspiration and re-injection, and (4) features reset. Embalming analysis is an ongoing process from the beginning of the embalming until disposition of the body.

In this third phase of analysis, an evaluation of the preservation of the body is necessary. Areas that are still lacking solution must now be treated using the supplemental preservative treatments of hypodermic injection or surface embalming. Some of the following considerations are evaluated during this third phase of the analysis:

1. What body areas have not received arterial solution after primary and multipoint injections are completed?
    a. Look for the absence of fluid dyes, little or no firming of the tissues, and the presence of intravascular discolorations.
    b. Treatment now must be hypodermic injection of the area or surface embalming or a combination of both.
2. Should cavity embalming be done immediately after arterial injection or delayed several hours?
    a. This may depend on the time at which the body must be ready for viewing.
    b. In thin, emaciated bodies, an attempt may have been made to fill out the tissues with a humectant—restorative co-injection; this chemical should be given time to ensure the tissues are firmed before aspiration is done.
    c. If a body is dead from an infectious disease, the embalmer may wish to delay aspiration to help ensure that any blood removed in the aspirated material will have time to mix with the arterial solution injected. Consider injecting a bottle of cavity fluid and waiting several hours before aspirating; this helps to ensure disinfection of the aspirated materials.
3. Are the features set properly?
    a. Be certain that the mouth is dry. Remove moist cotton and replace it with dry cotton if purge developed during arterial injection.
    b. Lips and eyelids should be set at the proper line of closure to produce natural appearance.
    c. If the eyelids are soft, cotton can be used for eye closure, and a drop of cavity fluid can be placed on the cotton to make an internal compress before adhesive is applied to the eyelids. A coating of surface embalming gel can also be applied externally.
    d. If residual air is present in the mouth after gluing, the lips can be parted slightly to release the air; limited aspiration of the thorax will remove the air.
4. Did purge develop during embalming?
    a. Remove packing material from the nasal and oral cavities.
    b. Purge may be aspirated from the throat and nasal passages using a nasal tube aspirator.
    c. Anal purge can be corrected after cavity embalming; manually apply pressure to the pelvic region to force as much of the fecal material from the orifice; pack the anal orifice with cotton saturated with cavity fluid, phenol cautery fluid, or a chemical solution used for treatment of skin lesions. Install a closure device such as an AV plug if necessary. Pants and coveralls or an adult incontinence brief can be used to protect clothing from soiling and control odors.
5. Is the body well-groomed? Trim fingernails and hair per instruction. Photos are helpful.
6. Are the body and hair clean and dried? The body must be turned on its side to check for clots or debris that were not cleaned away. Turning the body allows it to be dried on all sides.
7. Have decubitus ulcerations been treated? Compresses should be removed from decubitus ulcerations or skin lesions and replaced with clean compresses and fresh chemical or embalming powders. Plastic stockings, pants, or coveralls can be placed on the body to hold the compresses in position.
8. Is there any leakage? Intravenous line punctures can continue to leak after arterial injection. They should be properly sealed with a trocar button or superglue.
9. Are tracheostomy and colostomy openings closed? A pursestring suture can be used to close these openings. They should be packed with a cautery chemical and cotton. The tracheostomy can also be filled with incision seal powder. Apply glue and cotton after the suturing is completed.
10. Are incisions sutured? Sutures should be tight and not allow seepage. If leakage is present, remove sutures, apply incision seal powder or a mastic compound, and replace with tighter sutures.

| TABLE 10–4. Embalming Technique Variables | |
|---|---|
| Description | Variation |
| Setting of features | Before embalming, during embalming, after embalming |
| Method of mouth closure | Needle injector, musculature suture, mandibular suture, dental tie |
| Method of denture replacement | Cotton, mouth former, kapoc, mastic compound |
| Method of eye closure | Cotton, eye caps |
| Time for raising vessels | Before setting features, after setting features |
| Artery for primary injection | Right common carotid, right femoral, right axillary |
| Vein for drainage | Right internal jugular, right femoral, right axillary, right atrium of heart |
| Method of injection/drainage | One-point, multisite, split injection, restricted cervical, six-point |
| Method of drainage | Continuous, intermittent, alternate |
| Drainage instrument | Drain tube, angular spring forceps, trocar for direct heart drainage |
| Body treated with pre-injection | Used, not used |
| Arterial fluid strength | Low index, medium index, high index |
| Arterial solution injected | Mild solution, moderate solution, strong solution |
| Co-injection fluid | Used, not used |
| Fluid dye | Used, not used |
| Fluid dye color | Various shades of pink or tan |
| Use of fluid dye | Added to all solutions, added only to final solution |
| Humectant co-injection | Used, not used |
| Time usage of humectant | Added to all solutions, added only to final solution |
| Arterial solution strength | Same strength for all solutions, mild initial strength increased to stronger |
| Pressure for injection (pounds per square inch) | Low (2–10 psi), medium (10–20 psi), high (20 or more psi) |
| Rate of flow (ounces per minute) | Slow (5–10 opm), medium (10–15 opm), fast (more than 15 opm) |
| Change of pressure | Not changed during injection; begin low then increase |
| Change of rate of flow | Not changed during injection; begin slow then increase |
| Volume of solution injected | Based on various factors, i.e., weight, postmortem interval, edema, and dehydration |
| Method of aspiration | Hydroaspirator, electric aspirator |
| Time of aspiration | Immediately after arterial injection, delayed |
| Re-aspiration | Performed, not performed |
| Method of trocar closure | Trocar button, sutured |
| Method of cavity fluid injection | Gravity injector, embalming machine |
| Cavity fluid re-injected | Done, not done, done only if gases are present |
| Signs of fluid distribution | Clearing of livor, tissue firming, presence of dye |
| Features glued after embalming | Performed, not performed |
| Types of glue to set features | Rubber-based, super adhesive |
| Treatment for lack of fluid | Local arterial injection, surface compress, hypodermic injection |

Table 10–4 illustrates variations in embalming techniques, fluids, instruments, and other considerations.

## POST-EMBALMING MONITORING

Periodic monitoring allows the embalmer to make adjustments and perform treatments necessary to ensure ongoing stability of the body after embalming. The following conditions must be addressed and treated appropriately to serve this purpose.

- *Dehydration.* Evaluate the scope and severity of the affected area. Dehydration can be caused by (1) excessive embalming solution strength, (2) gravitation of tissue fluids from the face and neck into dependent tissues, (3) moisture loss to the surrounding environment exacerbated by direct currents from air conditioning or heating systems, and (4) inadequate distribution of embalming solution to an area. Surface tissues may be corrected with cosmetics and waxes. Feature dehydration may require hypodermic injection of tissue builder, cosmetics, and waxes. Resetting of the features may be necessary.
- *Purge.* Requires immediate correction. Evaluate to determine the origin of the purge. Re-aspiration of the cavities and repacking of the orifice are necessary. Evaluate the need to re-inject cavity fluid. Clothing may be soiled; remove and launder or dry clean.

- *Odor.* Evaluate to determine the origin of the odor. Untreated tissues continue to decompose. Re-embalming may be absolutely necessary. The same or additional arteries can be injected. A waterless solution is recommended. Re-aspiration of the cavities and repacking of orifices is likely to further reduce odors.
- *Leakage.* Evaluate; the source of leakage may be edema or possibly an embalming incision that was not tightly sutured. Identify the source and treat the affected area. Soiled garments may need to be laundered or dry cleaned. Plastic garments are recommended to contain minor leakage. Add preservative and absorbent powders inside the garment.
- *Softening of visible tissues.* Evaluate; tissue softening occurs with continued decomposition. Discolorations, blebs, and desquamation are common. Re-embalming may be necessary: arterial, hypodermic, and/or surface corrections.
- *Tissue gas.* Requires immediate correction. Foul odor, intense tissue swelling, and **crepitation** are classic signs of tissue gas. Crepitation is the crackling sensation produced by gases trapped in the tissues. Re-embalming is necessary. Tissue gas accelerates quickly.

## BIBLIOGRAPHY

American Board of Funeral Service, *Course Content Syllabus,* 2016.

Chemotherapy and embalming results. In: *Champion Expanding Encyclopedia.* Springfield, OH: Champion Chemical Co., 1986: No. 570.

Frederick JF. *Effects of Chemotherapeutic Agents.* Boston, MA: Dodge Chemical Co., 1968.

Shor M. Knowledge of effect of disease simplifies embalming. *Casket and Sunnyside,* September 1960.

Shor M. Conditions of the body dictate the proper embalming treatment. *Casket and Sunnyside,* November 1972.

Slocum RE. *Pre-embalming Considerations.* Boston, MA: Dodge Chemical Co., 1958.

---

### CONCEPTS FOR STUDY

Define the following terminology:
- Embalming analysis
- Extrinsic factors
- Intrinsic factors
- Post-embalming monitoring

1. Discuss historical methods of embalming analysis and relate these to current practices.
2. List the four steps outlined in embalming analysis.
3. Give several examples of topics that may be discussed during professional communication between the embalmer and arranging funeral director.
4. Give several examples of intrinsic factors and extrinsic factors.
5. Explain the purpose of embalming analysis.
6. Describe the four categories of information used in embalming analysis.
7. Discuss why the conditions present are more important than the actual cause of death.
8. List several effects of long-term drug therapy.
9. Recall the treatment for post-embalming purge.
10. Recall the treatment for post-embalming tissue gas.

CHAPTER 11

# Preparation of the Body Prior to Arterial Injection

## CHAPTER OVERVIEW
- Authorization to Embalm
- General Pre-embalming Treatments
- Shaving and Grooming
- Setting Facial Features
- Treatments for Pathological Conditions
- Removal of Invasive Medical Devices

Secure authorization to embalm prior to embalming. Permission to embalm is obtained from the next-of-kin or authorizing party responsible for final disposition decisions. Best practice is to obtain written documentation of the authorization for permanent record. In some states, written permission for embalming is required by law.

Embalming is separated into three phases: pre-arterial injection (before), arterial injection (during), and post-arterial injection (after). Included within each phase are the procedures routinely performed during that time period. As an example, the primary reason for positioning the body prior to embalming is that tissues become firm and extremities become less flexible after embalming.

Evaluation of the body is ongoing during each of these time periods. A four-step approach is helpful: (1) observation and evaluation of postmortem conditions, (2) proposed methods of treatment, (3) implementation of treatments, and (4) observation and evaluation of treatment results.

Effective embalming is achieved when these functions are successful: distribution, diffusion, and retention of embalming chemicals. In other words, embalming solution must distribute uniformly throughout the vascular system, diffuse deeply into structures such as tissues and cells, and a sufficient volume of a sufficient strength solution must be retained within the body (**Fig. 11-1**).

---

**THREE PHASES OF EMBALMING**

Phase 1. Pre-arterial injection (before)
Phase 2. Arterial injection (during)
Phase 3. Post-arterial injection (after)

---

## PRELIMINARY PREPARATION

The embalming process actually begins when the deceased is transferred from the mortuary cot to the preparation table. Mechanical lifting devices may be used when additional assistance is needed. The body is centered on the table. Clothing, sheeting, and body bags should be sprayed with a topical disinfectant prior to removal. Standing at the side of the embalming table, gently roll the body toward you by placing your hands on the shoulder and the hip of the deceased. After the body is rolled to one side, the sheet or body may be pushed beneath the center of the body. Next, roll the body back to the supine position. Move to the opposite side of the table, repeat the rolling process, and remove the sheeting or body bag from beneath the body.

Clothing should be removed without cutting whenever possible. Inventory and document all personal effects. Affix an identification tag or label to the items and securely store them until return to the family or authorized party. Do not dispose of any items unless you are directed to do so. Best practice is to document in writing the directive for disposition of personal effects. Glasses, jewelry, watches, and religious articles should be removed during embalming.

During body transfer, best practice is to **pull rather than push** the body. For example, transfer of the body from the mortuary cot to the embalming table can be accomplished in three steps: (1) place the cot next to the embalming table; (2) stand on the opposite side of the table and reach across toward the cot; and (3) pull the legs and buttocks onto the table first, then pull the trunk and shoulders. If the body has been placed on a sliding device such as a backboard, pull the board along with the body onto the preparation table.

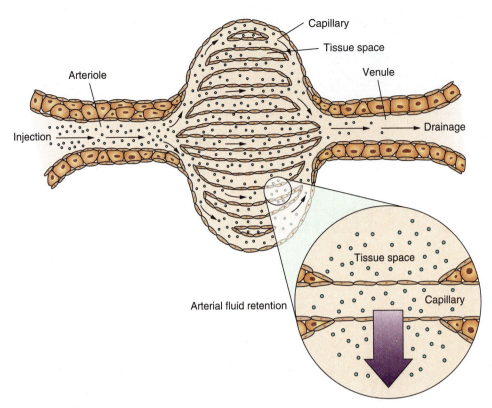

**Figure 11–1.** Arterial solution retention.

## BEST PRACTICES FOR LIFTING AND TRANSFERRING

### Know Your Limits

Evaluate the situation first.

Do not attempt to lift or transfer a body that is too heavy by yourself.

Request assistance for team lifting.

Use a mechanical device.

### The Squat Lift (Lift from a Lower Surface to a Higher Surface)

Stand close to the body, feet slightly apart.

Straighten your back and square your shoulders.

Bend your knees and squat down to the position of the body.

Keep the weight of the body close to you as you lift.

Bend your knees, not your back while lifting.

Avoid twisting your back when lifting; change direction with your feet.

### Transfer from Surfaces That Are Level and Abut One Another

Lock wheels on tables and stretchers before the transfer.

Straighten your back and square your shoulders.

Bend your arms, not your back.

Pull instead of push.

## PRIMARY DISINFECTION OF THE BODY

After the sheeting or clothing has been removed and the body is placed in the center of the table, a modesty cloth is draped to cover the genitalia (**Fig. 11–2**). All body surfaces and orifices are treated with a topical disinfectant. The surface disinfectant should be sprayed onto the body with particular attention to all body orifices. Follow manufacturer's instructions as to surface contact time. A droplet-type spray is preferred over-pressurized sprays, which lose too much of the disinfectant to the surrounding air and can then be inhaled by the embalmer.

Disinfection of the body should also include the destruction of body lice or mites (scabies). If scabies is suspected, a commercial pediculicide should be applied to the skin and the hair of the deceased. The embalmer should carefully handle these bodies so that the insects do not infest the skin of the embalmer. Carefully check for fly eggs or maggots, especially in the months of summer or in warm climates. Fly eggs appear as yellowish clusters in the corners of the eyes, nostrils, or ears or within the mouth. If present, these eggs can develop into the eating larval stage known as maggots in 24 hours. Great care should be taken to remove all eggs. If the larval stage has begun, a mortuary larvicide can be used.

Maggots also feed upon embalmed tissue, so it is very important to remove and destroy them. To prevent flies from depositing eggs, keep the body covered. Nostrils can be packed in the months of summer, and small pieces of cotton can be placed in the nostrils (extending outside the nostril) when the body is left in the preparation room or is shipped. In the months of summer, some funeral homes make a habit of covering the face of

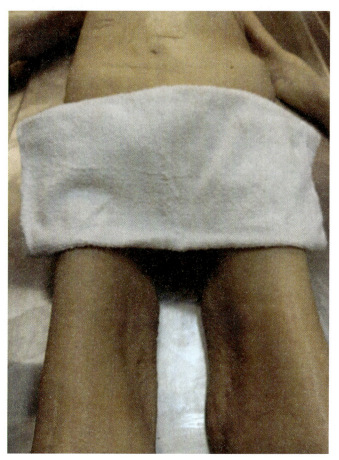

**Figure 11–2.** Modesty cloth.

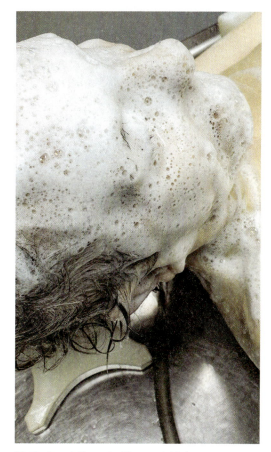

**Figure 11–3.** Face lathered with germicidal soap.

the body at night. Outside windows and doors of the preparation room should be screened. In addition, insecticides should be used if flies are present in the preparation room. Once fly eggs develop into the larval stage, the problem becomes very difficult, if not impossible, to control.

## BATHING THE BODY

The entire body is thoroughly bathed with warm water and germicidal soap. Special attention is given to the viewable areas, the face and hands (**Fig. 11–3**). These areas must be free of dirt and body oils for good cosmetic application after embalming. Scaling skin between the fingers, in facial creases, and around the hairline can be removed with a solvent. Massage cream applied to these areas helps to cleanse facial pores. After thorough washing and rinsing, the body should be dried with toweling. Flexing and rotating the limbs while bathing helps to relieve rigor mortis.

When household bleach (sodium hypochlorite) is used in the solution for washing the body, it is important that the chemical be washed away with water before any contact is made with formaldehyde. Sodium hypochlorite and formaldehyde, combined in large amounts, can potentially produce a toxic product.

Fingernails can be scrubbed with a nail brush to remove debris beneath the nails. Or, an instrument may be used to gently release materials from under the nails. A solvent is used to remove surface discolorations, such as grease or tobacco stains, from the fingers or fingernails. Nail polish is removed with polish remover or acetone. It is beneficial to leave polish on one fingernail to later match the color. Nails are trimmed and shaped after cleaning.

## CARING FOR THE HAIR

Hair is washed at the beginning of embalming to remove bacteria, dirt, oils, and odors from the hair (**Fig. 11–4**). The hair can be washed a second time to remove any blood or chemical odors that remain after the embalming procedure.

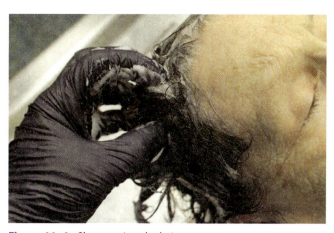

**Figure 11–4.** Shampooing the hair.

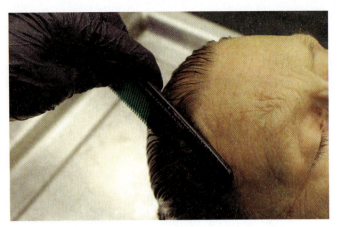

**Figure 11–5.** Combing the hair.

The following are best practices for hair care:
- Consult with the authorizing party before removing braids.
- Comb through hair prior to shampooing.
- Wash the hair with warm water and germicidal soap, or shampoo.
- Use cool water to remove dried blood from the hair.
- Use hair conditioner to detangle long hair and aid in styling.
- Apply a dry wash solvent to remove dandruff.
- Comb or brush hair back from the forehead (**Fig. 11–5**).
- Retain natural curls by kneading the hair with a towel after combing.
- Avoid overbrushing hair when it is falling out.
- Towel dry and/or blow dry the hair.

## SHAVING FACIAL HAIR

Facial hair is removed according to the wishes of the family and after permission has been obtained (**Fig. 11–6**). When instructions are not available prior to embalming, shaving can occur after embalming. However, shaving is more difficult after embalming when the tissues are less flexible. But much easier than restoring facial hair that has been mistakenly shaved.

Shaving creates smooth skin for the application of cosmetics. Cosmetics will stick to stubble hair making it more noticeable and creating an unpleasant appearance. Therapeutic drugs can cause facial and forehead hair growth on individuals who have never had facial hair. This type of facial hair is easily removed by lightly passing a razor over the facial tissues. After shaving the forehead, apply massage cream.

Note the following points during shaving of the face:
1. Use a good, sharp blade; more than one blade may be needed to shave dense growth.
2. Apply warm water to the face with a washcloth first.
3. Use shaving cream to lather the face.
4. When there is doubt about the length of sideburns, mustache, or beard, consult the family. If they cannot be reached, these areas can always be shaved after arterial embalming.
5. When using a new blade, it is wise to begin shaving on the left side of the face or in the neck area to slightly dull the blade.
6. Shave in the direction of hair growth; bodies vary, and sometimes shaving must be directed against or perpendicular to the growth.

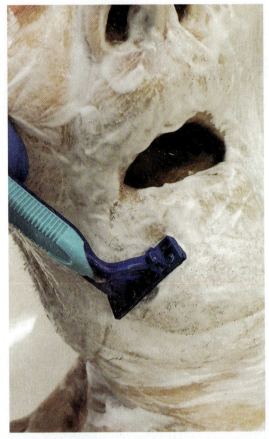

**Figure 11–6.** Shaving the face prior to closure of the mouth.

7. Use small, short, repeated strokes over an area to achieve the closest shave; an area can be shaved repeatedly or from one or several different directions.
8. Clean the razor frequently with warm water.
9. Try to shave an area without lifting the razor off the face; apply pressure on the razor and slide the razor over the area being shaved.
10. Use cotton or a washcloth to pull the skin taut for shaving; this is helpful in shaving beneath the mandible and the upper neck area.
11. After shaving, wash the face with a washcloth and warm water; a thin layer of massage cream may be applied. Trim hair from nostrils and ears at this time.

Razor abrasions occur from nicking the epithelial tissues. Application of massage cream helps to prevent the area from dehydrating and darkening. During arterial injection, arterial solution may leak through these nicked areas. It may be necessary to apply wax over these areas after cosmetics have been applied. This prevents further drying.

If facial hair must be shaved *after* arterial injection, lather the face with shaving cream and allow the lather to remain several minutes. Use a new razor blade. To avoid nicking the tissue, shave in small areas and keep applying lather to the area being shaved. When completed, apply a thin film of massage cream. An electric razor over a dry face is also effective.

To shave thick or long facial growth, first trim the hair to the manageable length with barber shears or hair clippers. Follow with razor shaving directed from the cheek downward over the face. Heavy growth may necessitate the use of several blades. After the body has been shaved, massage cream may be applied. A minimal amount is adequate to protect the skin. Massage cream has several advantages:

1. Protects the face and hands from surface dehydration.
2. Prevents broken skin areas such as razor abrasions from dehydrating and darkening.
3. Acts as a lubricant during facial massage to relieve rigor mortis.
4. Acts as a skin cleanser.
5. Protects the face from acidic purge from the mouth or nose.
6. Provides a base for cream cosmetics.

## RELIEVING RIGOR MORTIS

The embalmer manipulates the limbs of the decedent while removing clothing and bathing to relieve rigor mortis. The stiffened muscles caused by rigor prevent proper body positioning during embalming. Bending, flexing, rotating, and massaging limbs to relieve rigor can damage capillaries, which leads to tissue swelling during arterial injection. Avoid excessive exercise of the muscles in relieving rigor mortis. Relieving the rigor also relieves extravascular resistance upon the circulatory system. Relief of the rigor results in better arterial solution distribution and also better drainage. A routine procedure for relieving rigor mortis is as follows:

1. Firmly rotate the neck from side to side.
2. Flex the head.
3. Push the lower jaw up to begin to relieve the rigor in the muscles of the jaw. Repeat this several times. If the mouth is firmly closed begin by pushing the mandible upward; then firmly push on the chin to attempt to open the mouth. Massage the temporalis and the masseter muscles on the sides of the face. This may help open the mouth.
4. Flex the arm several times, then extend it. Finally, rotate the arm at the shoulder.
5. Grasp the fingers on the palm side of the hand and extend them (**Fig. 11–7**).
6. Grasp the foot and rotate it inward. Repeat several times. Attempt to flex the legs at the knee. Raise and lower the legs several times.

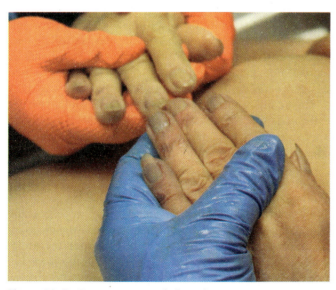

**Figure 11–7.** Fingers are extended to relieve rigor mortis.

## POSITIONING THE BODY

The objective of pre-embalming positioning is to create a comfortable and restful appearance. Preservative arterial solution will firm muscle tissues in the position they are set by the embalmer. It may not be possible to reposition the body after embalming. The positioning of the body as it rests on the embalming table should approximate the desired positioning of the body when casketed (**Fig. 11–8A,B**).

Three positioning levels are desired:
1. The highest level is the head.
2. The middle level is the chest (anterior thoracic wall).
3. The lowest level is the abdomen (anterior abdominal wall).

The body should be placed in a supine position in the center of the embalming table with the head located near the top of the table. This position allows adequate room for positioning devices for the head and arms. The carotid vessels can then be raised by the embalmer standing at the head of the table.

Establish the three levels of positioning. Rest the buttocks on the table or upon a **body bridge** to establish the abdominal level. Next, place a body bridge under the shoulders. Elevation of the head and shoulders helps to promote drainage from the head and neck areas. A variety of positioning devices can be used for shoulder supports. The chest and the head are also elevated to prevent blood that remains in the heart after embalming from gravitating into the neck and facial tissues and graying these tissues. This discoloration is often referred to as **formaldehyde gray** or **embalmer's gray.**

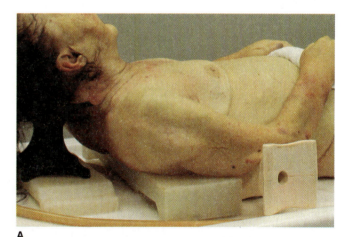

A

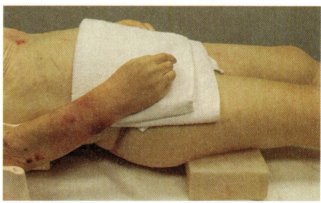

B

**Figure 11–8.** **A.** Positioning of the head and chest. **B.** Positioning of the abdomen.

Elevating the shoulders also helps to dry the body; air can easily pass between the body and the embalming table. This elevation helps to keep any water on the table from contacting the skin of the back and the neck. It is also easier to clean under the body. When the body is obese, a higher shoulder elevation will be needed to establish the three levels of positioning. The higher shoulder support allows the embalmer to slightly lower the height of the head. By doing so, the chin is elevated, to expose the neck.

If facial swelling from edema is present, elevation of the head and the shoulders is important for drainage of the edema from the tissues of the face and the neck. At the conclusion of the aspiration phase of cavity embalming, an **operative aid** such as a trocar can be passed under the clavicles to channel the neck tissues. This establishes routes for the drainage of edema into the thoracic cavity. As a **manual aid,** a pneumatic collar or elastic bandage can be applied to the external tissues of the neck to remove edema and reduce swollen tissues.

Shoulders are elevated to (1) assist drainage, (2) keep water from contacting the back and shoulders, (3) prevent gravitation of blood into facial tissues after embalming, (4) assist in drying the body by allowing air to pass beneath the body, (5) assist in draining edema from the facial and neck tissues, and (6) position the head and chest higher than the abdomen.

A head block can be used to stabilize a body with arthritic limbs. Place a head block under the thigh of the dependent leg to prevent the body from turning side to side.

The head is adjusted on the headrest after the shoulders have been elevated. If the shoulders have to be elevated greatly, the headrest will need additional elevation. Place a folded towel between the head and the headrest to elevate the head to the desired position. The head can be slightly tilted to the right, approximately 15 degrees for viewing. Or, the head may not be tilted at all out of necessity or in observance of local, cultural, or religious custom.

At the start of arterial injection, the hands can be placed at the sides of the body or lowered over the sides of table. This forces the blood in the veins of the arms to gravitate into the capillaries of the hands and expand the capillaries. Once the embalmer establishes fluid distribution into the arms and hands, the hands can be positioned upon the abdomen. Placement of the hands upon a towel will prevent them from slipping (**Fig. 11–9**). The elbows should be elevated from the embalming table with a head block or an arm positioning device. Raising the elbows prevents interference with blood drainage along the sides of the table. Keep the elbows close to the sides of the body. Cultural and religious custom may dictate the positioning of the hands.

## POSITIONING CHALLENGES

Care should be taken to ensure that the fingers remain together and do not separate or splay. A relaxed positioning of the fingers, slightly cupped, produces a natural appearance. Cotton can be placed in the palm of the hands and the fingers curved around the cotton. Webbed cotton can also be wrapped around the fingers to bind them during embalming. A drop of super adhesive glue between each finger will keep them together when other methods are unsuccessful.

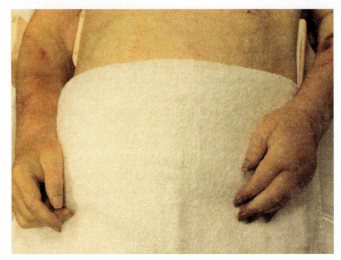

**Figure 11–9.** Placement of hands upon a towel to prevent slipping.

Place the feet close together and elevate them using a positioning device during embalming. When body height prevents proper fit into a casket of standard length, the knees can be slightly bent during embalming. The feet can also be manipulated to keep them at right angles to the leg. Omitting shoes may allow additional room in the casket. Every attempt should be made to avoid the need for an oversized casket.

Also, take a measurement from elbow to elbow to determine the width of the body for proper fit in the casket. Width can be reduced during preliminary body positioning by keeping the elbows close to the sides of the body or by elevating the elbows to the height of the abdomen and bringing the arms across the abdomen. The arms and hands will not cover one another; they will remain adjacent. This draws the upper arms together and decreases width. Turning the body slightly after placement into the casket will also help to reduce body width.

Conditions such as stroke and arthritis can contribute to positioning challenges of the extremities. Arms and legs appear drawn to the body trunk; the fingers can be tightly clenched. Spinal curvature is a condition caused by severe forms of arthritis and osteoporosis. Arthritis cannot be relieved like rigor mortis; the joints are no longer flexible. Avoid overmanipulation of the joints; damage to bones, tendons, and soft tissues can result. Numerous positioning devices will be necessary to maintain natural positioning during embalming. A **manual aid,** such as splinting and wrapping a limb, can be used to secure a limb in the desired position.

Use of the common carotid and internal jugular vein for embalming the legs is indicated when the femoral vessels are impractical. Supplemental hypodermic injection of the limbs after arterial injection ensures optimal results.

## SETTING THE FEATURES

The features are customarily set during the pre-embalming period. Once tissues are embalmed, features may be less flexible for adjustments. **Mouth closure** and **lip closure** are two distinct procedures. Mouth closure raises and holds the lower jaw into position; lip closure brings and holds together the mucous membranes of the lips.

## Mouth Closure Sequence

1. Relieve the rigor mortis present.
2. Disinfect the oral and nasal cavities and swab them clean.
3. If applicable, remove and clean dentures.
4. Pack the throat area.
5. Clean and replace dentures, when applicable.
6. Close the mouth to observe the natural bite.
7. Secure the mandible by one of the methods of mouth closure.
8. Place the lips in the desired position.
9. Embalm the body.
10. Inspect the mouth for moisture or purge material.
11. Seal the mouth.
12. Apply massage cream to the lips and facial tissues.

One of the four conditions exists when the mouth is set: (1) natural teeth are present; (2) natural teeth are present but several are missing; (3) dentures are present (complete set—well fitting, lower denture only—no upper denture, upper denture only—no lower denture, old and very loose-fitting dentures, new ill-fitting dentures, partial plates); and (4) neither dentures nor natural teeth are present.

Dentures are personal property, and many hospitals and nursing homes return them to the family with the belongings. When death occurs at home, the personnel transferring the body should ask for the dentures. It is possible to open the mouth after embalming and insert dentures, but this task is more difficult when tissues are firm, and the jaw is tightly set.

Relieve rigor in the jaw prior to cleaning the oral cavity. If purge is present, a nasal tube aspirator can be used to aspirate purge material. Following aspiration, disinfect inside of the mouth and nasal cavity. The throat and nasal cavities can be packed with cotton to control purge and odors exiting the stomach or lungs. The cotton used for packing material can be coated with massage cream first. This prevents the cotton from absorbing purge materials from the stomach or the lungs.

Achieving the most natural expression for the mouth of the deceased is subjective. Several photographs of the deceased are valuable in posing this feature appropriately. During life, the mouth is capable of infinite expression; choosing the final expression, one most recognizable by family and friends, is challenging.

First examine the condition of the lips. Observe the current closure as well as the contour of each lip. The following treatments may be applied:

- Remove loose skin, scabs, or any other debris with massage cream, solvent, or warm water.
- Open and drain fever blisters.
- Remove tight scabbing with a scalpel or leave in place for post-embalming treatment.
- Observe the weather line to determine the natural line of closure. The upper mucous membrane is often slightly longer and thinner than the lower mucous membrane.
- Observe for dental prognathism; caused by improper alignment of the teeth resulting in a protrusion of the mandible.

### Securing the Mandible for Mouth Closure

#### Method 1: Needle Injector

An alternate to suturing is the method of mouth closure using the needle injector. A barb attached to a wire is driven by a manual device into the center of the maxilla (upper jaw); another barb is driven into the mandible (lower jaw) in an opposing position (**Fig. 11-10**). The two wires are then twisted together to hold the mandible in position (**Fig. 11-11**). The

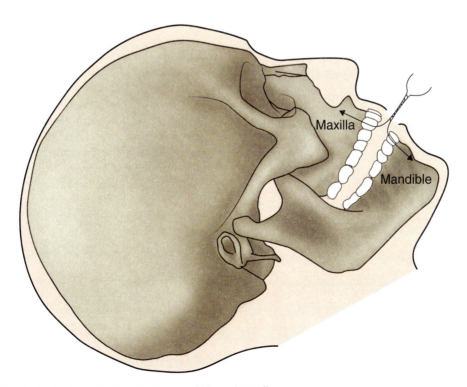

**Figure 11-10.** Needle injector barbs embedded in the mandible and maxilla.

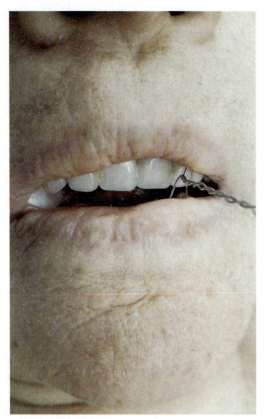

**Figure 11-11.** Needle injector wires twisted together to secure the jaw.

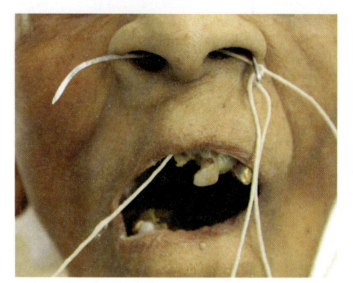

**Figure 11-12.** Needle passed through septum of nose.

barb imbedded into the maxilla should be placed at the center where the two maxillae fuse. This is called the **nasal spine**, and the bone is generally quite strong.

When dentures are available, insert them before using the needle injector. Upper dentures have a small notch in the center; drive the barb into the maxilla at this location. Atrophy of the maxilla and mandible is common with prolonged denture wear. The needle injector is not effective when bones are porous; the barbs will not stay embedded in soft bone. Tenuous fit may result in the barbs coming loose and the mouth reopening. Suturing is the best method when the bones are soft. The manual needle injector should be held at a right angle to the bone for best placement of the barb; an adjustment on the side of the device lessens the effort required to operate the injector. Electric needle injectors are also available.

If the jaw bones have been fractured, four injector wires can be used. Place one on each side of the fractured mandible and repeat for the maxilla. Cross the wires on the diagonal, making an ×. Twist the wires together until the bones are properly aligned.

### Method 2: Musculature Suture
*Best practice is to use an instrument instead of fingers; a hemostat can grasp and pull the needle from the nostrils. Needlesticks can be a source of injury during suturing.*

1. Open the mouth and raise the upper lip. Insert the threaded needle at a point where the upper lip joins the maxilla under the left nostril. Guide the needle against the maxilla to prevent the needle from entering the tissues of the upper lip. *If the soft tissues are caught by the thread, a pucker will result and this will alter the appearance of the mouth.* Slide the needle along the bone until the tip is visible in the left nostril. Grasp the tip of the needle *with a hemostat* and pull the needle and thread completely from the left nostril.
2. Reinsert the needle into the left nostril. Keep the needle in the base of the nostril to prevent a thread from being visible. Direct the needle through the nasal septum into the right nostril and pull the needle and thread completely from the right nostril (**Fig. 11-12**). Best practice is to use a hemostat for pulling the needle from the nostril.
3. Reinsert the needle into the base of the right nostril, direct the needle toward the mouth. Keep the needle against the maxilla and push the needle into the area where the upper lip joins the maxilla. Pull the needle and thread completely from the mouth *using a hemostat*.
4. When dentures are available, insert the lower denture into the mouth first, then place the upper denture. Keep the thread on the outside of the denture.
5. Pull to extend the lower lip and insert the needle on the right side of the mandible at a point where the lower lip joins the gum. Keep the needle against the bone. Make a very wide stitch through the superficial tissues, across the mandible, from right to left. Pull the needle *using a hemostat* completely from the left side at the identical position, where the lower lip joins the gum (**Fig. 11-13**).
6. Tie both threads together like tying a shoe except, wrap the thread twice instead of once. The second wrap will hold the thread in place and keep the mandible secure while completing the knot.
7. Align and adjust the lips for a pleasing appearance.

### Method 3: Sublingual Suture
Use a half-curve needle. Pass the needle, from right to left, behind the lower set of teeth, through the musculature and tissues of the lingual frenulum. The frenulum is the thin tissue that anchors the tongue to the floor of the mouth. The needle is directed toward the maxilla and the upper portion of the suture is completed in the same manner as the musculature suture. The mandible is raised to the desired height and the suture is secured.

### Dental Tie Variation

Tie the thread around the base of one tooth of the lower set. Thread the needle and direct it toward the maxilla. The upper portion of the suture is completed in the same manner as the musculature suture. Raise the mandible to the desired height and tie the thread around the base of a tooth in the lower set to complete the closure.

### Method 6: Drill and Wire

This method is used extensively for trauma restorations of the skull. Fractured and missing bone is replaced and aligned piece by piece and secured into place with wire. A small hole is drilled through the right side of the mandible and the left side of the maxilla. A wire is passed through both holes and twisted together in the same manner as the needle injector wires.

### Method 7: Gluing the Lips

This method is common for mouth closure of infants and children. This closure can be used when the jaw is firmly set and cannot be opened before or after arterial embalming. The disadvantage is that this method does not guarantee that the jaw will not separate over time.

### Method 8: Chin Rest (Historical)

The chin rest is a historical device. The device consists of two small prongs that are inserted into the nostrils. Attached to the two prongs is a sliding support, which is placed beneath the chin to secure the chin in the desired position. This method depended on the overly firm tissues obtained with early embalming fluids. These fluids rapidly and rigidly firmed the tissues. Once the tissues of the face and jaw were completely firm, the device was removed.

## Modeling the Mouth

Natural teeth create the foundation for natural facial expression. The mouth is an essential part of overall expression. When several teeth are missing, appearance is altered. Several materials are used to fill areas where teeth are gone to establish the natural curvature of the mouth.

When all of the natural teeth are missing, and dentures are unavailable, pack the throat and oral cavity. Select a method of mouth closure. A mouth former can be placed to create contouring of the mouth and align the lips. Some mouth formers have holes through which the needle injector wires or the suture thread can be passed. Mouth formers are available in a variety of materials and can be trimmed to fit. Numerous materials can be used in place of a mouth former, such as cotton or mortuary putty.

If cotton is used to replace missing teeth, apply long strips to cover the mandible and the maxilla. Add strips of cotton to recreate natural form and contour. Model the upper integumentary lip first.

When there are dentures but no natural teeth, insert the dentures prior to using the needle injector. The dentures should be cleaned and disinfected first. Cotton placed on the tongue can help to hold the dentures in position. The mandibular suture can be used to secure the lower denture into position. If the lower denture does not fit well, use the upper denture and vice versa. The upper denture gives the best foundation for the curvature of the mouth. It can be held in position by placing cotton

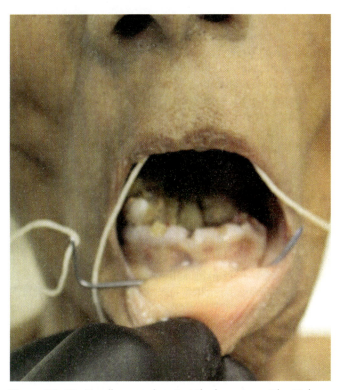

**Figure 11–13.** Needle passed against the bone in a wide stitch.

### Method 4: Mandibular Suture

The suture is passed completely around the mandible. This method is ideal when the deceased is shipped to a different location; the jaw will not separate during transport.

1. Open the mouth and insert the needle behind the lower set of teeth, beneath the tongue near the lingual frenulum. Push the needle downward into the base of the mouth, through the soft tissues, and exit below the chin. Pull the needle with a hemostat completely from the tissue; allow a length of thread to remain in the mouth.
2. Reinsert the needle into the hole at the base of the chin where the needle first exited. Pass the needle upward just in front of the center of the mandible, where the lower lip meets the gum. The suture has passed completely around the mandible. Pull the thread taut and exercise each thread in a back-and-forth motion until the thread reaches the mandible. Keeping the tip of the needle as close as possible to both the anterior and posterior sides of the mandibular bone for this suture minimizes any resulting dimple. The small exit hole beneath the chin created by the needle is easily concealed with restorative wax.
3. Complete the upper portion of the suture in the same manner as the musculature suture.

### Method 5: Dental Tie

A full set of natural teeth is necessary for this method of mouth closure. A thin thread or dental floss is tied around the base of one front tooth of the upper set and one front tooth of the lower set. The thread or floss is tied to secure the jaw in position. Opposing incisor teeth are commonly used. The dental tie is ideal for aligning a fractured jaw. Numerous dental ties can be placed.

or mortuary putty in the area normally occupied by the lower denture. If the denture does not fit at all, do not use it. When placing dentures in the mouth, always insert the lower denture first. After it is in position insert the upper denture. In most people, the line of mouth closure where the two mucous membranes meet is located at the inferior margin of the upper teeth. Establishing the curvature of the upper integumentary lip is the key to a natural appearance.

There are occasions when rigor is so intense that the jaws cannot be opened. It is still wise to use some form of mouth closure. In these instances, if dentures are in the mouth, it is impossible to remove them for cleaning. Spray a disinfectant into the mouth and dry and clean the buccal cavity with cotton swabs.

### Positioning and Closing the Lips

After the mouth has been closed, the natural line of closure is established. The mouth is convex in curvature from corner to corner. In the bilateral view of the mouth, looking from the chin upward to the forehead the convex, or horseshoe curvature of the mouth is easily observed (**Fig. 11–14**). Retaining this curvature avoids making the mouth look flat with a straight line of closure. The center of the mouth is the highest projection. The line of closure is along the inferior margin of the upper teeth. A small amount of cotton inserted high on the maxillae, on a line from the corner of the mouth to the center of the closed eye, helps to raise the area surrounding the corners of the mouth (angulus oris eminences) (**Fig. 11–15**).

The corner eminences can also be defined with tissue builder following arterial embalming. The upper lip, or superior mucous membrane, is usually thinner and longer than the lower lip, or inferior mucous membrane. This appearance can later be highlighted when cosmetics are applied. The weather line, the line of demarcation between the moist and dry portions of each lip, determines the line of closure. Proper lip closure allows the lips to abut, not overlap. Remove any debris on the lips prior to embalming. To hold the lips in position during embalming the following products can be used: lip seal creams (very thick massage creams), petroleum jelly, and lip glue. A super adhesive glue is not customarily used for temporary closure; use this method for challenging situations when the lips will not remain closed.

Application of a lip cream to the lips during embalming will hold them in position and also help to smooth wrinkles on the lips. Natural wrinkles or lines in the mucous membranes are vertical, but lines from dehydration are horizontal. Place a very thin film of lip cream on each lip, and then bring the lips into contact. They will pull away from each other slightly. In doing so, the horizontal wrinkles will be removed as the lips stretch. After embalming, wrinkled lips can be corrected by gluing, tissue building, or waxing. Once the lips have been brought into contact the embalmer creates a pleasing and acceptable form of mouth closure (**Fig. 11–16**).

The same methods can be used if the lips are slightly separated after embalming. Some embalmers find it helpful to keep the lips slightly separated during arterial injection. This allows the mucous membranes to contour as they expand with arterial solution, and prevents the lip closure from appearing tight or pursed.

If the lips are glued temporarily, they should be reopened after embalming to release any material present. Air from the lungs can be forced into the mouth during aspiration of the body and can be released when the mouth is open. The lips can be permanently glued once the buccal cavity is cleaned and dried.

### Eye Closure

In establishing the line of eye closure, the upper eyelid, or superior palpebra, forms two-thirds of the closed eye; the lower eyelid, or inferior palpebra, forms one-third of the closed eye. The line of closure is located in the inferior one-third of the **eye orbit**. The line of closure is curved. The inner corner of the eye, the **inner canthus**, is slightly higher and larger than the outer corner, the **outer canthus** (**Fig. 11–17**).

Best practices for eye closure:
1. Eye closure is customarily done prior to arterial injection.
2. The eyes can be cleaned with moist cotton. Like all areas of the body, the eyes should be sanitized using a topical nonastringent disinfectant. In addition to cleaning the surface and corners of the eyes, clean and align the lashes.
3. Cleaning the eyes also helps to relieve rigor mortis in the muscles of the eyelids. If the face is emaciated or dehydrated, the eyelids may have to be stretched slightly to improve flexibility for proper closure. This can be done by inserting the smooth handle of an instrument, such as an aneurysm hook beneath the lid, and gently stretching the tissue (**Fig. 11–18A**).
4. Establish the anterior projection of the closed eye and secure lid closure by inserting cotton and/or an eye cap (**Fig. 11–18B,C**). Close the inner canthus to prevent

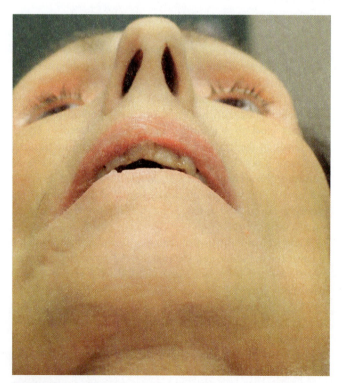

**Figure 11–14.** Bilateral view shows convex curvature of the mouth.

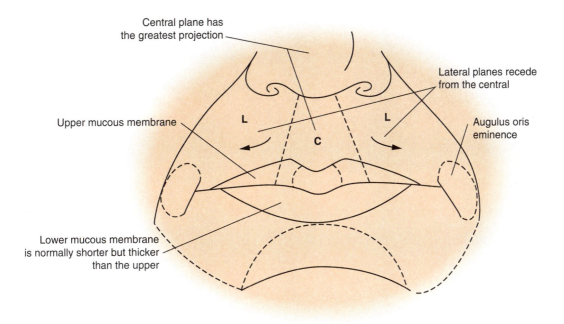

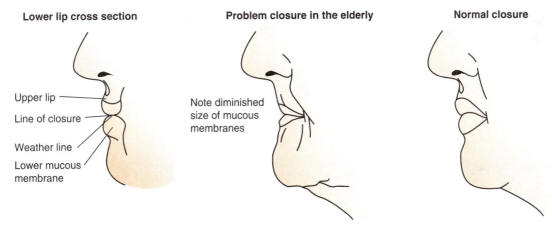

**Figure 11-15.** Positioning the lips. Profiles show various closures.

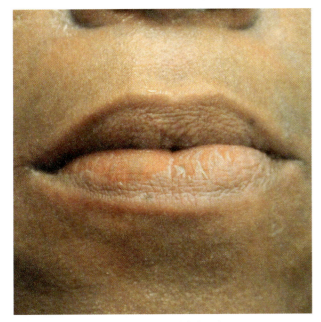

**Figure 11-16.** Pleasing and acceptable lip closure.

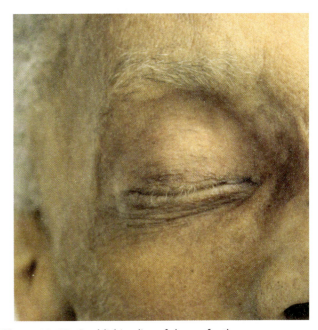

**Figure 11-17.** Establishing line of closure for the eye.

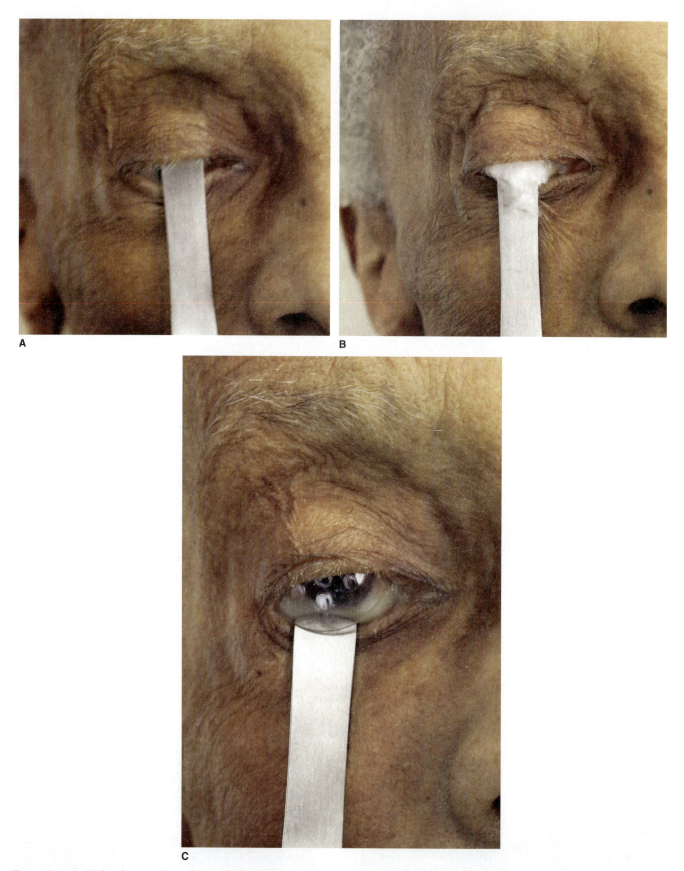

**Figure 11–18. A.** Gentle stretching of the eyelid to improve flexibility. **B.** Insertion of cotton to establish proper projection. **C.** Insertion of an eye cap to maintain closure.

dehydration in this area. The moist tissue of the inner canthus will shrink and darken if not properly closed.

a. *Eye cap.* Eye caps resemble a contact lens. They are designed to cover a larger surface area than a contact lens. Eye caps may be perforated; the perforations hold the lids closed. The convex shape of the cap helps to maintain the convex curvature of the closed eye. The cap maintains contour of the closed eye. Should the eyes be sunken, use several caps or two caps with mortuary putty or a piece of cotton sandwiched between to elevate the closed eyelids.

b. *Cotton.* Cotton may be placed under the closed eyelids to keep the lids closed, elevate the lids, and establish the convexity of the closed eye. Lift the upper lid and insert the cotton under the upper eyelid with the handle of an aneurysm needle or forceps. Lift the upper eyelid over the cotton and place it in its proper position. Evert (turn outward) the lower eyelids and insert the cotton into the area covered by the lower eyelid. Lift the lower eyelid into position.

After arterial injection if the eyelids do appear too soft, several drops of cavity fluid can be placed on the cotton used for eye closure.

### Difficult Eye Closure

In cases of extreme emaciation, postmortem dehydration, or if the vitreous (gel-like fluid) was removed from the eye globe during autopsy, the eyes can be sunken and the globe dehydrated. The globe can be rounded, or inflated by the direct injection of tissue builder. Apply a drop of super adhesive glue to the site of needle entry to prevent loss of fluids. To bring the eyelids together, the lids may need to be exercised and stretched to secure closure. After stretching the lids, temporary pre-embalming gluing of the lids may be helpful. The margins of the lids abut, they do not overlap. For difficult closures, overlapping may be necessary.

To control dehydration, place a massage or stay cream on the cotton or eye caps. Cotton can also be saturated with a supplemental humectant fluid.

## PACKING THE TRUNK ORIFICES

A topical spray disinfectant is reapplied to the areas surrounding the anal and the vaginal orifices prior to treatment. Long strips of saturated cotton are inserted with packing forceps into the orifices. Phenol solution, undiluted cavity fluid, or autopsy gel may be used to saturate the cotton. This treatment may be repeated after embalming if discharge of fecal and other materials occurs during embalming. A threaded closure device may be inserted following the cotton packing to prevent further discharge.

## REMOVAL OF INVASIVE MEDICAL DEVICES

Invasive medical devices may be removed by the embalmer before, during, or after embalming. Any device that poses a hazard or interferes with arterial embalming is removed prior to embalming, disinfected, and properly disposed in the biohazard waste container. Devices that could potentially mark the tissues of the face are also removed.

## Implantable Devices: Defibrillators and Pacemakers

Implantable devices can be removed before or after embalming. Implantable devices containing batteries must be removed prior to cremation. Risk of explosion can result in injury to crematory personnel and damage to equipment during the cremation process. Implantable cardioverter-defibrillators (ICD) and pacemakers are usually visible in the upper chest. The device is easily palpated beneath the skin. A small semilunar incision is made with a scalpel along the superior border of the device (**Fig. 11–19A**). As the device is removed from the incision, two electrical leads are exposed. A best practice is to cut each lead independent of the other, with surgical scissors (**Fig. 11–19B**). A strong magnet can interrupt the device mode but will *not* turn off the device. Proper removal and disposal of medical devices should follow the instructions of the authorizing agent or next-of-kin. Disposal instructions may be contained in the language of embalming and cremation authorization forms. Medical devices that should be discarded are placed in approved biohazard sharps or waste containers. The incision is sutured after the device is removed (**Fig. 11–19C**). Bonding agents and super adhesive glues may also be used to seal the incision. Electrical leads that pass through the subclavian or cephalic vein can interfere with blood drainage during embalming.

## Surgical Incisions

Recent surgical incisions can be a source of infection. Liberally disinfect the area during the initial bathing. Surgical staples or sutures can remain in place when secure and no leakage is noted. Hypodermically inject a cautery solution into the marginal tissues, and apply a cotton compress overtop. Plastic wrap is used to contain chemical fumes while the pack is in place. If the incision must be opened, add sealing powder to prevent leakage before resuturing. Apply a surface sealant after final bathing.

## Types of Air Passageway Tubes

Tubes that enter the mouth or the nostrils should be removed, or extubated, in the pre-embalming period. These tubes, if left in place for any time, can mark the corners of the mouth or nose. When the tubes have been in the patient's mouth or nose for several weeks, the surrounding skin may be compromised. Massage of these areas during arterial injection may help to restore them to their natural contour.

Cotton saturated with a disinfectant or cautery agent can be placed in the surgical opening to disinfect the respiratory passages. Close these openings after arterial embalming. Should any purge develop in the lungs or stomach, the surgical opening provides an outlet for the purge material. After packing with cotton and incision seal powder, a small purse-string suture can be made to close the opening. Restorative wax or tissue builder and cosmetics are used to conceal the closure.

## Endotracheal Tubes

An endotracheal tube is placed into the mouth, then into the trachea to assist breathing. The tube is connected to a ventilator, which delivers oxygen to the lungs. Endotracheal tubes should be removed, or extubated, in the pre-embalming period and the area should be disinfected (**Fig. 11–20**).

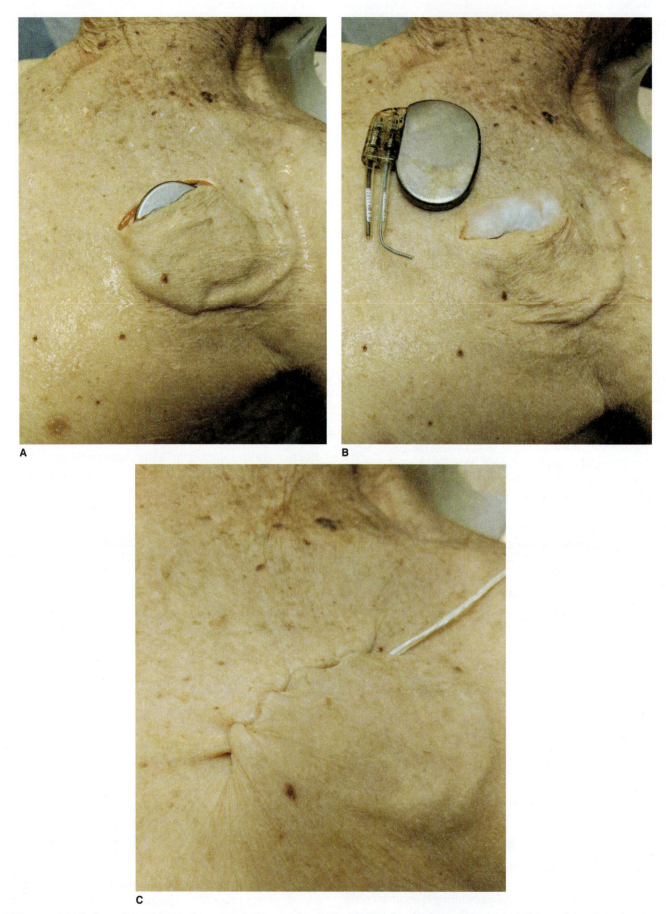

Figure 11–19. A. A semilunar incision for removal of pacemaker. B. Electrical leads cut and device removed. C. Inversion suture closes incision.

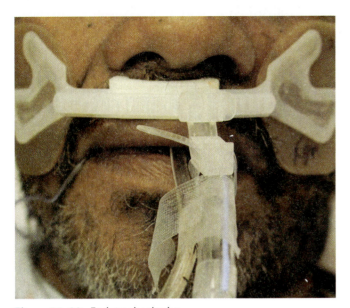

Figure 11-20. Endotracheal tube.

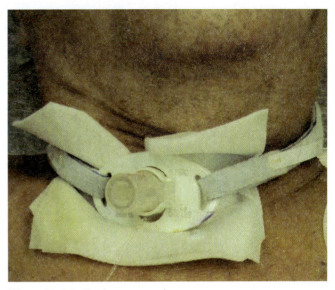

Figure 11-22. Tracheostomy tube.

### Nasopharyngeal Tubes

The tube is inserted into the nasal passageway to secure an open airway. The distal tip rests in the nasopharynx. Nasopharyngeal tubes should be removed, or extubated, in the pre-embalming period and the area should be disinfected (**Fig. 11-21**).

### Tracheostomy Tubes

A small metal or plastic tube that keeps the stoma and the trachea open to assist breathing (**Fig. 11-22**). Tracheostomy tubes should be removed in the pre-embalming period and the area should be disinfected.

### Abdominal Feeding Tube

The abdominal feeding tube is inserted into the stomach through a small incision in the abdominal wall (**Fig. 11-23**). Feeding tubes can be removed before or after arterial embalming. Wrap the tubing first with cotton; pressure is released when the tube is cut and material contained in the tube may discharge. The tubing may be extracted fully or a segment may remain internally. Disinfect the area after the tubing is withdrawn. Insert cotton saturated with phenol, autopsy gel, or undiluted cavity fluid into the opening using a forceps.

Close the opening with a purse-string suture or large trocar button.

Depending on the location of the feeding tube, the opening may be used for cavity aspiration and introduction of cavity fluid following arterial embalming. This also holds true for colostomy stomas.

### Surgical Drains

Surgical drains can be removed before or after arterial embalming. Drain openings should be packed with cotton saturated with phenol, autopsy gel, or undiluted cavity fluid. A small purse-string suture or large trocar button is used to close the opening. This should be done prior to cavity embalming.

### Colostomy

Colostomy is a surgical procedure that diverts a section of the colon to an opening in the abdominal wall. Stool drains into the collecting bag from this opening, called a *stoma*. The collecting bag can be removed either before or after arterial embalming. Once the collecting bag is removed, the stoma is visible (**Fig. 11-24**). Irrigate any remaining fecal material and

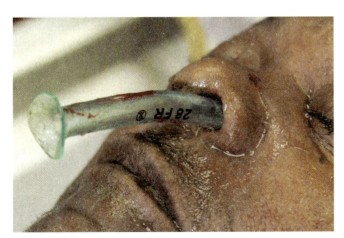

Figure 11-21. Nasopharyngeal tube.

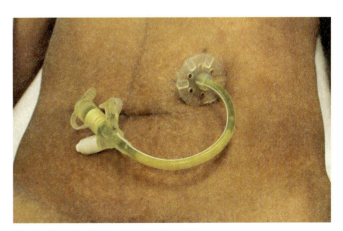

Figure 11-23. Abdominal feeding tube.

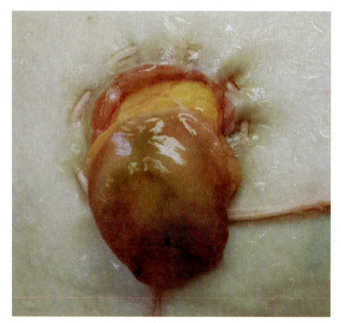

**Figure 11–24.** Stoma exposed.

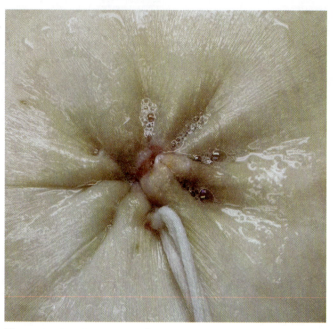

**Figure 11–26.** Purse-string closure.

thoroughly disinfect this area. Place saturated cotton over the stoma and push it back into the abdominal opening (**Fig. 11–25**). Close the opening with a purse-string suture (**Fig. 11–26**). Surface glue and cotton can be applied to prevent any leakage. Disinfect the collecting bag prior to disposal. Pour a few ounces of undiluted cavity fluid or other mortuary disinfectant into the bag and discard in an approved biohazard container.

### Intravenous Catheters (I.V.)

Intravenous catheters can remain in place until arterial embalming is completed. These invasive devices did not hamper circulation during life, and leaving them in place will not interfere with arterial injection or blood drainage. They can be removed after arterial and cavity embalming is completed. When these tubes are removed from the areas that will not be seen after the body is dressed, their openings can be enlarged with a scalpel and a trocar button can be inserted to prevent leakage. Super adhesive glue can be applied to these openings, especially in visible areas such as the back of the hands or the neck. Alternatively, cauterant can be injected with a fine needle (small gauge) and syringe directly into the opening to prevent leakage.

### Urinary Catheter

A catheter can be inserted into the urinary tract through the urethra or the abdominal wall. It can be removed prior to arterial embalming. Cut a small side vent into the catheter tubing with scissors to collapse the balloon dilated within the bladder. Then pull the catheter from the body: If the catheter was inserted through the abdominal wall, a small purse-string suture or large trocar button can be used to close the opening. In females, the urethra can be packed with the cotton saturated with cavity fluid, autopsy gel, or a phenol cautery chemical after the catheter is removed. Be certain to dispose the catheter in a biohazard container.

### Casts

The two most common types of casting material are plaster and fiberglass. A vibrating cast-cutting saw is used to remove the cast. Casts should be removed prior to arterial embalming whenever possible. This allows inspection of the casted area. Leaving a cast in place means the embalmer cannot ensure that embalming solution is distributed to the area covered by the cast. When the cast must remain, elevate and cover the cast with plastic to protect from soiling by blood drainage.

## EXTERNAL ORTHOPEDIC DEVICES

External orthopedic devices used for fixation of traumatic bone injuries may be removed before or after embalming (**Fig. 11–27**). Tools are needed to remove the hardware from these devices; pliers may be necessary to securely grip and unscrew the nuts from the bolts. The metal rods penetrating the bone are firmly set. This type of activity poses an injury risk to the embalmer. Extra caution

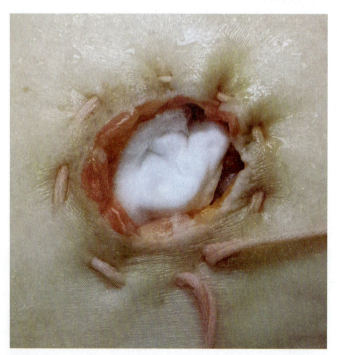

**Figure 11–25.** Cotton inlay.

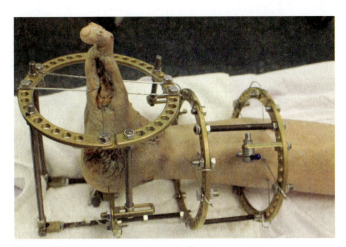

**Figure 11–27.** External orthopedic fixator.

must be exercised. A team approach is recommended so that one embalmer can stabilize the device and extremity, while the other removes the hardware.

## GENERAL PRE-EMBALMING TREATMENTS

Most of the treatments that follow employ concentrated solutions that contain either formaldehyde or phenol. Personal protective equipment should be worn when handling these chemicals. When formaldehyde, phenol, bleaching surface compresses, or surface preservative gels are used, cover them with plastic to (1) control odor, (2) prevent evaporation, and (3) prevent inhalation of toxic fumes by the embalmer.

Hypodermic syringes should be flushed with tissue builder solvent after each use. When injecting the face with chemicals other than tissue builder, the point of entry, when possible, should be inside the mouth or a hidden point of entry should be used, since unlike tissue builder, these chemicals can leak. Injection of the backs of the hands can be done by entering the hypodermic needle into the webbing between the fingers. Some leakage can be expected and this should stop in a short period of time. Seal the needle entry points with super adhesive glue.

### Visible Discoloration—Livor Mortis, Postmortem Stain, Ecchymosis, Purpura

Discolorations of the face, arms, and hands should be carefully examined before arterial injection. Livor mortis is an intravascular blood discoloration; once hemolysis occurs, postmortem stain is extravascular. Stain cannot be cleared by arterial injection but can be bleached and lightened. Livor can be distinguished from stain by applying digital pressure to the discoloration. If the discoloration lightens, the discoloration is intravascular and can be cleared. If it does not lighten, the discoloration is stain. Livor mortis can also be removed from an area by elevating the affected tissues. Livor and stain can occur in the same tissues; livor precedes stain. Refrigeration, blood thinners, and carbon monoxide all speed hypostasis of the blood and the resulting livor mortis and postmortem stain.

Elevation of the shoulders and head will prevent the occurrence of livor mortis. If already present, elevation will promote drainage of livor mortis from the facial tissues.

Ecchymosis and purpura are localized antemortem, extravascular blood discolorations. These conditions are frequently seen on the backs of the hands. The discolorations cannot be removed but can be bleached. The treatments that follow ensure good preservation of the affected areas. Optional treatments include the following:

1. Subcutaneous hypodermic injection using a phenol bleaching chemical or undiluted cavity fluid before or after arterial injection.
2. Application of a surface preservative gel or compress of a bleaching solution before, during, and following arterial injection.
3. A combination of surface and hypodermic treatments before or following arterial injection.

### Skin Lesions and Ulcerations

Observe and evaluate any rashes, lesions, infected areas, decubitus ulcers, and skin cancers. After cleansing the body, the embalmer should begin treatment of these areas immediately to (1) disinfect the affected area, (2) preserve the tissues surrounding the lesion, (3) dry the tissues, and (4) deodorize the tissues. These areas should be of concern to the embalmer for the following reasons:

1. They can be a source of contamination to the embalmer, such as staph and herpes infections.
2. The tissues can be necrotic: decomposition of the superficial and deep tissues is in progress.
3. Blood supply to the necrotic tissues is poor; little or no contact between arterial solution and the diseased tissue.
4. Odors may be present. Tissues left untreated can produce offensive odors, may be noticeable after embalming, dressing, and casketing.
5. Necrotic tissue can contain the anaerobic gas bacillus that produces gas gangrene.

A common example of necrotic and infected tissue is the decubitus ulcer, also called a *pressure sore* or *bedsore*. These ulcerations result from limited circulation into an area that receives constant contact pressure. The bony areas: hips, buttocks, elbows, shoulders, and heels are commonly affected by pressure sores. Prolonged contact pressure is anticipated in bedridden patients. Staph infections accelerate tissue death, and the area becomes necrotic. Treat the affected area with a topical disinfectant or swab with undiluted cavity fluid or a cautery chemical.

Topically treat bandages or coverings before removal. Dispose of these materials in the biohazard waste container. Treat the area hypodermically and apply saturated compresses or autopsy gel prior to embalming. This helps to control odors, to preserve the necrotic tissue, and to destroy any bacteria present.

Apply fresh compresses after embalming. Dress the body in a suitable plastic garment. When the hips or buttocks are affected, an adult incontinence brief can be used. Add absorbent and preservative powders to the garment or brief.

### Lacerations and Fractures

A **laceration** is defined as a jagged tear in the skin. In the pre-embalming period, a laceration should be cleaned of any blood or debris. This is easily done with germicidal soap and cool water. After the edges of the laceration are cleaned, the torn skin should be aligned. Several small bridge sutures can be placed along the laceration to hold the edges in position during embalming. If the laceration is in an area of the body that will be seen, massage cream can be placed around the area after the

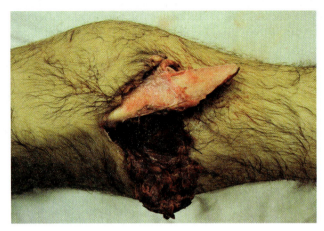

**Figure 11–28.** Compound fracture of the femur.

bridge sutures are in place. This protects the unaffected skin. If the laceration is in a body area that will not be viewed after arterial injection, the laceration can be closed with a baseball suture. During embalming, arterial solution may leak from the laceration. Place a compress over the lacerated tissues to contain the solution as an effective means of surface preservation.

Compound fractures (**Fig. 11–28**) pose risk of injury to the embalmer. Injuries to viewable areas do require restoration; nonviewable injuries require containment to prevent leakage, but do not need to be restored. Evaluation of each case is recommended.

## Abrasions

An **abrasion**, also known as *excoriation*, is a wearing away of the upper layer of skin as a result of applied friction force. The embalmer encounters two types of abrasions:

- **Dry Abrasion**—Dry abrasions are dehydrated. The area resembles a scab formation. The tissue is dark and feels rough and firm to the touch. Dry abrasions do not present preservation issues. The area can be concealed after embalming.
- **Moist Abrasions**—The underlying tissue of a moist abrasion is wet and appears shiny. Preservation is necessary; cauterizing the wet tissue will dry the area for restoration and concealment.

In the pre-embalming period, inspect and evaluate abrasions and clean the affected area. Moist abrasions can be covered with a compress of undiluted cavity fluid, phenol cautery solution, or autopsy gel. During embalming, arterial solution may pass through the abraded tissues. After embalming, the objective is to dry these abrasions. A hair dryer can be used to force-dry wet tissue and expedite the process when there is inadequate time for chemicals to work.

## Skin-Slip, Torn Skin, Blisters, Pustules, and Scabs

Pre-embalming treatment begins with the application of a topical disinfectant. All loose and damaged skin is debrided (removed). Blisters and pustules are opened and drained. Apply a surface preservative gel or surface compress to the affected area. In visible areas protect unaffected tissues by applying a light coating of massage cream. Allow surface treatments to remain in place during embalming; arterial solution may seep through the affected areas. After embalming remove surface chemicals and air or force-dry the tissues. Dry areas will darken. Conceal visible discolorations with restorative waxes and cosmetics.

## Gases

There are three sources of gas in the dead human body. When gases are present in the tissues, distension and swelling can occur. Gases can be palpated (examined by touch). **Crepitation** is the crackling sensation produced by the presence of air in the subcutaneous tissues. **Table 11-1** outlines the characteristics of these gases.

| TABLE 11–1. Gases Causing Distension | | | |
|---|---|---|---|
| Type | Source | Characteristics | Treatments |
| Subcutaneous emphysema | Puncture of lung or pleural sac; seen in CPR treatments; puncture wounds to thorax; rib fractures; tracheotomy | No odor; no skin-slip; no blebs; gas can be extreme, present even in toes; can create intense swelling; rises to highest body areas | Gas will escape through incisions; establish good arterial preservation; channel tissues after arterial injection to release gases |
| True tissue gas | Anaerobic bacteria; C. perfringens | Very strong odor of decomposition; skin-slip; skin blebs; the condition and amount of gas increase with time; spore-forming bacteria may be passed by cutting instruments to other bodies | Use of special "tissue gas" arterial solutions; localized hypodermic injection of cavity fluid; channel tissues to release gases |
| Gas gangrene | Anaerobic bacteria; C. perfringens | Foul odor; infection | Strong arterial solutions; local hypodermic injection of cavity chemical |
| Decomposition | Bacterial breakdown of body tissues; autolytic breakdown of body tissues | Odor may be present, skin-slip in time; color changes; purging | Proper strong chemical in sufficient amounts by arterial injection; hypodermic and surface treatments; channel to release gases |
| Air from embalming apparatus | Air injected by embalming machine (air-pressure machines and hand pumps are in limited use today) | First evidence in eyelids; no odors; no skin-slip; amount would depend on injection time—most would be minimal | If distension is caused, channel after arterial injection to release gases |

### Subcutaneous Emphysema

Subcutaneous emphysema results from penetration or tearing into the pleural cavities or lung tissues. When gas is detected in the tissues and neither odor nor skin slip is present, examine the body for external punctures near the lungs, recent tracheostomy, or fracture of the clavicle, sternum, or ribs. Subcutaneous emphysema can be widespread in a body. Subcutaneous emphysema is a common condition after blunt force trauma to the chest and the administration of cardiopulmonary resuscitation (CPR).

### Gas from Decomposition

Signs of decomposition are discoloration, odor, purge, skin slip, and gas. Gases can accumulate in the viscera, body cavities, or skeletal tissues.

### True Tissue Gas

The source of this gas is Welch's bacillus (*Clostridium perfringens*), an anaerobic spore-forming bacillus that thrives on necrotic tissue. Tissue gas can be passed between bodies by contaminated cutting instruments. A very strong odor of decomposed tissue is characteristic (foul amines). The condition may begin in the agonal and early postmortem periods. Tissue gas will accelerate until chemically arrested. Tissue distension may begin in the abdomen. Severe distension may restrict the flow of arterial solution and the drainage of blood. The abdomen should be punctured and the gas allowed to escape prior to embalming. Make a puncture with a scalpel near the standard point of trocar entry, 2 inches superior and 2 inches to the left of the umbilicus (**Fig. 11–29**). Follow with the insertion of a trocar to relieve tissue gas.

When facial tissues and the upper chest are affected, make a semilunar incision, from the center of the right clavicle to the center of the left clavicle to allow gases to escape. Embalm using restricted cervical injection. After embalming, channel tissues and apply pressure to the distended areas to force the removal of gases. Disinfect all instruments thoroughly after embalming. Immerse the trocar in a cold chemical sterilant.

## Ascites

When the abdomen is tightly distended, the embalmer must determine if the distension is caused by gases or edema. Either way, extravascular pressure is created and must be relieved before arterial embalming. Insertion of the trocar into the upper abdominal region will allow both edema and gases to escape. Generalized edema and tortuous (twisted) veins visible in the superficial abdominal tissues is indicative of ascites. Edema within the abdominal cavity does not dilute the arterial solution but it will dilute the cavity fluid.

### CONCEPTS FOR STUDY

Define the following terminology:
- Convex curvature
- Crepitation
- Dental tie
- Lip closure
- Mandible
- Mandibular suture
- Manual aid
- Maxilla
- Mouth closure
- Musculature suture
- Needle injector
- Operative aid
- Prognathism
- Sublingual suture

1. Explain best practices for lifting and transferring.
2. List several uses of massage cream.
3. Name the three levels of positioning of the body.
4. Recall several reasons for supporting the shoulders with positioning devices.
5. Compare the various methods of mouth closure.
6. What is the difference between lip closure and mouth closure?
7. How can pre-embalming gas distension be treated?
8. Explain the process for relieving rigor mortis.
9. Describe one method of treating decubitus ulcers prior to embalming.

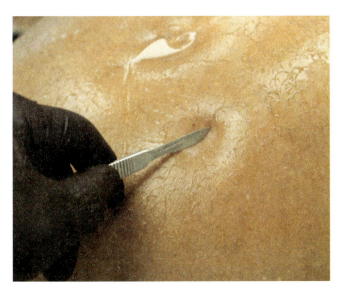

**Figure 11-29.** Scalpel puncture to abdomen to relieve tissue gas.

### FIGURE CREDIT

Figures 11–2, 11–6, 11–11, 11–19A-C, 11–23, 11–24, 11–25, 11–26 are used with permission of Sharon L. Gee-Mascarello.

Figures 11–3, 11–4, 11–5, 11–7, 11–8A,B, 11–9, 11–12, 11–13, 11–14, 11–16, 11–17, 11–18A-C, 11–20, 11–21, 11–22, 11–27, 11–28, 11–29 are used with permission of Kevin Drobish.

### BIBLIOGRAPHY

American Board of Funeral Service, *Course Content Syllabus*, 2016.

*From Alpha to Omega in the Preparation Room*, 4th ed. Dallas, TX: Professional Training Schools, 1999.

Mayer JS. *Restorative Art*, 13th ed. Dallas, TX: Professional Training Schools, 1993.

Thomas CL. *Taber's Cyclopedic Medical Dictionary*, 19th ed. Philadelphia: F.A. Davis, 2001.

# CHAPTER 12

# Injection and Drainage Techniques

### CHAPTER OVERVIEW
- Arterial (Vascular) Embalming Processes
- Injection Sites and Techniques
- Drainage Sites and Techniques
- Purpose and Contents of Drainage

Arterial embalming has two primary functions: injection of preservative solution and drainage of blood and other fluids from the blood vascular system. A total of four distinct processes are actually occurring simultaneously during arterial embalming:
1. **Injection** of the embalming solution from the embalming machine into the artery(ies).
2. **Distribution** of the embalming solution throughout the blood vascular system.
3. **Diffusion** of the embalming solution into the cells and tissues of the body.
4. **Drainage** of the contents of the blood vascular system.

The proper selection of vessels and corresponding injection and drainage methods is critical to achieve uniform preservation and sanitation. Ideal vessels and methods will ensure:
- A sufficient volume of embalming solution is delivered and retained in the tissues.
- Adequate drainage removes intravascular blood discolorations, edema, and cellular waste.
- A proper moisture balance is established to prevent tissue dehydration.
- The appearance of the deceased is acceptable.

| One-point Injection | Injection and drainage from a single site. |
| Multipoint Injection | Injection from two or more sites. |
| Six-point Injection | Injection from six sites. |
| Split Injection | Injection at one site and drainage from a different site. |
| Restricted Cervical | Injection of the trunk with restriction of solution entering the head using both common carotid arteries. |
| Instant Tissue Fixation | High strength solution injected into a specific region using short bursts under high pressure. |

## ARTERIAL (VASCULAR) INJECTION TECHNIQUES

### One-Point Injection Technique

A one-point injection uses the same site for both arterial injection and blood drainage (**Fig. 12–1A–C**). Same site injection and drainage is suitable when the embalmer anticipates uncomplicated distribution of embalming solution and favorable blood drainage. This method is customarily selected as the primary injection technique. The method selected for incising the artery will determine whether both arterial tubes can be placed simultaneously into that artery.

The most frequently selected vessels for one-point injection include the right common carotid artery and right internal jugular vein, the right femoral artery and right femoral vein, and the right axillary artery and right axillary vein. The left common carotid artery is often raised as a secondary site to supplement the injection of solution and/or clear blood discolorations from the left side of the face; the left internal jugular vein is also raised as a secondary drainage site. When additional vessels are raised, this becomes a multipoint injection.

#### One-Point: Right Common Carotid Artery and Right Internal Jugular Vein
- Insert an arterial tube into the right common carotid artery directed toward the trunk of the body
- Insert a drainage instrument (angular spring forceps or jugular drain tube) into the right internal jugular vein directed toward the heart
- Inject toward the trunk of the body
- Insert an arterial tube into the right common carotid artery directed toward the head
- Inject toward the right side of the head

#### One-Point: Right Femoral Artery and Femoral Vein
- Insert an arterial tube into the femoral artery directed toward the right foot

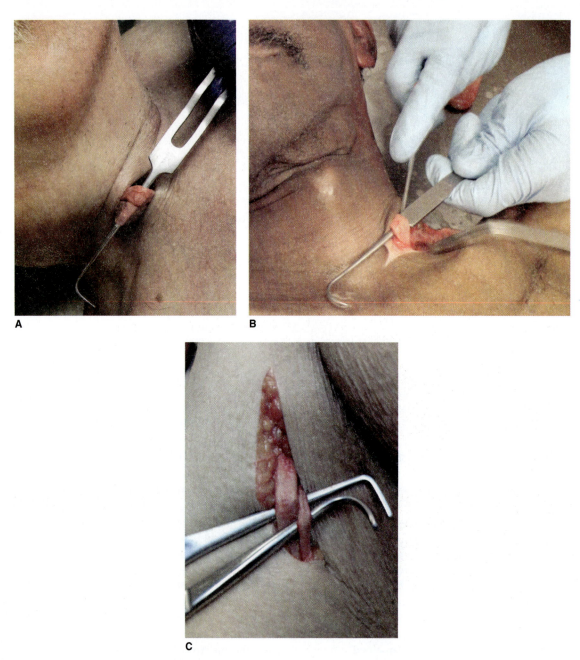

**Figure 12–1. A.** One-point injection: right common carotid artery and right internal jugular vein. **B.** One-point injection: left common carotid artery and left internal jugular vein. **C.** One-point injection: right femoral artery and right femoral vein.

- Insert a drainage device (femoral drain tube or straight spring forceps) into the femoral vein directed toward the heart
- Inject toward the right leg
- Insert an arterial tube into the femoral artery directed toward the trunk and head
- Inject toward the trunk and head

### One-Point: Right Axillary Artery and Axillary Vein

- Insert an arterial tube into the axillary artery directed toward the right hand
- Insert a drainage instrument (axillary drain tube or straight spring forceps) into the axillary vein directed toward the heart
- Inject toward the right arm
- Insert an arterial tube into the right axillary artery directed toward the head and trunk
- Inject toward the head and trunk

## Disadvantages of One-Point Injection

### Short-Circuiting of Arterial Solution

Embalming solution tends to follow the most direct route from the point of injection, through the arterioles and capillaries into the venules, to exit as drainage. This can account for a great amount of arterial solution loss. Short-circuiting can be decreased by restricting drainage to create intravascular pressure.

### Path of Least Resistance

Embalming solution follows the path of least resistance to enter the network of capillaries nearest the injection site. Skin has a greater presence of capillaries compared to the deeper body tissues. The result is that the skin surrounding the injection site can easily swell when over embalmed. Injection from a more distant site is warranted when the neck and facial features are affected.

### Shell Embalming

Short-circuiting and paths of least resistance cause embalming solution to reach only the skin and the superficial tissues. Shell embalming is the result of inadequate preservation to the deeper tissues. Tissue massage combined with manipulation of extremities and restriction of drainage will encourage movement of arterial solution into the muscles and deep tissues to prevent shell embalming.

### Multipoint Injection Technique

Multipoint injection is the injection from two or more sites. An additional site, or multiple sites, is identified to supplement the primary injection site when arterial solution cannot reach a particular area or when the area is insufficiently preserved. Suitable arteries are located closer to the area insufficiently embalmed. For example, injection begins with the right femoral artery (primary site) but embalming solution does not adequately supply the right lower leg and foot. To supplement embalming of the right lower leg and foot, raise and inject the right anterior tibial artery (secondary site) and right dorsalis pedis artery (tertiary site). Multiple injection sites (three in total) are used in this example to ensure thorough preservation of the lower leg and foot.

### Advantages of Multipoint Injection

Injection from multiple points increases the overall effectiveness of embalming. Each additional site is used to inject a specific region or section of the body, called **sectional embalming**. Military regulations require the use of multiple sites for long-term preservation. Multipoint injection is recommended to address lengthy postmortem time intervals between death and embalming, and between embalming and funeral rites, and between embalming and final disposition. The use of multiple injection sites is beneficial in the following conditions:

- Autopsy
- Blood cancers and malignancies
- Contagious diseases
- Decomposition
- Difficult to firm tissues
- Generalized edema (anasarca)
- Organ and tissue donation
- Poor peripheral circulation
- Purge (embalming solution)
- Refrigeration
- Ruptured aortic aneurysm
- Shipping the body to a different location
- Trauma
- Tissue gas

### Six-Point Injection Technique

A six-point injection isolates each extremity (both arms; both legs) and both sides of the head. Embalming following a complete autopsy (cranial and trunk) is an example of a six-point injection (**Fig. 12–2**). A six-point injection is also

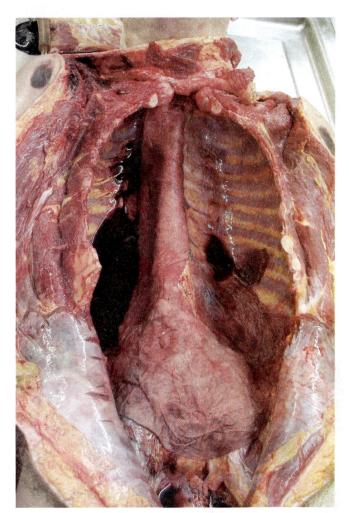

Figure 12–2. A six-point injection is used for embalming a complete autopsy.

used for nonautopsied cases. The anticipation of embalming challenges such as poor distribution of solution, incomplete blood drainage, increased probability of tissue distension, and lengthy postmortem delays validates six-point embalming. A different solution strength may be used in each region. Drainage can be taken from the accompanying vein at each injection site, or all drainage can be taken from the right internal jugular vein. Customarily the extremities of the body are injected prior to the head. When the right side of the face is the most visible (viewable) side, the left side is injected before the right side. This order of injection allows the embalmer to make adjustments prior to injecting the most visible side of the face. In the following examples, injection alternates from the left to right throughout the procedure to establish a consistent routine. The order of injection is based upon professional judgment.

### Chronology for Six-Point Injection (Nonautopsy)

- Left leg—inject the left femoral artery (or external iliac) toward the foot
- Right leg—inject the right femoral artery (or external iliac) toward the foot
- Left arm—inject the left axillary artery (or brachial or subclavian) toward the hand

- Right arm—inject the right axillary artery (or brachial or subclavian) toward the hand
- Left side of the head—inject the left common carotid artery toward the head
- Right side of the head—inject the right common carotid artery toward the head

### Chronology for Six-point Injection (Autopsy)
- Left leg—inject the left femoral artery (or external iliac) toward the foot
- Right leg—inject the right femoral artery (or external iliac) toward the foot
- Left arm—inject the left axillary artery (or brachial or subclavian) toward the hand
- Right arm—inject the right axillary artery (or brachial or subclavian) toward the hand
- Left side of the head—inject the left common carotid artery toward the head
- Right side of the head—inject the right common carotid artery toward the head

## Split Injection Technique

Split injection is the injection of solution from one site with drainage from a different site (**Fig. 12–3A,B**). This method reduces short-circuiting of the solution and establishes a uniform distribution of the arterial solution. The most frequently used combination of vessels in the split injection method is the right internal jugular vein (drainage) and the right femoral artery (injection).

Choice of a single site of injection can lead to the split injection method (two sites) when drainage is difficult to establish. For example, the initial site of injection is the right femoral artery and right femoral vein. When inadequate drainage is recognized, the right internal jugular vein is raised to solve the poor drainage.

### Split Injection: Right Femoral Artery and Right Internal Jugular Vein
- Insert a drainage instrument into the right internal jugular vein directed toward the heart
- Insert an arterial tube into the right femoral artery directed toward the right foot
- Insert an arterial tube into the right femoral artery directed toward the trunk and head
- Inject the right leg and foot first
- Inject the trunk and head
- Drainage is taken from the right internal jugular vein

### Split Injection: Right Common Carotid Artery and Right Femoral Vein
- Insert a drainage instrument into the right femoral vein directed toward the heart
- Insert an arterial tube into the right common carotid artery directed toward the right side of the head
- Insert an arterial tube into the right common carotid artery directed toward the trunk
- Inject down the right common carotid artery first to embalm the trunk and left side of the face
- Inject the right side of the head
- Drainage is taken from the right femoral vein

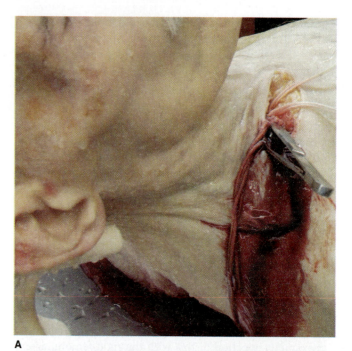

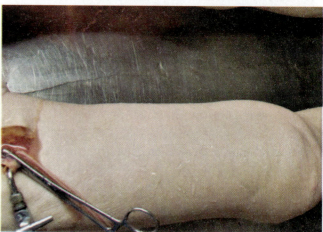

**Figure 12–3.** **A.** Split injection. Right internal jugular vein is used for blood drainage. **B.** Split injection. Right femoral artery is used for arterial solution injection.

### Advantages of Split Injection Using the Femoral Artery as the Primary Injection Site

Split injection is a valuable method for enhancing facial features during arterial embalming. Injection from the right femoral artery, directed toward the head, allows solution to distribute simultaneously through both left and right common carotid arteries. The injection pressure is slowed by the distance between the injection site and the head. The result is a gradual and symmetrical contouring of the face. Additional feature enhancement using a hypodermic syringe and needle may not be necessary after embalming. (See Selected Readings, "Enhance Emaciated Features Arterially Using Split Injection and Restricted Drainage".)

### Restricted Cervical Injection Technique

**Restricted cervical injection (RCI)** effectively controls (restricts) the volume of arterial solution entering the head and the face (**Fig. 12–4A–D**). Restricted cervical injection is

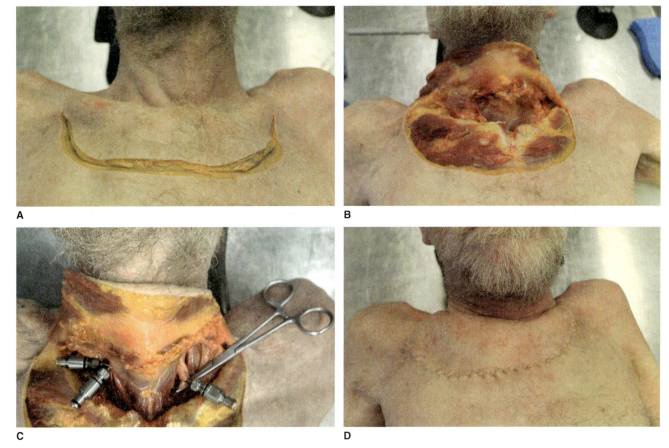

**Figure 12–4.** Restricted Cervical Injection. **A.** Semilunar incision to raise both right and left common carotid arteries and right internal jugular vein. **B.** Semilunar skin flap reflected. **C.** Placement of three arterial tubes and one hemostat. **D.** Semilunar incision sutured.

the primary embalming technique practiced by a large number of embalmers. The RCI method is standard at many establishments. The RCI method affords the greatest control over entry of arterial solution into the head. Because the tubes that are directed toward the head remain open while the trunk is injected, excess solution that reaches the face and head via the collateral circulation will drain from the carotid arteries through the open arterial tubes. This method prevents facial distension and dehydration when large volumes of strong solution are required to meet the preservative demands in the trunk of the body.

## Advantages of the Restricted Cervical Injection Method

- The carotid arteries are large.
- The carotid arteries are very elastic and have no branches, so they are easy to elevate.
- The carotid arteries are accompanied by the largest veins.
- The carotid arteries are rarely sclerotic.
- Clots or coagula present in the arterial system will be pushed away from the head.
- Embalming solution can be directed exclusively toward either the trunk or the head.
- RCI allows the best control over the volume of arterial solution entering the head.
- Two strengths of arterial solution can be used: one for the trunk and another for the head.
- Two rates of flow can be used: one for the trunk and another for the head.
- Two pressures can be used: one for the head and another for the trunk.
- Large volumes of solution can be injected into the trunk without overinjecting, swelling, or dehydrating the facial features.
- Features may be set after the trunk is both embalmed and aspirated; especially with the occurrence of purge during injection.

### Restricted Cervical Injection Method

1. Raise the right common carotid artery and insert an arterial tube directed toward the trunk of the body. Insert an arterial tube directed toward the right side of the head and **leave the stopcock open.**
2. Insert a drainage instrument into the right internal jugular vein directed toward the heart.
3. Raise the left common carotid artery and insert an arterial tube directed toward the left side of the head; tie off the lower portion of the left common carotid artery and leave the stopcock open.
4. Inject the trunk of the body **first**; drainage is taken from the right internal jugular vein. (Solution entering the head by collateral circulation exits through the two open stopcocks. Only the trunk of the body is embalmed.)
5. Inject the left side of the head.
6. Inject the right side of the head.

The restricted cervical injection is recommended in several situations.

### Nonautopsied Body
This technique allows the embalmer greater control over the amount of arterial solution entering the head. It allows large volumes of fluid, increased pressures, and faster rates of flow to be used for embalming the body trunk and the limbs without over injection of the head and the face. A separate solution can be prepared for injection of the head and the face.

### Bodies with Facial Trauma
With restricted cervical injection a minimum volume of a very strong solution can be injected into the head to preserve and firm tissues with a minimum amount of tissue distension.

### Bodies in Which Facial Distension Is Anticipated
Delayed embalming, refrigerated, frozen, and bodies exhibiting early signs of decomposition are all examples where the face can easily swell during arterial injection. Restricted cervical injection allows the trunk to be saturated with large amounts of strong solution, while the head and facial tissues are injected separately to control distension.

### Bodies in Which Eye Enucleation Has Been Performed
Restricted cervical injection allows complete control over the strength, amount of solution, pressure, and rate of flow of arterial solution entering the facial tissues and thus helps to control distension of the eyelids.

### Bodies with Generalized Edema
A large volume of solution can be injected into the trunk areas. Frequently, if facial tissues are not edematous, a milder solution can be used for injection of the head to prevent distension and/or dehydration of the tissues.

### Difficult-to-Firm Bodies
With many of the drugs used today protein levels in the body can be low. Restricted cervical injection allows the embalmer to inject large quantities of preservative solutions without overembalming the facial tissues.

### Bodies with Distribution Problems
Restricted cervical injection allows the use of high pressures and high rates of flow without distending the facial tissues.

### Bodies with a High Formaldehyde Demand
Burned bodies and bodies dead from renal failure require large amounts of preservative. Restricted cervical injection allows the embalmer to inject strong solutions of special purpose high-index fluids without overembalming the facial tissues.

### Bodies in Which Purge Is Expected
In a body that purges prior to arterial injection, the purge often continues during the embalming process. Examples include bodies with esophageal varices (as in alcoholism); bodies that suffered pneumonia, tuberculosis of the lungs, and ulcerations of the upper digestive organs; and bodies that show decomposition changes. Restricted cervical injection allows the embalmer to embalm the limbs and the trunk areas, then **aspirate the body,** set the features, and embalm the head. This eliminates the necessity to reset the features if purge occurs.

### Jaundiced Bodies
The head can be embalmed with a jaundice fluid preparation or other jaundice treatment. Restricted cervical injection allows thorough distribution of the solution to the facial tissues. The remainder of the body can be injected using arterial solutions suitable to the body conditions. First, inject the body, then inject the head and the face.

> **ADVANTAGES OF COMMON CAROTID ARTERY USE FOR RCI**
> 1. Arteriosclerosis is rarely seen in the carotid arteries; they are very large vessels and very elastic.
> 2. The common carotid arteries have no branches (except their terminal branches) and thus are easily raised to the surface.
> 3. Clots present in the right or left carotid artery can be identified and removed.
> 4. The carotid arteries allow direct injection of the head and facial tissues.
> 5. The carotid arteries are accompanied by the large internal jugular veins, which directly drain the head and the face.

## Instant Tissue Fixation Technique

**Instant tissue fixation** is an embalming technique that combines with restricted cervical injection. Strong solution under high pressure is injected in a burst-suppression pattern. A minimum volume of preservative creates maximum firming without tissue swelling. This embalming technique is used primarily for the injection of the head (other areas can be similarly treated) with a limited volume of a very strong (hypertonic) arterial solution. Use of the instant tissue fixation method is beneficial in the following conditions:

- Early decomposition when facial swelling is anticipated.
- When facial trauma is present.
- When facial tissues must be dried and firm for restorative treatments.
- When facial excisions are necessary, cancers, etc.
- Reembalming of the face.

Both right and left common carotid arteries are raised and usually drainage is taken from the right internal jugular vein. In this method of injection, very little drainage is taken as only a minimal volume of arterial solution is injected. A very strong arterial solution is prepared, and in extreme cases, a waterless solution is used. For example, 16 ounces of a high-index arterial fluid (25-index or above), 16 ounces of a coinjection chemical, 16 ounces of water, and 1 to 1½ ounces of arterial fluid dye. This hypertonic solution is designed to quickly preserve, dry, and firm the tissues.

## Method of Injection

Insert an arterial tube into the left common carotid artery. Select large diameter arterial tubes; as large as the arteries will allow. Turn the machine **on** with the rate-of-flow valve **closed**. Set the pressure at 20 pounds (psi). Open the rate-of-flow valve a full turn and immediately turn it **off**. Or, open and close the stopcock to create the burst-suppression method of injection. Repeatedly turn the rate-of-flow valve on and off, or open and close the stopcock, until sufficient solution has been injected. Only a minimum volume of solution is needed because of its strength. The dye will indicate the presence of the solution in the tissues. In addition, the dye helps to prevent graying of the tissues. Next, the right side of the head is injected in the same manner.

## BLOOD DRAINAGE

Drainage is brought about by displacement. As the arterial solution fills the vascular system the contents of the vascular system are displaced. There are 5–6 quarts of blood in the vascular system of the 160-pound body. This accounts for approximately 8% of the body weight. At death, there is generally a wave contraction of the arterial system. This contraction forces the greatest volume of blood into the capillary and the venous portions of the blood vascular system.

It has been estimated that after death, 85% of the blood is found in the capillaries, 10% in the veins, and 5% in the arteries. Amounts of blood in the vascular system vary depending on the cause and the manner of death. In addition, the blood will gravitate (postmortem hypostasis) into the dependent body regions over time. This engorges the dependent capillaries with blood (livor mortis) and leaves the less-dependent tissues free of most of the blood.

## LYMPHATIC CIRCULATION

The lymphatic vessels originate as blind-end tubes called lymph capillaries (**Fig. 12–5**). These tubes are located in the spaces between the cells. The lymph capillaries are larger and more permeable than the blood capillaries. They converge to form lymph channels called the lymphatics. These lymphatics have valves similar to those of veins and contain lymph nodes along their routes. Their fluid eventually enters the blood vascular system by flowing into the thoracic and the right lymphatic ducts. The thoracic duct empties lymph into the junction of the left subclavian vein and the left internal jugular vein. The lymph from the right lymphatic channel empties into the junction of the right subclavian vein and the right internal jugular vein.

In life, the lymph is composed of the fluids that pass from the blood through the walls of the capillaries. Here it is called tissue or interstitial fluid. More fluid enters the interstitial spaces from the blood than is directly reabsorbed back into the bloodstream by the capillaries. This excess fluid is drained by the lymph system. Once the interstitial fluid enters the lymph capillaries it is called lymph. At the time of death these lymph channels can be the site of large numbers of microbes. The lymph system is part of the defense system for protecting the body from pathological microbes. Embalming solution will diffuse from the interstitial spaces into the lymph channels. Massage and manipulation of the body during injection combined with the use of restricted drainage help to move embalming fluid throughout the lymph system.

Embalming solution can be diffused through the lymphatics in the following order: lymphatic capillary → lymphatic vessel → lymph nodes → lymph vessels → lymphatic trunk → subclavian veins.

### Contents of Drainage

Drainage is composed of blood and blood clots, interstitial and lymphatic fluid, and embalming solution. As arterial solution flows into the capillary, a portion of the solution passes through the walls of the capillary and is retained by the body. This retained preservative is the portion of the embalming solution that preserves, sanitizes, moisturizes, and colors the body tissues. Some of the embalming solution moves through the capillaries, into the venules and veins, and exits as part of the drainage. It has been estimated that 50% or more of the drainage taken during embalming is actually embalming solution.

The color and consistency of the drainage changes during arterial injection of the body. During injection of the first gallon of embalming solution, drainage contains more blood than during subsequent injections. As the blood in the vascular system is gradually displaced and replaced with embalming solution, the drainage lightens in color and becomes thinner. The initial drainage is the most dangerous; however, all drainage should be carefully controlled and splashing should be avoided. Embalming the body raised on body bridges allows

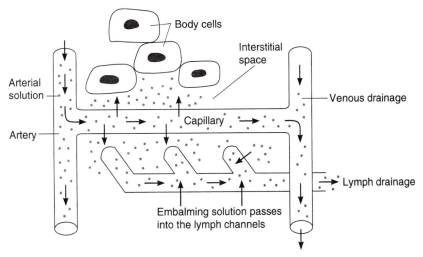

**Figure 12–5.** Lymphatic circulation.

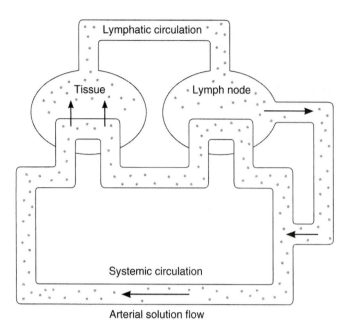

**Figure 12-6.** Lymphatic and systemic circulation.

the drainage to fall onto the preparation table where it can be washed into the sanitary sewer system. Closed drainage (a clear plastic hose attached to a drain tube and the open end placed in the sanitary drain) will not expose the embalmer to the contents of the drainage.

As the embalming solution passes through the capillaries, some of the interstitial fluid in the tissue spaces is drawn into the capillaries by osmosis because of the high concentration of the embalming solution, especially when strong arterial solutions are used. Some interstitial fluid will also enter the drainage through the lymphatic system (**Fig. 12–6**). Dehydration can result when too much interstitial fluid is removed. In bodies with skeletal edema, this is how the edema is removed from the tissue spaces.

Bacteria and microbial agents and their products that have entered the blood vascular system before or after death are also removed in the drainage. In bodies with skeletal edema, the edematous fluid may be part of the drainage. Venous coagula are included in the contents of the drainage. Several types of clotted materials present in the drainage; however, all clotted materials come from the **veins** or from a heart chamber. It is impossible for any arterial coagula to pass through the capillary beds and enter the venous side of the circulatory system.

The following coagula can be identified:

- **Postmortem coagula**—These coagula are not actual clots, but simply blood inclusions that have congealed and stuck together; they can be large and dark.
- **Postmortem clots**—These clots are multicolored. The bottom portion of the clot is dark, for it was formed by red blood cells that gravitated to the dependent part of a vessel. The clear layer on the top of the clot is a jelly-like layer of fibrin.
- **Antemortem clots**—Clots such as thrombosis form in layers—a layer of platelets, followed by a layer of fibrin, followed by another layer of platelets, and so on.

The viscosity of the blood can vary depending on the cause of death and the time between death and embalming. As the body gradually dehydrates after death, the viscosity of the blood increases. Bodies that have been refrigerated for very short periods after death, have been administered anticoagulant drugs such as heparin or dicumarol, or have died from carbon monoxide poisoning, exhibit low blood viscosity.

The volume of drainage is not equal to the volume of embalming solution injected. A large portion of the blood vascular system, particularly the arteries, is empty at death. This entire area must be filled, which accounts for the delay often noted between the start of the injection and the start of the drainage. At the conclusion of the embalming, the arterial system is filled; some of the injected solution is found in the capillaries and the veins, and some has passed through the capillaries to be retained by the tissues and the cells.

In some bodies, there will be little or no drainage. As long as the solution is distributing and there is no swelling or discolorations in the tissues, drainage need not be a concern. The following examples illustrate cases that present little to no drainage:

- In cases of esophageal varices and ruptured ulcerations of the digestive tract (blood has been lost to the lumen of the esophagus, stomach, or intestines), drainage actually occurs within the intestinal tract.
- Accidental death could cause the spleen or other internal organ to rupture; blood is lost from these sites and drainage also occurs at these ruptures.
- Traumatic death may result in a large loss of blood outside the body. This hemorrhage decreases the volume of blood available for drainage.
- Insertion of the drainage tube into the femoral or external iliac vein may tear the vein, allowing drainage to flow into the abdominal cavity.
- When a preinjection embalming solution is used, a portion of the blood is removed. At the time of arterial solution injection, there is less blood to drain.
- Pathological lesions such as with tuberculosis may account for a blood loss in life and will create an internal site of drainage at the time of arterial solution injection.
- Bloodstream infections frequently cause extensive clotting, and anemic diseases reduce blood volume; these factors contribute to poor distribution and low drainage volume.

Often in bodies in which hemorrhage into the digestive tract or abdominal cavity occurred prior to death, there may be a gradual swelling of the abdomen as the arterial solution is injected because some of the drainage (and arterial solution) will fill the digestive tract or abdominal cavity. This drainage can later be removed with a trocar. Likewise, hemorrhage into the stomach, esophagus, or lung tissues can result in a purge during injection. The purge will take the form of drainage. It is actually possible to drain from the mouth if a stomach ulcer has ruptured large veins! Aspiration can later remove these fluids. Some medications cause gastrointestinal bleeding. If this bleeding was intense, a major portion of the drainage may flow into the intestinal tract during arterial injection.

The bodies just described may demonstrate two forms of drainage: internal, into a cavity or hollow organ, and external, through the drainage tube or exit as purge.

Good drainage may be expected under the following conditions:

1. The interval between death and preparation is short; the body retains some heat.

2. The body shows early evidence of livor mortis, indicating that the blood has a low viscosity and can easily be moved.
3. Death was not the result of a febrile disease or a bloodstream infection.
4. Skeletal edema is present.
5. The body is jaundiced.
6. The person had been treated with blood thinners or anticoagulants (e.g., heparin, dicumarol, aspirin), resulting in low blood viscosity.
7. The body was refrigerated shortly after death but not for a long period.
8. Death was due to carbon monoxide poisoning.

## Purpose of Drainage

The bodies used for dissection are often embalmed but not drained and most are swollen to the point where they could not be viewed for funeral purposes. Bodies dead for long periods of time can be slowly embalmed without draining and are often suitable for viewing. Drainage is taken for a number of reasons:

1. *To make room for the arterial solution.* Distension would result without removal of some of the blood (especially today, when 3–5 gallons of preservative solution is injected into the average body).
2. *To reduce a secondary dilution of the arterial fluid.* The blood in the capillaries along with the interstitial fluids can dilute the embalming solution.
3. *To remove intravascular blood discolorations.* Livor mortis is a postmortem intravascular blood discoloration. Discolorations such as carbon monoxide and capillary congestion are antemortem blood discolorations. Injection of arterial solution accompanied by blood drainage should greatly reduce or remove these discolorations.
4. *To remove a tissue that rapidly decomposes.* Blood is a liquid tissue that rapidly decomposes after death, and decomposition of the blood can result in discolorations, odors, and formation of gas.
5. *To remove an element that speeds decomposition.* Blood, a portion of which is liquid, can hasten hydrolysis and the decomposition of the body tissues. Moisture is needed for decomposition and blood can provide that medium.
6. *To remove bacteria that is present in the blood.* With some diseases, the microbes normally found in the intestine can translocate to the bloodstream. After death, this translocation greatly increases. Removal of blood as drainage helps to reduce microbial agents in the body.
7. *To prevent discolorations.* When the blood in the body (hemoglobin) mixes with the formaldehyde of the arterial solution methyl-hemoglobin can form, which produces a gray color in the tissues (formaldehyde gray).
8. *To reduce swollen tissues.* When pitting edema is present in the skeletal tissues, it is possible to remove some of the edematous fluid via the blood drainage from the body.

Drainage, from some bodies, is most important in clearing very pronounced discolorations, especially when the face, the neck, and the hands are affected. If a primary purpose for drainage must be stated, it would be that the drainage makes room for the arterial solution so it can be evenly distributed to all tissues of the body with a minimum distension.

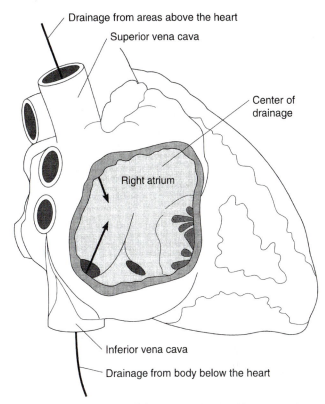

**Figure 12–7.** The center of drainage in the dead human body is the right atrium of the heart. The superior vena cava returns blood to this chamber from the head and upper extremities. The inferior vena cava returns blood from the visceral organs, trunk, and legs.

## Center of Drainage in the Dead Human Body

The center of drainage in the dead human body is the right atrium of the heart (**Fig. 12–7**). The superior vena cava returns blood to this chamber from the head and the upper extremities. The inferior vena cava returns blood from the visceral organs, trunk, and legs. If the internal jugular vein is used as a drainage point, all blood from the lower extremities and visceral organs must pass through the right atrium to be drained. Likewise, if drainage is to be taken from the femoral vein, blood from the arms and the head must pass through the right atrium. After death, the blood in the right atrium frequently congeals. This condition warrants drainage from the right internal jugular vein where an instrument, such as angular spring forceps, can be placed directly into the right atrium to fragment this coagulum. Drainage instruments are inserted into the vein and directed toward the heart.

## Above and Below Heart Drainage

Some embalmers also use two locations for drainage. A second drainage point is often used when the femoral vein is used as the beginning injection and drainage point. If there is a blockage in the inferior vena cava, right atrium, or the jugular veins, the neck and the face can begin to discolor. The veins of the neck and possibly the tissues of the neck can distend. The right internal jugular vein should be raised and opened as a second drainage site.

## Drainage Sites

The primary drainage site is the location from which drainage is first taken. In the unautopsied body, the veins most commonly used for drainage are the right internal jugular vein, the femoral vein, or the external iliac vein.

Axillary and basilic veins can be used, but their small size and the need to extend the arm make these veins an impractical choice. **Any vein can be used for drainage whether it is large or small or on the right or left side of the body.** In unusual circumstances, even the external jugular vein can be used if the internal jugular vein is obstructed by a cancerous growth or a large attached thrombosis. A broken vein can still be used as a drainage site; if an instrument such as angular forceps cannot be inserted, a grooved director may be used. Following injection, the area can be dried and the ends of the broken vein are ligated.

Should a vein tear while it is being raised, the following steps can be taken to attempt to place an instrument in the portion of the vein leading to the heart:
1. Force as much blood from the vein as possible.
2. Clean the area using an absorbent material.
3. Observe where blood is seeping from the broken portion of the vein.
4. Clamp an edge of the wall of the broken vein with a small serrated or rat-toothed hemostat, or place the hemostat across the entire broken portion of the vein.
5. Gently insert a drainage device toward the heart; if the vein has been torn into two pieces, do not remove the hemostat.
6. After embalming, pass ligatures and tie off the severed ends of the vein (holding them with hemostats).

In Chapter 9, the advantages and the disadvantages of the various veins for drainage are discussed, as are the incision locations and the relationships of veins to arteries. The internal jugular vein is the most valuable drainage point. It is the largest systemic vein that can be raised in the unautopsied body. The right internal jugular vein leads directly into the right atrium of the heart. **Figure 12–8** illustrates why the **right** and not the left internal jugular vein is most frequently used for drainage. Should there be a complication with the right internal jugular vein, the left can be used, but note that the vein turns to the right, often making insertion of a drainage instrument difficult.

### Direct Heart Drainage Technique

The right atrium of the heart is the center for venous drainage in the dead human body. Routinely, a drainage device is inserted into the right internal jugular vein and guided into the right atrium. A different method involves piercing the right side of the heart with a trocar and guiding the tip of the instrument directly into the right atrium (**Fig. 12–9**). **Direct heart drainage** was first practiced when embalming was done at the residence of the deceased.

Today, direct drainage from the right atrium is recommended for infectious cases to eliminate contact with blood and bodily fluids. The drainage is contained within the tubing leading to the aspirator instead of freely flowing along the sides of the embalming table. The direct method is also beneficial when drainage is difficult to establish from a vein and to clear stubborn facial discolorations.

- Inject one-half to one full gallon of arterial solution against closed drainage.
- Connect the trocar to the clear tubing on the aspirator and engage the aspirator.
  - Set the aspirator at low to moderate suction.
- Insert the trocar through the abdominal wall at the standard point of entry near the umbilicus: 2 inches to the left and 2 inches superior.
- Direct the trocar into the mediastinum area and intersect a line extending from the lobe of the right ear to the left anterior superior iliac spine.
- Guide the tip of the trocar into the right atrium of the heart and stop.
  - The first appearance of drainage in the tubing indicates proper positioning of the trocar tip.

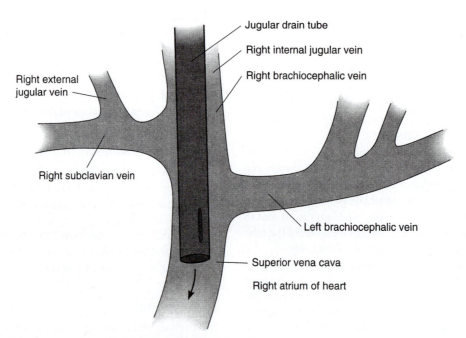

**Figure 12–8.** Drainage instrument placed in the right internal jugular vein.

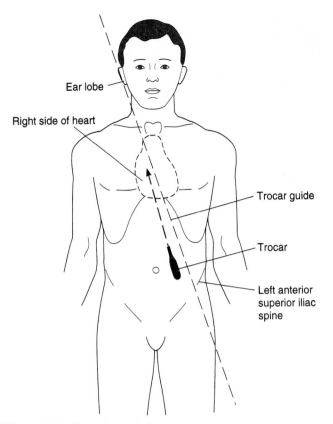

Figure 12–9. Direct heart drainage.

- Discontinue operation of the aspirator; drainage will continue by gravity siphonage.

Mastery of this technique is critical to prevent the tip of the trocar from breaching the heart muscle. In doing so, a six-point injection would become necessary. Practice trocar placement during routine cavity aspiration to reinforce the location of the right atrium and master the technique.

## Drainage Instrumentation

A large variety of drainage devices are available. The standard drainage instruments are the drain tube and the angular spring forceps. Drainage instruments are inserted into veins and directed toward the heart. Some embalmers prefer to lubricate these devices with massage cream to facilitate their entry into the vein. Drain tubes contain an internal mechanism called a stirring rod, which can also be lubricated with massage cream. After each use, drain tubes should be disassembled, flushed with water, cleaned, and disinfected.

The **grooved director** is used to guide a drainage instrument, such as an angular spring forceps or drain tube, into the right internal jugular vein. The grooved director is inserted into the vein first with the grooved side facing downward, away from the embalmer. The director is lifted upward as the drainage instrument is placed into the groove and guided toward the right atrium. Once the drainage instrument reaches the atrium, the grooved director is removed.

Many times, a drain tube cannot be fully inserted into the vein; it should not be forced. As long as a portion of the tube can be inserted, it will keep the vein expanded. Changing the position of the tube in the vein often assists with the drainage. Tubes should be tied into a vein, but loosely enough so that their position can be changed.

Drain tubes come in a variety of lengths and diameters. Those for use in the internal jugular vein (**Fig. 12–10**) are very large in diameter and short in length. Axillary drain tubes are long and slightly curved for insertion into the axillary vein. Axillary drain tubes are not very large in diameter. A variety of drain tubes are made for the femoral vein; they come in a wide range of diameters and lengths. One type of iliac drain tube is designed to be inserted into the external iliac vein, and the tip of the tube reaches into the right atrium of the heart; they are approximately 20 inches in length and made of plastic, metal, or rubber. Drain tubes, with very small diameters, are also available for embalming unautopsied infants.

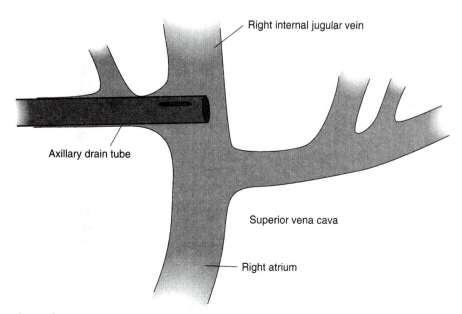

Figure 12–10. Axillary drain tube insertion.

| Advantages of the drain tube | Disadvantages of the drain tube |
|---|---|
| The tube keeps the vein expanded. | The size of the opening is limited to the diameter of the tube. |
| The stirring rod helps to fragment coagula. | The tube can block the opposite portion of the vein. The tube can block other veins. |
| Drainage can be stopped to build intravascular pressure. | Coagula cannot be grasped. The tube may mark the face or interfere with positioning of the head. |
| Closed drainage technique can be used. | The tube can easily be pushed through the vein into a body cavity. |

Angular spring forceps can be used to assist drainage from any vein.

| Advantages of angular spring forceps | Disadvantages of angular spring forceps |
|---|---|
| Provides a very large opening for the drainage. | May require removal to close the vein for intermittent drainage. |
| The head can be positioned to the right. | Drainage may splatter. |
| Forceps will not mark the face. | Embalmer contact with the drainage is increased. |
| Coagula can be manually grasped. | |
| Does not block other venous tributaries. | |

The angular spring forceps is convenient to use for drainage from the right internal jugular vein. It does not block drainage from the left innominate vein, right subclavian vein, or upper portion of the right internal jugular vein. These tributaries can be blocked if the jugular drain tube is used. It provides a wide opening for the passage of coagula and it allows the right side of the head to drain. Large masses of coagula can be broken and easily removed from the superior vena cava and the right atrium. The head can easily be positioned without the forceps marking the side of the face.

## Methods of Drainage

Many embalmers use a combination of drainage methods. They might begin the injection using continuous drainage and then restrict the drainage (using intermittent drainage) after the blood discolorations clear. There are three basic types of drainage in relationship to arterial injection.

### Alternate Drainage

In alternate drainage, the arterial solution is never injected while drainage is being taken. A quart or two of the arterial solution is injected; then the arterial injection is stopped and venous drainage commences. This is allowed to continue until drainage subsides; then the drainage instrument is closed. The process is then repeated. Injection and drainage are alternated until the embalming is completed. Because 1 or 2 quarts of fluid is constantly injected into a confined system, it is believed that a more uniform pressure is developed in all parts of the body. More complete distribution of arterial solution is achieved and more complete drainage results. Fluid diffusion is enhanced, for pressure filtration is increased. This method increases preparation time and care must be taken to avoid distension.

### Concurrent (Continuous)

In concurrent drainage, injection and drainage are allowed to proceed at the same time throughout the embalming. Because of the open drainage, it may be difficult to attain a pressure sufficient to saturate tissues throughout the body. Clots (in the venous system) may not be dislodged when the concurrent method is used. Fluid will follow the path of least resistance and more embalming solution may be lost to the drainage. This method of drainage may dehydrate and wrinkle body tissues. It has value in the preparation of bodies with high moisture content to the tissues (edema), for which dehydration is encouraged.

### Intermittent Drainage

In this process, the injection of the embalming solution continues throughout the embalming and the drainage is shut off for selected short periods. Some embalmers stop drainage until a particular amount of solution is injected (1 or 2 quarts); others stop drainage until surface veins are raised. It is important that surface intravascular blood discolorations clear before intermittent drainage is begun. This method is less time-consuming than the alternate method, encourages fluid distribution and pressure filtration, helps to prevent short-circuiting of the embalming solution and its loss to the drainage, and promotes retention of the embalming solution by the tissues (**Fig. 12–11**). Intermittent drainage helps the body to retain tissue fluid (which provides a proper moisture balance) and is recommended when colloidal fluids such as humectants or restorative fluids are used to slightly distend emaciated tissues.

## Techniques for Improving Drainage

Drainage (1) makes room for the arterial solution in the vascular system, (2) allows for a thorough distribution of the embalming solution, (3) prevents distension of the body tissues, and (4) prevents adverse discolorations. Creation of good drainage can be done in two periods, prior to injection of the preservative solution and during the injection.

Preembalming techniques include the following:

- *Selection of a large vein.* Preference is generally the internal jugular or the femoral, or external iliac vein.
- *Selection of a large drainage instrument.* An angular spring forceps or drainage tube is used.
- *Injection of a preinjection fluid.* Follow the manufacturer's dilution of the chemical and volume of the chemical injected. If a preinjection chemical is not used, a mild arterial solution

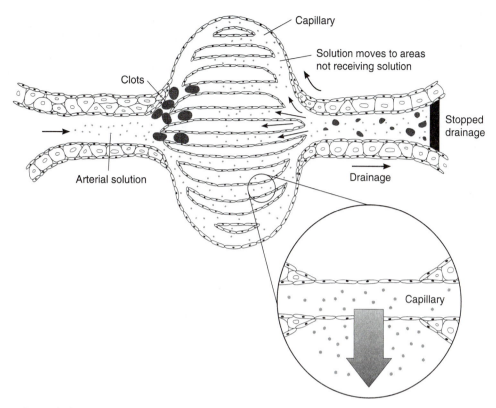

**Figure 12–11.** Intermittent drainage.

can be injected to clear blood discolorations and establish circulation.
- *Removal of extravascular pressure such as gas and fluids in the abdomen.*

The following techniques are included during injection:
- Use of drainage devices to fragment clots.
- Use of massage and pressure applied over the heart and/or liver to move venous clots.
- Increase in the rate of solution injection or increase in the pressure of the solution being injected.
- Intermittent and alternate forms of drainage techniques.
- Selection of another drainage site if necessary.

## Disinfection of the Drainage

The initial drainage, also called *first drainage* presents the greatest risk to the embalmer when the cause of death was due to a bloodborne pathogen. The Centers for Disease Control and Prevention mentions several bloodborne pathogens, including hepatitis B (HBV), hepatitis C (HCV), human immunodeficiency virus (HIV), malaria, and syphilis. HBV, HCV, and HIV are the three specific diseases addressed by the OSHA bloodborne pathogens standard. At present, OSHA permits bulk blood, suctioned and aspirated fluids to be carefully drained into a sanitary sewer system. Drainage from embalming consists of blood, interstitial fluids, lymph, and arterial solution. The arterial solution will to some degree sanitize the blood and body fluids present in the drainage. Upon entering the sanitary sewer system, drainage is further diluted by running and flushing water. The embalmer can minimize contact with blood drainage by using a drain tube instead of angular spring forceps; attach the device to a generous length of tubing that reaches the drain of the flush sink or other basin.

### Closed Drainage Technique

This technique is also recommended for embalming bodies dead from highly infectious or contagious diseases. A strong arterial solution (or waterless solution) is injected at a very slow rate of flow without taking any blood drainage from a vein. Aspiration should be delayed as long as possible to allow the embalming solution to diffuse to all regions of the body. Should facial discoloration be noted, direct heart drainage can be employed to remove congested blood and prevent formaldehyde gray (putty gray discoloration). Direct heart drainage is taken from the right atrium of the heart using the trocar (see Chapter 12).

### Embalming Solution Tracing Problems

| ONE-POINT INJECTION AND DRAINAGE | |
|---|---|
| Skeletal tissues | Trace arterial solution from the femoral artery (tube directed downward) to the right great toe; drain from the right femoral vein |
| Skeletal tissues | Trace arterial solution from the right femoral artery to the left side of the upper lip; drain from the right femoral vein |
| Visceral tissues | Trace arterial solution from the right femoral artery to the fundus of the stomach; drain from the right femoral vein |

| SPLIT INJECTION AND DRAINAGE | |
|---|---|
| Skeletal tissues | Trace arterial solution from the right femoral artery to the right great toe; drain from the right internal jugular |
| Skeletal tissues | Trace arterial solution from the right common carotid to the left upper lip; drain from the right femoral vein |
| Visceral tissues | Trace arterial solution from the right common carotid to the appendix; drain from the right femoral vein |
| **RESTRICTED CERVICAL INJECTION** | |
| Skeletal tissues | Inject the right common carotid down to reach the left lower lip; drain from the right internal jugular |
| Skeletal tissues | Inject the right common carotid down to reach the right upper lip (with the stopcock directed upward closed); drain from the right internal jugular |
| Visceral tissues | Inject down the right common carotid to the tissues of the left lung; drain from the right internal jugular |

## CONCEPTS FOR STUDY

1. List the advantages of the following injection techniques:
   One-point injection
   Multipoint injection
   Six-point injection
   Restricted cervical injection
   Split injection
   Instant tissue fixation
2. List the advantages of the following drainage techniques:
   Alternate drainage
   Concurrent (continuous) drainage
   Intermittent drainage
   Direct heart drainage
3. List the purposes for, and contents of, drainage.
4. List several techniques for stimulating drainage.

## FIGURE CREDIT

Figures 12–1A-C, 12–2, 12–3A,B are used with permission of Sharon L. Gee-Mascarello.

Figure 12–4A-D is used with permission of Kevin Drobish.

## BIBLIOGRAPHY

Collison K. Creutzfeldt-Jakob disease—fact and fiction: Part 2. *The Dodge Magazine*. January 2002; 94(1).

Investigating factors relating to fluid retention during embalming, Parts I and II. In *Champion Expanding Encyclopedia*, Nos. 499 and 500. Springfield, OH: Champion Chemical Co., August/September 1979:2013–2020.

Johnson EC. A study of arterial pressure during embalming. In *The Champion Expanding Encyclopedia*. Springfield, OH: Champion Chemical Co., 1981:2081–2084.

Kroshus J, McConnell J, Bardole J. The measurement of formaldehyde retention in the tissues of embalmed bodies. *Director*. March/April 1983:10–12.

Mechanics of proper drainage. In *Champion Expanding Encyclopedia*, No. 442. Springfield, OH: Champion Chemical Co., November/December 1973:1785–1788.

Removal of blood via the heart. In *Champion Expanding Encyclopedia*. Springfield, OH: Champion Chemical Co., May 1976:1885–1888.

Shor M. An examination into methods old and new of achieving greatest possible venous drainage, *Casket and Sunnyside*. July 1964:20.

CHAPTER 13

# Distribution and Diffusion of Arterial Solution

## CHAPTER OVERVIEW
- Distribution of Arterial Solution
- Diffusion of Arterial Solution
- Resistances: Intravascular and Extravascular
- Injection Pressure and Rate of Flow
- Signs of Arterial Solution Distribution, Diffusion, and Retention

Arterial embalming could be referred to as capillary embalming. The capillaries comprise the smallest network of blood vessels and create the necessary link for embalming solution to reach the cells. As embalming solution passes from the capillaries to the tissues, the solution makes contact with the cellular proteins. The preservatives in the solution stabilize the cell proteins and create a condition of temporary preservation. This chapter discusses the intravascular movement of arterial solution through the blood vascular system into the extravascular tissues and ultimately, into the cells. At the capillary level, embalming solution permeates the cell membrane, aided by a series of mechanisms called *passive physical transport systems*. The transport mechanisms require no cellular energy.

Movement of embalming solution from an intravascular to extravascular location is called **fluid diffusion**. Embalming solution that does not diffuse into the tissues, remains in the venous system and exits with blood drainage. Drainage is comprised of a mixture of blood, tissue fluids, lymph, and some of the arterial solution. Blood discolorations also are cleared through drainage.

Once blood is evacuated and discolorations clear, the embalmer focuses on retaining as much embalming preservative solution as possible within the tissues. Retained solution, without causing visible distension of the tissues, is a key factor in thoroughly preserving and sanitizing the body.

Vascular, or arterial embalming is a **unified process** that can be divided into four functions: (1) **Delivery** of the arterial solution from the embalming machine through the tubing and arterial tube into the artery. Also referred to as injection. (2) **Distribution** of the arterial solution from the point of injection throughout the arterial system and into the capillaries. Also referred to as perfusion. (3) **Diffusion** of arterial solution from within the vascular system through the capillary walls and into the tissue spaces. (4) **Drainage** of blood, interstitial and lymphatic fluids, and residual embalming solution.

This simple diagram illustrates the unified process of preservative solution delivery (**Fig. 13–1**). All four phases: delivery, distribution, diffusion, and drainage occur at the same time. These processes work similarly to a lawn sprinkler. Arterial solution fills the vascular system, much like water fills the hose to reach the sprinkler. Some of the arterial solution flows through the walls and pores of the capillaries into the tissue spaces, as water passes through the holes in the sprinkler to reach the grass. The major difference is that all of the water is sprayed out of the sprinkler. In embalming, a portion of the arterial solution stays inside the capillaries and flows into the veins to be removed as drainage.

As much as 50% of arterial solution can be lost with drainage because the vascular system is **not a closed** system. Arterial solution is allowed to pass through the walls and small pores of the capillaries to enter the interstitial spaces. In these tissue spaces, a fluid surrounds and bathes the cells of the body. In life, this tissue fluid serves to transport the nutrients and oxygen carried by the blood to the cells, as the blood remains in the blood vascular system and does not have direct contact with the cells. The tissue fluid also carries the wastes of cell metabolism to the blood vascular system, where they

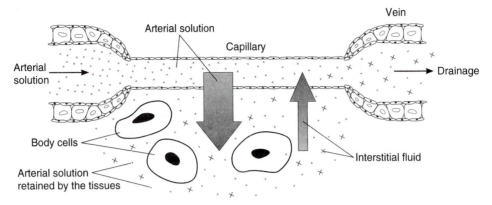

**Figure 13–1.** Drainage and retention of arterial solution.

are carried to the organs of the body that dispose of these wastes.

> In the embalming of a body that has been dead a long time and in which decomposition has begun, injection can result in the immediate swelling of tissues. This swelling occurs because the capillary walls (only one cell in thickness), after being decomposed, can no longer hold arterial solution. Arterial solution thus flows from the large arteries into the small arterioles and then directly into the interstitial spaces. As almost all the arterial solution enters the interstitial spaces, the tissues become distended. In embalming this type of body, it is important to inject a strong arterial solution, so that the maximum amount of preservation is achieved with minimum tissue distension. This is particularly important for the face and hands when the body is presented for viewing.

A similar process occurs in arterial embalming. Arterial solution flows through the arteries into the capillaries. A portion of the solution leaves the capillaries and passes into the fluid in the tissue spaces. Eventually it moves toward and enters the cells to make contact with the cell proteins. In this manner, the cells of the body are preserved. The embalming solution that passes through the pores or walls of the capillaries and eventually embalms the cells is the **retained arterial solution**. It is this retained arterial solution that stabilizes the body proteins and brings about the temporary preservation of the dead human body.

The arterial solution that remains in the capillaries is pushed ahead into the venules and veins to eventually be drained from the body. In this way, the arterial solution serves only to clear the vascular system of blood. This solution can embalm only the walls of the vascular system along the delivery route. The vascular system is extensive and the preservation of arteries, capillaries, and veins would diminish, but not arrest decomposition. Muscle cells and connective tissue cells account for the bulk of the body, and their preservation is essential if decomposition is to be halted and a thorough and extended preservation of the body achieved.

Drainage is a combination of **blood**, **arterial solution**, **interstitial fluids**, and **lymphatic fluids**. It is easy to see how blood and embalming solution are elements of the drainage, but interstitial fluid becomes part of the drainage through two routes. In living bodies, excess interstitial fluid is carried away from the spaces between the cells by the lymph system. This system empties into certain large veins of the body. In the embalming process, some embalming solution diffuses into the interstitial fluid and is removed by the lymph system. Even more importantly, embalming solution is present in the capillaries, and as it moves through the capillaries it draws some tissue fluid with it into the drainage. This explains why dehydration often occurs in areas such as the lips and the fingers during injection—more tissue fluid is being removed than is being replaced by embalming solution.

Arterial embalming involves both physical and chemical applications. Filling the arterial system by forced injection with some apparatus that pushes solution into the body under pressure involves physical procedures. Control of the drainage is a physical process. Some of the injected solution is forced through the walls of the capillaries simply by the physical process of filtration.

The arterial fluid is chemical in nature. When properly diluted, it makes a homogeneous solution that is described as hypotonic. Through the physical transport processes of osmosis and dialysis, this hypotonic solution passes from the capillaries into the interstitial spaces. The preservatives in the solution chemically combine with the proteins in the body cells and the protein in microorganisms and their products to form new compounds and alter the proteins in such a manner that the tissues are preserved and sanitized.

## ARTERIAL SOLUTION INJECTION

Arterial embalming begins with the injection of a preservative solution, under pressure, into an artery of the body. *Arterial, or vascular embalming can be defined as the injection of a suitable arterial embalming solution, under pressure, into the blood vascular system to accomplish* **temporary preservation**, **sanitation**, *and* **restoration** *of the dead human body*. The solution moves from the arteries to the capillaries and then passes through the capillaries to come into contact with the body cells. A portion of the embalming solution remains in the capillaries to remove the blood and its products from the vascular system in the form of drainage. This drainage is taken from a vein of the body.

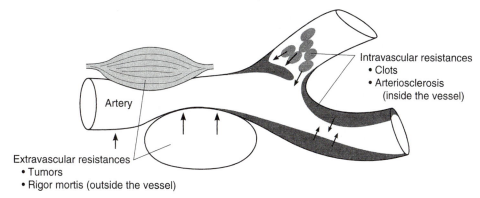

**Figure 13–2.** Extravascular resistance outside and intravascular resistance within the vessel.

It is necessary to inject an embalming solution under pressure. Early embalming injection apparatus (the gravity percolator) consisted of a simple receptacle filled with arterial solution and elevated above the body. The pressure required to distribute the solution throughout the body was created by gravity. The process required no electricity and was aptly called *gravity embalming*. However, numerous types of resistance occur within the body during injection. Resistances are described by relationship to the vascular system. Resistances within the blood vessels are called **intravascular resistances**; resistances outside the blood vessels are called **extravascular resistances** (Fig. 13–2).

Resistances affect arterial solution distribution and diffusion. Poor distribution of the arterial solution results in poor diffusion. Motorized, or pressurized injection, such as the centrifugal pump embalming machine, overcomes the resistances that interfere with arterial solution distribution. As embalming solution travels from the large central trunk of the arterial system (the aorta) into the arterial branches (arterioles and capillaries), the diameter of the arterial system actually **expands** because of the innumerable branches of the vessels. The injection pressure needed to force the solution through the narrow arteries **decreases** by the time the solution reaches the capillaries. Pressurized injection creates a passive physical transport system known as "pressure filtration." Pressure filtration is responsible for a portion of the **diffusion** of the arterial solution.

The arterial solution at the microcirculatory level can take three routes: (1) A portion flows through the capillaries, where some of the embalming solution passes through the walls of the capillaries to embalm the tissues. (2) The portion that remains in the capillaries flows on to the venules. This embalming solution helps to remove the blood from the capillaries and the veins and eventually exits as drainage. (3) The remaining embalming solution flows through direct connections that link arterioles and venules. It eventually exits as drainage.

Intravascular pressure (IVP), which brings about pressure filtration that moves the embalming solution from the capillaries into the interstitial spaces, is created by the pressure from the machine and the expansion of the elastic arteries. This pressure effects embalming solution filtration through the walls of the capillaries. Pressure filtration is one of the major processes by which embalming solution enters the tissue spaces.

IVP also remains with the embalming solution that flows into the venous system. This is what helps to create the small (approximately one-half pound) pressure that the drainage exhibits. A great amount of the drainage pressure is brought about by arterial solution flowing directly through connecting routes—directly from arterioles to venules and not passing through the capillary routes.

During life, some capillaries are not blood-filled as a result of vasoconstriction. Other capillaries are engorged with blood due to physical activity of the body that causes vasodilation. For example, when a person is running, more blood is concentrated in the muscles being used than in the muscles not being used. At death, the vascular system relaxes but its capacity had been increased due to vasodilation during the predeath physical activity. As a result, the embalmer can inject a large volume of solution without causing immediate distension of the tissues or drainage.

Blood drainage from the average body equals one-half or more of the total volume of arterial solution injected. The goal of embalming is to retain more than one-half of the arterial solution injected. The embalmer controls numerous variables to promote uniform distribution of the embalming solution throughout the body so that the tissues retain as much embalming solution as possible. Injection pressure and speed of delivery are two variable controls to achieve this. *An "old rule" of general practice suggested injection of 1 gallon of sufficient strength embalming solution for every 50 pounds of body weight (1:50 ratio). This original practice serves as a starting point, though it is an overgeneralization that does not consider the individual preservative demands for each body to be embalmed. The practice of considering embalming analysis along with ongoing evaluation for each body is the professional standard used to determine the volume and strength of solution needed. Individual analysis during embalming ensures optimal preservation every time.*

Extravascular and intravascular resistances are responsible for nonuniformity in distribution of the embalming solution. The diameters of the artery, the arterial tube, and the delivery hose from the machine to the arterial tube, all produce resistance. As a point for injection, the artery with the largest diameter, generally the common carotid or the femoral artery, should be selected. An arterial tube of appropriate size should be inserted into the artery. The arterial tube should not damage the inner wall of an artery.

# INTRAVASCULAR RESISTANCE

Intravascular resistances can be caused either by narrowing or obstruction of the lumen of a vessel. This narrowing or obstruction is brought about by conditions found either within the lumen of the vessel or within the walls of the vessel. The **lumen** can be **obstructed** by blood, antemortem emboli, antemortem thrombi, and postmortem coagula and thrombi.

As the embalming solution flows from the aorta into the narrowing branches of the arterial tree, the lumen of the arteries also narrows. A coagulum that is loosened and moved along with the solution will eventually clog a small distributing artery (**Fig. 13–3**). Arterial coagulum could never be reduced to a size where it could pass through arterioles and capillaries. When a coagulum reaches an arterial branch through which it can move no farther, distribution of solution beyond this point is stopped. The only way tissues beyond this point can receive embalming solution is through the collateral circulation.

Intravascular resistance resulting from **narrowing of the lumen** can be caused by arteriosclerosis, most frequently seen in the arteries of the lower extremities; vasoconstriction, frequently seen on one side of the body as a result of a stroke; arteritis, brought about by inflammation of the artery; and intravascular rigor mortis, postmortem narrowing caused by rigor mortis of the smooth muscles in the arterial walls. Unlike extravascular resistance, the embalmer can do little to remove intravascular resistance.

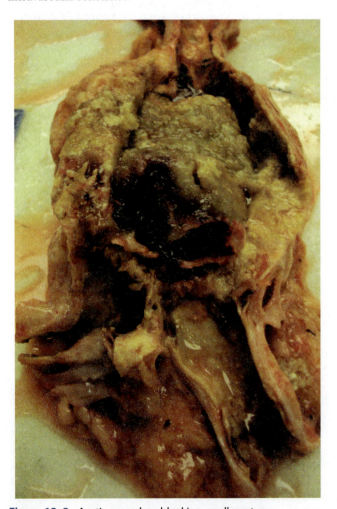

**Figure 13–3.** Aortic coagulum blocking smaller artery.

# EMBALMING PROCEDURES FOR INTRAVASCULAR CHALLENGES

The following embalming techniques can be used when intravascular problems are anticipated:

1. Use sufficient pressure and rate of flow to uniformly distribute the arterial solution. A slow rate of flow can help to prevent coagula in the arteries from floating free and clogging smaller branch arteries. Once circulation is established, a faster rate of flow can be used.
2. If arterial coagula are anticipated (i.e., bodies dead for long periods, gangrene evidenced in distal limbs, and death from infections) inject from the right common carotid artery (or restricted cervical injection). This pushes arterial coagula away from the arteries that supply the head and arms (the areas to be viewed). The legs can be injected separately, if necessary, or treated by hypodermic and/or surface embalming.
3. Avoid using a sclerotic artery for injection. The common carotid is rarely sclerotic, whereas the femoral and iliac arteries are frequently sclerotic.
4. Use the largest artery possible for the primary injection point. This is usually the common carotid, external iliac, or femoral artery.
5. Use an arterial tube of proper size so that it will not damage the walls of the artery.

# EXTRAVASCULAR RESISTANCE

Extravascular resistance is pressure placed on the outside of a blood vessel. This pressure is sufficient to collapse or partially collapse the lumen of the vessel. The embalmer is better able to reduce or remove extravascular resistance than intravascular resistance. Therefore, the following discussion of extravascular resistances includes techniques that can be used to reduce or remove the pressures that these resistances place on blood vessels.

## Rigor Mortis

The postmortem stiffening of the voluntary skeletal muscles is a strong extravascular resistance. Rigor mortis is not a uniform condition. It may be present in some muscles and absent in others. This can cause a very uneven distribution of arterial solution. Embalming prior to or during the onset of rigor is generally recommended. When rigor is present, gentle but very firm manipulation and massage of the muscles helps to reduce the rigor. The massage and manipulation can be done prior to and during arterial injection. During the injection of the first gallon of arterial solution, firm massage and exercise of the extremities can be very important in establishing good distribution. Massage should be done especially along the arterial routes (e.g., axilla, wrist, sides of fingers, groin, and popliteal space).

## Gas in the Cavities

Decomposition gases in the abdominal cavity can exert enough pressure to push the large abdominal aorta and inferior vena cava against the spinal column, thus causing these vessels to narrow or collapse. Most frequently, this pressure can be removed at the beginning of the embalming by puncturing the abdominal wall with a trocar or scalpel and releasing some of the gasses. It may also be necessary to puncture some of the large and small intestines. This can easily be done without fear of interrupting the circulation.

### Expansion of the Hollow Viscera During Injection

Too rapid an injection of arterial solution, especially in bodies dead for long periods, can result in expansion of the hollow visceral organs. This expansion causes the abdomen to swell and places sufficient pressure on the aorta and vena cava so as to collapse their lumens. Stomach purge often accompanies this abdominal distension. Insert a trocar into the abdominal cavity, keeping the point just beneath the anterior abdominal wall, and puncture some of the distended intestines.

### Tumors and Swollen Lymph Nodes

These distended growths and organs can place pressure on the blood vascular system, creating distribution and drainage problems. Sectional injection may be necessary. A higher injection pressure and pulsation may help to obtain good distribution. Massage and manipulation may also help to encourage solution distribution and drainage.

### Ascites and Hydrothorax

Enough fluid may accumulate in the thoracic and abdominal cavities to interfere with blood drainage and arterial solution distribution. Drainage from several sites may be necessary. The ascites can be removed or relieved by inserting a trocar into the abdominal cavity or inserting a drainage tube through a puncture made in the abdominal wall.

### Contact Pressure

Portions of the body that push against the embalming table or against positioning devices (such as shoulder blocks) may not receive enough arterial solution. Contact pressure can restrict the flow of solution into the shoulders, buttocks, and backs of the legs. During embalming, these areas should be manipulated and massaged to relieve the pressure from the contact with the embalming table.

### Visceral Weight

In all bodies, abdominal viscera create some resistance. In obese bodies, however, there can be sufficient visceral weight on the large vessels in the abdomen to restrict drainage and possibly solution distribution. Higher pressures, pulsation, and a more rapid rate of flow may help to overcome this resistance. Manipulation and massage of the abdominal area may also assist distribution and drainage.

### Bandages

Medical dressings and bandages applied to an extremity should be removed prior to arterial injection (**Fig. 13–4**). Such bandages can disrupt drainage from the hands and feet. During injection, even a patient identification band can be a source of vascular resistance.

### Skeletal Edema

Skeletal edema occurs in the body appendages, trunk, and head. This edema can be so intense that it exerts extravascular resistance to the distribution of embalming solution as well as

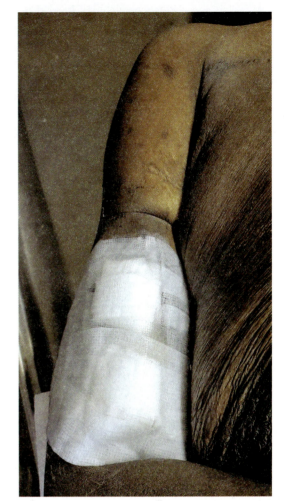

**Figure 13–4.** Medical dressings or bandages are removed prior to arterial injection.

a resistance to blood drainage. Numerous conditions, from pathological disorders to drug treatments, can cause skeletal edema. These intense edemas are frequently seen postoperatively, particularly after open heart or vascular surgery. Higher injection pressures, pulsation, manipulation, and massage assist in distribution and drainage. Sectional vascular embalming may be necessary.

### Inflammation

Inflamed tissue can swell to the extent that vascular constriction results. Higher injection pressures, pulsation, and massage may assist in distributing arterial solution into these body areas. Sectional vascular and hypodermic embalming may be necessary.

## COMBINED RESISTANCE

Extravascular and intravascular resistances rarely exist in a vacuum, in other words, *in and of themselves.* During embalming the "average" body, exhibits a combination of resistances. For example, an individual in their sixties, whose sudden death is attributed to myocardial infarction, may present with resistances caused not just from heart disease. Rigor mortis, arteriosclerosis, contact pressure with the embalming table, and blood in the dependent portions of the vascular system may also be noted.

These various sources of resistance demonstrate that even in a sudden death, numerous vascular resistances are present that can restrict good arterial distribution and blood drainage. In the preceding example, the rigor may be intense enough to reduce distribution to the point that sectional embalming is necessary. On the other hand, if anticoagulant drugs were on board, the blood would remain in a liquid form and postmortem clotting would be diminished. Arterial distribution and blood drainage would be improved.

At the time of death, invasive treatments and administered drugs could cause extensive ecchymoses on the backs of the hands, or extreme antemortem subcutaneous emphysema resulting in gross distension of the tissues of the neck and face. Delays between death and preparation greatly increase postmortem coagula in the vessels.

All these hypothetical factors demonstrate that the embalmer must prepare each body on the basis of the conditions exhibited by the individual body. The embalming analysis considers each of these individual body conditions. As the embalming progresses, ongoing analysis considers such factors as the extent of arterial distribution, volume of drainage, clearing of discolorations, amount of tissue distension, degree of firming, and so on.

## NEED FOR RESISTANCE

Complete resistance would be a negative embalming factor. Total arterial resistance would prevent distribution of embalming solution; total venous resistance would prevent blood drainage. If arterial resistance was not present, the inability to establish venous drainage would cause tissue distension. During embalming, some resistance is always found throughout the vascular system. The injection pressure is greatest on the arterial side of the capillaries. This pressure overcomes arterial resistances and helps to distribute the embalming solution. The resistance in the capillary network slows the embalming solution and helps to hold it within the capillaries, giving the solution an opportunity to diffuse (to pass from the capillary to the interstitial spaces). This brings about a more uniform distribution of the embalming solution, reduces short-circuiting of the embalming solution, and helps the tissues to retain more embalming solution. If there were no resistance at all, the embalming solution would pass directly through the capillaries and into the drainage. Consider another example when no resistance exists, death from a ruptured aneurysm of the abdominal aorta. Solution will distribute until it reaches the ruptured tissue; without any resistance, the embalming solution will follow the path of least resistance, exit the rupture, and fill the abdominal cavity.

During injection and drainage of the body, embalmers create resistance to effect better penetration of the embalming solution and reduction of the loss of solution. Intermittent or alternate methods of drainage are used to restrict drainage and increase intravascular resistance. Drainage can also be stopped completely as the final volume of solution is injected, to increase resistance. Inject the remaining one-fourth to one-half gallon, with the vein closed. Aspiration can also be delayed several hours. This technique helps the expanded capillaries to retain the embalming solution longer, allowing time for the solution to diffuse.

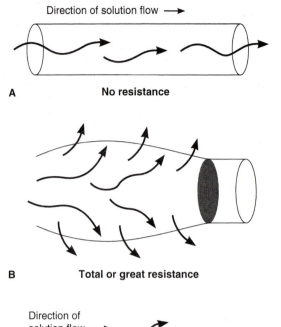

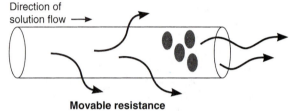

**Figure 13–5.** **A.** No resistance. **B.** Total or great resistance. **C.** Movable resistance.

**Figure 13–5** illustrates the need for some degree of resistance. **Figure 13–5A** shows little or no resistance. The solution rushes through the tissues, resulting in tissue dehydration. Filtration is reduced, solution can easily short circuit, and the uniformity of distribution is reduced.

**Figure 13–5B** demonstrates total resistance; such as an extensive blood clotting condition. Once the system is filled with solution, tissue distension occurs and uniformity of distribution is reduced.

**Figure 13–5C** represents a movable resistance, such as low viscosity blood in the venules and veins or the use of intermittent drainage. Blood removal is more complete, distribution is more uniform, and, most important, more embalming solution is retained by the body with a minimum of tissue distension.

## PATHS OF LEAST RESISTANCE

When vascular resistances are present in a body, the arterial embalming will distribute to areas where little or no resistance exists. As a result, some areas receive too much solution and others do not receive enough. The following three questions serve to analyze solution distribution and can be repeated throughout the arterial injection process:

1. Is the embalming solution distributing through the blood vascular system?
2. What areas are receiving sufficient solution?
3. What areas are *not* receiving sufficient embalming solution?

The following three indicators are signs of arterial solution distribution:

1. Solution volume in the embalming machine is decreasing.
2. When the rate-of-flow valve is opened, the reading on the pressure gauge lowers, or drops. This drop in pressure is called the **differential pressure**. The greater the drop in pressure, the greater the rate of flow (speed of delivery). The differential reading of 10 (**Fig. 13-6B**) indicates that the embalming solution is being injected twice as fast as it would if the differential reading were 5 (**Fig. 13-6A**). The fact that the reading dropped to 5 or 10 from the initial reading of 15 when the rate-of-flow valve was closed indicates that solution is entering the body. As the solution fills the vascular system, the reading may rise. This shows that more resistance is being created by the filling of the vascular system. To maintain the rate of flow at the original delivery speed, the pressure or the rate of flow setting has to be increased.

   *Example.* The machine is turned on with the rate-of-flow valve (or the in-line stopcock) in the closed position. (**No** solution is entering the body.) The pressure is set to 20 pounds per square inch (psi). The rate-of-flow valve is now opened and the reading drops to 15 psi. The differential reading is 5. After a gallon and a half is injected, the reading increases to 18. This indicates the system has been filled and more resistance is being encountered. To establish the original rate of flow, open the rate-of-flow valve until the reading drops to 15. If this does not happen, increase the pressure to 23 psi. If the reading remains at 18 the differential is again 5, and this was the original rate of flow. Differential pressure is a good indicator of the resistance in the body. However, it can also indicate that an arterial tube is clogged. Checked arterial tubes prior to use by flushing water through the device.

3. Drainage should be evident when solution is entering the body and making the proper circuit through the arteries, capillaries, and veins.

Once it has been determined that the arterial solution is entering the body at a rate of flow and pressure that do not cause distension, the embalmer determines which body regions are receiving arterial solution and which areas are not. A group of indicators known as the signs of arterial solution distribution and diffusion help to make this determination. Most of these indicators, such as the presence of fluid dye in the tissues, demonstrate only the presence of embalming solution in skin regions.

The dermis, the deep layer of the skin, is very vascular and offers little resistance to the flow of embalming solution, as the solution flows rapidly and easily into the surface areas of the body. The embalmer can easily detect the presence of embalming solution in the skin. Concern must be given to the deep tissues and the muscles. It is very important that solution distribute to these body tissues, which offer more resistance. To achieve this deeper penetration of solution, the drainage can be restricted and massage must be very firm. Penetrating agents in the arterial solution also promote the passage of solution into the deeper tissues.

The skin areas offer little resistance to the flow of solution; also, some localized areas can receive large amounts of arterial solution. These areas are generally in the vicinity of the artery injected. Solutions will establish pathways where they quickly pass through a group of capillaries near the artery being injected. The solution then passes rapidly into the drainage. This frequently happens when injection and drainage occur at the same location. This short-circuiting reduces the total volume of solution available for saturation of other body areas.

Many direct connections exist between arterioles and venules in the microcirculation of the blood. Here, again, is a route that offers little resistance to the flow of fluid. Embalming solution can rapidly pass from the arterial system to the veins without distributing to the tissues. Restricting the drainage can reduce the amount of arterial solution lost in these direct routes.

Once the embalmer determines that solution is entering the body and where it is within the body, it must be determined which body areas have received sufficient solution. There is no one positive test for determining if a body area has sufficient arterial solution. If there is any doubt about solution distribution, the embalmer should raise an artery that supplies the area and sectionally inject. Hypodermic or surface embalming may be necessary. With local injections, it may be wise to increase the strength of the injected chemical to help ensure good preservation. It is better to slightly overembalm an area than to risk the chance that an inadequate amount of preservative has reached the area.

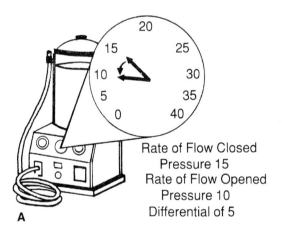

A
Rate of Flow Closed
Pressure 15
Rate of Flow Opened
Pressure 10
Differential of 5

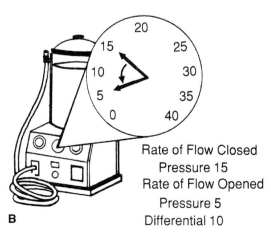

B
Rate of Flow Closed
Pressure 15
Rate of Flow Opened
Pressure 5
Differential 10

**Figure 13-6.** Pressure-flow differentials. **A.** Slower rate of flow. **B.** Faster rate of flow.

## INJECTION PRESSURE AND RATE OF FLOW

**Injection pressure** is the amount of pressure produced by an injection device to overcome initial resistance within the vascular system. Injection pressure is needed to overcome intravascular and extravascular resistances. The pressure needed is created by the embalming machine.

**Rate of flow** is the amount of embalming solution injected in a given time period, also called the *speed of delivery*. The rate of flow is generally measured in ounces per minute (opm). A device called a rate-of-flow meter can be installed on the embalming machine to measure the speed of embalming solution delivery (**Fig. 13–7**).

Injection pressure and rate of flow are related, but not identical. Of the two, the rate of flow is the factor of most concern to the embalmer. The ideal rate of flow can be as much arterial solution as the body can accept as long as (1) the solution is evenly distributed throughout as much of the body as possible, and (2) there is little or no distension of the tissues. The ideal pressure is the amount needed to establish this rate of flow.

Use of a centrifugal pump embalming machine makes it possible to have a set pressure with the rate-of-flow valve closed. It is then possible to open the rate-of-flow valve to a certain point and establish the desired rate of flow. The pressure set with the rate-of-flow valve closed is called the **potential pressure**. When the rate-of-flow valve is opened, the resultant pressure reading is called the **actual pressure**. The difference between actual pressure and potential pressure is the rate of flow or the **differential pressure**.

There are many theories as to the amount of pressure and rate of flow that should be used. Keep in mind that these factors vary in different ways:

1. *From body to body*. Bodies injected shortly after death when rigor is not present can be injected much faster than bodies that have been dead for a long period of time with rigor fully established. A low pressure can be used to establish a high rate of flow in a recently deceased body.
2. *In different body areas*. Fluids always follow the path of least resistance. Areas such as the skin and vascular visceral organs and glandular tissues easily accept fluid. Resistance is greater in tissues where arteriosclerosis is present in the arteries or in body areas where blood has clotted or coagulated in the vessels.
3. *As embalming proceeds*. As embalming proceeds, resistance increases: (1) when vessels are empty and the solution rapidly enters (after the vessels fill, more resistance is created); (2) when the preservative in the solution acts on the capillaries, allowing less solution to flow into the tissue spaces (more solution will then be directed into the drainage); (3) when the tissue spaces become filled to capacity with arterial solution; and (4) when arterial clots move and block small arteries and venous coagula are hardened by the preservative solution, making more difficult to remove.

It can easily be seen that the needed pressure and rate of flow can vary from body to body and at different times in the embalming process.

After death, and depending on the cause of death, large arteries may collapse because the volume of circulating blood has decreased. Increase in the pressure or rate of flow may well promote filling of the vessels and start good distribution. When this has been accomplished, the amount of pressure can be reduced. The pressure used at that time should be sufficient to maintain a rate of injection that is slightly greater than the amount of drainage. (On average, the total drainage will equal approximately one-half of the total volume of solution injected.)

**Ideal pressure** is then defined as the pressure needed to overcome the vascular resistances of the body to distribute the embalming solution to all body areas. The **ideal rate of flow** is defined as the rate of flow needed to achieve uniform distribution of the embalming solution without distension of the tissues.

There are two schools of thought about the ideal injection rate. Some embalmers prefer a low pressure and a rapid rate of flow. Others prefer a high pressure and slow rate of flow. A moderate injection rate suggests delivery of 1 gallon of solution over 10–15 minutes with a pressure setting between 2 and 10 pounds to achieve ideal rate of flow.* Slower rates of injection may prevent arterial coagula from blocking smaller distal arteries and diminishing or completely stopping the distribution of arterial solution.

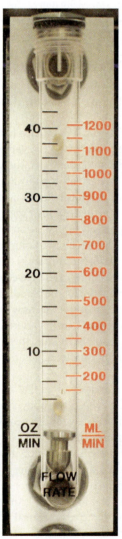

**Figure 13–7.** Rate-of-flow meter measures speed of embalming solution delivery in ounces per minute (opm).

---

*See Selected Readings: Guidelines Submitted to OSHA from the National Funeral Directors Association *Committee* on Infectious Diseases (Summer 1989).

Not all bodies can be injected within the same time allowance at the same rate of flow and injection pressures. As soon as distension is evident, injection should be stopped and the cause evaluated. The injection pressure can be reduced, the rate of flow can be reduced, or sectional embalming can be done. Likewise, if arterial solution is not entering some areas of the body, the rate of flow can be increased, the pressure can be increased, or sectional embalming may be necessary.

Three factors combined: sufficient pressure, adequate rate of flow, and restricted drainage should produce the following results: a removal of blood from the main and collateral circulation; saturation of the soft tissues with the injected arterial solution; a buildup of intravascular pressure (IVP); restoring of moisture to the tissues if a proper solution is injected; and a retention of a sufficient amount of arterial solution within the tissues to provide sufficient preservation without tissue distension.

For the injected embalming solution to accomplish its function of preservation, it must reach and penetrate **all** tissue areas. Merely flushing the solution through the blood vascular system and out the drain tube does not achieve the intended purpose. It requires time for the preservative solution to diffuse out of the capillaries and penetrate, and saturate tissues.

Clinical studies have demonstrated that as much as 50–55% of the embalming solution can be lost through the drainage, regardless of the pressure set for embalming. Techniques such as restricted drainage may help to retain more embalming solution within the body.†

The foregoing would be true under ideal conditions. The **ideal rate of flow** and the **ideal pressure** will vary from body to body. The ideal values of these two factors are the pressure necessary and the rate of flow necessary to overcome the resistances and evenly distribute the preservative solution throughout the entire body, while at the same time the body retains as much of the preservative solution as possible without distension or dehydration of the body tissues.

## CENTER OF ARTERIAL SOLUTION DISTRIBUTION

During life, blood is returned to the heart. During embalming, blood also flows in the direction of the heart. *The ascending aorta and arch of the aorta are the center of arterial distribution.* The arch is a continuation of the ascending aorta and gives off three large branches from its superior surface. From right to left, these are the brachiocephalic artery, which supplies the right side of the head, right shoulder and right arm; the left common carotid artery, which supplies the left side of the head and face; and the left subclavian artery, which supplies the left shoulder and left arm. The arch continues also as the descending thoracic aorta, through which the embalming solution is distributed to all other parts of the body.

The arch of the aorta is a continuation of the **ascending aorta**, which begins at the left ventricle. The embalming solution is injected into the arteries of the body because of the valve

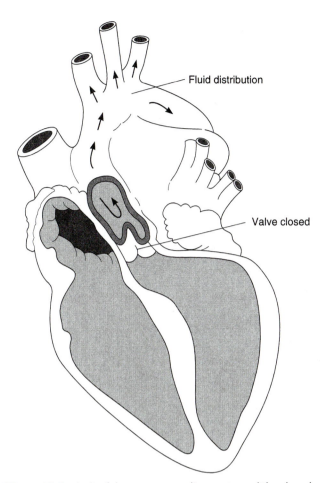

**Figure 13–8.** Arch of the aorta, ascending aorta, and the closed semilunar valve.

at the beginning of the ascending aorta called the **aortic semilunar valve**. This valve is situated between the left ventricle of the heart and the ascending aorta. As embalming solution is injected, the ascending aorta fills and causes the aortic semilunar valve to close (**Fig. 13–8**). Once the semilunar valve closes, the arteries of the body begin to fill with the embalming solution. If the valve fails to close, or leaks, the left ventricle fills with embalming solution. When this happens, the cusps of the left atrioventricular (bicuspid) valve will close, and the arteries of the body will fill.

If both valves fail to close, arterial solution will flow to the lungs through the pulmonary veins and can cause lunge purge. Or, the solution could flow into the right ventricle through the pulmonary artery, and from the right ventricle to the right atrium. In this case, the solution will exit as drainage. Injection of solution by excessive pressure and rapid rate of flow can cause both valves to remain open. Lung purge in both scenarios would consist primarily of arterial solution.

## SIGNS OF ARTERIAL SOLUTION DISTRIBUTION AND DIFFUSION

There are a number of indicators that can be used to tell if the arterial solution is present in an area. In addition to the presence of the solution, there needs to be a sufficient amount of the solution; and the solution needs to be at a strength where

---

†Kroshus J, McConnell J. The measurement of formaldehyde retention in the tissues of embalmed bodies. Director March/April 1983; 10–12 (See Selected Readings).

the tissues will be stabilized. Most of the signs of distribution and diffusion are surface indicators.

> **SIGNS OF ARTERIAL SOLUTION**
> Dye is evident in the tissues
> Distension of superficial blood vessels
> Blood drainage
> Clearing of intravascular blood discolorations

> **SIGNS OF ARTERIAL SOLUTION DIFFUSION**
> Dye is evident in the tissues
> Firming of the tissues
> Loss of skin elasticity (firming is evident)
> Drying of the tissues
> Rounding of fingertips, lips, and toes
> Mottling of the tissues (bleaching)
> Fluorescent dye observed using a blacklight (Ultraviolet lamp)

## Dyes

The most reliable sign of arterial distribution and diffusion is the presence of an active fluid dye in the tissues (**Fig. 13–9**). As active fluid dyes stain the tissues, they act not only as a sign of solution distribution, but also clearly demonstrate solution diffusion. The dyes help to prevent formaldehyde gray and provide an excellent internal cosmetic. They are available in pink and suntan. Many arterial fluids contain active dye, but additional dyes may be added separately to the arterial solution.

## Fluorescent Dye

Historically, fluorescent dyes were present in embalming fluids and could only be observed with an ultraviolet lamp, or blacklight. When the lights of the embalming room were turned off, the blacklight would reveal the presence of dye in the tissues as a bluish-white glow. Importantly, the dyes would only indicate the presence of embalming solution in the superficial tissues. At present, active dyes serve the same purpose.

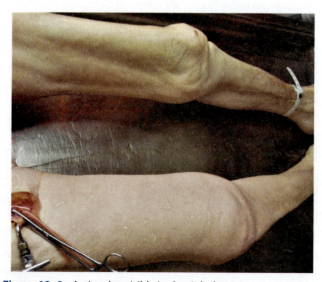

**Figure 13–9.** Active dye visible in the right leg.

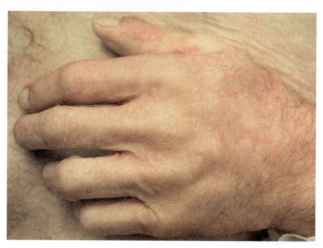

**Figure 13–10.** Livor mortis cleared from fingers of left hand.

## Clearing of Intravascular Blood Discoloration

Livor mortis is observed during pre-embalming analysis. Livor mortis is usually seen in the dependent body areas. The presence of livor mortis can indicate which areas of the body were dependent at death; a method common in death investigation. When an area with livor mortis is manually pressed, the discolored tissues will lighten as blood is gravitated from the area. This can be demonstrated by squeezing your own fingertip for several seconds. After squeezing, the tissues will appear lightened. Blood is returned to the area through capillary refill. The rapid removal and return of blood to your fingertip indicates that blood is intravascular; the gravitation of postmortem livor mortis indicates the blood discoloration is also intravascular. During injection, intravascular blood discolorations are removed through blood drainage. Clearing of livor mortis is easily observed (**Fig. 13–10**). Massage can help to stimulate clearing of livor mortis.

## Distension of Small Surface Vessels

When embalming solution reaches certain areas, such as the hands, feet, or temple of the forehead, superficial small vessels can be observed by their distension (**Fig. 13–11**). This is an indication of embalming solution distribution and and intravascular pressure (IVP). Gravitated blood can also cause veins in the hand to distend when they are placed on the embalming table.

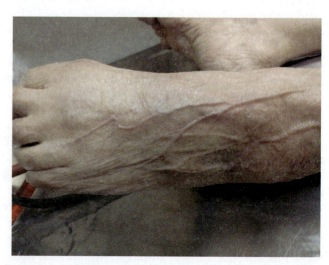

Figure 13–11. Distension of superficial vessels in the left foot.

Gas in the cavities can cause small vessels to distend. Observe these areas prior to and during arterial injection. Slight distension is favorable. If the distension becomes too pronounced, modifications to embalming should be made.

### Loss of Skin Elasticity

As embalming progresses, the preservative solution will begin to firm the tissues. Tissues will also become less flexible or less elastic. When embalmed tissue is gently pulled upward, it will not extend far before settling back into position. Unembalmed tissue is more elastic and will stretch farther. Dehydrated tissues will remain in the drawn position, sometimes not settling at all. This illustrates the benefit of interaction with the tissues during arterial injection. Decisions can be made to adjust dilutions to attain proper moisture balance.

### Firming (Fixation) of the Tissues

Rigor mortis can easily be mistaken for firming of the tissues by the arterial solution. It is most important that in making the pre-embalming analysis of the body, the **presence of rigor** be noted. Some bodies exhibit little or no firming after embalming, usually due to disease conditions. Most bodies exhibit some degree of firming. Firming, although not a fool-proof sign of embalmed tissue, is nevertheless an indicator that embalmers rely upon as a sign of arterial distribution. Some embalming chemicals are designed to produce tissues that are only slightly firm or that exhibit no firming. Different embalming chemicals can also affect the degree and speed of tissue firming.

### Drying of the Tissues

As arterial solution reacts with the tissues, they will lose some degree of moisture and feel drier to the touch when compared to observation before embalming. Dry tissues are a positive indication of embalming. The degree of dryness is tempered to achieve a natural moisture balance. Tissues not reached by the embalming solution have more luster, or appear shiny and even moist to the touch.

### Bleaching of the Tissues

Some arterial fluids produce a mottled effect of the skin when the solution is present. This mottled coloring is caused by the bleaching quality of some arterial fluids. Dyes in the embalming solution often mask this bleaching effect.

### Blood Drainage

The presence of blood drainage indicates that embalming solution is being distributed to the tissues and organs of the body. It does not, however, indicate what specific areas of the body are receiving arterial solution. As a sign of distribution, it does not account for short-circuiting of arterial solution. Some body areas might be receiving too much and other body areas might not be receiving any solution. Excellent preservation can be accomplished in some bodies with little or no drainage. Restricting the drainage can often help in the distribution of the arterial solution.

### Rounding of Features

Fingertips and facial features, especially the lips, will fill and expand as arterial solution reaches these areas. Injection and drainage methods, strength and volume of embalming solution affect the natural contour of these areas. Ideally, features are restored to acceptable appearance. Excessive drainage and astringent solutions can cause the reverse to happen; features will show signs of dehydration and unacceptable appearance.

> The presence of numerous signs of both embalming solution distribution and diffusion is needed to measure the effectiveness of embalming. A single sign is not a reliable measure of embalming solution distribution.

## OBSERVATIONS PRIOR TO INJECTION

Postmortem changes can present false signs of arterial solution distribution and diffusion. Thorough observation and documentation of all conditions present before embalming begins can prevent errors that negatively impact the success of the procedure. Observe and document the following postmortem conditions:

### Presence or Absence of Livor Mortis in All Body Areas

Also examine the nailbeds as some degree of livor is usually present. However, postmortem positioning of the hands may gravitate the livor from the nailbeds. When the presence of livor is not noticed prior to embalming, the absence could be mistaken during embalming as clearing due to arterial solution injection and blood drainage.

### Degree of Rigor Mortis

Attempt should always be made to relieve rigor prior to injection. This is not always possible in arthritic limbs. The jaw may also be firmly set by the muscle contractions during rigor. Rigor can easily be mistaken for firming of the tissues during embalming.

### Distension of Veins or Small Arteries

Veins on the backside of the hands can be distended before arterial solution is injected as a result of gravitation of the blood. Distension of veins in the forehead and temples can indicate intravascular pressure (**Fig. 13-12**). Gases in the cavities or conditions such as ascites or hydrothorax can put pressure on

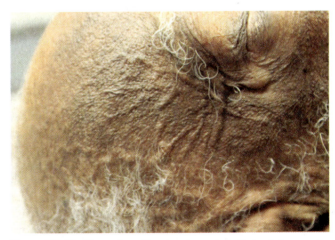

**Figure 13–12.** Distension of temporal vessels indicates intravascular pressure.

the diaphragm and heart and cause small vessels to fill with blood. This distension or its absence should be noted prior to arterial injection.

### Skin Discolorations

Skin of cooled or frozen bodies may have a pinkish hue; bodies dead from carbon monoxide poisoning may appear cherry-red. It is important to note these discolorations (resulting from hemolysis) prior to arterial injection. The pinkish tissue can be mistaken for the presence of arterial solution dye in the tissues.

### Tissue Firmness

Mortuary refrigeration will firm the subcutaneous fatty tissues; creating a false sign of preservation. True tissue firmness is created by the cross-linking of proteins caused by embalming chemical preservatives.

## IMPROVING ARTERIAL SOLUTION DISTRIBUTION

During arterial injection, several mechanical and manual procedures can be followed to improve the distribution of the arterial solution.

1. Increase the rate of flow of the arterial solution being injected.
2. Increase the pressure of the arterial solution being injected.
3. Inject the arterial solution using pulsation.
4. Restrict the drainage; use intermittent drainage and the alternate method of drainage.
5. Massage along the pathway of an artery toward the area not receiving solution. For example, massage the axillary space toward the hands.
6. Inject an adequate volume of embalming solution. Areas initially not receiving solution may receive solution during subsequent injections.
7. Relieve extreme abdominal extravascular pressures caused by gas or abdominal edema (ascites) using a trocar. Insert the trocar in the left inguinal region and direct superficially along the anterior abdominal wall. Pierce the transverse colon.
8. When solution distributes, but there is little drainage, select another drainage site.

Treatments for specific areas may also be applied. For facial tissues, massage the neck along the common carotid arteries. For the arms and hands, lower them below the sides of the embalming table to create capillary expansion (**Fig. 13–13**). This method expands the vessels and promotes better arterial solution distribution. For the fingers, massage the radial and ulnar artery areas of the forearm and then massage the sides of the fingers; pressure can also be applied to the nail beds. For the legs, massage along the femoral arteries, flex the legs, and turn the foot inward to "squeeze" the muscles of the legs.

Gentle pressure applied to the lips and eyelids will attract solution to these tissues. Avoid over manipulation which can cause swelling, dehydration, and desquamation.

Body areas that receive no solution or inadequate amounts of arterial solution should be injected separately (sectional embalming). If distribution is still an issue, restricting drainage from the limb, massaging, increasing the pressure or rate of flow of injection, or using pulsation with higher pressures may all help to distribute solution into a particular body area.

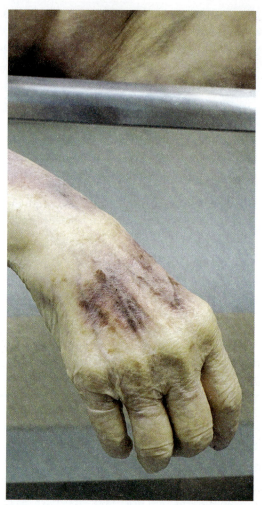

**Figure 13–13.** Hand lowered below the table to create capillary expansion.

A preservative solution must enter a body region or area before it can reach a specific location. Arterial solution cannot enter the fingers when it is not entering the arm.

> When doubt exists as to whether a body area has received any, or an adequate amount of arterial solution, raise the artery that supplies the area in question and separately inject that area until adequate preservation is evident.

## DIFFUSION OF THE EMBALMING SOLUTION

One of the keys to arterial embalming is arterial fluid **diffusion** (**Fig. 13–14**). Fluid diffusion can be defined as *the passage of some elements of the injected embalming solutions from within the capillary (intravascular) to the tissue spaces (extravascular).*

Capillaries are the smallest blood vessels. They link the smallest arteries (arterioles) to the smallest veins (venules). They are actually the extensions of the inner linings of these larger vessels. Their walls are composed of endothelium, which lines the entire vascular system and is made up of flat, single-layered cells called **squamous epithelium**. These very thin-walled cells form the semipermeable membranes through which substances in the blood must pass to reach the body cells.

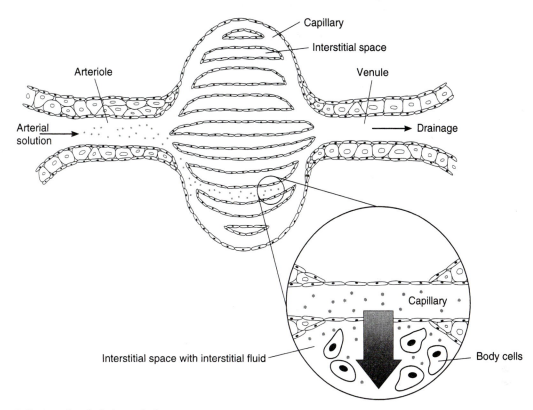

**Figure 13–14.** Diffusion of embalming solution.

In the living body, the blood does not have direct contact with body cells. All of the cells (e.g., muscle cells, nerve cells) are surrounded by a liquid called interstitial (tissue) fluid. Blood nutrients and oxygen must pass through the walls of the capillaries and into the interstitial fluid. These products diffuse through the tissue fluid to reach the body cells. This same movement occurs in embalming. The arterial solution must pass from within the capillary, through the walls of the capillary, into the interstitial fluid, and finally to the body cells. It must then enter the cells of the body and react with the protoplasm protein. The preservative will also act on the proteins in the membranes surrounding the cells.

The capillary network of the blood vascular system is so vast that a pinprick to living tissue will damage a sufficient number of blood vessels to cause bleeding.

## MECHANISMS OF ARTERIAL SOLUTION DIFFUSION

In the living cell, **active transport** is one mechanism that moves material across the cell membrane: nutrients are moved into the cell and waste is removed from the cell. Energy for active transport is produced by the living cell. Active transport does not function in the dead human body.

**Passive physical transport mechanisms** are responsible for the movement of embalming solution from within the capillaries to the tissue spaces. The energy needed to move the solution through the walls of the capillary originates from a nonliving mechanism. Passive mechanisms move materials (embalming solution) through dead cell membranes. The main passive mechanisms in the dead body include pressure filtration, osmosis, and dialysis.

### Pressure Filtration

**Pressure filtration** caused by intravascular pressure, is one of the most important passive physical transport systems. Pressure filtration moves embalming solution from the capillaries to the tissue fluids. In this process, both the solute and solvent portions of the embalming solution pass into the interstitial fluid. Penetrating agents (wetting agents, surface tension reducers, or surfactants) in the concentrated embalming fluid lower its surface tension. The reduction of surface tension makes the embalming solution "wetter," and it can more easily pass through the minute pores and the cell membranes of the capillaries.

IVP places enough pressure on the embalming solution to force it through the pores between the cells of the capillary walls. This is similar to the effect of a lawn soaker hose. Some of the solution enters the tissue spaces to mix with the interstitial fluid. The embalming solution that remains in the capillary pushes on to remove the blood and exits as part of the drainage.

In the agonal period, respiration can become difficult and shallow. Sufficient oxygen is not delivered to the blood. As a defense mechanism, the pores between the cells of the capillaries expand in an attempt to get more oxygen. It is theorized that at death the capillaries are permeable, for their pores are still expanded. As a result, embalming solution can easily be filtered (or pushed) through these pores (caused by IVP). In some bodies, the capillaries may have begun to decompose. The injected solution can now easily flow through the broken capillaries into the tissue spaces. When this happens, the body tissues easily distend. This is seen in bodies that have been dead for long periods. These bodies easily swell and there is little or no drainage.

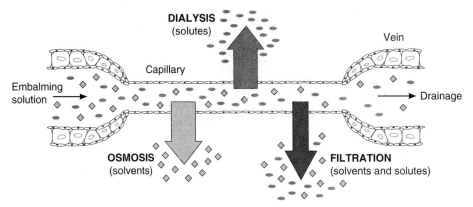

**Figure 13–15.** Summary of solution diffusion: pressure filtration, osmosis, and dialysis.

Likewise, when the limbs are exercised to break up rigor mortis, many capillaries may be torn. The muscle tissues can rapidly swell on injection and, again, drainage is minimal. In bodies in which decomposition is evident or rigor is present, stronger solutions should be used so preservation can be achieved with a minimal amount of solution. This keeps swelling at a minimum. Pressure filtration is, no doubt, one of the primary mechanisms by which embalming solution comes into contact with the interstitial spaces and fluids (**Fig. 13–15**).

## Osmosis

**Osmosis** is the passive transport mechanism involved with liquid (or solvent) movement. It involves the passage of a solvent (such as water) through a semipermeable membrane from a dilute to a concentrated solution. Embalming solutions are more dilute (or less dense) than the interstitial fluids that surround the body cells. The interstitial fluids and the embalming solution are separated by the walls of the capillaries, which are semipermeable. Some of the chemical compounds found in the interstitial fluid cannot move through the capillary walls into the blood vascular system. The more dilute solution, in this case, the embalming solution, is described as hypotonic, meaning it is more dilute or less dense than the interstitial fluid. For example, in mixing a 1-gallon solution of embalming solution, assume that 8 ounces of concentrated fluid is added to 120 ounces of water; for every ounce of embalming fluid, 15 ounces of water is used to dilute the solution.

Some of the hypotonic embalming solution will easily pass through the walls and minute pores of the capillary to enter the interstitial spaces and mix with the interstitial fluid. It will then travel through the interstitial fluid and come into contact with the cells. Again, the process of osmosis will occur. This time the mixture of interstitial fluid and embalming solution will pass through the cell membrane and the preservatives will enter the cytoplasm of the cell. All along this route, contact of the preservative solution is made with proteins whether they are in the walls of the capillaries, in the interstitial fluid, in the membranes of the cells, or in the cytoplasm of the cell. New substances are being produced from the reaction between the protein and the preservative. In this manner, the process of preservation occurs.

When embalming solutions are too weak (too dilute), these solutions will rapidly pass through the capillaries into the tissue fluids. Not only can swelling occur, but inadequate preservation will result. Tissues become waterlogged by weak solutions. Water accelerates decomposition. A reverse condition can be created by mixing solutions that are too concentrated. Concentrated solutions can cause the moisture in the interstitial fluid to move into the capillaries, causing dehydration. This is desired in conditions such as edema.

**Primary dilution** is when the embalmer dilutes the concentrated arterial fluid from the bottle, with water. Coinjection fluids, humectants, and water softeners are commonly used for dilution. These solutions are described as being hypotonic for embalming the average body under normal moisture conditions. They allow some moisture to be added to the tissues and assist in retaining tissue moisture.

Within the tissue spaces, where the interstitial fluid is present, dilution of the arterial fluid continues. This dilution of the embalming solution that occurs in the tissues of the body is called the **secondary dilution**. The moisture found in the tissues dilutes the fluid. In addition, the fluid that remains in the capillaries and exits with the drainage is also diluted by the liquid portion of the blood. The secondary dilution of the fluid can be very great in bodies with skeletal edema.

During embalming analysis, the embalmer evaluates the moisture conditions of the body. Three questions are asked: (1) Are tissues dehydrated? (2) Are the tissues edematous? (3) Is tissue moisture ideal? The primary dilution is prepared according to the evaluation.

## Dialysis

**Dialysis** is mechanism responsible for the diffusion of the dissolved crystalloid solutes of a solution through a semipermeable membrane. Interstitial fluid, cytoplasm of the body cells, and embalming solutions are composed primarily of the solvent water. Dissolved in these solutions are very small solutes called **crystalloids** and very large solutes called **colloids**.

The embalming solution in the capillary is separated from the interstitial fluid by the semipermeable membrane of the capillary wall. The cytoplasm within the cell is separated from the interstitial fluid by the semipermeable **cell membrane**. In dialysis, small crystalloids can diffuse through the semipermeable membranes, but large colloids in the solutions cannot. Water is the primary solvent in embalming solutions; alcohols and glycerine are other examples. The solutes in embalming fluids are various crystalloids such as salts, preservatives, and germicides and colloids (humectants). Interstitial fluid is comprised of the solvent water and various crystalloid salts and colloids (proteins, enzymes, etc.). Crystalloids in the embalming solution can diffuse through the capillary semipermeable membrane into the interstitial fluid. These preservatives, germicides, dyes, and so on then spread through the interstitial fluid and again pass through the cell membrane to enter the cytoplasm of the cell.

To repeat, dialysis is the diffusion of crystalloids across a semipermeable membrane that is impermeable to colloids. It is the process of separating crystalloids (smaller particles) from colloids (larger particles) by the difference in their rates of diffusion through a semipermeable membrane.

## MOVEMENT OF EMBALMING SOLUTIONS FROM OUTSIDE THE CAPILLARIES TO INSIDE THE CELLS

Fluid diffusion is defined as the movement of embalming solution from within the capillary (intravascular) to the interstitial fluid (extravascular). Embalming solution does not stop moving once it leaves the capillary and enters the interstitial space to mix with the interstitial fluid. The interstitial fluid (intercellular or tissue fluid) is a viscous solution similar to the cytoplasm found inside the cells of the body. It contains inorganic chemicals, proteins, carbohydrates, and lipids dissolved in water. This fluid surrounds the cells of the body and is the connection between the blood vascular system (capillaries) and the body cells. Embalming solution must pass from the capillaries into the interstitial fluid, spread through the interstitial fluid, and finally enter the cells of the body (**Fig. 13-16**). Once inside the body cells, the embalming solution again diffuses to come into contact with all portions of the cell.

The concentrated embalming elements are spread through the interstitial fluid by the passive transport systems called **diffusion** and **filtration gravitation**. Passage of embalming solution into the body cells is brought about by the passive transport systems of **absorption, osmosis,** and **dialysis**.

### Diffusion

Diffusion means scattering or spreading. Small particles such as molecules are always moving in all directions. For example, place a drop of fluid dye into a gallon of water and let the solution of dye and water set without stirring. In a short period, the entire gallon of water is slightly and evenly colored by the dye. The concentrated drop of dye has spread through the water. Diffusion occurs from a region of high concentration to a region of lower concentration. In a similar manner, once the embalming solution passes into the interstitial fluid, it spreads (or diffuses) through the interstitial fluid to come into contact with the cells of the body. By the processes of dialysis, adsorption, and osmosis, it passes into the cell and, once in the cell, spreads through the cytoplasm by diffusion.

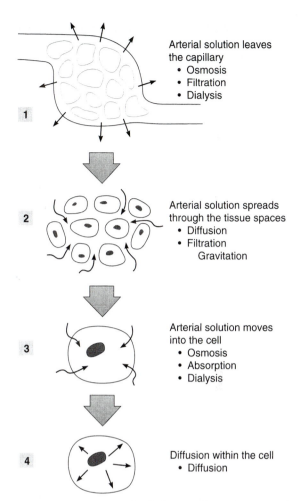

**Figure 13-16.** Movement of embalming solution from outside the capillaries to inside the cells.

### Absorption

The cytoplasm of the body cells is composed of a continuous aqueous solution (cytosol) with all the organelles (except the nucleus) suspended in it. The fluid inside the cells of the body is called **colloidal dispersion**. The large colloid molecules, because of their large surface area, tend to **absorb** molecules. Colloidal dispersions in cells absorb molecules from the surrounding interstitial tissue fluids. In this manner, some of the embalming solution present in the interstitial fluid is absorbed into the body cells.

### Gravity Filtration

Gravity filtration is the extravascular settling of embalming solution by gravitational force into the dependent areas of the body. This passive transport system helps to move embalming solution throughout the interstitial fluid. In the embalmed body, gravity filtration is responsible for the movement of embalming solution into the dependent tissues—lower back, buttocks, and backs of arms, legs, and shoulders. It may be of some value in moving embalming solution into those areas that are in contact with the embalming table. This slow movement continues for some time after the injection of solution. This is *not* a gravitation of fluids through the vascular system. It is extravascular movement of the solution through the interstitial fluid.

## CONCEPTS FOR STUDY

Define the following terminology:
- Absorption
- Active transport
- Actual pressure
- Aortic semilunar valve
- Arch of the aorta
- Ascending aorta
- Combined resistance
- Delivery of arterial solution
- Dialysis
- Differential pressure
- Diffusion of arterial solution
- Distribution of arterial solution
- Drainage of blood
- Extravascular resistances
- Gravity filtration
- Injection pressure
- Intravascular resistances
- Left ventricle
- Osmosis
- Passive transport systems
- Potential pressure
- Pressure filtration
- Primary dilution
- Rate of flow
- Retained arterial solution
- Secondary dilution

1. Name the four functions of arterial embalming.
2. Explain the significance of the ascending aorta and the arch of the aorta to arterial embalming.
3. Why is some form of resistance within the vascular system necessary during embalming?
4. How can rigor mortis be relieved?
5. Discuss several postmortem conditions that can give false signs of arterial solution distribution.
6. List the components of drainage during embalming.
7. Restate several signs of arterial solution diffusion.
8. Recognize the areas of the body affected by skeletal edema.
9. Describe the role of the aortic semilunar valve in arterial solution distribution.
10. Name and give the function of the three main passive physical transport mechanisms.

## FIGURE CREDIT

Figures 13-3, 13-10 are used with permission of Kevin Drobish.
Figures 13-4, 13-7, 13-9, 13-11, 13-12, 13-13 are used with permission of Sharon L. Gee-Mascarello.

## BIBLIOGRAPHY

Anthony CP. *Textbook of Anatomy and Physiology.* St. Louis, MO: CV Mosby, 1979:40–53.

Arnow LE. *Introduction to Physiological and Pathological Chemistry.* St. Louis, MO: CV Mosby; 1976:66–73.

Dhonau CO. *The ABCs of Pressure and Distribution, File 86.* Cincinnati, OH: Cincinnati College of Embalming.

Dhonau CO. *Manual of Case Analysis,* 2nd ed. Cincinnati, OH: Embalming Book Co., 1928.

Frederick JF. The mathematics of embalming chemistry, Parts I and II. *The Dodge Magazine.* October–November 1968.

Johnson EC. A study of arterial pressure during embalming. In *Champion Expanding Encyclopedia.* Springfield, OH: Champion Chemical Co., 1981:2081–2084.

Kroshus J, McConnell J, Bardole J. The measurement of formaldehyde retention in the tissues of embalmed bodies. *Director.* March/April 1983:10–12.

Zweifach BW. The microcirculation of the blood. *Scientific American.* January 1959.

# CHAPTER 14

# Cavity Embalming

## CHAPTER OVERVIEW

- Purposes for Cavity Embalming
- Body Cavities and Contents
- Trocar Guides
- Sequences: Aspiration–Injection–Re-aspiration

The oldest methods of embalming, dating back to the Egyptians, included treatment of the viscera. Until the modern era of embalming, most embalming techniques involved not only removal of the viscera (evisceration) from the thoracic and abdominal cavities but also removal of the brain from the cranial cavity. Embalmers using these early embalming processes recognized the difficulty in preserving the body if some method of visceral treatment was not practiced. Upon introduction of the trocar in the late nineteenth century, embalmers moved away from the direct incision approach to preserve and sanitize the contents of the body cavities.*

There is a need to continue the preservation and sanitation processes after arterial embalming because:

1. Purulent materials, blood, and edematous fluids within the body cavities along with unembalmed tissues continue to decompose and remain an excellent medium for bacterial growth. Untreated microbes become a source of gases and odor and can create purge from an external body orifice.
2. The contents *within* the hollow visceral organs, the stomach, intestines, and urinary bladder are not reached by the arterial solution.
3. There is no external method for verifying if the walls and tissues of the visceral organs have received the arterial solution.

The aspiration procedure and subsequent perfusion with cavity fluid is designed to reach the substances and microbial populations found within the thoracic, abdominopelvic, and when necessary, the cranial cavities. Those materials found within the hollow viscera and portions of the visceral organs themselves, which are not supplied by arterial injection, are treated in the process of cavity embalming.

Cavity embalming is a two-step process: aspiration of the cavities and their contents, followed by the injection of a strong preservative/disinfectant chemical. This process takes place *after* the arterial embalming. Depending on the condition of the body, the process involves subsequent steps of re-aspiration and re-injection of the cavities.

There may be occasions when cavity treatment is *not* employed in preparation of the body. For example, when the body is bequeathed to a medical school or when the hospital or medical examiner allows the body to be arterially embalmed prior to autopsy or postmortem examination.

There are also situations in which arterial embalming is not feasible. Cavity embalming, surface, and hypodermic embalming would be the principal means of preserving and sanitizing the remains. These cases include badly decomposed and badly burned bodies.

## CHRONOLOGY OF CAVITY TREATMENT

1. Arterial embalming
   a. Limited treatment of the abdominal cavity prior to, or during arterial injection when the abdomen is distended.
      (1) Drainage of ascites.
      (2) Removal of gases.
   b. Limited aspiration of the thorax when subcutaneous emphysema is present.
2. Aspiration of the cavities
   a. Time of treatment.
      (1) Immediately after arterial injection.
      (2) Several hours after arterial injection.
   b. Suggested order of aspiration.
      (1) Thoracic cavity and its contents (**Fig. 14–1A**).
      (2) Abdominal cavity and its contents (**Fig. 14–1B**).
      (3) Pelvic cavity and its contents (**Fig. 14–1C**).
3. Injection of cavity chemicals into the body cavities.
4. Closure of the trocar point of entry.
5. Washing and drying of the body.
6. Possible re-aspiration.
7. Possible re-injection.

Not all microorganisms die with the host. Many survive and continue to multiply after somatic and cellular death. During the agonal and postmortem periods following somatic death, microbes from the hollow intestinal organs enter the bloodstream and lymph channels where they translocate to the skeletal tissues and interstitial fluids. In tissues not reached by arterial treatments, the decomposition cycle continues to

---

*Inventor of trocar: Samuel Rodgers, U.S. Patent No. 207551, New York City, August 27, 1878.

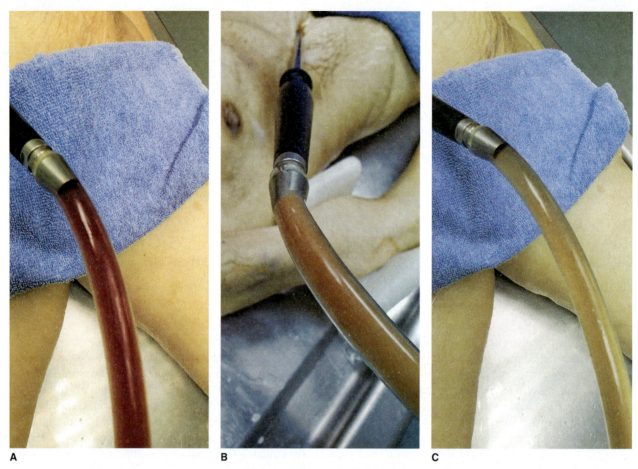

**Figure 14–1.** **A.** Aspiration of blood from the thoracic cavity. **B.** Aspiration of undigested food abdominal cavity. **C.** Aspiration of urine from pelvic cavity.

produce undesired effects. Cavity treatment destroys microbes and inactivates the medium upon which these microbes grow and multiply.

Cavity embalming treats the (1) **contents** of the hollow viscera (**Table 14–1**), (2) **walls** of the visceral organs not embalmed by arterial injection, and (3) **contents** of the spaces between the visceral organs and the walls of the cavities.

| TABLE 14–1. Contents of the Hollow Viscera That Must Be Treated | |
|---|---|
| Organ | Contents to Be Aspirated or Treated |
| Lungs, trachea, bronchi | Blood, edema, purulent material, gases |
| Stomach | Hydrochloric acid, undigested food, blood, gases |
| Small intestine | Gases, undigested foods, partially digested foods, blood |
| Large intestine | Gases, fecal material, blood |
| Urinary bladder | Urine, pustular material, blood |
| Gallbladder | Bile |
| Pelvis of the kidney | Urine, pustular material, blood |
| Heart | Blood |
| Inferior vena cava, portal veins | Blood |

The contents of the **hollow** portions of the viscera are not perfused during arterial injection. Materials within these spaces continue to decompose when untreated, and the resulting products of decomposition can produce **odors, gas formation, and purge.** Gases can move into the skeletal tissues and cause distension of viewable areas, such as the face and hands.

It is not possible to externally determine which visceral organs did or did not receive arterial solution. The embalmer cannot inspect these organs for signs of arterial distribution; cavity embalming must **ensure** that the walls and parenchyma of the hollow viscera and the **stroma** and **parenchyma** of the solid organs are embalmed. The stroma comprises the blood vessels, connective tissue, ducts, and nerves; the parenchyma is the functional tissue that comprises the bulk of the organ.

The solid organs treated by cavity embalming are the pancreas, spleen, kidneys, liver, and lungs. When cranial cavity treatment is performed, the solid brain and brain stem will also undergo aspiration and injection of a preservative solution.

Partially digested food material within the stomach and small intestines, as well as the gases and liquids resulting from the breakdown of these materials, are removed by the aspiration process. Materials not removed are treated by the injection of cavity fluid (**Table 14–2**). If these materials are not removed or treated, gases can form and produce sufficient pressure upon the stomach and diaphragm to create purge from the oral or nasal cavities.

| TABLE 14-2. Cavity Contents That Must Be Treated | |
|---|---|
| Cavity | Material to Be Treated |
| Thoracic | Blood, edema, purulent material, gases |
| Pericardial | Blood, edema |
| Abdominal | Blood, edema, purulent material, gases |
| Pelvic | Blood, edema, purulent material, gases |
| Cranial | Blood, edema, gases |

Liquids within the cavities will not only decompose, but they will also serve as a medium for bacterial growth and will dilute cavity chemicals.

Purge exiting the **mouth, or the oral cavity** originates from the **lungs**, the **stomach**, or the **throat** (Table 14–3).

Purge from the **nose, or nasal cavity** can also originate from the lungs, stomach, or throat. When fecal material is not evacuated or treated with cavity fluids, sufficient gas can form within the abdomen to cause lung or stomach purges. In addition, purge from the **anal orifice** is probable. Rectal hemorrhage can be a source of bloody purge exiting the anal orifice.

Cranial purge (brain purge) is rare. Gases within the cranial cavity can spread into the facial tissues through the various foramina that lead from the cranial cavity to the soft facial tissues. Generally, a liquid or semisolid purge from the cranial cavity is the result of a fracture of the temporal bone. The point of exit for brain purge is the ear. Gas formation in the cranial cavity can produce sufficient pressure to distend the eyes; gases within the palpebral tissues (eyelids) also cause swelling.

Infection or inflammation of the brain or meninges can lead to formation of gases and edema within the cranial cavity. Hemorrhages from stroke can cause blood and edema to accumulate in the cranial cavity. Advanced decomposition can produce sufficient pressure to cause purge from the cranial cavity.

**Foramina** near the eye serve as pathways for gas accumulation in the tissues surrounding the eye orbit: the optic foramen, superior orbital fissure, inferior orbital fissure, infraorbital foramen, supraorbital foramen, anterior ethmoidal foramen, and posterior ethmoidal foramen.

After recent cranial surgery (such as gunshot or trauma to the head) or advanced decomposition, aspiration and injection of a few ounces of cavity fluid into the cranial cavity may prevent the buildup of gases.

| TABLE 14-3. Description of Purge | | |
|---|---|---|
| Source | Orifice | Description |
| Stomach | Nose/mouth | Liquids, semisolids, dark brown "coffee ground" appearance; odor; acid pH |
| Lungs | Nose/mouth | Frothy; any blood present is red in color, little odor |
| Brain | Nose/ear/eyelids | Gases can move into tissues of the eye, fractures can cause blood to purge from the ears, creamy white semisolid brain matter may exit through a fracture or the nasal passage |

Arterial embalming supplies sufficient solution to the brain and cerebrospinal fluid through both the internal carotid and vertebral arteries. Routine aspiration and injection of the cranial cavity of an adult are usually unnecessary. Cranial treatment is often necessary for infants; the brain decomposes very rapidly. Cavity fluid can be introduced into the cranial cavity with a large hypodermic needle through the nostril of the nose and through the cribriform plate of the ethmoid bone to reach the cranial cavity.

## INSTRUMENTATION AND EQUIPMENT REQUIRED

A trocar with a length of tubing attached to an aspiration device (electric or hydroaspirator) is needed to perform aspiration. After aspiration, a cavity fluid injector is connected to the trocar to manually inject the cavity fluid. The trocar entry site, in the abdominal wall, can be closed using a postmortem needle and ligature or a trocar button. (inserted with a trocar button applicator). An instrument tray filled with disinfectant solution is used to disinfect all instruments used during the process.

### Devices Used to Create a Vacuum for Aspiration
*Hydroaspirator*
The hydroaspirator is a device installed in the preparation room on the supply line for the cold water. A vacuum is created by turning on the water supply. The creation of optimal vacuum is dependent upon water pressure within the supply line. A vacuum breaker is installed on the drinking water supply line for the facility in which the preparation room is located to prevent reverse siphonage, or backflow. Municipal ordinances require antisiphonage devices to prevent aspirated materials from entering the drinking water supply in the preparation facility.

The trocar frequently clogs when large masses of organic material are aspirated. There is a distinct change in the sound of the device when this happens. Water in the tubing will **reverse** flow, aspiration will stop, and water will fill the body cavities. When this happens, leave the trocar inserted into the body cavity and shut off the water source immediately. Remove the trocar, place the tip of the instrument into the sink drain, and turn the control lever of the device to allow water to flow from the tubing. Slowly increase water pressure. Raise the tip of the instrument just above the sink drain to inspect the organic material clogging the trocar tip. Remove material from the sharp trocar tip with an instrument instead of your fingers. High water pressure creates a forceful spray from the trocar; low pressure will push the aspirated material into the holes of the trocar point for removal. Once material is cleared, switch the control lever on device back to aspiration and continue the process.

Clear plastic tubing is recommended for cavity aspiration; aspirated material can be seen in the tubing as it is withdrawn. Some trocars have a *sight glass* built into the instrument to view aspirated material. The color and composition of aspirated material indicates the source of the material.

*Electric Aspirator*
Electric aspirators are stand-alone motorized devices. The motor is encased in a metal or plastic housing. An inlet for the water supply leads to the impeller on the motor shaft; the impeller spins to create the suction. Electric aspirators are recommended when low water pressure exists.

### Hand Pump (Historical)

A dual-purpose handheld device used for both arterial solution injection and cavity aspiration. A glass jar with a rubber stopper, called a *gooseneck* was commonly paired with the hand pump. The gooseneck fits snugly into the jar opening, making the jar airtight. The two openings in the gooseneck were for the attachment of two hoses to the hand pump. One hose created air pressure; the other hose created a vacuum. Neither arterial solution nor aspirated material flowed through the hand pump.

### Air Pressure Machine (Historical)

The air pressure machine operated on the same principle as the hand pump. The machine provided either air pressure or vacuum; arterial solution and cavity aspirate did not pass through the machine. The machine had two outlets. One created a vacuum for aspiration; the other forced air into the jar. The gooseneck was also used. Aspirated material was collected in the jar. Special jars were designed for this purpose; thick glass prevented implosion during use. The contents of the jar were treated before disposal into the sewer system.

## Instruments Used in Aspiration

### Trocar

A trocar is a long hollow needle with a removable sharp point that is available in varying lengths and bores. Whetstones or other sharpening devices can be used to keep the points honed, or dull points can be discarded in the biohazard sharps container and replaced by a new blade. The trocar is used to pierce the wall of the abdomen and the walls of the internal organs in the thoracic and abdominal cavities. The trocar, attached to the suction device, is used to withdraw the contents of the organs and residual fluid that has pooled in the cavities. The trocar is also used to introduce the disinfectant/preservative solution over and into the internal organs.

The **infant trocar** is smaller in both length and diameter than the standard adult size. The smaller trocar is designed for cavity treatment in infants and children. The infant size trocar is commonly used for hypodermic injection of preservative chemicals into areas of the limbs or trunk not reached by arterial embalming.

Complete disinfection/sterilization of the trocar after each use is extremely important. Microorganisms can be transferred from one body to another by a contaminated or improperly cleaned trocar. For example, an improperly cleaned trocar can harbor the spore-forming microorganism, **Clostridium perfringens, responsible for true tissue gas.** Instrument trays of sufficient size and length for the trocar are needed for hard chemical disinfection. The autoclave method is also used for trocar sterilization.

### Tubing

Clear plastic or rubber tubing approximately 6–8 feet in length and $3/8$ to $1/2$ inch in diameter is used to connect the trocar to aspiration devices. The wall of the tubing must be thick enough to prevent collapse when suction is generated. Clear or semi-clear tubing permits visual examination of the material being removed and aids in determining which organ or cavity space is being aspirated. The embalmer should be very careful to ensure that the tubing is securely fastened to the trocar during aspiration and cavity treatment. Otherwise, the tubing can detach from the trocar exposing the embalmer to biological and chemical substances. Proper personal protective equipment (PPE) is necessary during cavity treatment.

### Nasal Tube Aspirator

The nasal tube aspirator is designed for aspiration of the nasal and oral cavities. The instrument is inserted into the nares of the nose to reach the nasal cavity and back of the throat; also into the oral cavity to reach the throat. The small diameter holes in the tip of the instrument can readily clog when thickened material is aspirated. The nasal tube aspirator can be unclogged using the same method for clearing the trocar.

### Autopsy Aspirator

The autopsy aspirator is used for aspiration of the trunk cavities of the autopsied body. Large-sized openings at the working end of the instrument lessen the chance of clogging with aspirated material. The aspirator can be placed on the floor of the cavity for passive operation during embalming.

## VISCERAL ANATOMY

### Cranium

The interior of the cranial vault comprises anterior, middle, and posterior cranial fossae in which portions of the brain and brainstem are located. The frontal lobes of the cerebrum rest on that portion of the cranial floor created by the anterior cranial fossa. The temporal lobes, hypothalamus, and midbrain cover the floor of the middle fossa. The large, posterior fossa houses the medulla, pons, and entire cerebellum.

### Thorax

Although the lungs are properly described as contents of the thorax, their apices extend above the level of the first rib into the neck. The right lung comprises three lobes and the left lung two lobes, although this is subject to some variation. The left lung is further characterized by the presence of a cardiac notch or impression to accommodate the ventricles of the heart. Medially, both lung surfaces relate to the contents of the mediastinum and contain the hilar structures, that is, the pulmonary vessels and the main-stem bronchi. Inferiorly, the lungs are related to the diaphragmatic pleura and the diaphragm.

The heart lies retrosternal (behind the sternum, or *breastplate*), in the middle mediastinum and extends from the second intercostal space inferiorly to the fifth. The lateral cardiac margins extend beyond the lateral margins of the body of the sternum. The great vessels arise from the base of the heart at the level of the second intercostal space, behind the upper portion of the body and the manubrium of the sternum.

### Abdomen

The majority of abdominal viscera consist of some part of the digestive apparatus, which is mainly tubular with some modifications and specializations of this basic structure in various locations. As the straight-tubed esophagus passes through the diaphragm and enters the abdomen, it quickly gives rise to the stomach. The remainder of the alimentary or digestive tube, in order, consists of the duodenum, jejunum, ileum (small intestine), cecum, ascending colon, transverse colon, descending colon, sigmoid colon, rectum (large intestine), and anus.

Organs that facilitate digestion include the gallbladder, liver, and pancreas.

A rather peripatetic (moving) organ, the stomach is one whose location varies with changes in the position and orientation of the body. It is, therefore, difficult to describe specific relationships of the stomach. Similarly, the shape of this organ is dependent on the amount and type of food-stuffs contained therein as well as the extent to which the digestive process has progressed. A "typical" stomach possesses greater and lesser curvatures, a fundic region that extends above the level at which the esophagus enters, and a pyloric region at the junction of the stomach and the duodenum.

The small intestine is divided into three segments—continuing from the stomach; the C-shaped **duodenum** is the first part of the small intestine, about 10 inches in length and is the shortest part of the small intestine. It merges to become the second part of the small intestine, the **jejunum**, approximately 8 feet in length; the jejunum merges into the third portion of the small intestine called the **ileum** and measures approximately 12 feet in length and terminates at the cecum of the large intestine. These organs occupy much of the abdomen and both are suspended by a fan-shaped mesentery from the posterior body wall.

The large intestine can be distinguished grossly from the small bowel by (1) its larger diameter, (2) the presence of three longitudinal muscle bands, the taenia coli, (3) haustra sacculations, and (4) fatty appendages called *epiploic appendices*, none of which is found on the small intestine.

A diverticulum (sac or pouch), the **cecum**, marks the beginning of the large intestine and extends inferiorly beyond the level at which the ileum joins the ascending colon. The cecum is situated in the right iliac and hypogastric regions. Opening from it is the vermiform appendix. Extending superiorly from the cecum is the retroperitoneal **ascending colon**, which continues to the right colic or hepatic flexure, inferior to the liver in the right lumbar region. Here, the colon turns sharply to the left in the umbilical region, as the **transverse colon**. This is a freely movable portion of the large bowel, suspended by the transverse mesocolon from the posterior body wall and extending to the left colic or splenic flexure in the left hypochondriac and lumbar regions. Here, the colon again becomes retroperitoneal and descends to the level of the iliac crest as the **descending colon**. In the left iliac region, the descending colon forms the **sigmoid colon** which is once again freely movable, being suspended by the sigmoid mesocolon. Anterior to the third sacral vertebra, the sigmoid colon gives way to the **rectum**.

The largest glandular organ in the body is the liver, which develops as an outgrowth of the digestive tract and retains a functional and anatomical relationship with it. It rests primarily in the right hypochondriac and epigastric regions. The upper surface of the liver is higher on the right than on the left. The upper surface rests against the inferior surface of the diaphragm from which it is suspended by the coronary ligaments. On the inferior surface of the liver is the gallbladder, whose cystic duct is joined by the common hepatic duct from the liver to form the common bile duct that empties the duodenum. The gallbladder and the lower portion of the right lobe of the liver lie anterior to the right hepatic flexure in the right lumbar region.

The pancreas lies cradled in the C-shaped duodenum and extends across the midline from right to left at about the level of the second lumbar vertebra. The major subdivisions of the pancreas include the head, neck, body, and tail. The main duct of the pancreas typically joins the common bile duct immediately as they both enter the duodenum.

The remaining unpaired organ in the abdomen is the spleen, which is located in the left hypochondriac region. Lying in the umbilical left and right lumbar regions are usually paired kidneys. These lie along the posterior body wall, with the right slightly lower than the left because of encroachment by the large right lobe of the liver. Both kidneys lie at the level of the umbilicus and both are retroperitoneal. In its own separate capsule at the superior pole of each kidney is a suprarenal gland.

### Pelvis

Internal pelvic viscera in the male include the prostate gland, seminal vesicles, urinary bladder, and rectum. The last structure was already discussed. The prostate gland is situated at the base of the urinary bladder, surrounding the prostatic or initial portion of the male urethra.

The urinary bladder is situated behind the pubic symphysis in the midline and its shape and size are dependent on the volume of urine contained within it. This muscular, distensible structure receives urine from the kidneys via the paired ureters, which open posterolateral into the bladder.

In the female, the urinary bladder occupies a position similar to that in the male but is separated from the rectum by the intervening uterus and its adnexa. In addition to the uterus and bladder, other visceral structures in the female pelvis include the ovaries, uterine tubes, and vagina. The muscular unpaired uterus is positioned in the midline and is supported by a double layer of peritoneum called broad ligament. The uterus is divided into several parts, including the fundus, body, and cervix.

Through the cervix, the cavity of the uterus communicates with the vagina, which is a distensible tube, flattened anteroposterior. The uterine tubes communicate with the opening directly into the abdominal cavity and the uterine cavity. The abdominal cavity, therefore, opens to the external environment via the uterine tubes, the cavity of the uterus, the cavity of the cervix, and the vagina. The paired ovaries are located on the posterior aspect of the broad ligament on either side of the uterus. The uterus, tubes, and ovaries are supported by an elaborate system of ligaments derived from reflections of the peritoneum.

## TOPOGRAPHICAL DIVISIONS OF THE ABDOMEN

The following topographical systems of dividing the abdomen guide the embalmer to the approximate location of the various abdominal organs. The embalmer must have a working knowledge of visceral organ location to effect thorough preservation (**Fig. 14–2**). This understanding is important: (1) in the process of cavity embalming, (2) when one or more organs have been removed for transplant, and (3) when partial autopsies have been performed. Working knowledge of the relationship of the vascular system to the visceral organs is vital.

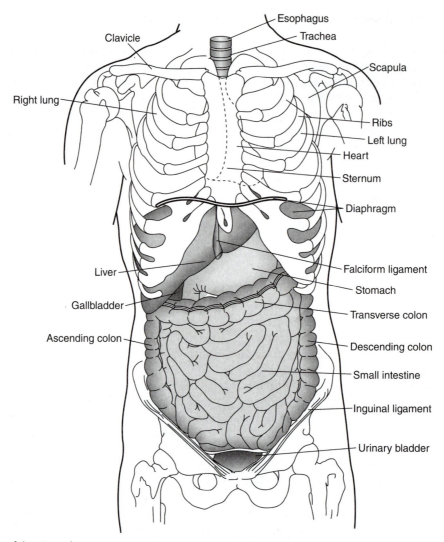

**Figure 14–2.** Anatomy of the visceral organs.

### The Nine-Region Method

To establish the nine abdominopelvic regions (**Table 14–4**), extend two **vertical** lines upward from a point midway between the anterior superior iliac spine and the symphysis pubis. Draw two **horizontal** lines. Join the upper line to the lowest point of the costal margin on each side, at the level of the inferior margin of the tenth costal cartilage. Join the lower horizontal line to the tubercles on the respective iliac crests (**Fig. 14–3**).

### The Quadrant Method

To establish the four abdominopelvic regions, or quadrants, a **horizontal** line is drawn from left to right through the **umbilicus**. A **vertical** line is drawn down the midline of the body (**Fig. 14–4**).

### Trocar Guides

The efficiency of using the trocar to pierce the internal organs and aspirate their contents is enhanced by the use of trocar guides (**Fig. 14–5**). **The main trocar guides reach the stomach, cecum, urinary bladder, and heart.** The guides originate at the common insertion point: 2 inches to the left and 2 inches superior to the umbilicus. The point of the trocar is inserted into the abdomen and kept close to the anterior abdominal wall until the target organ is reached.

### Guide for the Right Side of the Heart

Direct the trocar to intersect a line drawn from the left anterior–superior iliac spine and the right earlobe. After the trocar has passed through the diaphragm, depress the point and enter the heart.

### Guide for the Stomach

Direct the trocar point toward the intersection of the fifth intercostal space and the left midaxillary line (established by extending a line from the center of the medial base of the axillary space inferiorly along the rib cage) continue until the trocar enters the stomach.

### Guide for the Cecum

Direct the trocar toward a point one-fourth of the distance from the right anterior-superior iliac spine to the pubic symphysis; keep the point of the trocar well up near the abdominal wall until within 4 inches of the right anterior-superior iliac spine; then dip the point 2 inches and insert it forward into the colon.

| TABLE 14-4. The Nine Abdominopelvic Regions | | |
|---|---|---|
| **Right Hypochondriac** | **Epigastric** | **Left Hypochondriac** |
| Part of the liver | Stomach including cardiac and pyloric openings | Part of liver |
| Part of right kidney | Portion of liver | Stomach, fundus, and cardiac regions |
| Greater omentum | Duodenum, pancreas | Spleen |
| Coils of small intestine | Suprarenal gland and parts of kidneys | Tail of pancreas |
| Gallbladder | Greater omentum | Left colic splenic flexure<br>Part of left kidney<br>Greater omentum |
| **Right Lumbar** | **Umbilical** | **Left Lumbar** |
| Lower portion of liver | Transverse colon | Part of left kidney |
| Ascending colon | Part of body kidneys | Descending colon |
| Part of right kidney | Part of duodenum | Coils of small intestine |
| Coils of small intestine | Coils of small intestine | Greater omentum |
| Greater omentum | Greater omentum | |
| Right colic (hepatic) flexure | Bifurcation of the abdominal aorta and inferior vena cava | |
| **Right Inguinal (Iliac)** | **Hypogastric** | **Left Inguinal (Iliac)** |
| Cecum, appendix | Bladder in adults if distended | Part of descending colon |
| Part of ascending colon | Uterus during pregnancy | Sigmoid colon |
| Coils of small intestine | Coils of small intestine | Coils of small intestine |
| Greater omentum | Greater omentum | Greater omentum |

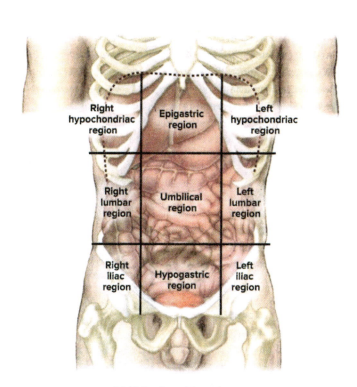

(a) Abdominopelvic regions

**Figure 14–3. The Nine-Region Method.** (Used with permission from McKinley M et al. *Human Anatomy*. 5th ed. New York, McGraw Hill, 2017, Fig. 1.11A.)

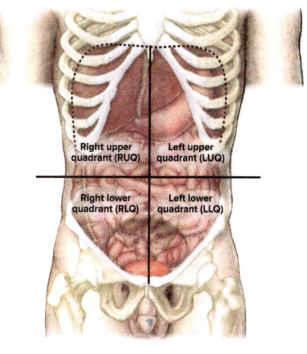

(b) Abdominopelvic quadrants

**Figure 14–4. The Quadrant Method.** (Used with permission from McKinley M et al. *Human Anatomy*. 5th ed. New York, McGraw Hill, 2017, Fig. 1.11B.)

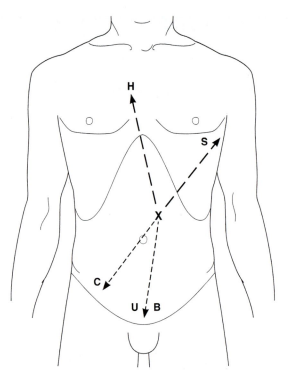

**Figure 14–5. Trocar Guides.** X is the insertion point for the stomach, cecum, urinary bladder, and heart.

### Trocar Guide for the Urinary Bladder

Keep the point up near the abdominal wall directing the trocar to the median line of the pubic bone (symphysis pubis) until the point touches the bone. Retract the trocar slightly, depress the point slightly, and insert into the urinary bladder.

## PARTIAL ASPIRATION PRIOR TO OR DURING ARTERIAL TREATMENT

Cavity embalming, complete aspiration, and injection of cavity fluids, **follows** arterial injection and drainage. There is one exception to this rule: When the abdomen is tightly distended with gas or edema, this pressure should be relieved **prior to or during** arterial injection. The presence of edematous fluid, as in ascites or gases in the abdomen can cause **extravascular resistance**. The pressure exerted upon the vessels can interfere with distribution of arterial solution and drainage of blood.

Extravascular pressure is relieved by making a scalpel puncture into abdomen at the standard point of trocar entry 2 inches left and 2 inches superior to the umbilicus. Insert a trocar or large drain tube into the cavity to release the edema or gases. The entry site may also be in the lower portion of the abdomen; the right or left inguinal or hypogastric region. From this point, edema will gravitate from the abdomen. The **transverse colon may be pierced** to relieve gas accumulation (**Fig. 14–6**).

## ANTEMORTEM SUBCUTANEOUS EMPHYSEMA

A condition where there is a noticeable amount of gas in the tissues **prior to embalming** is antemortem subcutaneous emphysema. Many times, the facial tissues will be quite distended, the tongue will protrude, gases may be felt all along the thoracic walls, and, in the male, the scrotum may be distended with gas.

**If there is no odor and if there are no signs of decomposition**, palpate for a broken rib or examine the body for a puncture wound to the thorax or a very recent tracheotomy opening. Look for large needle punctures over the skin of the rib cage. This condition is brought about by a rupture or by the puncturing or tearing of the pleural sac of the lung. Air was forced into the tissues as the person struggled to breathe air. If the condition is severe enough, try and remove some of this gas **prior to arterial embalming**.

Insert the trocar into the abdomen at the standard point of entry, then direct the point through the diaphragm, keeping the point just under the rib cage so as not to damage any of the large vessels. This should help to relieve some of the gases. Likewise, using a carotid incision will help to relieve gases from the neck tissues. Removal of these gases can be better accomplished by channeling and/or lancing the tissues after the arterial injection is completed.

## TIME PERIOD FOR CAVITY TREATMENT

There are two periods during which cavity aspiration and injection can take place: (1) immediately following arterial injection and (2) several hours following arterial injection. This time delay will allow the intravascular pressure to assist the diffusion of the arterial solution from the capillaries into the interstitial spaces. Some embalmers inject the last quarter gallon of arterial solution with the drainage closed, being careful to remove the arterial tubes

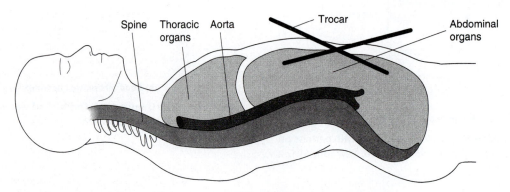

**Figure 14–6.** Trocar levels to relieve abdominal distension caused from ascites and gas accumulation.

and drainage devices quickly and to tie off the vessels so as much pressure as possible remains within the vascular system.

Begin aspirating **prior to suturing incisions that were made for the arterial injection**. Aspiration takes the pressure off the vascular system and thus decreases the possibility of leakage from the incision should some small vessels leak.

Some embalmers do not perform the cavity embalming until the time of dressing and casketing, while others perform the cavity embalming immediately at the conclusion of the arterial embalming. The theory of aspiration shortly after arterial injection has the following advantages:

1. Large numbers of microbes that can easily multiply and accelerate decomposition are removed as soon as possible.
2. Removal of the microbes prevents the possibility of translocation of the microbes to the skeletal tissues.
3. Removal of these microbes prevents or minimizes the possible production of gases that could cause purge.
4. Immediate aspiration removes materials that could purge if sufficient gases were generated during the delay.
5. Removal of the contents of the hollow viscera and cavities eliminates a bacterial medium.
6. Removal of blood from the heart, liver, and large veins helps to prevent blood discolorations and the condition known as embalmer's gray or formaldehyde gray caused by inadequate blood removal.
7. If there has been some distension of the neck or facial tissues during arterial injection, immediate aspiration decreases the swelling. This is often seen in bodies dead from pneumonia when hydrothorax is present.

The second theory is to have a long delay prior to aspirating the body. Some embalmers delay aspirating for 8–12 hours. The theory is to allow a maximum time for the arterial solution to penetrate into the tissue spaces and into the walls of the visceral organs. This will then make the walls easier to pierce with the trocar when the aspirating is done. When a humectant coinjection is supplemented to recontour emaciated tissues, inject the last half-gallon against closed drainage. Delay cavity aspiration. The delay allows time for the facial tissues to contour and firm.

## ASPIRATION TECHNIQUE BY TROCAR

The standard point of trocar entry is located 2 inches to the left of and 2 inches superior to the umbilicus. This point is used for the standard trocar; from it, the embalmer is able to reach all areas of the thoracic, abdominal, and pelvic cavities. The trocar should also be able to reach above the clavicle into the base of the neck. A second reason for using this point, especially with infants and children, is that the liver is on the right side of the body. At the location where the trocar is inserted, it is easier to move the instrument from point to point. If it were inserted on the right side, the trocar would be entangled in the solid tissues of the liver.

During the aspiration of the cavities, the trocar can be withdrawn enough to let air pass through the instrument. This helps to clear materials from within the trocar and the tubing. Some embalmers withdraw the trocar several times during aspiration and plunge it into a container of water to flush out the tubing and trocar.

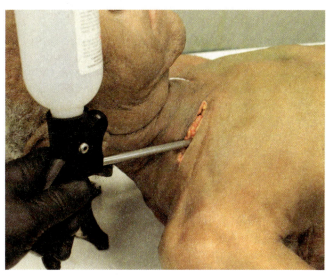

**Figure 14–7.** Cavity fluid introduced through carotid incision using the Evolution injector.

An orderly method of aspiration should be employed. Gases are usually found in the anterior portions of the abdominal and thoracic cavities. Liquids gravitate to the posterior portions of the cavities. If each cavity is "fanned" from right to left, most of the viscera are pierced. This "fanning" can be done in about three levels of depth.

Begin by inserting the trocar and aspirating the most anterior portions of the cavity. Then progress from right to left within the middle portion of the cavity, and finally from right to left through the deepest portions of the cavity. Treat both abdominal and thoracic cavities in this manner.

Cavity fluid can be introduced through the incisions used for arterial injection (**Fig. 14–7**). This method can be used in combination with the standard site of entry. If used as a replacement for abdominal trocar entry, the incision site method is limited only by the length of the trocar.

## RECENT SURGERY OR ORGAN REMOVAL

If the deceased was an organ donor or died during the course of an operation and no autopsy was performed, the surgical incision or the incision used to remove the organ(s) may or may not have been loosely closed by the hospital. For such bodies, the following protocol simplifies the treatment of the cavities:

1. Disinfect the surgical incision with a phenol solution.
2. Arterially embalm the body.
3. Remove loose sutures, surgical staples, and so on, and open the incision.
4. Swab the edges of the incision with a phenol solution.
5. Suture closed the incision using a tight baseball suture. If possible, use sufficient quantities of incision seal powder.
6. Aspirate the cavities and inject cavity fluid.

> Surgical drainage openings may be closed by suture or trocar button **prior** to aspiration of the cavities.

## PARTIAL AUTOPSIES AND ORGAN DONATIONS

After a partial autopsy on an adult, the unautopsied cavity can be difficult to treat from the cavity that has been opened. It is much simpler to treat the walls of the autopsied cavity by hypodermic treatment and painting with autopsy gel. Fill the cavity with an absorbent material and saturate the material with a cavity fluid. Suture the cavity closed. Now treat the unautopsied cavity by aspirating the cavity and its visceral contents. Inject a sufficient quantity of cavity fluid.

## DIRECT INCISION METHOD

In the treatment of bodies that have recent surgical incisions or from which organs were removed after death, resuturing followed by aspiration and injection with the trocar is recommended.

An alternate method can be used where a body cavity (or cavities) has been opened by surgery or a partial autopsy or removal of a donated organ. **The direct incision method** uses this incision to lance and drain the various organs and aspirate the cavity. Cavity fluid can be injected after the body is resutured. This method is unsanitary and can be time consuming. Often, there is no access to both the abdominal and thoracic cavities.

## ORDER OF TREATMENT

A suggested order might be thoracic cavity, abdominal cavity, and pelvic cavity. Likewise, when injecting cavity fluid, inject the thoracic cavity first, then the abdominal and pelvic cavities.

## ASPIRATION OF THE THORACIC CAVITY

At the standard point of entry, direct the trocar into the thoracic cavity. A good point at which to begin aspiration is the right side of the heart, using the trocar guide as an imaginary line running from the left anterior superior iliac spine to the lobe of the right ear. Intersect this line with the trocar in the mediastinal area. This technique also provides practice for those occasions on which the trocar may have to be used as a drainage instrument (which will have to be inserted into the right atrium of the heart). Next, aspirate the anterior chambers of the right and left pleural cavities. Direct the trocar a little lower and pierce the central portions of the lungs and the heart.

> Observe and identify what is being aspirated. Clear tubing suggested.

Finally, aspirate the deep areas of the pleural cavities. If hydrothorax is present, edematous liquids will be found, often in great quantities. Be certain that the trocar is directed to either side of the vertebral column where the great vessels enter and leave the lungs. This also aspirates the bronchial tubes leading to the trachea.

## ASPIRATION OF THE ABDOMINAL CAVITY

After aspiration of the thorax, the trocar can be withdrawn and the stomach aspirated. Use the trocar guide. Move the trocar toward a point established along the left midaxillary line, at about the level of the fifth intercostal space. As the trocar moves toward this point, it should pierce the stomach.

Several passages can be made through the stomach wall. Aspiration not only removes gases, liquids, and semisolids from the organs, but also pierces the viscera so that cavity fluid can better penetrate the visceral organs. Next, the cecum and bladder can be aspirated again using the trocar guides.

In similar "fanning" movements, aspirate the entire abdominal cavity again. Try to establish three levels. Remember, gases, when they can move, will be in the anterior portions and liquids in the posterior portions of the cavities.

In aspiration of the abdomen, the small intestines and the greater omentum have a tendency to cling tightly to the small holes located in the point and shaft of the trocar. For this reason, it is best to keep the instrument in constant motion, except when a large amount of liquid such as edema in bodies with ascites is being drained. Removing the trocar from time to time helps to prevent the clogging of these small holes.

Pay special attention to the posterior of the liver. It is here that the great vessels enter and leave this organ. The liver is very difficult to preserve. Therefore, numerous passes with the trocar should be made through the solid portions of this organ. Also, give special attention to the large intestine, especially the **transverse colon**. Check the previous charts to observe the location of this intestinal organ. The large intestine, especially the transverse portion, should be thoroughly pierced to allow the escape of gases and to assist later in penetration of the cavity fluid.

To assist the trocar in piercing the abdominal organs, apply external pressure gently on the abdominal wall. Never direct the tip of the trocar toward the hand applying the pressure; this could result in an accidental injury to the embalmer. To facilitate passage of the trocar through the coils of the small intestine, in addition to applying pressure on the abdomen, pass the trocar to a bony part such as the ilium or pubic bone. In this way, the point of the trocar will pass through the intestine rather than push it aside or slip around it.

Another method that can be used in aspirating the abdomen and inferior portion of the thorax is to insert the trocar in the center of the right or left inguinal region of the abdomen. Long passes can be made with the trocar, which will pass through the lumen of the intestines as the point forges ahead through the diaphragm. Many embalmers feel they can better pierce the large and small intestine from this point of trocar entry.

## TREATMENT OF THE MALE GENITALIA

Following aspiration of the pelvic and abdominal cavities, if the shaft of the penis and the scrotum have not received sufficient arterial solution, introduce cavity fluid through the following procedure. To enter the scrotum, direct the point of the trocar to the most anterior portion of the symphysis pubis. Draw back slightly on the trocar and direct the point over the top of the symphysis pubis into the penis and scrotum. In cases of hydrocele (edema of the scrotum), make several passes to channel the tissues of the scrotum. Using a cloth placed around the scrotum, force excess fluid into the pelvic cavity. Inject undiluted cavity fluid into the scrotum.

Less frequently encountered is a hernia that forces a portion of the intestines into the scrotum. This condition can severely enlarge the scrotum. The trocar is directed into the scrotum to pierce the loops of the intestine and withdraw as much of the content as possible. Later, this area should be injected with cavity fluid. The embalmer can also use the trocar to pull the intestine back into the abdominal cavity. This is slowly accomplished by pulling on the intestine with the point of the trocar. Gradually, the intestine can be manipulated into the abdominal cavity.

## CRANIAL ASPIRATION

The point of entry in cranial aspiration is the right or left nostril (nares). A small trocar is introduced into the nostril and pushed through the **cribriform plate of the ethmoid bone**. At this point, the instrument enters the anterior portion of the cranial cavity (**Fig. 14–8**). It is not possible to move the trocar into the posterior portion of the cavity; therefore, any gases present must be removed from this anterior position.

Inject only a few ounces of concentrated cavity fluid. This is done by using a hypodermic syringe with a long needle. After injection, tightly pack the nostrils with cotton to prevent leakage.

## INJECTION OF CAVITY CHEMICALS

After the complete aspiration of the thoracic and abdominal cavities, preservative/disinfectant cavity chemicals are placed within the cavities over the viscera. **Cavity fluid** is not diluted; it is used in concentrated form. In cases of hydrothorax or ascites or where blood has escaped during arterial injection or during aspiration of the organs, the fluids—blood and edema—dilute the cavity fluid.

The volume of cavity fluid is determined by the mass of tissues to be treated; relative to body size and weight. A total of 32–48 ounces of undiluted cavity chemical is recommended for treating the three cavities of the adult: thoracic, abdominal, and pelvic. Larger bodies may require additional volumes of cavity fluid while infants and smaller bodies, need less.

Prior to cavity chemical injection, flush the trocar thoroughly to remove any aspirated materials. Undiluted cavity chemical is injected by the gravity method, using a cavity fluid injector. The injector fits into the bottle and is turned until the threads in both the injector and the bottle are secure. The opposite, hub end of the injector connects to the hosing. The hosing connects to the trocar. The higher the bottle is raised, the faster the cavity fluid flows into the body. A small opening on the side of the gravity injector allows air to flow into the cavity fluid bottle and acts as a throttle. By placing a finger over this opening, the embalmer stops the flow of cavity fluid. This can be done when the trocar must be withdrawn to change its position within a body cavity. After use, the gravity injector, tubing, and trocar should be flushed with cold water to remove residual chemicals. Immerse the trocar in a cold steriliant solution. The Evolution injector is used for cavity fluid injection only, not used for aspiration. The Evolution injector attaches directly to the bottle of cavity fluid; hosing is unnecessary.

The chemicals are sprayed or made to flow over the **anterior surface** of the viscera close to the anterior wall of the thoracic and abdominal cavities. The cavity chemicals gravitate through the openings in the viscera made by the trocar and are absorbed by or rest on the posterior surface of the cavity walls.

After the cavity fluid is injected, some embalmers make several passes with the trocar through the abdomen and thorax to release gases that may have been displaced to the surface of the cavities. This movement of the trocar helps to distribute the cavity fluid. Cover the open end of the trocar with a cloth saturated with disinfectant so formaldehyde fumes and/or body gases are not released into the air.

After the trocar puncture has been closed and during the post-embalming washing and drying of the body, **turn the body on its sides** not only to wash and dry the back and sides of the body, but also to distribute the cavity fluid and bring any trapped gases to the surface of the cavities.

The cavity chemicals should be kept in the body and not be allowed to spill or run onto the surface of the abdominal wall. Use a wet cloth to wrap the trocar and cover the opening in the body as the fluids are injected. If cavity chemicals accidentally flow onto the surface of the body, immediately flush with cold running water.

It is possible to inject cavity fluid into the trachea or esophagus. If the nasal passages or throat have not been tightly packed with cotton when the features were set, this fluid can exit when the body is turned to be dried after it is washed. Limited aspiration can be done with the nasal tube aspirator after the body is placed into a supine position. The nasal passages can be tightly repacked with cotton. Open the lips and, using dry cotton, make certain all the liquid is dried from the mouth. If the embalmer feels that cavity fluid purge may be a problem during dressing and casketing, reaspirate the thoracic cavity at this time, giving special emphasis to the posterior of the neck, where the trachea and esophagus are located. Packing the throat and nasal passages with an abundant amount of cotton prior to embalming can help reduce the chance of cavity fluid purge.

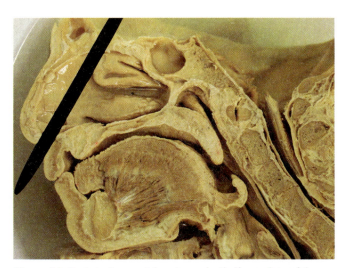

**Figure 14–8.** Anterior cranial cavity and cribriform plate of the ethmoid bone.

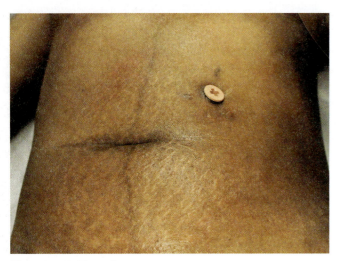

Figure 14–9. Trocar button.

## CLOSURE OF THE ABDOMINAL OPENING

Several methods can be used to securely close the opening used for aspiration. A threaded trocar button provides a secure closure (**Fig. 14–9**). A variety of styles and sizes of trocar buttons are available. Trocar buttons are inserted with a trocar button applicator. To flush cavity chemical and fumes, the water hose can be positioned above the site during insertion of the trocar button (**Fig. 14–10**). Trocar buttons are easily removed for re-aspiration and re-injection, as needed.

Two sutures are commonly used to close the trocar opening: the **purse-string suture** (**Fig. 14–11A**) and the **reverse suture, also called the N- or Z-suture**. To reduce exposure and minimize cavity fluid leakage, the suture can be placed at the onset of cavity injection. Insert the trocar and place sutures by circling the instrument (**Fig. 14–11B**). After injection of chemical, pull upward on the suture thread with one hand while withdrawing the trocar with the other. Secure the thread by tying a complete knot (**Fig. 14–11C**). Apply glue and cotton overtop the closure.

The barrel of the trocar can enlarge the abdominal opening if there is poor integrity to the abdominal skin to a size where a trocar button would be impossible to use. This condition necessitates the use of sutures for closure.

Some embalmers do not close the trocar openings but allow them to remain open for the escape of any gases. If this is done, the opening should be covered with cotton and the cotton covered with plastic to prevent any soilage of the clothing. This technique is not recommended when the body is being shipped.

## RE-ASPIRATION AND REINJECTION

Several hours, following the embalming of the body, it may be necessary to again aspirate the body cavities. This is called **re-aspiration**. In most circumstances, this is sufficient treatment. However, if an abundant amount of gas appears to be present in the cavities or if the trocar indicates to the embalmer that the viscera appear soft in texture, a **re-injection** of one or more bottles of concentrated cavity fluid is recommended. Under certain circumstances, such as advanced decomposition, the presence

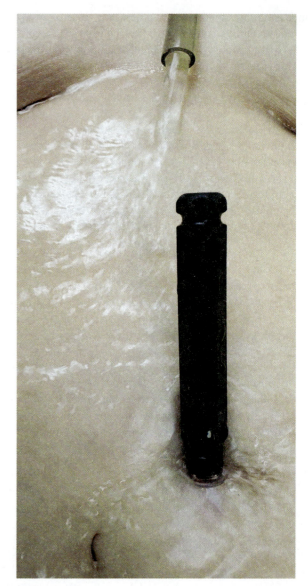

Figure 14–10. Running water during trocar button insertion.

of true tissue gas or a death by drowning, re-aspiration, and re-injection may need to be repeated several times.

Some funeral firms have a rule that **all** bodies must be re-aspirated prior to dressing and casketing or the transportation of a body. This is a precaution against the possibility of purge. It is possible for gases to develop in the cavities following embalming if all of the contents of the body cavities were not treated by the first aspiration and injection of cavity fluid. Handling of the body during transportation can cause liquids and gases to relocate and increase the possibility or actually cause a post-embalming purge.

Re-aspiration is strongly advised under certain conditions, these would include but are not limited to the following:

1. When prior to dressing, the trocar button is removed and a noticeable amount of gas appears to be present in the abdomen
2. When the body is to be transported **to** another funeral establishment (Ship-out)
3. When the body is received **from** another funeral establishment (ship-in)
4. When decomposition is present

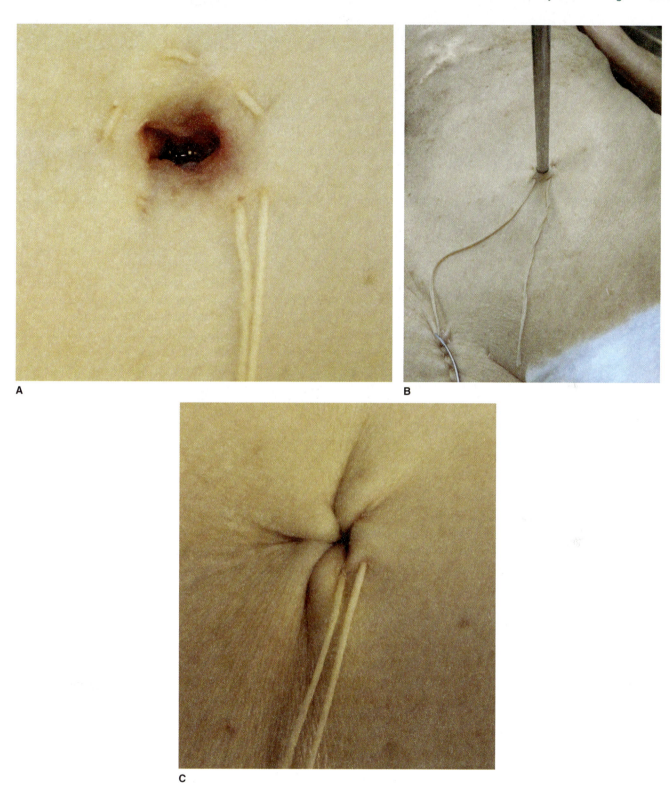

**Figure 14–11. A.** Purse-string suture. **B.** Purse-string suture is placed while the trocar remains inserted. **C.** Completed closure. The ligature is knotted securely and the remaining thread is cut closely to the skin's surface..

5. In the case of recent abdominal surgery
6. When the embalmer is dealing with an obese body
7. When the body shows evidence of gas—distension of the veins of the neck or backs of the hands
8. When purge is present
9. When death involved blood infection or infection of the abdominal cavity (e.g., sepsis, peritonitis, or pneumonia)
10. When death occurred from drowning
11. In the case of bodies with ascites

Re-aspiration is also used when the facial tissues have been distended with edema or gases. The neck can be channeled with the trocar during cavity embalming. Repeated aspiration can assist in the removal of liquids and gases out of the tissues of the face and neck.

## CONCEPTS FOR STUDY

Define the following terminology:

- Air pressure machine
- Autopsy aspirator
- Electric aspirator
- Hand pump
- Hydroaspirator
- Main trocar guides
- Nasal tube aspirator
- Nine-region method
- Purulent materials
- Quadrant method
- Re-aspiration
- Reinjection
- Trocar

1. Under what circumstance can tissue gas be transferred from one decedent to another during cavity aspiration?
2. Explain the process of cavity embalming.
3. Name the characteristics of stomach purge and lung purge.
4. Recall the nine-region method; list the name of each region.
5. List the names of each of the four quadrants.
6. State the trocar guides for the following organs:
   a. Right side of the heart
   b. Stomach
   c. Cecum
   d. Urinary bladder
7. Present two methods of closing the trocar opening in the abdominal wall.
8. Give the standard point of trocar entry; defend the choice of this location.
9. List conditions that necessitate re-aspiration of the body cavities.
10. Explain why partial aspiration may be necessary prior to or during arterial injection.

## FIGURE CREDIT

Figures 14–1A-C, 14–9, 14–10, 14–11A-C are used with permission of Sharon L. Gee-Mascarello.

Figure 14–7 are used with permission of Kevin Drobish.

## BIBLIOGRAPHY

American Board of Funeral Service, *Course Content Syllabus*, 2016.

Burke PA, Sheffner AL. The antimicrobial activity of embalming chemicals and topical disinfectants on the microbial flora of human remains. *Health Lab Sci* 1976;13(4):267–270.

Cavity fluids. In: *Champion Encyclopedia*, No. 454. Springfield, OH: Champion Chemical Co., 1975:1833–1836.

Dorn JM, Hopkins BM. *Thanatochemistry*. Upper Saddle River, NJ: Prentice-Hall, 1998.

Grant ME. Cavity embalming. In: *Champion Encyclopedia*. Springfield, OH: Champion Chemical Co., 1987:2338–2341.

Proper cavity treatment. In: *Champion Encyclopedia*, No. 449. Springfield, OH: Champion Chemical Co., 1974:1813–1816.

Rose GW, Hockett RN. The microbiological evaluation and enumeration of postmortem specimens from human remains. *Health Lab Sci* 1971;8(2):75–78.

Tortora GJ. *Principles of Human Anatomy*, 3rd ed. New York: Harper & Row, 1983.

Trocar and its proper use. In: *Champion Encyclopedia*, No. 422. Springfield, OH: Champion Chemical Co., 1971:1705–1708.

Weed LA, Baggenstoss AH. The isolation of pathogens from tissues of embalmed human bodies. *Am J Clin Pathol* 1951;21:1114.

Weed LA, Baggenstoss AH. The isolation of pathogens from embalmed tissues. *Proc Soc Mayo Clin* 1952;27:124.

CHAPTER 15

# Treatments after Arterial Injection

## CHAPTER OVERVIEW
- Post-embalming Treatments
- Removal of Medical Devices
- Types of Suture Methods
- Plastic Garments
- Terminal Disinfection and Embalmer Hygiene
- Periodic Monitoring Until Final Disposition

## POST-EMBALMING TREATMENTS

Post-embalming treatments are routinely carried out after completion of arterial and cavity embalming. Numerous variables, including preferences of the embalmer, influence the order in which each treatment is performed.

1. Supplemental preservative and corrective treatments.
2. Adjustments to feature setting.
3. Closure of incisions.
4. Packing of orifices.
5. Removal of invasive medical devices.
6. Final bathing and inspection of all bodily areas.
7. Application of adhesives to incisions.
8. Applying plastic garments.
9. Terminal disinfection of instruments and preparation room surfaces.
10. Removal and disposal of personal protective equipment (PPE).
11. Handwashing and related personal hygiene.
12. Preparation of documents.

## SUPPLEMENTAL EMBALMING

Insufficient preservation can exist following arterial embalming when solution does not adequately distribute within the vascular system. Additional arteries are raised and injected closest to the unaffected areas. Unembalmed areas that remain after these attempts will be treated by supplemental embalming methods. There are two supplemental methods of embalming: surface embalming and hypodermic embalming.

### Surface Embalming

Surface embalming is the *application of an embalming chemical directly to the surface of the tissues*. Surface embalming chemicals and compresses (packs) are applied to both **external** and **internal** body surfaces. External compresses are applied directly to the exposed skin surfaces. Internal surface compresses are called **inlays.** Inlays are applied to the unexposed surface tissues of the buccal cavity (inside of the mouth), beneath the eyelids, inside the nasal cavity, beneath the autopsied scalp, and to the interior walls of the autopsied trunk. There are numerous other applications for inlays. Applications to intact skin areas are made anywhere on the body. Areas of broken skin such as abrasions, skin slip, burned tissues, and lesions respond favorably to surface embalming. Following treatment, cover chemicals and compresses with plastic sheeting to reduce fumes and to prevent the chemical from evaporating.

**Accessory chemicals** formulated for surface embalming include liquids (phenol cautery agents, cavity fluid), preservative formalin creams and gels (autopsy gel), preservative powders, and drying and hardening compounds. Accessory chemicals are specifically formulated to preserve, cauterize, dry, deodorize, and bleach tissues on contact. Many of these formulations contain phenol. For treatment of severe conditions, products may need longer application times. Where a phenol compress is removed, the area can be rinsed with alcohol to stop further bleaching and drying action.

Creams and gels are applied directly to the skin using a wide-bristled brush or poured onto cotton and applied as a surface pack (compress). Gels are available in two choices: low viscosity (semiliquid) or in high viscosity form (gelatinous). Creams and gels are designed to rapidly penetrate the tissues. They can remain in place on nonviewable areas, covered with plastic sheeting or a plastic garment.

Arterial fluid is not recommended as a surface embalming chemical; cosmetic dyes in the fluid can stain the skin. The penetrating action of arterial fluids is slower compared to cavity fluid and accessory surface chemicals. An arterial fluid designed to penetrate rapidly would not distribute within the vascular system. After the surface compress is removed, rinse and dry the area before cosmetic application.

## Hypodermic Embalming

Hypodermic embalming is the *subcuticular injection of preservative chemicals using a hypodermic needle and syringe or a small-gauge trocar.* This method is used to treat both small localized body areas and larger areas, such as the trunk walls of the autopsied body, a limb that did not receive sufficient arterial fluid, or an area that cannot be arterially injected.

Hypodermic needles are available in varying gauges and lengths. Smaller bores needles (18–22 gauge) are ideal for tissues of the face and hands; large-bore needles (10–16 gauge) are used for greater surface areas. Larger needle entry sites may be closed using a trocar button; smaller sites can easily be sealed with glue. An infant trocar or hypovalve trocar can be connected to the centrifugal embalming machine for the injection of large body areas.

The arterial solution used for arterial injection can be used for hypodermic injection. It is recommended that it be strengthened with a high-index arterial fluid. Arterial solution should only be used on areas that will not be viewed, as the dye in the fluid can blotch the skin. Cavity fluid as well as specially designed accessory embalming chemicals may be used for hypodermic embalming. Phenol solutions should be reserved for localized treatments of discolored areas or tissues when bleaching of tissues is necessary. The phenol solutions would not be used for routine supplemental hypodermic embalming. Be advised that cavity fluids and fluids containing phenol may void the manufacturer's warranty when used in the embalming machine.

## Treatments for Visible Areas

Well-preserved tissues will not dehydrate at the rate of poorly embalmed tissues. Application of glue to the eyelids and lips reduces the effects of dehydration; the marginal tissue membranes of both lids and lips are moist and will rapidly dry, shrink, and discolor. Visible areas treated by surface inlays or compresses can be coated with a massage cream or spray after the chemical is removed. The creams and sprays may also provide a good base for cosmetic application.

### Mouth, Lips

Cotton can be placed over the teeth or dentures and moistened with cavity fluid. Use a hypodermic needle and syringe to apply a few drops of fluid. The lips can then be glued; the preservative works from inside the oral cavity to preserve the tissues of the lips and mouth. Cosmetic treatment can be immediate using this method of preservation.

### Eyelids

Insert a small amount of cotton independently or in combination with an eye cap. Draw a small amount of cavity chemical into the hypodermic syringe. Moisten the cotton with a few drops (**Fig. 15–1**). Close the eyes and seal the lids with an adhesive.

In facial areas, where hypodermic needles would be used, most of the injections can be made from inside the mouth. In

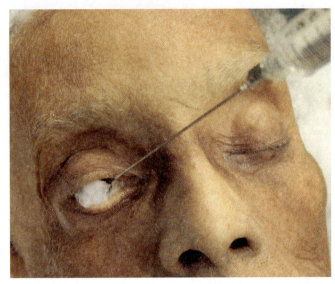

**Figure 15–1.** Cotton placed beneath eyelids and moistened with a few drops of cavity fluid.

this manner, leakage will not exit onto the face. Unlike tissue builder, these chemicals have a tendency to seep from the point of puncture. In the autopsied body, large portions of the face can be reached through scalp incisions.

The hands can be injected from either the palmar or dorsal surface. The needle is directed between the fingers (**Fig. 15–2**). The thumb and fingers are injected directly by guiding the

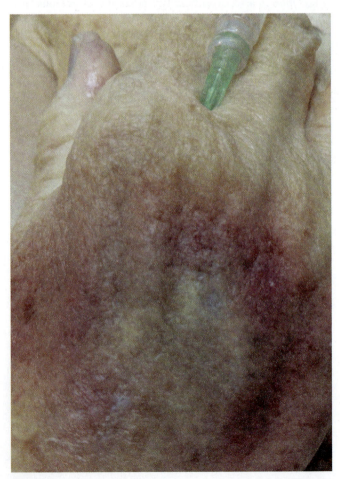

**Figure 15–2.** Hypodermic injection of the hand to bleach blood discolorations.

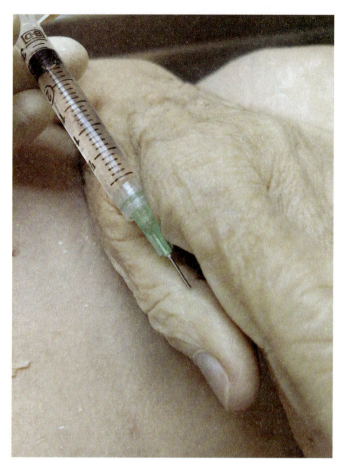

**Figure 15–3.** Hypodermic injection of the thumb (and fingertips) to create natural contour.

needle toward the tip of the digit (**Fig. 15–3**). Super adhesive can be applied to the needle puncture after injection to prevent leakage from the site.

The nose can be treated hypodermically by inserting the needle inside the mouth. The ear can be reached by hypodermic injection from behind the ear.

For larger areas, such as the arm and leg, the infant or hypovalve trocar can be inserted into the area of the cubital fossa of the arm to reach the arm and forearm. If the elbow area contains edema, the trocar can also be entered from the upper pectoral region to reach the distended area. The leg can be treated by inserting a small-gauge trocar just inferior or superior to the knee. From this point, both the thigh and lower leg can be reached (**Fig. 15–4**). Trunk walls, hip, and buttock can be reached by inserting a trocar into the center of the lateral trunk wall.

### Nose

Cotton saturated with preservative fluid can be inserted into the nostrils. Later, push the cotton further into the nasal cavity so that it will not be noticeable. A small-gauge hypodermic needle can be used to inject a preservative solution from inside the nostrils into various areas of the nose. If hypodermic treatment is used, expect some leakage from the injection sites. Cotton can be placed within the nostrils to absorb residual leakage and later removed. The bridge of the nose, nasal septum (columella nasi), tip, and wings often need contouring for natural appearance.

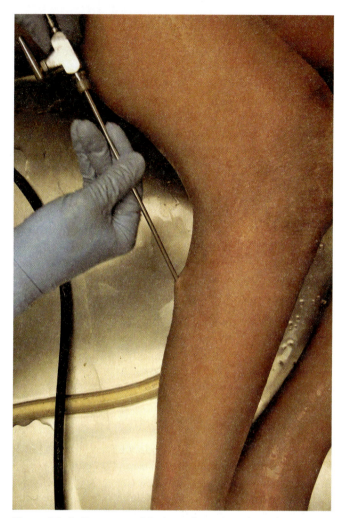

**Figure 15–4.** Treatment of the lower leg using a hypodermic trocar.

Careful handling and directing of the needle will prevent injury to the embalmer during hypodermic injection.

### Treatments for Nonvisible Areas

For areas that will not be seen, such as the legs or feet, supplemental treatments can be used to enhance preservation. Surface embalming powders have been used for many years. Diapers can be used to contain the powder, or the powder can be placed in plastic garments such as stockings, coveralls, or pants after the garments are in position. Powders can also be used to treat the interior walls of the abdomen and thorax in the autopsied body. Powders are not as effective as gels or liquids. Read the label to be certain the powder is a preservative and not just a deodorant or absorbent.

### Treatments for Larger Areas

Certain conditions, such as arteriosclerosis, gangrene, and edema, require additional injection of the legs. A combination of supplemental embalming methods (hypodermic and surface) can be used. If arterial treatment has been unsuccessful, the legs can be injected hypodermically. The solution injected can be undiluted arterial or cavity chemical. The legs can also be painted with autopsy gels and embalming powder can be placed into the plastic stockings.

In the trunk area, hypodermic injection can be used when the tissues have received insufficient arterial fluid. Coveralls, pants, or a Capri garment can be used and embalming powder or autopsy gel painted over the areas being treated. When edema is a problem in the elbow area, hypodermic treatment can be used (inject from the upper arm), paint with autopsy gel and wrap with gauze. A plastic sleeve can then be placed over the treated area.

In nonviewable areas where the infant trocar or hypovalve trocar has been used, the punctures can be sealed with a trocar button. When machine injection and a trocar are used, phenol products should be avoided. Phenol can be damaging to injection machines. When injection is completed, the embalming machine must be thoroughly flushed and cleaned; clear ammonia run-through the machine will help to eliminate formaldehyde residue.

# CLOSURE OF INCISIONS

Two methods are commonly used to close incisions, sutures and super adhesive glue. Best practices prior to incision closure:

1. Do not suture until after cavity aspiration; aspiration relieves pressure on the vascular system and helps to prevent leakage.
2. Be certain all vessels are securely tied. This prevents any further leakage.
3. If there is edema in the surrounding tissues, force as much liquid out of the incision as possible.
4. Dry the incision.
5. Cotton saturated with a cautery solution can be placed into the incision. This compress can remain within the incision (**Fig. 15–5**). The addition of incision seal powder, will also help to prevent leakage.
6. Make several sutures before adding the incision seal powder to the incision. Pull upward on the suture thread to create a "pocket"; direct the powder into the pocket.
7. After suturing, apply a liquid or spray sealant to the area to prevent leakage.

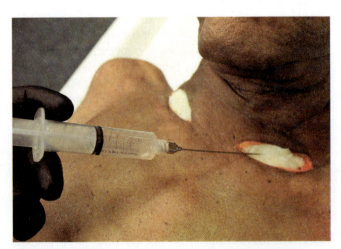

**Figure 15–5.** Cotton saturated with cautery solution prior to suturing the incision.

## Suturing

### Cotton or Linen Thread

Linen thread is stronger than cotton thread and is recommended for autopsy, long bone donors, and vessel incision sutures. For restorative sutures, which are located on visible areas, dental floss is an excellent material to use.

### A 3/8-inch Circle Needle

The 3/8-inch circle needle is used for restorative sutures and to suture incisions made to raise vessels.

### Double-Curved (S-Curve) Postmortem Needle

The double-curved autopsy needle is easy to grip with the gloved hand. It is used to close autopsy incisions, long-bone donor incisions, surgical incisions, and incisions made to raise vessels.

Postmortem needles come in a variety of sizes and shapes: half- and double-curved, circle, and Loopuypt styles. Some have a patented "spring-eye" for easy threading of the needle. Regardless of the size or the shape of the needle, it is most important to keep it sharp. Suturing can be very dangerous if the needles are dull, as extra pressure must be applied. In doing so, the embalmer increases the chance of the needle breaking or piercing her or his skin. A sharp needle makes suturing much easier, safer, and faster.

To tighten the suture, pull on the thread and not on the needle. Pulling on the needle weakens the suture thread where it passes through the eye of the needle, and breakage can occur.

The embalmer can suture using single- or double-stranded thread. This depends on the strength of the suture thread or on the type of suture. It is wise to double the thread when cotton thread or three- or four-twist linen thread is used. Single-strand suture thread works best with five- and six-twist linen thread (dental floss).

## Direction of Suturing

To make suturing more efficient, follow these directions for the various sutures.

- *Common carotid artery*. If using the parallel incision, suture from the inferior portion of the incision superiorly. Suture from the medial portion of the incision laterally if using a supraclavicular incision.
- *Axillary artery*. Suture from the medial area of the incision laterally (with the arm abducted).
- *Brachial artery*. Suture from the medial portion of the incision laterally with the arm abducted).
- *Radial and ulnar arteries*. Suture from the distal portion of the incision medially.
- *Femoral artery*. Suture from the inferior portion of the incision superiorly.
- *Autopsies (trunk standard "Y" incision)*. Use bridge sutures to align the skin into position. Begin the trunk suturing at the pubic symphysis and suture superiorly.
- *Popliteal artery*. Begin the suture at the inferior (or distal) portion of the incision and suture superiorly.
- *Anterior and posterior tibial arteries*. Begin the sutures distally and suture superiorly.

CHAPTER 15 • Treatments after Arterial Injection 227

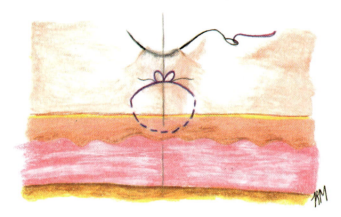

Figure 15–6. Bridge, or individual suture.

## Sutures

### Bridge, or Individual Sutures

Bridge sutures temporarily align tissue margins and secure them in position until permanent sutures replace them (**Fig. 15–6**). Numerous bridge sutures are placed to align the tissue flaps of the Y-incision created during autopsy.

### Baseball Suture

The baseball is the most commonly used suture to close incisions (**Fig. 15–7**). It is considered the most secure and leakproof. In addition to the closure of incisions at the injection site, it is suited for closure of lengthy incisions, as in autopsy, surgery, and long-bone donation. To make this stitch, pass a suture needle and thread from beneath the incision up through the integument, and cross the needle from side to side with each stitch (**Fig. 15–8**). The resulting lacing pattern is similar to the stitching on a baseball. As each stitch is pulled tightly,

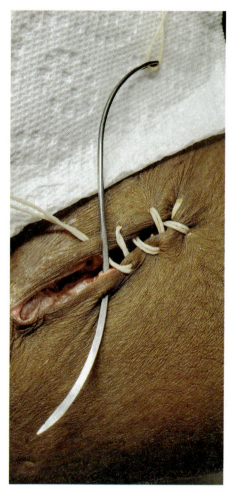

Figure 15–8. Baseball suture. The suture needle is directed side to side in a lacing pattern.

the tissues adjacent to the incision pucker and create a visible ridge on the skin surface (**Fig. 15–9**).

When the baseball suture is used for the closure of lengthy incisions, the thread can be knotted, or locked down every few inches. This prevents the thread from unraveling should it break. If the thread does break, it will not be necessary to start the entire suture over again. To lock the suture, pass the needle through both sides of the incision and tie a knot as though the suture were completed. *Do not* cut the ligature; use the same thread to continue suturing. Locking down the suture will also relieve tension from the thread, minimizing fatigue to the embalmer's hand during suturing.

### Interlocking (Lock) Suture

The interlocking suture continues throughout the closure; unlike the occasional lock down practice above. A tight, leak-proof closure is created. The disadvantage is the visible ridge on the surface of the incision. To begin, direct the needle through both epithelial margins of the incision. Keep the thread tight with the hand not holding the needle. Lock the stitch by looping the thread and passing the needle through the loop. Pull the thread tight. Insert the needle on the same side of the incision each time the process is repeated until the incision is closed.

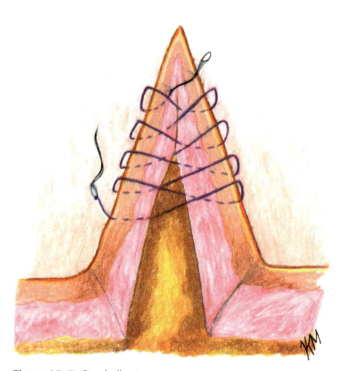

Figure 15–7. Baseball suture.

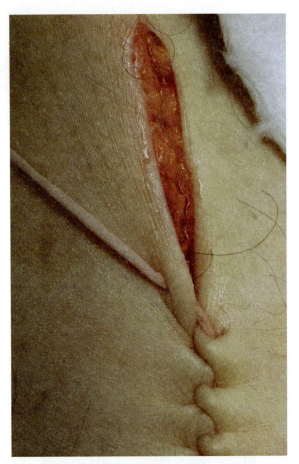

**Figure 15–9.** Tightened baseball sutures create a visible ridge.

### Single Intradermal (Hidden) Suture

The single intradermal suture is made entirely within the dermal layer, traversing the needle side to side within the incision. The needle does not pass through the epidermal tissues, the thread is hidden from view (**Fig. 15–10**). To begin the closure, insert the needle deep into the dermal tissues at one end of the incision. Make a knot in the thread a short distance from the end and pull the knot to the position of the needle entry in the integument. Direct the needle in a back-and-forth pattern from one side of the incision to the other. Align the margins of the incision as the thread is drawn to prevent gaps and tissue misalignment. To complete the closure, direct the needle through the integument as far as possible from the end of the incision. Draw the margins of the incision together by pulling on the free end of the thread. Puckering will result if the thread is pulled too tightly. Pull upward on the thread and cut the thread at the tissue surface; the excess thread disappears into the incision.

### Double Intradermal Suture

The double suture is knotted at each end, creating greater holding strength than the single intradermal. This is also a dermal layer suture. The same thread is used for two needles; one needle is threaded at each end. One of the needles is directed through the tissues of one side of the incision; the other needle on the opposite side. Maintain parallel stitches that resemble the lacing pattern of a shoe. Continue the process until the incision is completely sutured. After drawing the margins tight, knot the two ends together. Relieve any tissue puckering by smoothing the incision with digital pressure. To end the suture, pass both threads through the eye of one needle. Insert the needle beneath the skin at the end of the incision and pass it approximately one-half inch. Pull upward and cut the thread at the tissue surface; excess thread disappears into the incision.

### Inversion, or Worm Suture

The inversion suture gathers and turns under excess tissues (**Fig. 15–11**). Inverted tissues create a flat closure; a visible ridge on the skin surface is avoided. The incision is easily concealed. After completion, the knot can be pulled into the incision and the excess thread cut closely to the surface. No thread is visible. The lacing pattern is similar to the single intradermal.

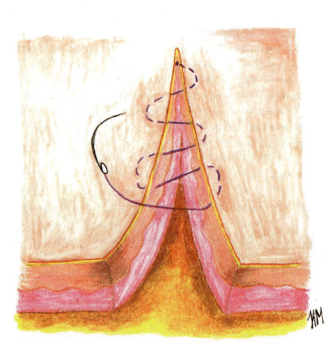

**Figure 15–10.** Single intradermal, or Hidden suture.

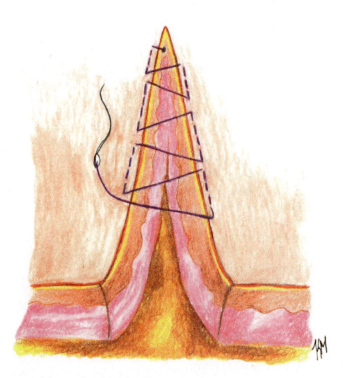

**Figure 15–11.** Inversion, or Worm suture.

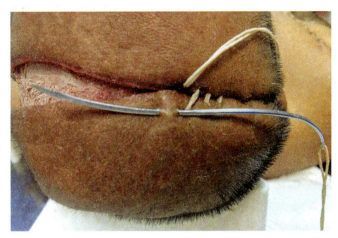

**Figure 15–12.** Inversion or Worm Suture. The needle runs parallel to the incision.

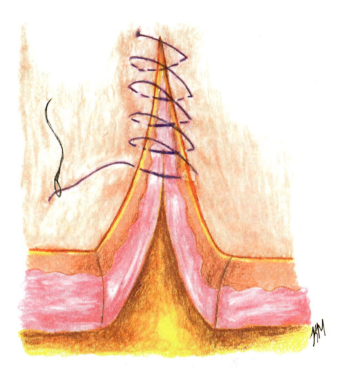

**Figure 15–14.** Continuous, or Whip suture.

Stitches are made on the surface only; the needle passes back-and-forth overtop the skin surface rather than into the dermal tissues. Each stitch is made parallel and close to the margin of the incision (**Fig. 15–12**). Stitches that are uniform in length and drawn moderately tight produce an optimal closure. The inversion is ideal for suturing the cranial autopsy incision and the smaller incisions used for arterial injection (**Fig. 15–13**). The inversion suture is not drawn as tightly as the baseball and may not be suitable for trunk autopsy incisions.

### Continuous, or Whip Suture

The continuous suture is used to temporarily close lengthy incisions (**Fig. 15–14**). Disadvantages include a visible tissue ridge, visible suture thread, and leakage potential. The exposed thread can draw, or *wick* body fluids; the thread will remain wet. Surface glues may not adhere and clothing can be soiled. Routinely, the whip stitch is used by autopsy and organ procurement technicians to temporarily restore the body cavities for transfer to the funeral home. To make this stitch, direct the needle through both epithelial margins of the incision. Reverse direction of the needle and pass overtop the skin surface, back to initial needle entry site. Place the next stitch one-half to one full inch beyond the previous stitch. Repeat the process until the closure is complete.

### Concealing the Suture Thread and the Knot

The final length of thread and the knot can be completely hidden when suturing is complete. This practice prevents any exposed thread from wicking moisture from the incision and remaining wet. The incision can be easily concealed when the clothing provided does not hide the incision. Application of cosmetics and restorative waxes can be used for concealing.

At the completion of suturing, place a knot in the thread. Move the knot as close as possible to the surface of the skin. Do not cut the thread. Place the needle beside and directly against the knot. Drive the needle into the incision 2 or 3 inches away from the knot and exit the incision. Pull the thread taut, with a quick snap on the thread the knot will disappear. Excessive force will pull the knot too deeply. The objective is to hide the knot just below the epithelium yet keep it embedded in the dermal tissues. Cut the tail of the thread close to the skin surface and it will disappear into the incision. Both thread and knot are no longer visible. Apply adhesive glue to the exit hole. See **Fig. 15-15A–D**.

### Super Adhesive Glue and Bonding Agents

Super adhesive glues and bonding agents can be used for some closures in place of sutures. A variety of types are available. Some are suitable for bonding in the presence of moisture. These adhesives are a good choice for sealing jagged tissues that cannot be sutured. Routinely, glues are applied to sutured incisions to prevent leakage. The tip of the applicator can be used to apply the glue directly, or glue can be applied first to an instrument for application. Clean the instrument or applicator tip after use to prevent buildup.

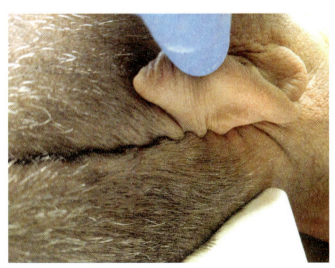

**Figure 15–13.** Completed inversion suture for the cranial autopsy incision.

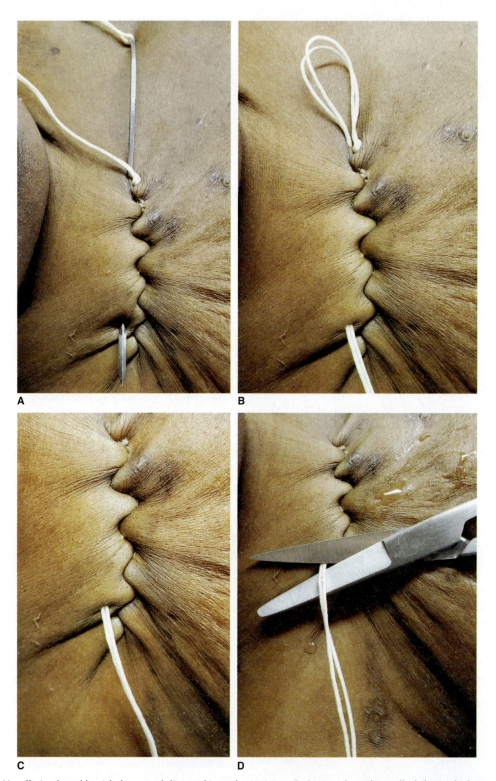

**Figure 15–15** **A.** Needle is placed beside knot and directed into the incision. **B.** Suture thread is pulled through the incision. **C.** Knot is hidden. Only tail of the thread is exposed. **D.** Thread is cut close to the surface of the skin. Thread and knot are no longer visible.

## REMOVAL OF INVASIVE MEDICAL DEVICES

### Pacemakers and Defibrillators

Devices containing batteries must be removed when cremation is the method of final disposition; batteries create explosion and injury hazards during the cremation process. Remove the device through a small semilunar incision. Best practice is to cut wire leads independently with surgical scissors. A strong magnet can interrupt the device mode but will not turn off the device. Close the incision by suturing or application of a bonding agent or super adhesive glue.

### Colostomy

A colostomy is the opening of the colon through the abdominal wall to the skin surface. The **stoma** is the exposed portion of the bowel. Remove and disinfect the colostomy collecting

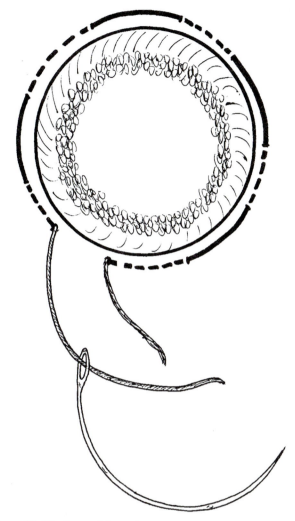

**Figure 15–16.** Purse-string suture.

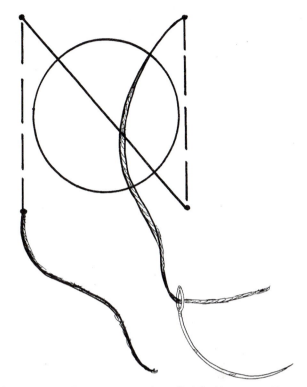

**Figure 15–17.** Reverse suture, also called the N-suture or Z-suture.

bag before disposal in a biohazard waste container. Topically treat the area with a compress of cavity fluid or a phenol solution. The stoma can be reinserted in the body cavity using firm pressure. Either of the purse-string suture (**Fig. 15–16**) or the reverse suture, also called an *N-suture* or *Z-suture* (**Fig. 15–17**) can effectively close the colostomy. Seal the closure with glue to prevent leakage.

### Surgical Drains

Surgical drains are placed postsurgically to prevent the accumulation of blood, pus, and infected fluids; to prevent accumulation of air; and to identify the type of fluid leakage. Remove surgical drains and close the openings using a purse-string suture.

## TREATMENT OF DISCOLORATIONS AND ULCERATIONS

Additional treatments for discolorations and ulcerations continue after embalming. Discolorations may be bleached at this time in preparation for cosmetic and restorative applications. Ulcerations may be treated a second time to ensure sanitation before dressing.

## TREATMENT OF PURGE

After arterial and cavity embalming, the possibility of purge exists from any of the orifices. Tightly packing the throat prior to mouth closure and arterial injection can decrease any purge from the mouth. Packing the nose prior to arterial injection can create a blood or fluid purge from the nostrils during arterial injection.

The mouth, nose, and anal orifice can also be packed after embalming is completed. This allows the evacuation of purges and fecal matter during the embalming and the cavity treatment.

When anal purge is present after embalming, force as much purge as possible from the rectum by firmly pressing on the lower abdominal area. Pack the rectum using cotton saturated with cavity fluid, autopsy gel, or a phenol solution. Dry packing should be inserted into the anal orifice after the moistened cotton. Leave a portion of the dry cotton so that it can be seen. This will help to fully block the anal orifice. An AV plug device may also be used to seal the orifice.

When purge is present from the mouth or nose immediately following arterial injection and cavity treatment, it may be necessary to reaspirate and reinject cavity fluid. Clean out the orifices and be certain they are tightly packed with plenty of dry cotton or cotton webbing. If possible, repack the throat area.

## TREATMENT OF DISTENSION

Visible areas such as the face, neck, and hands that are distended may need to be reduced for viewing of the body. These treatments can be carried out during the post-embalming period. Some swellings, such as edema, can be treated by specific arterial solutions during arterial injection. It is necessary to know the cause of the distension to perform the best corrective treatment. Swellings present before arterial injection should be documented on the Embalming and Decedent Care Report. Examples of such conditions include edema, tumors, swellings caused by trauma, distension from gases of decomposition in the tissues or cavities, tissue gas produced by *Clostridium perfringens*, distension caused by allergic reactions, distension brought about by the use of steroid drugs, and gases in the tissues from subcutaneous emphysema.

Distension of facial tissues, the neck, or glandular tissues of the face or the tissues surrounding the eye orbit during embalming of the body can be caused by an excessive amount of arterial solution in these tissues. Some of the causes of this swelling are very rapid injection of solution, use of too much injection pressure, poor drainage from these areas, breakdown of the capillaries due to trauma or decomposition, excessive massage, and use of arterial solutions that are too weak. It is essential during embalming of the body that the embalmer is alert to any tissue distension. Injection should be immediately stopped and the situation evaluated and remedied.

In pitting edema, excess moisture is present in the tissue spaces. In solid edema, the excess moisture is within the cells. Pitting edema can be moved by mechanical aids such as gravitation, massage, channeling of the area, and application of pressure using a pneumatic collar, weights, elastic bandage, water collar, or digital pressure to move the moisture to another area. Elevation of the head and firm digital pressure slowly drain pitting edema from the facial tissues. During cavity aspiration, the trocar can be used to channel the neck, which may allow some of the edema to drain from the facial tissues into the thorax.

Edema of the eyelids can be treated in several ways: (1) weighted surface compresses, (2) cavity fluid on cotton under the eyelids, during and after injection, (3) hypodermic injection of phenol compound or cavity fluid after embalming, and (4) by use of a tissue reducing spatula after embalming.

After preservation of the lids is accomplished, channels can be made under the skin from within the mouth or temple area. Carefully apply external pressure to the distended tissues and massage as much of the edema from the tissues as possible. A side effect of removing edema from the facial tissues or hands is that the skin may become very wrinkled. Tissue preservation must always be the primary concern. The tissue-reducing spatula may also be used to remove wrinkling from the eyelids.

Subcutaneous emphysema is air trapped in the subcutaneous tissues. Cardiopulmonary resuscitation, a traumatic event, or surgical procedure can puncture the lung and allow gas to escape into the subcutaneous tissues. As the individual struggles to breathe, more air is forced into the body tissues. Gases can easily be detected after death by palpating the tissues. The term **crepitation** is used to describe the spongy feel of the gas as it moves through the tissues when they are pushed upon. Arterial injection and blood drainage may remove a small portion of the gas, but gas that is trapped in the facial tissues must be removed by channeling. Channeling can be done post-embalming. A scalpel or hypodermic needle is used to channel the affected facial tissues from inside the mouth. Once the channels are made, the gas can be manually squeezed from the tissues. The lips can be lanced to release trapped gases. If the eyes are affected, the lids can be everted and the underside of the lids incised with a suture or hypodermic needle. Cotton can be used to close the eyes; it will also absorb any leakage.

Subcutaneous emphysema can be differentiated from true tissue gas. True tissue gas has a very distinct foul odor that worsens progressively and is caused by an anaerobic bacterium. Blebbing and skin-slip develop with true tissue gas. (See Chapter 24 for treatments of true tissue gas.)

## RESETTING AND GLUING THE FEATURES

The features can be corrected after embalming. Additional cotton or mastic compound can be inserted to fill out sunken and emaciated cheeks. If the cotton that was originally used to set the features becomes moist during the embalming, as a result of contact with purge or blood and fluid from the suture or needle injector used for mouth closure, it should be replaced with dry cotton.

The dentures are not always available at the beginning of the embalming. The mouth can be reopened and the dentures inserted afterward. These procedures are more difficult when the tissues are firm and less pliable. Eyes can be closed or reset after arterial injection. (Refer to Chapter 18 for post-embalming procedures after eye enucleation.)

After the features have been properly aligned, the features can be secured with glue. Adhesive applied to the lips and eyelids helps to avoid separation caused by dehydration. The area where the adhesive is to be applied should first be cleaned with a solvent. The skin of the lips and margins of the eyelids should be clean, dry, and free of moisture or oils. Super adhesive glue works very well for securing the eyelids. It ensures good closure of the inner canthus, which dries quickly and darkens. Apply glue to the mucous membranes behind the weather line.

If the body was transferred from another funeral establishment, the lips may separate during travel or during a flight. During the delay, the tissues have additional time to become very firm. In such cases, the lips can be stretched or exercised with the blunt handle of an aneurysm needle or a pair of forceps. If the eyelids separate, they may also have to be exercised or stretched to obtain closure. Super adhesive glue is more effective in securing the mouth and eyes when the tissues are very firm.

## FINAL INSPECTION, BATHING, AND DRYING

After final inspection of the entire body, shampoo the hair and bathe all areas to remove dried blood and chemical odors. Thorough drying eliminates the potential for mold growth on the skin surface, especially in warm climates. Apply a massage cream or spray to face and hands and cover the body completely with a full sheet. A layer of plastic sheeting to cover the face will decrease surface evaporation.

## PLASTIC GARMENTS

Prior to dressing, protective plastic garments can be placed on the body to contain any minor leakage and odors (**Fig. 15–18**). Adult incontinence garments may also be used if minor leakage is anticipated.

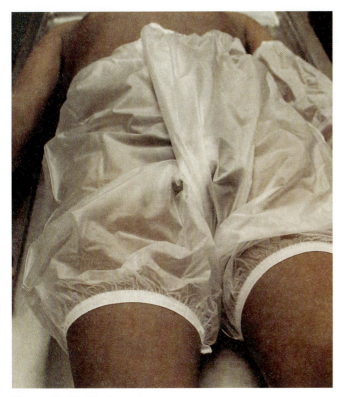

**Figure 15–18.** Plastic pants.

Be certain the body is thoroughly dried before using a plastic garment. Pants or coveralls can be placed on the trunk when the leakage from the orifices, ulcerations, or traumatic injuries is present. The capri garment is ideal for coverage of the full lower extremities, from the hips to the feet. Plastic stockings are used after surface treatment of the legs. Plastic sleeves may be applied over broken skin at the elbows or on the arms. Place embalming and absorbent powders into the garment to control leakage, mold growth, and odor. If general edema, tissue decomposition, or extensive burns are present, a unionall may be necessary to protect clothing and casket fabric from soiling. The unionall is a plastic garment which covers the entire body, except for the neck and head. Plastic garments are available up in a variety of sizes. Best practice is to use a garment slightly larger than necessary.

## Terminal Disinfection

Terminal disinfection practices are carried out after the embalming process to comprehensively clean all of the preparation room surfaces. The floors, countertops, cabinets and drawer handles, mortuary equipment, and any other soiled surfaces are included. Instruments are cleaned, placed into cold sterilant, dried, and returned to countertops or drawers.

### Disinfectant Checklist

In selecting a disinfectant for instruments and other preparation room paraphernalia, keep in mind the characteristics of a good disinfectant:

- Has a wide range of activity (works against viruses, bacteria, and fungi)
- Is of sufficient strength (active against spore-forming organisms of bacilli and fungi)
- Acts in the presence of water
- Is stable and has a reasonably long shelf-life
- Is noncorrosive to metal instruments
- Fast-acting
- Is not highly toxic to living tissues or injurious to the respiratory system

## Care of the Embalming Machine

After use, the embalming machine is flushed with warm water. Fluids that contain a humectant such as lanolin or silicon often leave a thick residue in the tank. Ammonia and lukewarm water flushed through the machine removes the residue. A water softener or a dishwasher detergent is also effective. Embalming machine cleaners are available from embalming chemical suppliers. After cleaning, fill the embalming machine one-third with fresh water to keep the silicone used to seal the tank wet. This prevents drying and shrinking of the seal and prevents leakage. Dissolved gases such as the chlorine found in tap water also have time to release before the next use of the machine. The later addition of embalming fluid to the water decreases the release of formaldehyde fumes. Place the lid on the tank of the machine in between use.

## Surfaces

All preparation room surfaces should first be cleaned with cool water and a small amount of antiseptic soap to remove organic debris. A preliminary wash removes any debris and chemical residue present. Remember that many disinfectants, such as bleach contain chlorine, and this chemical should not come into contact with formaldehyde. Bleach and warm water make a very good cleaning solution. The table, countertops, and drains can be wiped clean and disinfected with this solution. Many commercially available products are also good disinfectants. Be certain to clean the area under the table surrounding the drainage outlet. Tops of overhead lighting should also be given attention. Tubing used for aspiration should be soaked in a disinfectant solution. Pay attention to handles on cabinets and drawers. Commercial products used for cleaning the preparation room contain dilution instructions. (Refer to Chapter 3 for a review of disinfection practices.)

## Instruments

### Clean Instruments Prior to Disinfection

Removing organic material from the instrument makes disinfection more effective. Immerse all instruments including trocars in a cold sterilant solution according to product usage guidelines. Dispose of used cutting blades in a biohazard sharps container. Take special care with nondisposable cutting instruments when gas gangrene or tissue gas has been encountered. The causative agent of this condition, *C. perfringens*, is a spore-forming bacillus and can easily be passed via contaminated cutting instruments. They should remain in this solution several hours. After disinfection, instruments should be rinsed, dried, and properly stored (**Fig. 15–19**).

## Personal Hygiene

Personal hygiene practices apply to the embalmer. Removal and disposal of PPE, handwashing, bathing and showering, laundering of washable garments, and other modes of hygiene are practiced after embalming. Best practice is to wear surgical scrubs

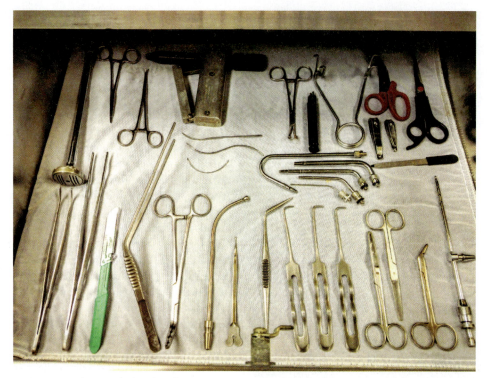

**Figure 15–19.** Instruments properly stored after disinfection.

instead of work attire beneath PPE. Include the cleaning of the nostrils of the nose where odors can linger. Nose hairs act as a natural filter, preventing the entry of foreign particles, such as dust and pollen, bacteria, spores, and viruses. Particles stick to the wet surfaces inside the nose to prevent inhalation. Harmful particles that are inhaled into the lungs may cause respiratory infections.

## DOCUMENTATION AND SHIPPING PREPARATION

Complete the appropriate **Embalming and Decedent Care Report** for every deceased. The report should contain specific information related to the pre-embalming conditions of the deceased and personal effects received with the body. Inventory and document all personal items. Document all decedent care treatments performed.

The report must accompany all bodies being prepared and shipped to another funeral facility. When the body has been autopsied before shipping, the report should indicate whether the viscera was retained by the postmortem examiner or returned with the body. Organs and tissues recovered for donation must also be noted. When viscera are treated during embalming and returned to the body cavities, note the method and chemicals used. Bodies should never be shipped without some form of covering. Place undergarments, hospital gown, plastic coveralls, or pants on the body.

When positioning instructions have not been given by the receiving funeral home, make certain hands are not placed on top of one another. Place the hands separated, upon the abdomen. Resting one on top of the other can create indentations. The receiving establishment may prefer to reverse the hands for custom or preference. A light coating of massage cream or spray can be applied to the face and hands to prevent surface dehydration during shipping. Live floral arrangements that are placed inside of casket or shipping container can cause excess moisture. Certain flowers also have staining properties. All memorial items and personal effects placed into the container should be documented. Inform the receiving funeral home of the items and indicate where they will be found.

## PERIODIC MONITORING UNTIL FINAL DISPOSITION

Periodic monitoring of the deceased and performance of the treatments necessary to maintain post-embalming stability is an ethical duty. Periodic surveillance is also called **custodial care**. The dignified care of all human remains is expected of all professional death care providers.

Extended periods of storage prior to final disposition create additional opportunities for adjustments and corrections. These may include cosmetic and feature setting adjustments, treatments for discolorations, leakages and purges, the presence of mold, and infestations by insects.

Potential areas of leakage could include:
- Any area of trauma to the face or hands where the skin was broken or torn
- Cranial autopsy incisions
- Autopsy sutures
- Surgical sutures
- Sutures at sites where vessels were raised for arterial injection
- Areas where edema is present
- Intravenous punctures
- Punctures used for drawing postmortem blood samples
- Any point where the skin has been broken

Minor seepage (e.g., intravenous puncture) may be corrected by wiping away the accumulated liquid, injecting a phenol compound to cauterize the area, and sealing the puncture with a super adhesive. Where the skin has been torn, a phenol compound surface compress (or a cavity fluid compress) can be applied; later the area can be cleaned with a solvent, dried with a hair dryer, and sealed with a super adhesive glue.

Clothing can be protected by sheets of plastic. The casket interior, pillow, and clothing should be inspected for any signs of leakage. If leakage is judged severe, the body should be removed from the casket and carefully undressed. Incisions can be opened, dried, checked to be certain vessels are ligated, and resutured using large amounts of incision seal powder within the incisions. Plastic garments can be placed on the body and, if necessary, edges sealed with mortuary tape. Interior damage may be severe enough to require replacement. Casket pillows can be reversed for minor leakage. Blankets and clothing may need to be replaced.

## Purge

If purge has occurred, it will be necessary to reaspirate the body. No doubt the body will have to be taken back to the preparation room for this procedure. Not only should the body be thoroughly reaspirated, but the cavities should also be reinjected with undiluted cavity fluid. If gases were noted when the trocar button was removed, leave the body in the preparation room, if possible, for several hours and repeat the treatments again before redressing the body. The mouth and nasal cavities should be checked for dryness and tightly repacked with cotton or cotton webbing. The lips can then be resealed and cosmetics reapplied. Distended eyelids may indicate the presence of gases in the tissues. It may be necessary with this condition to aspirate the cranial cavity and inject some cavity fluid into the anterior cranial cavity. The presence of true tissue gas may necessitate reembalming of the body.

## Maggots

Infestation of the body with maggots is a nightmare experienced by few embalmers today. In the summer months, bodies should be carefully examined for fly eggs, in particular the corners of the eyes, within the mouth, and the nostrils. If maggots are present, they can be picked from the surface of the body with cotton saturated with a hydrocarbon solvent. To stimulate maggots to emerge to the surface from areas beneath the skin or from the mouth or nostrils, the areas can be swabbed with a petroleum product. They should be placed in plastic bags before being discarded. The challenge with maggots is not knowing if all have been found. Maggots found on the clothing and hair can be vacuumed; properly clean the collecting canister on the vacuum.

## Mold

In warm climates, mold can be a problem when bodies are being held for long periods. Bodies should be thoroughly dried to discourage mold growth. Mold needs to be carefully removed with a scalpel or spatula. The area is then swabbed with a phenol compound chemical and later thoroughly dried before cosmetics are applied. Placing embalming powder inside plastic coveralls, pants, and/or stockings helps to control mold growth.

### CONCEPTS FOR STUDY

Define the following terminology:

- Accessory chemicals
- Baseball suture
- Bridge (individual) suture
- Capri pants
- Continuous (whip) suture
- Coveralls
- Crepitation
- Custodial care
- Double intradermal suture
- Hypodermic embalming
- Interlocking (lock) suture
- Inversion (worm) suture
- Pants
- Personal hygiene
- Shirt jacket
- Single intradermal (hidden) suture
- Stockings
- Surface embalming
- Terminal disinfection
- Tissue gas
- Unionall

1. Recall several post-embalming treatments.
2. Name the two types of supplemental embalming methods.
3. List several types of accessory chemicals.
4. Describe the internal hypodermic treatment method for reaching facial tissues.
5. Relate two methods of closing an incision.
6. Express the advantage of locking down a suture when closing a lengthy incision.
7. Explain the process for hiding the suture thread and knot at the completion of the closure.
8. Summarize terminal disinfection practices and personal hygiene for the embalmer.
9. State the benefits of plastic garments and body coverings for shipment of a deceased to another funeral establishment.
10. Define custodial care and defend its importance as a professional ethic of death care providers.

## FIGURE CREDIT

Figures 15–1, 15–5, 15–18 are used with permission of Kevin Drobish.

Figures 15–2, 15–3, 15–4, 15–8, 15–9, 15–12, 15–13, 15–15A-D, 15–16, 15–17, 15–19 are used with permission of Sharon L. Gee-Mascarello.

Figures 15–6, 15–7, 15–10, 15–11, 15–14 are used with permission of Kristine Miller.

## BIBLIOGRAPHY

American Board of Funeral Service, *Course Content Syllabus,* 2016.

Grant ME. Chronological order of events in embalming. In: *Champion Expanding Encyclopedia*, No. 571. Springfield, OH: Champion Chemical Co., October 1986.

Venes D. Taber's Cyclopedic Medical Dictionary, 19th ed. Philadelphia: F.A. Davis, 2001.

CHAPTER 16

# General Age Considerations

## CHAPTER OVERVIEW

- General Age Categories
- Considerations
- Degenerative Diseases

Age is just one of the many factors considered during the pre-embalming analysis; numerous intrinsic and extrinsic conditions influence the selection of embalming methods. However, the embalmer can expect to modify treatments with respect to age. Embalming considerations such as vessel selection, injection and drainage techniques, strength and volume of embalming solution, and injection pressure and rate of flow are all influenced by the age of the decedent.

The particular age of a decedent can also cause the embalmer to expect conditions common to a particular age category. For instance, to list a few: the hands and the head of an infant are positioned differently than those of an adult; arterial tubes needed for infant embalming are much smaller in diameter; a majority of infants, children, and young adults are autopsied; methods of mouth closure differ with respect to age, and severe arthritic conditions in advanced age may present positioning challenges.

| | |
|---|---|
| Preterm | Live birth before 37 weeks gestation |
| Stillborn | Death occurs before or during delivery |
| Infant | Birth to 18 months |
| Toddler | 18 to 48 months |
| Child | 4 to 12 years |
| Adolescent | 12 to 18 years |
| Young adult | 18 to 25 years |
| Adult | 25 years to the mid-seventies |
| Advanced | Mid-seventies and beyond |

## CONSIDERATIONS FOR PRE-EMBALMING ANALYSIS OF INFANTS

Body water ratios and fat content are higher in infants. Recognize the relationship of body water and body fat, as both contribute to total body weight. At birth, the body water present is approximately 75% of total body weight. At 1 year of age, water weight declines to around 60%, similar to an adult. Body fat in the newborn is approximately 12% of total body weight and doubles to 25% at 6 months of age. This increases to about 30% at age 1.

Infant skin is delicate and can easily distend, wrinkle, and dehydrate when arterial solutions are too harsh, injected too rapidly, and under high pressure. Arteries and veins are small; a variety of arterial tubes in different diameters and lengths are necessary. Small bore sizes will easily clog. Best practice is to insert a needle injector wire through the barrel to clear any debris. The wire can remain for instrument storage. Most infants are autopsied.

In addition to moisture, congenital disease processes and medications can further increase moisture and waste products in the tissues. Renal and liver failure can cause accumulation of waste products. Both greatly increase the preservative demand of the body. Pre-injection is not recommended as an embalming solution for embalming infants; the preservative content is low or none at all. Despite assumptions, infants may require higher solution strengths. Modify the harshness of strong formulations with supplemental fluids, such as coinjections. Volume in solution injected will vary according to body size.

All treatment should begin with topical disinfection and bathing. Gentle extension and manipulation of the head and the extremities will aid in positioning. Remove medical dressings for inspection and medical devices for disposal. Placing the infant on a bath towel will prevent slippage on the embalming table. Leave the towel in place throughout the procedure.

### Feature Setting

Eye caps may be trimmed with scissors to fit beneath small eyelids. Cotton may be used in place of eye caps. Apply a thin film of massage cream or spray to maintain eye closure and prevent tissue dehydration. The needle injector method of closure is impractical due to the unossified jaw bones. The barb will not properly embed in the soft bone. A musculature or other suture method can be used effectively.

An adhesive glue applied to the lips can substitute for suturing. The lips can remain slightly parted. When this is done, massage cream should be placed on the tongue and buccal cavities inside the mouth to prevent dehydration. Only the corners of the mouth are glued. Create a relaxed mouth closure to produce a comfortable expression.

## Positioning

Positioning varies considerably. The arms can be positioned at the sides of the body or the forearms and hands placed upon the abdomen. A toy or stuffed animal is often placed in the hands. The head may be turned slightly to rest on the right cheek for a relaxed or sleeping pose. Cotton or toweling can be placed beneath the head and shoulders to substitute for a head block. Attention is also given to the positioning of the legs. Infant-sized caskets are customarily full couch design and the legs are visible.

## Vessel Selection in Nonautopsied Infants

### Common Carotid Artery

All arteries should be usable; size is the varying factor. The common carotid is the largest, easily accessible, and very shallow. The common carotid artery is accompanied by a large vein, the internal jugular vein. Placing a support under the shoulders and lowering the head will bring vessels closer to the surface for ease in raising them. Keep in mind, that the thymus gland can be quite large in the infant. Turn the head in the direction **opposite** that of the vessels being raised. Place a horizontal incision in one of the wrinkles in the neck. This type of incision is easily concealed after closure. Seal the incision with adhesive, subcutaneous suture, or the inversion (worm) suture. When drainage is insufficient, raise the left internal jugular vein.

### Femoral or External Iliac Artery

The second largest nonaortic vessels are the external iliac and femoral arteries. The external iliac is slightly larger than the femoral. The accompanying veins are relatively large and may be used for drainage. If a small drain tube is not available, these veins can be expanded by inserting a small forceps into the vessels. **Always inject the distal leg first.** This allows the embalmer to observe the effects of the embalming solution in the tissues of the leg to determine if too much or too little dye has been used. When drainage is difficult to establish from the femoral vein, the right internal jugular vein can be raised.

### Axillary Artery

Use of the axillary artery may be impractical for efficient embalming of the entire body. The vessel is very small.

### Abdominal Aorta

*Use of the aorta for embalming an unautopsied infant requires the embalmer to make an external incision that resembles an autopsy.* The abdominal aorta is very large artery for use as an injection point. Both artery and vein are deep-seated, resting on the anterior surface of the spine. A small incision can be made just to the left of the midline in the middle of the abdomen, and inferior to avoid the liver. The liver is usually large in the infant. The omentum is a large flat adipose tissue layer nestling on the surface of the intraperitoneal organs. The omentum must be opened and a portion of the small and large intestines resected from the spine to visualize the vessels. The aorta is held in position by its parietal branches, four pairs of lumbar arteries. Once located, the aorta can be opened and a large diameter arterial tube placed in the direction of the legs; a second tube placed and directed toward the head. The vein can be opened and the blood passively drained into the cavities. Use of a drainage instrument placed into the vein is unnecessary. The lower portion of the body should be injected first, then the upper portion. During injection, the intestines can greatly expand. Release any fluids by clipping the intestines with surgical scissors. The entire body can be embalmed using this one-point injection method.

### Ascending Aorta

*Use of the aorta for embalming an unautopsied infant requires the embalmer to make an external incision that resembles an autopsy.* The ascending aorta is also used as an injection point. Drainage can be taken from the right auricle of the heart (the small ear-like appendage of the right atrium of the heart). Clip open the auricle to allow drainage.

The incision can be made down the midline of the sternum. Because the sternum is not yet ossified and remains a cartilage, a scalpel or surgical scissors can be used to make the incision. The incision must be held open with some form of retraction to allow injection of the aorta. Another type of incision, the U-incision can be used. This incision is directed inferiorly from a midpoint of the clavicle to the base of the sternum, and then directed superiorly to the mid-point of the opposite clavicle. The tissue is bluntly dissected to expose the sternum. The sternal cartilage is incised at its junction with the ribs and freed of its lateral attachments. Reflect the tissue flap toward the head. The embalmer must open the pericardium and expose the heart and its great vessels. The ascending aorta is observed as it rises from the left ventricle of the heart. Open the ascending aorta or the arch of the aorta to insert an arterial tube. The internal thoracic arteries must be clamped during arterial injection. The entire body can be embalmed using this one-point injection method.

## Cavity Treatment

An infant trocar is selected for aspirating and injecting the cavities. Infant trocars are shorter in length and inside diameter than a standard trocar. The customary point of entry or a lower point such as the right or the left inguinal abdominal area may be used. Cavity embalming can immediately follow arterial injection or be delayed for several hours. Injection of undiluted cavity chemical follows. The volume of cavity chemical varies with respect to the size of the infant. The entry site is closed by a purse-string or reverse suture, or by a trocar button.

## Preparation of the Autopsied Infant

Various types of postmortem examinations are performed on infants:
- *Complete autopsy.* Both cranial and trunk cavities are opened and internal organs removed for examination (**Fig. 16–1A,B**).
- *Partial autopsy.* Specific cavities are opened for examination.
- *Local autopsy.* Specific organs are targeted for examination. The spine may be examined by dorsal approach.

CHAPTER 16 • General Age Considerations

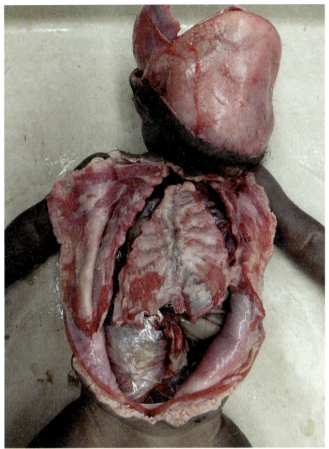

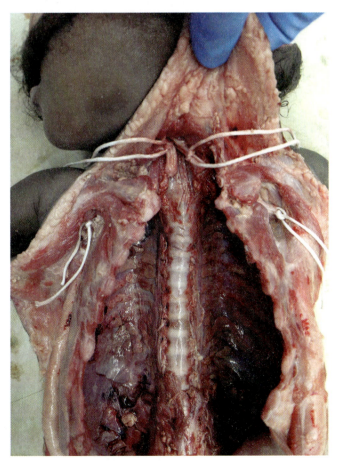

**Figure 16–1.** **A.** Complete autopsy; cranial and trunk cavities. **B.** Sternum and viscera bag removed.

interval between death and embalming. Mortuary refrigeration can produce a variety of complications. Solution strengths similar to those used for adult bodies are practical when supported by the pre-embalming analysis. Harsh tissue reactions can be reduced by the addition of supplemental fluids such as humectants and other types of coinjection chemicals. Arterial fluids designed for infant use are available. The addition of trace amounts of dye to enhance complexion color is recommended. Volume is determined per case.

Best practice is to raise and ligate all arteries prior to injection of embalming solution (**Fig. 16–2**). The additional time necessary to raise arteries during arterial injection unnecessarily exposes the embalmer to chemical fumes. Inject the legs and arms prior to injecting the head so that solution adjustments can be made (**Fig. 16–3A–C**). Clear intravascular blood discolorations and confirm uniform distribution throughout the tissues. The tissues will expand and contour as evidence of distribution. Massage to encourage favorable distribution. Apply digital pressure to the fingertips and the lips to clear these areas of blood discolorations. If facial tissues begin to wrinkle or swell, it is recommended that injection be stopped and the solution modified. Hypotonic (weak) arterial solutions easily distend tissues.

### Supplemental Embalming

#### Hypodermic Embalming

Hypodermically treat the back, shoulders, trunk walls, buttocks, and external genitalia to ensure thorough preservation

Note: Organ and tissue donation vary widely in scope. Postmortem care is specific to the nature of the recovery. Treatments may be similar to preparing the autopsied infant.

### Embalming Solution

There are many suggested chemical combinations, strengths, and dilutions for infant arterial embalming. One false theory is that infants must always be embalmed with very mild solutions and low-index arterial fluids. Infant tissues contain a higher percentage of water compared to adults. Additionally, disease processes and drug therapies can increase tissue moisture and the accumulation of waste products. Autopsy increases the time

**Figure 16–2.** Raise and ligate all six arteries prior to injection. Vessels in the legs not shown

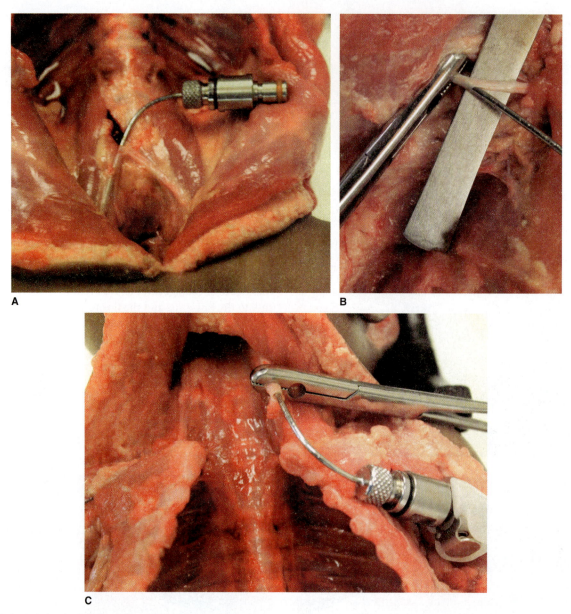

**Figure 16–3. A.** Injection of the right common iliac artery. **B.** Injection of the right axillary artery. **C.** Injection of the left common carotid artery.

in these areas (**Fig. 16-4**). An infant trocar or large-diameter hypodermic needle is ideal. The head may be injected hypodermically from within the incision made for carotid artery injection, from the natural openings of the mouth and nostrils, or from beneath the autopsied scalp. Arms and legs may be injected from within the open trunk cavities or from external points.

### Surface Embalming

Internal compresses, referred to as inlays, are first saturated with chemical. Inlays can be placed into the interior of the neck, the cranium, and the trunk cavities. Inlays can also be inserted under the pectoral chest flaps (over the sternum) before suturing the trunk. Preservative gels can be brushed onto surfaces such as the calvarium of the skull and the anterior chest and abdominal skin flaps prior to suturing. Cover compresses with plastic sheeting to prevent evaporation and release of fumes. External compresses of cotton saturated with undiluted cavity fluid or a topical preservative may be used to preserve areas as small as the ears or, in other cases, the entire body. Compresses should be left in place long enough to accomplish complete preservation. Cover with plastic sheeting to prevent chemical evaporation and release of fumes into the air.

### Closure of the Cranial and Trunk Incisions

Coat the interior of the cranial vault with preservative autopsy gel and apply absorbent and preservative powders (**Fig. 16-5**). Add a quantity of cotton to fill the cranial cavity to absorb residual fluids and stabilize the calvarium once it is replaced (**Fig. 16-6**). Often, infants are held during the memorial event. To recreate weight in the head, form a ball with a small amount of modeling clay, wrap tightly in cotton, and place into the cranial cavity. Several methods are used to secure the calvarium, such as calvarium clamps, drill and wire, and suturing. The inner surface of the reflected scalp and surface of the calvarium is likewise coated with preservative gel or mastic compound (**Fig. 16-7**). The scalp is drawn back to its normal position and sutured.

CHAPTER 16 • General Age Considerations

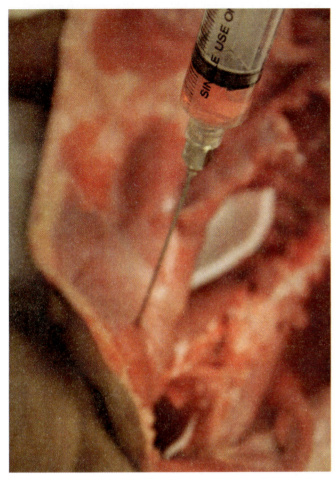

Figure 16–4. Supplemental hypodermic injection of the trunk walls.

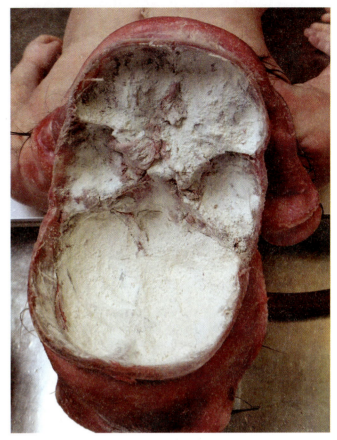

Figure 16–5. Preservative powder applied overtop the preservative gel in the cranial vault.

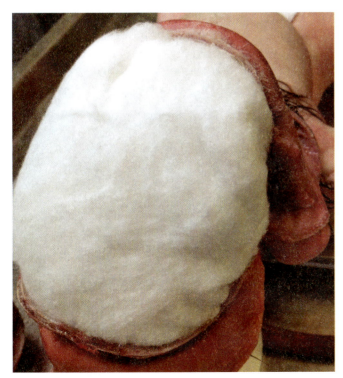

Figure 16–6. Cotton packing in cranial vault.

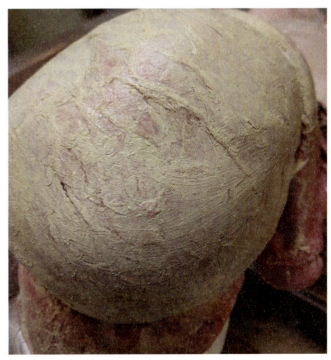

Figure 16–7. Preservative mastic compound applied to calvarium.

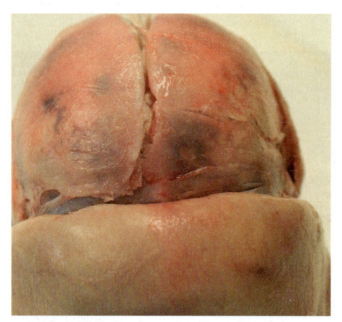

Figure 16–8. Fontanelles present in the unossified cranium.

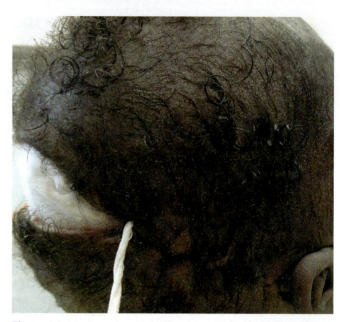

Figure 16–10. Inversion suture begins on the right side of the scalp.

The fontanelles are the spaces between the bones of the skull in the fetus and young infant. Bone ossification is not complete and the sutures of the cranium are not fully formed (**Fig. 16–8**). When the fontanelles are still present, fill the cranial cavity with cotton to create natural contour (**Fig. 16–9**). The soft bone plates are aligned and sutured together with fine thread or dental floss and a small postmortem needle. Apply mortuary putty to cover the fontanelles. This mastic material will hold the soft cranial plates in place and prevent leakage. The mastic will also adhere to the interior surface of the scalp and prevent slippage during suturing.

Begin suturing on the right side of the cranium and end on the left side (**Fig. 16–10**). Select thin suture material and a small postmortem needle. The inversion (worm) suture is ideal to invert the scalp tissues for a clean line of closure that may easily be concealed by hair, mortuary wax, or cosmetics. Super adhesive glue provides a leakproof closure. A tight baseball or intradermal suture may also be used for closure.

The abdominal, thoracic, and pelvic cavities should be coated with autopsy gel or a preservative absorbent compound following aspiration and drying of the cavities (**Fig. 16–11**). Fill the cavities with absorbent material, such as cotton; saturate the material with a preservative chemical (**Fig. 16–12**). The sternum (breast plate) is properly oriented before replacing it to cover the open cavity (**Fig. 16–13**). Webbed cotton can be applied to overtop the sternum and saturated with

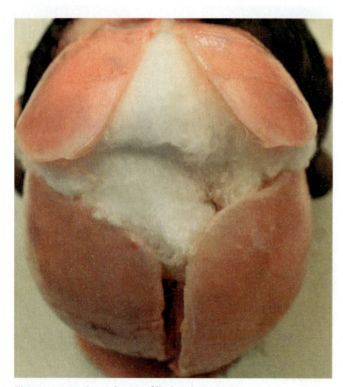

Figure 16–9. Cranial cavity filled with cotton.

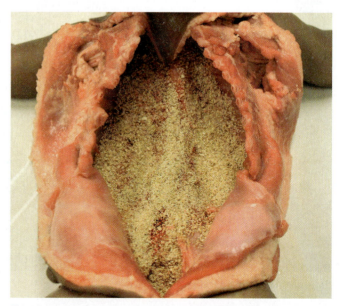

Figure 16–11. Absorbent compound placed into cavities.

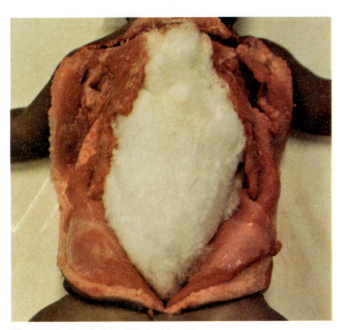

Figure 16–12. Cavities filled with cotton.

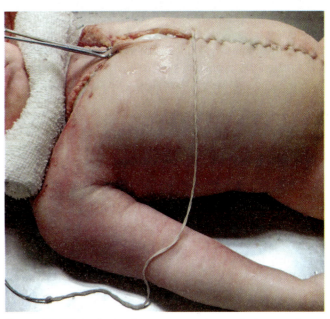

Figure 16–14. Gathering forceps secure tissues during suturing.

preservative chemical. The skin flaps are held together with gathering forceps to ensure proper alignment; suturing begins at the pubic symphysis and is directed superiorly (**Fig. 16–14**). A tight baseball suture provides a good closure. The body is bathed and the skin surfaces are thoroughly dried. Sutures are sealed with surface glue. The trunk area can be covered with thin plastic sheeting to protect clothing.

### Fetuses and Preterm Infants

Decedent care is provided to all human beings after death, regardless of age. Fetuses should be preserved by supplemental hypodermic and surface methods; arterial injection is likely impractical. Supplemental treatments are effective to stabilize the fetus until final disposition. Viewing the fetus or preterm infant is an individual choice. Size of the preterm infant determines the embalming method. All three methods are suitable. Very small diameter arterial injection tubes are available.

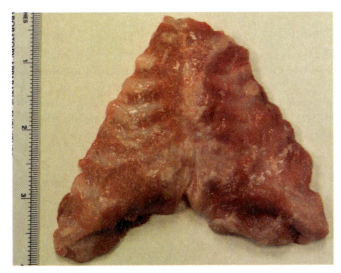

Figure 16–13. Size of infant sternum.

## CHILDREN

### Vessel Selection

The vessels of children are larger than those of the infant, but still smaller than those of the adult. Arteries should be in ideal condition and free of arteriosclerosis. The two major injection sites used in embalming the adult are also used for embalming the child: (1) the common carotid artery and the internal jugular vein and (2) the femoral artery and femoral vein. There is no need to consider use of the abdominal aorta or the arch of the aorta in this age group. Likewise, the many disadvantages of the axillary artery and vein do not make this a good primary injection site. Many in this age group are autopsied, so most of the embalming is done from the primary autopsy sites—right and left common carotid, right and left external and internal iliac, and right and left subclavian arteries.

In the unautopsied body, the right internal jugular vein is the largest vein that can be used for drainage. It also affords direct access to the right atrium of the heart. Whenever facial blood discolorations are present, this vein affords the best possible clearing of the facial tissues.

Some embalmers prefer the femoral vessels for this age group strictly because their location permits the use of clothing that can be opened at the neck. The possibility of leakage or visibility of the carotid incision should be of little concern if properly prepared, sutured, and sealed.

If there has been any trauma to the face or head or if there has been a long delay between death and preparation, the facial tissues may swell during injection. The best control over fluid flow into the head and the face is obtained by the use of restricted cervical injection.

### Fluid Strengths and Volume

Fluid strength is determined by the condition of the body. Tissues are more delicate than adults. A medium-index fluid in the index range 18–25 is most satisfactory. Two schools of thought exist as to embalming solution strengths: the first is to use one mixture strength throughout the entire operation; the second is to begin the injection with a mild solution, and after clearing intravascular blood discolorations, gradually strengthen the solution. Supplemental chemicals may be used to control harsh reactions of the embalming chemicals. Dye can always be used for its cosmetic effect and to indicate the distribution of arterial solution. In cases of trauma and the effects of diseases, such as edema and renal failure, appropriate fluid strengths should be used and, if necessary, special-purpose high-index fluids.

Children require a smaller volume of fluid than adults, but a greater volume than that used for infants. Intravascular blood discolorations should have cleared, some firming of the tissues should be present, and there should be evidence of good distribution as indicated by the presence of dye. All of these indicators help to establish the volume of the fluid to be injected.

Common causes of death in children include meningitis, pneumonia, viral, and systemic diseases such as leukemia and cystic fibrosis. When contagious or infectious disease is the cause of death, the arterial solution strength should be of sufficient strength to sanitize the body tissues without any adverse effect to the appearance of the body. A thorough aspiration of the cavities is necessary, followed by injection of sufficient concentrated cavity fluid to reach all areas of the cavities. Reaspiration and reinjection of the cavities may be necessary.

### Pressure and Rate of Flow

The rate of flow should be a greater concern than pressure to the embalmer, especially when embalming a child. If arterial solution is injected too quickly into the body, the tissues may distend. Injection must be slow enough that the drainage can be restricted at times during the injection. This helps to prevent a loss of the solution through low-resistance paths, especially those vessel connections located near the injection site.

Sufficient force is necessary to establish good distribution, especially in distal body areas such as the hands and the feet. By the use of intermittent drainage, short-circuiting of solution is reduced and retention of solution is increased. Rapid injection with continuous drainage often has the tendency to remove moisture from a child's tissues. This could lead to wrinkling of the skin. A sufficient pressure and rate of flow should be used to achieve a uniform distribution of the solution.

### Setting of Features and Positioning

The arms can be more relaxed than those of the adult and the head positioned with a similar slight tilt to the right. Mouth closure may also be more relaxed than an adult. Lips may be fuller than the adult. Some drugs stimulate the growth of facial hair; this fine hair can easily be shaved to prevent a negative impact on cosmetic application. Cosmetics can stick to fine facial hair and produce an unnatural appearance.

## ADOLESCENT THROUGH ADULT

It is important that the embalmer should remember that age is only one factor in the embalming analysis. Other factors to consider are vast: time between death and preparation, progress of decomposition, moisture content, discolorations, condition of the blood vascular system, protein and nutritional condition, traumatic or surgical considerations, time between preparation and disposition, weight, autopsy and organ donation considerations, and pathologic changes. Vessel selection and injection and drainage methods are always case specific.

### Supplemental Fluids

Supplemental chemicals can be used in the embalming of all bodies. These chemicals are designed to enhance the preservative and disinfecting qualities of the preservative fluids, control moisture, add color to the tissues, and adjust pH of the tissues as well as the arterial solution. Supplemental chemicals include pre-injection and coinjection fluids, humectants, dyes, and water conditioners. In addition, there are specialized supplemental fluids to control tissue gas, bleach internal discolorations, and remove edema from the tissues.

### Solution Strength and Volume

Age is not the single factor in determining the strength and the volume of the preservative solution to be injected. Intrinsic conditions (within the body) such as weight and body build; moisture in the tissues; effects of disease, surgery, or trauma; blood discolorations; and effects of long use of medications, all influence arterial solution strength and volume. Several extrinsic factors, such as time lapse between the death and the embalming, and time that lapse between embalming and the disposition of the body is considered. Sufficient strength and volume of the embalming chemical must be used to assure thorough sanitizing and preservation of all body areas. Fluid companies make a variety of arterial fluids; consider their recommendations. Some are formulated for infants and children, some for general use, and other formulations are specific to certain conditions such as edema, jaundice, and decomposition. When formaldehyde is the primary preservative chemical, various indexes and buffers in the fluids will produce varying degrees of firmness. For the average body, one that does not present embalming complications, a milder solution can be used at the start of the embalming. After good distribution of the solution has been established and the intravascular blood discolorations have been cleared, the solution can be strengthened. This can be accomplished by (1) adding more of the same concentrated arterial fluid or (2) adding a stronger arterial fluid to the original dilution.

### Pressure and Rate of Flow of Injection

An ideal speed of delivery, called *rate of flow*, is defined as the injection of 1 gallon of solution in a period of 10–15 minutes. Healthy body tissues can accept fluid at this rate of speed without distension. Sufficient pressure and rate of flow should be used to overcome the resistances within the vessels and to distribute the arterial solution without causing tissue distension. The greater the resistance in a body, the greater the pressure required. A pressure setting of 5–20 psi (measured in pounds per square inch or psi) is sufficient to overcome most body resistances. This range is variable and dependent upon conditions specific to the body and embalmer preference. Many prefer low pressures; others prefer high pressures; some inject with 140 psi as the standard pressure. Speed of delivery is just as variable. The first injection, while the vascular system is filling, should be slow to prevent arterial coagula from loosening and moving within the vessels. Coagula can block smaller arteries and prevent the flow of solution. Slow flow allows the solution to distribute overtop the coagula. After the first gallon, the speed of injection is increased.

Some embalmers prefer to inject at a rapid rate of flow initially. The theory is that this places greater pressure on the arterial side of the capillaries and increases filtration of the embalming solution through the capillaries. With this method, continuous drainage is used throughout the preparation. The body must be observed carefully to detect any facial or neck distension. This method can also loosen coagula in the arteries creating arterial emboli that can block smaller arterial branches. Multipoint injection and hypodermic embalming may then be necessary to effectively embalm tissues receiving insufficient preservation.

Pressure and rate of flow must be sufficient to evenly distribute the preservative solution to all body areas without distension of any tissues. Injection speed should be such that restricted drainage can be employed to assist with the solution distribution, penetration, and retention.

## ADVANCED AGE

Life expectancy in the United States in 2020: 75.1 years for men and 80.5 years for women. Embalmers customarily embalm greater numbers in the advanced age group. The number of persons living into their late eighties and nineties is expected to double within several years. It is useful to identify common conditions associated with advanced age.

### Arthritic Conditions

Degenerative physical changes occur naturally with age, such as arthritis, muscle atrophy, and osteoporosis. These conditions may be exacerbated in patients confined to a bed or otherwise incapacitated. Muscle atrophy causes reduced skeletal muscle mass. The muscles of the extremities remain contracted and resist being straightened (**Fig. 16–15**). Frequently the arms are drawn up to the chest and the fingers are clenched. Spine curvature results from atrophy of the spinal muscles. Arthritic conditions cause joint inflammation and stiffness. Osteoporosis causes bone brittleness and weakness, partly due to calcium and nutrient loss. Alzheimer's, Huntington's, and Parkinson's diseases and Amyotrophic Lateral Sclerosis (ALS), also known as *Lou Gehrig's disease*, are degenerative diseases of the nervous system.

Degenerative changes create numerous positioning challenges for the embalmer. It may be necessary to secure the body in position during embalming. Retracted limbs can cause abrupt positional changes during embalming. Positioning devices such as body bridges and head blocks placed beneath the thighs and shoulders provide adequate support. Rolled bath towels placed under the shoulders also help to achieve temporary position. The casket bedding and pillow later provide this support and create comfortable positioning. The neck may be difficult to position. Application of firm pressure to arthritic limbs and arms can alter their positioning. Unintentionally, it is possible to tear tendons and atrophied muscles while positioning cases with severe conditions. Leaving the arms and legs in the original positions may be acceptable to the family. It is not recommended that tendons or skin be cut to achieve good positioning. It is not possible to unclench severely arthritic fingers with causing harm. When the legs are drawn to one side or into the fetal position, use of the femoral vessels is limited.

The common carotid would be the best site for injection. If it becomes necessary to inject the legs, an attempt can be made to raise the femoral or external iliac artery. The popliteal artery may also be a choice. If these vessels are found to be sclerotic, an attempt should be made to inject using a small arterial tube; if this is not possible the legs should then be hypodermically injected using a small trocar and a dilute solution of cavity fluid injected through the embalming machine. In addition to hypodermic injection, the legs can be brushed with a preservative surface gel and placed in plastic stockings.

### Mouth Closure

Frequently a loss of weight is manifested in the facial tissues of the elderly. After mouth closure, place cotton or mortuary putty over the teeth or dentures to fill sunken areas of the cheeks. Consider natural and acquired facial markings to avoid overfilling tissues. Atrophy of the two maxillary bones, the maxilla and mandible may prevent use of the needle injector method of mouth closure. A method of suturing is advised for mouth closure (**Fig. 16–16**).

### Arteriosclerosis

Although not a problem exclusively to older age groups, sclerotic arteries are frequently encountered. The artery most frequently affected by sclerosis is the femoral artery. In a very thin individual, the condition can be felt, or palpated. Sclerosed vessels appear hard and irregular. The common carotid artery is the best primary choice when sclerosis is present in the femoral vessels. Rarely is the carotid found to be sclerotic. Arteriosclerosis during life can be attributed to poor peripheral circulation; tissues of the lower extremities are commonly affected. Arteriosclerosis can also result in amputation of a limb. Treat recent amputations by hypodermic injection. Place a plastic

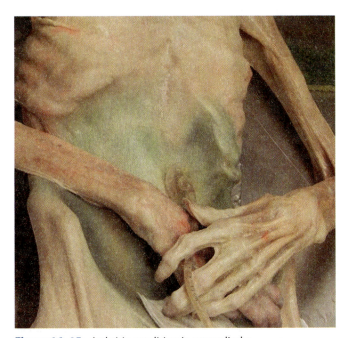

**Figure 16–15.** Arthritic condition in upper limbs.

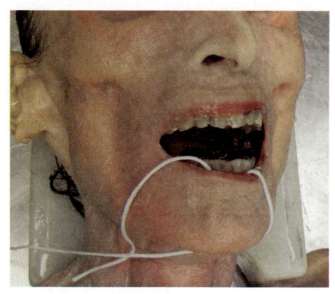

**Figure 16–16.** Musculature suture used for mouth closure.

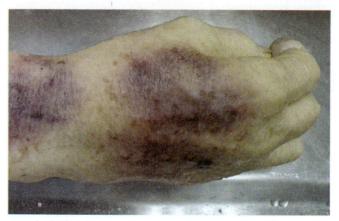

**Figure 16–17.** Senile purpura on the back of the hand.

stocking with the addition of absorbent and preservative powders to control any leakage.

Poor circulation also causes decubitus ulcers (bedsores) to develop in dependent tissues that receive prolonged contact pressure. Some ulcerations affect smaller areas such as the heels of the feet; others affect larger areas such as the buttocks and hips. Bacteria invade the tissues and produce odor and necrosis. It is important to properly disinfect these areas. Undiluted cavity fluid can be applied on cotton compresses to the ulcerated areas. Hypodermic treatments are effective. When bandages cover these areas, treat the bandage topically before removal and disposal. At the time of dressing, fresh cotton saturated with undiluted cavity chemical, a phenol solution, or autopsy gel is applied to the ulcerations; plastic garments should be used to cover these areas. Embalming powder is placed in the garment to control odors. Gangrene may also be present. Treat wet gangrene hypodermically with a cauterizing chemical, apply a compress covered with plastic sheeting. Gangrene of a limb can be dressed in a plastic garment.

Arteriosclerosis can also cause an aneurysm in a blood vessel. An aneurysm is an excessive bulging in the wall of a blood vessel, causing the wall to weaken. An aneurysm can burst (rupture), causing internal bleeding; often leading to death. Leakage of embalming solution during arterial injection will occur at the site of a ruptured aneurysm. Classic signs that an abdominal aortic aneurysm has ruptured: upon injection there is little to no blood drainage, the abdomen distends abruptly, and solution distribution is not observed. Damage to vascular continuity prevents any further circulation of embalming solution. A six-point injection is necessary. Following sectional injection, hypodermically treat the trunk walls to ensure preservation.

## Senile Purpura

Senile purpura (or ecchymosis) is an extravascular irregularly shaped blood discoloration that often appears on the arms and the backs of the hands (**Fig. 16–17**). The condition is brought about by fragility of the capillaries. In the elderly, excessive medications, blood thinning drugs, vitamin deficiencies, uremia, hypertension, thin skin, and slight bruising can easily lead to senile purpura. These discolorations vary greatly in size and do not clear during arterial injection. Often, the affected area becomes engorged with fluid and swells during arterial injection. Discolored areas can darken after embalming and are prone to separate from the underlying tissue. Handle areas of the hands affected by purpura with caution; tissues easily tear.

When senile purpura is present over the hands and the arms, and often the base of the neck, the arterial solution should be strengthened. A fast rate of flow is not recommended. A slower rate of flow helps to limit further rupture of capillaries. It may be necessary to use multiple injection points. If the arms are separately injected, a special-purpose high-index fluid can be used to dry these areas. Surface compresses of cavity fluid, phenol, or autopsy gel can be used. If the skin tears, remove all loose skin at the beginning of embalming. After surface compresses have had time to cauterize or bleach these discolored areas, the surface of the skin can be dried with a hair dryer and restorative and cosmetic treatments applied.

## Malignancy

Positive advances in medicine and patient care have influenced the increase in life expectancies. Longer life spans increase the probability of malignancies due in part, to the exposure to numerous and varied environmental factors. Cancers or neoplasms that begin as localized tumors can easily invade healthy tissues, spread via the blood vascular system, and invade organs. This can disrupt vital functioning to the point of death. The embalmer is concerned with the following systemic effects of a malignancy:

- Disseminated intravascular coagulation; clots scatter throughout the vascular system.
- Disruption of metabolism by uncontrolled secretion of hormones. Metabolic imbalance influences weight control, cell membrane activity, and the metabolism of sugars, fats, and proteins.
- Secretion of peptide and steroid hormones by tumors. Hormone secretions can result in sustained hypercalcemia; excessive calcium levels.
- Anemia results from a lack of healthy red blood cells leading to reduced oxygen flow to the body's organs. Skin pallor, fast heartbeat, tiredness, and weakness are common side effects.

- Cachexia or severe weight loss is caused by the tumor competing with the body for metabolites results in a wasting away of body tissues.

The local effects of a malignant tumor include invasion and destruction of normal tissues; obstruction of intestines, airways, urinary tract, and biliary tract; pathologic fractures; perforation of the hollow viscera; erosion of blood vessel walls, creating acute and chronic hemorrhage; and establishment of portals of entry for infections.

Both local and systemic effects of malignancy have an effect on embalming. Weight loss and emaciation produces unsupported, senile skin; loose and flabby. The skin can also be dry due to the inability of the body to retain proper water balance. Localized edema can result when local tumors exert pressure on veins and lymphatics. If the hormone balance has been interrupted and a condition such as sustained hypercalcemia exists, the excess calcium can easily create a barrier at the cell membrane, making it impermeable to embalming solutions. When embalming preservative cannot penetrate the cells, tissue firmness is difficult to establish. Senile tissues can appear firm following arterial injection due to rapid accumulation of fluids in the loose tissues. In time, as the embalming solution gravitates, the tissues become soft.

Cancer deaths are often attributed to pneumonia and respiratory arrest. Embalming solutions should be of moderate strength, at or above 2% and well-coordinated by the addition of supplemental chemicals such as coinjection. Coinjection will maintain solution strength, modify harshness, and increase distribution and diffusion of the arterial solution. Coinjection fluids increase cell permeability; promoting passage of arterial solution through cell membranes.

Metabolic disturbances and renal and respiratory failure, often accompany malignancy. The result is a buildup of metabolic wastes in the tissues. Waste products increase the demand for preservative. Use of a strong, well-coordinated arterial solution ensures satisfactory preservation. The rate of flow setting must be adequate to distribute the fluid throughout the entire body.

If the facial tissues are emaciated, restricted cervical injection is recommended. This allows for separate embalming of the head. A milder solution containing humectant can be used to restore lost moisture and contour the facial tissues.

If localized edema is present in the arms or the legs, use multiple sites for injection. When the femoral arteries are sclerotic, use supplemental preservation methods: hypodermic and surface embalming.

A colostomy may be present as a result of malignancies involving the intestinal tract. The collecting bag can remain in place during arterial injection and cavity treatment. After cavity treatment, the bag should be removed and disposed of properly in a biohazard waste container. Cotton inlays saturated with cavity fluid or a phenol solution can be inserted into the colostomy opening in the abdominal wall. Closure of the opening is easily achieved with a purse-string or reverse suture.

### Cardiac Disease

Cardiac disease may be treated by surgery such as heart bypass or valve repair. Incisions will be present when death occurs within days or a few weeks postsurgical. Edema in the facial tissues is common when postsurgical therapies involve large volumes of intravenous fluids. The common carotid artery and the internal jugular vein is the ideal primary injection and drainage technique. A moderate to strong arterial solution with the addition of dye helps to indicate the distribution of arterial fluid. When local obstructions exist, sectional embalming is necessary. If there is extensive edema of the facial tissues, restricted cervical injection should be used and strong solutions for the treatment of the edematous face should be employed. When recent incision closures leak during injection, suture overtop the existing staples or sutures, or remove them altogether and apply a new closure. Remove metal staples with a hemostat. Dry the incisions and hypodermically treat discolored or inflamed tissue margins; this can be a sign of infection.

Remove implantable devices, such as cardio-defibrillators and pacemakers, when cremation is the form of final disposition.

### Diabetes Mellitus

Diabetes mellitus is a group of diseases resulting in excess sugar in the blood. Insulin helps to regulate blood sugar level. Insulin therapy is a primary treatment for diabetes (**Fig. 16–18**). The principal manifestations of diabetes include **hyperglycemia** (excess sugar in the blood), **glycosuria** (sugar in the urine), and **ketosis** (acidosis characterized by the presence of ketones in the blood and the body tissues). A strong odor of acetone may be noted due to its presence in the urine and the perspiration. Pathologic changes include poor peripheral circulation, particularly in the lower extremities, and degenerative changes in small blood vessels. Kidney failure, enlargement of the liver (due to high sugar content), and fungal infestations of the lung can also be prevalent. Skin infections lead to pruritus, a

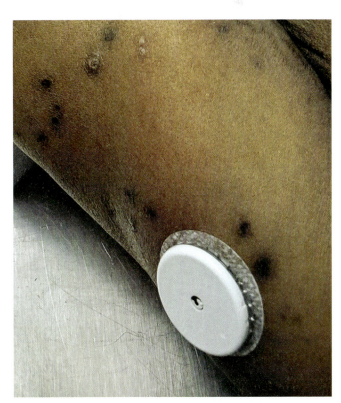

**Figure 16–18.** Transdermal insulin delivery system.

condition characterized by chronic itching of the skin. Visible scratches on the arms and legs are commonly observed.

Restricted cervical injection is recommended. Two different arterial solutions can be used for separate injection of the trunk and head. Supplemental methods, hypodermic, and surface treatments are also recommended. Cavity embalming should immediately follow arterial injection and be thorough. Fungal infections can be localized in the respiratory tract. Inject liberal amounts of cavity fluid into the liver and the lungs. Place plastic garments on the lower extremities when ulcerations are present.

The following list summarizes the recommended treatment:
1. Carotid vessels for primary injection.
2. Strong, well-coordinated arterial solutions.
3. Dye to trace distribution.
4. Massage limbs to stimulate distribution of solution during arterial injection.
5. Immediate and thorough cavity aspiration and injection.
6. Hypodermic and surface embalming treatments for areas receiving insufficient arterial fluid.
7. Plastic garments.

## CONCEPTS FOR STUDY

Define the following terms:

- Anemia
- Cachexia
- Disseminated intravascular coagulation
- Fontanelles
- Gathering forceps
- Glycosuria
- Hypercalcemia
- Hyperglycemia
- Ketosis

1. Define the various age categories.
2. Describe how an eye cap may be modified to fit beneath the eyelid of an infant.
3. Name a method, other than suturing, for infant mouth closure.
4. Recall how positioning for infants differs from adults.
5. Name several arteries suitable for arterial embalming of infants.
6. Explain the impact of making an external incision to raise an aortic vessel for embalming an infant.
7. State why it is a best practice to raise all six arteries prior to arterial injection of an autopsied body.
8. Name several areas of the autopsied body treated by supplemental embalming methods.
9. Describe one function of gathering forceps.
10. Give a reason for providing decedent care to a fetus.
11. Explain how strength and volume of embalming solution differs in children compared to adults.
12. List several degenerative diseases of the nervous system.
13. List several systemic effects of malignancies.
14. Explain why the careful handling of hands with senile purpura is important.

## FIGURE CREDIT

Figures 16–1A,B, 16–2, 16–4, 16–5, 16–6, 16–7, 16–10, 16–11, 16–12, 16–14, 16–15, 16–16, 16–17, 16–18 are used with permission of Sharon L. Gee-Mascarello.

Figures 16–3A-C, 16–8, 16–9, 16–13 are used with permission of Kevin Drobish.

## BIBLIOGRAPHY

Bickley HC. *Practical Concepts in Human Disease*. Baltimore: Williams & Wilkins, 1974:92–95.

The Elderly Case. In: *Champion Expanding Encyclopedia*, Nos. 413–415. Springfield, OH: Champion Chemical Co., 1971. Slocum RE. Type six classification. In: *Pre-embalming Considerations*. Boston: Dodge Chemical Co., 1969:79.

Smith AL. *Microbiology and Pathology*, 12th ed. St. Louis, MO: C.V. Mosby, 1980:513–514.

Spriggs AO. Preparation of children's bodies. In: *The Art and Science of Embalming Springfield*, OH: Champion Chemical Co., 1963: 127–128.

CHAPTER 17

# Preparation of Autopsied Bodies

## CHAPTER OVERVIEW
- Types of Postmortem Examinations
- Common Forensic Autopsies
- Outline for Preparation of Autopsied Bodies
- Restorative Treatments for Facial Trauma

---

Autopsy is the postmortem examination of the dead human body. There are two types of autopsy: the medical (hospital) autopsy and the medicolegal (forensic) autopsy. Most coroners and medical examiners *do not* want the body embalmed prior to the autopsy. However, some pathologists prefer that only arterial injection, not cavity treatment, is done prior to the autopsy.

In certain autopsies, particularly hospital autopsies, the family not only must give permission for the autopsy, but they also have the right to limit the extent of the autopsy. Where special instructions have been given, it is important that the pathologist follow the limitations established by the family. The partial autopsy may consist of external examination and/or removal of only one or two organs.

The embalmer should document in the Embalming and Decedent Care Report the type of autopsy performed and the disposition of the visceral organs.

## TYPES OF AUTOPSIES

### Medical or Hospital Autopsy

Permission for the medical or hospital autopsy is obtained from the person authorized to make final disposition decisions. Hospital autopsies can confirm or verify a diagnosis. Several additional reasons are given by the College of American Pathologists for the performance of the hospital autopsy*:

- When doctors have not made a firm diagnosis.
- When death follows unexpected medical complications.
- When death follows the use of an experimental drug or device, a new procedure, or unusual therapy.
- When death follows a dental or surgical procedure done for diagnostic purposes and the case does not come under the jurisdiction of medical examiner or coroner.
- When death occurs suddenly, unexpectedly, or in mysterious circumstances from apparently natural causes and the case does not come under the jurisdiction of medical examiner or coroner.
- When environmental or workplace hazards are suspected.
- When death occurs during or after childbirth.
- When there are concerns about a hereditary disease that might affect other members of the family.
- When there are concerns about the possible spread of a contagious disease.
- When the cause of death could affect insurance settlements.
- When patient care is questioned.

### Medicolegal or Forensic Autopsy

Reasons for a medicolegal autopsy ordered by a coroner or medical examiner include (1) determination of the **cause of death** (such as, but not limited to, blunt force trauma, multi-organ failure, myocardial infarction, pancreatic cancer, pulmonary embolism), (2) determination of the **manner of death** (such as accidental, homicide, natural, suicide), (3) establishment of the **time of death**, (4) recovery, identification, and preservation of evidence, and (5) provision of factual and objective information for legal authorities. The cases that come under the jurisdiction of a coroner or medical examiner vary from state to state and from county to county within a state. The following general list represents typical cases that would be reported to a coroner or a medical examiner.

- All sudden deaths not caused by readily recognizable disease or wherein the cause of death cannot be properly certified by a physician on the basis of prior, or recent medical attendance.
- All deaths occurring in suspicious circumstances, including those where alcohol, drugs, or other toxic substances may have had a direct bearing on the outcome.
- All deaths occurring as a result of violence or trauma, whether apparently homicidal, suicidal, or accidental (including those caused by mechanical, thermal, chemical, electrical,

---

*Adapted from recommendations of the College of American Pathologists headed by Dr. Hans J. Peters, *New York Times*, July 21, 1988.

or radiation injury, drowning, and cave-in), regardless of the time elapsed between injury and death.
- Any fetal death, stillbirth, or death of a baby within 24 hours of birth, where the birth mother has not been under the care of a physician.
- All therapeutic and criminal abortions, regardless of the length of pregnancy, and spontaneous abortions beyond 16 weeks gestation.
- All operative and perioperative deaths in which the death is not readily explainable on the basis of prior disease.
- Any death wherein the body is unidentified or unclaimed.
- Any death where there is uncertainty as to whether or not it should be reported to the coroner's office.
- Death within 24 hours of admission to a hospital is not considered a reportable death unless it falls into one of the specific categories defined.

## COMMON FORENSIC AUTOPSIES

This is not a complete list. Determination will vary from state to state and within counties of a particular state.
- Victims of homicide.
- Victims of deaths in the workplace.
- Motor vehicle drivers who have been involved in accidents.
- Pedestrians who have been involved in accidents.
- Passengers who have been involved in accidents but who lack clear evidence of trauma.
- Victims of intra- and perioperative accidental deaths.
- Epileptics.
- Possible victims of sudden infant death syndrome.
- Infants or children with evidence of bodily injury.
- Inmate fatalities in correctional facilities, nursing homes, or medical institutions.
- Victims of trauma.
- Victims of nontraumatic, sudden, unexpected deaths.
- Victims of anorexia nervosa.
- Multiple victims of coincidental, unexplained death at one location.
- Victims of possible poisoning or overdose deaths.
- Any other case in which the pathologist holds a bona fide belief that the death is unexplained and/or an autopsy is in the best interest of the public or that it is necessary for the proper administration of the statutory duties of the office of the coroner.

## AUTOPSY DEFINED

Autopsies are defined by the extent of the postmortem examination. The **partial autopsy** is limited to a specific cavity or region of the body and the incision is made accordingly. The **complete autopsy** examines the entire body. A standard Y-incision is used to examine the torso, or trunk of the body (**Fig. 17–1**); a cranial incision is used to examine the head.

The **complete autopsy** involves full physical examination, tissue and fluid sampling, and removal of both cranial and visceral organs for examination, including, *but not limited to*:
1. Cranial cavity and its contents:
    a. Brain
    b. Pituitary gland
    c. Structures of the inner ear

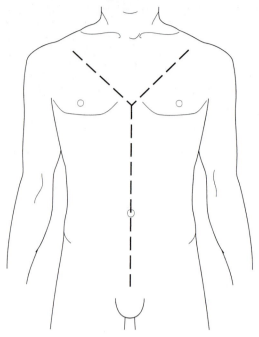

**Figure 17–1.** Standard Y-incision used in the trunk autopsy.

2. Vitreous of the eye
3. Organs located in the neck:
    a. Thyroid gland
    b. Larynx
    c. Esophagus and the trachea (cervical portion)
    d. Portions of the common carotid arteries
    e. Tongue
4. Thoracic cavity and its contents
5. Abdominal cavity and its contents
6. Pelvic cavity and its contents
7. Testes of the scrotum
8. Spinal cord
    a. *Dorsal* approach: examination of the vertebral column from the backside (**Fig. 17–2**).
    b. *Ventral* approach: examination of the vertebral column from within the body cavities; a wedge is removed from the vertebral column.
    c. *Cranial* approach: examination and removal from the foramen magnum.

## GENERAL CONSIDERATIONS

### Best Practices

1. When not in use, remove sharp instruments from the embalming table.
2. Cover sharp bones prior to placement of embalmer's hands into a body cavity.
3. Wash gloved hands when soiled and change gloves often during the embalming procedure.
4. Avoid high water pressure to flush blood and fluids from the embalming table.
5. Practice continuous aspiration of the cavities during arterial injection to remove drainage and excess arterial fluid.
6. Clamp leaking arteries and small veins to avoid excessive loss of embalming solution and to improve solution distribution during arterial injection.

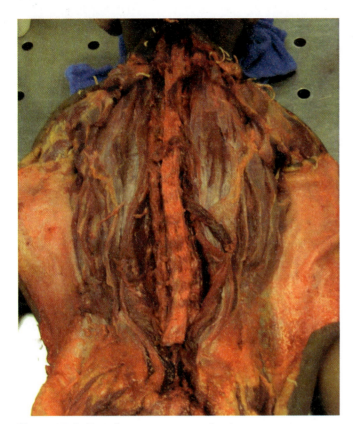

**Figure 17–2.** Dorsal postmortem examination.

7. Run water over the table continuously to flush blood and chemicals toward drainage.
8. Pack external orifices: esophagus, trachea, ears, rectum, and vagina.
9. During embalming, the calvarium and sternum can be soaked in preservative solution within a sealed bag or container.

## Fluid Strength

Preparation of the autopsied body is delayed. The delay may occur between death and autopsy or between autopsy, release of the body, and embalming. Mortuary refrigeration is routine before and following autopsy. Delays increase the probability of surface tissue dehydration, distension during arterial injection, and an increase in the preservative demand of the tissues. Evidence of decomposition is common with lengthy time delays. Time delays often necessitate the use of **stronger than average arterial solutions.**

## Use of Fluid Dyes

Delay also brings about rigor mortis and, if long enough, the passing of rigor. Rigor can cause poor arterial solution distribution and may also be a false sign of fluid firming. Fluid reactions with body proteins do not proceed normally when a body is in rigor mortis. Refrigeration can bring about hemolysis of the blood trapped in the superficial tissues. This hemolysis can create an appearance similar to that of the dye present in arterial solutions. The tissue thus appears embalmed. In addition, refrigerated tissues feel embalmed because the fats in the subcutaneous tissues have hardened. Use dye in the arterial solution to serve as an indication of arterial solution distribution. Keep in mind that dyes show only surface distribution of arterial solutions; not deeper tissue diffusion. Massage deep tissues, such as the muscles of the legs during rigor. Intermittent drainage increases intravascular pressure and promotes diffusion of embalming solution and drainage of blood from the vascular system.

### Pressure and Rate of Flow

Tissues can assimilate only a certain amount of fluid in a given period of time. Often, arterial solution is injected too fast into the body and swelling results. In preparation of the autopsied body, inject each section separately. During injection into a specific body region, such as an arm or a leg, higher pressures and faster rates of flow can be safely used to help establish good circulation. The embalmer can vary the rate of flow for each area and, if necessary, vary the pressure to overcome the resistances of a particular body region. In addition, intermittent drainage and pulsation can be used for each area to establish good distribution and diffusion.

### Drainage

During arterial injection it is not necessary to insert drainage devices into the veins. Drainage material will flow directly into the body cavities. Once in the cavities, an autopsy aspirator is used to evacuate drainage to reduce fumes and maintain visual inspection of the cavity interior. Autopsy aspirators are designed to not clog easily; large holes are present at the working end of the instrument. Clamping the vein with a hemostat or applying digital pressure with a piece of cotton temporarily stops the drainage. Intermittent and alternate drainage greatly assists in fluid distribution, diffusion, and retention of the arterial solution.

## OUTLINE FOR TREATMENT OF THE COMPLETE AUTOPSY

The order for treatment of all autopsied cases is determined by the judgment of the professional embalmer and based upon factors and individual conditions discovered during embalming analysis.

1. Apply a topical droplet spray to the surface of the body and the orifices. Bathe the body with germicidal soap. Relieve rigor mortis. Position the head and the shoulders.
2. Shave and set features before or after cranial injection.
3. Remove temporary sutures and open the cavities. Remove the bag containing the viscera. Disinfect the internal surfaces of the body cavities with a topical spray.
4. Locate and place ligatures around the six arteries needed for sectional arterial injection (**Fig. 17–3**):
    a. Right and left external iliac arteries (or common iliac, or internal iliac).
    b. Right and left axillary arteries (or subclavian).
    c. Right and left common carotid arteries.
5. Prepare the arterial embalming solution. Consider a variety of factors in determining the strength of the solution. Different solutions may be prepared for different sections of the body.
    a. Cause of death.
    b. Height and weight.
    c. Time interval between death and preparation.

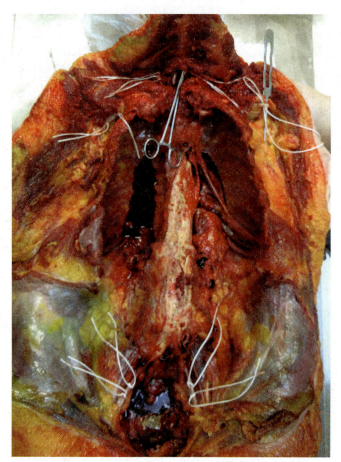

**Figure 17–3.** Arteries ligated for injection of the trunk autopsy.

d. Presence of decomposition changes.
e. Moisture content.
f. Protein content.
g. Refrigeration.
6. Inject using rates of flow and pressures that meet the demands of the various body areas. Drainage may be concurrent or intermittent.
   a. Inject the legs. Inject each leg separately or use a Y-tube to inject both legs concurrently.
   b. Inject the arms separately or with a Y-tube.
   c. Inject the head.
      (1) Inject the left side first.
      (2) Inject the right side (viewing side).
7. Use supplemental embalming: hypodermic and surface treatments of the trunk walls, the shoulders, the neck, and the buttocks.
8. Treat internal surfaces with accessory chemicals: drying and hardening compounds or preservative powders.
9. Prepare abdominal and thoracic cavities and neck area:
   a. Return the viscera bag and add preservative chemical or replace viscera directly into the body cavities. Add hardening compound to the viscera bag or directly to the viscera that have been replaced into the body cavities.
   b. If viscera are not returned, fill cavities with absorbent material such as cotton and saturate with preservative chemical.
   c. Contour the neck area with cotton and saturate with preservative chemical or autopsy gel.

10. Suture thoracic and abdominal cavities.
11. Dry cranial cavity. Treat walls with preservative powder or gel and attach calvarium.
12. Suture scalp.
13. Wash and dry body.
14. Apply glue to incisions of the thoracic and abdominal cavity.
15. Select plastic garments as needed; place embalming powders into the garment.
16. Prepare the Embalming and Decedent Care Report.

## PREPARATION OF THE AUTOPSIED BODY

Transfer the body to the embalming table. Open the zippered pouch and apply liberal amounts of a topical disinfectant to all body surfaces and the interior of the body bag. Roll the body to one side and roll the body bag to the middle of the table. Rest the body back on the table. Move to the other side of the table and roll the body to the opposite side. Roll the body bag to the center and gently pull the remainder of the bag free. Place the bag into the biohazard waste container. Bathe the body with a disinfectant solution. Let this topical solution remain on the body for at least 10 minutes. The body can then be rinsed and dried. Relieve any rigor mortis present and proceed to positioning of the body:

1. Remove the pathologist's temporary sutures and reflect the skin flaps to expose the thoracic, abdominal, and pelvic cavities. Apply a broad-spectrum disinfectant droplet spray. Remove the sutures from the cranial incision, reflect the scalp, and remove the calvarium to expose the cranial vault. Disinfect the cranial cavity with topical spray. During arterial injection, support the reflected scalp with cotton to avoid causing a crease across the forehead. The scalp can also be returned to its natural position and massaged to assist distribution of fluid through the scalp tissues.
2. Inspect the arteries needed for injection.
3. Shave the face before injecting the head; although shaving may be completed after injection.
4. Set features before injecting the head and make necessary adjustments upon completion of injection.
5. *Mix arterial solution.* If there has been a delay between death and preparation and the body has been refrigerated, a stronger arterial solution is needed. Add some tracer dye to indicate the distribution of arterial solution in the body. Fluid selection is determined by the conditions present in the area of the body being injected. (*Example: the legs may have edema, but the arms and the hands have no edema.*)
6. Inject the lower extremities:
   a. The ideal vessels for injection of the legs are the right and the left common iliac arteries (**Fig. 17–4**). Any leakage from the internal iliac branch can be clamped where the vessels were cut for removal of the pelvic organs. Arterial solution will reach the legs by the external iliac; the internal iliac artery will supply solution to the tissues of the buttocks and perineum. Injection of the common iliac would also supply solution to the trunk walls through branches of the external iliac artery. In some autopsies, the common iliac and the internal iliac arteries have been excised. In this situation, the embalmer will use the external iliac artery to inject each leg. Injecting each

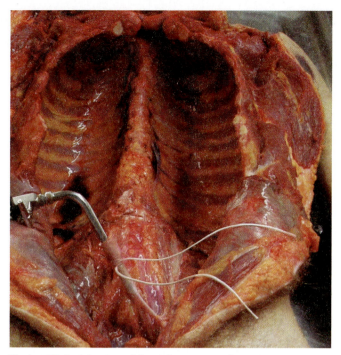

**Figure 17–4.** Injection of the right common iliac artery.

common iliac artery or external iliac artery separately permits more control over the flow of the solution into the extremity being injected. The embalmer can control the pressure, rate of flow, and strength of the solution used for each leg. Separate direct injection of the internal iliac artery accompanied by massage to the buttocks and the upper thighs can bring about a noticeable amount of arterial solution distribution to these areas. It should always be attempted; leakage may need to be controlled with hemostats.

b. During autopsy, the technician may completely cut through the external iliac artery directly beneath the inguinal ligament. It is important to remember that arteries remain open when cut. The artery can be retrieved to use for injection by placing the nose of a hemostat into the lumen of the artery. Gently tighten the hemostat to secure the artery while an arterial tube is inserted. Place a ligature around the artery to secure the arterial tube in place during injection. An arterial hemostat can also be used to secure the tube in the artery. Best practice is to use a ligature along with the arterial hemostat. After injection, the hemostat is removed and the remaining ligature is used to tie the vessel closed. Ligatures are also used by the embalmer to lift the vessels for easier use.

c. When a sufficient volume of solution does not reach the leg, raise the femoral artery to inject the lower extremities. *When the vessels of the leg are sclerotic, use supplemental embalming methods: inject the legs hypodermically with a small gauge trocar and brush the legs with autopsy gel.*

d. Allow drainage to enter the abdominopelvic cavity. If intermittent drainage is desired, use a hemostat to stop drainage for intervals.

e. If the fluid does not reach the foot, institute the following procedures:

(1) Firmly massage the leg, pushing along the arterial route (femoral, popliteal, and anterior and posterior tibial arteries). Rotate the foot medially. This squeezes all of the muscles of the lower leg.
(2) Use a higher injection pressure and pulsation.
(3) Limit drainage by using intermittent drainage.

7. Inject the upper extremities:
   a. As a general rule, the embalmer should always use the artery closest to the center of circulation. If the arch of the aorta and its branches remain intact, use it to inject both the head and upper extremities. Often the arch of the aorta is removed during autopsy and the embalmer utilizes the subclavian arteries to inject the upper extremities. In the complete autopsy, the following vessels must be clamped if the subclavian artery is injected:
      (1) Vertebral artery (if a cranial autopsy has been done).
      (2) Internal thoracic artery.
      (3) Inferior thyroid artery (when neck organs have been removed).
   
   The right subclavian is a branch of the brachiocephalic artery. It can be distinguished from the right common carotid artery, because the subclavian is usually larger in diameter. Follow the direction of the insertion of an arterial tube to determine if the right subclavian artery has been entered; it heads laterally toward the arm. The left subclavian branches off the arch of the aorta. If, after clamping off the leakage from the severed branches of the subclavian, leakage still continues, it may be necessary to raise and inject the axillary artery. Note that when using the axillary is that the shoulder, the upper portions of the back, and the deep muscles of the neck do not receive arterial solution distribution.
   
   b. The axillary artery can be raised by incising the pectoralis major and minor muscles (**Fig. 17–5**). Raise the artery just as it leaves the cervicoaxillary canal. If the axillary artery is raised at this point, all its branches can be used to distribute fluid to the trunk walls and the shoulder areas. In addition, the arm can be placed in a natural position. Use of the axillary artery avoids many of the leakage problems seen with the subclavian artery, and the axillary can be raised from the incision

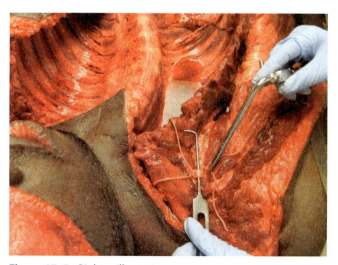

**Figure 17–5.** Right axillary artery.

the pathologist has already made (if that incision rises to the shoulder area). *If the fluid does not flow easily down the arm, pull back on the arterial tube. This usually frees the tube of any blockage.*

c. Drainage can be taken from the subclavian vein. If intermittent drainage is desired, place a hemostat on either the subclavian or the axillary vein.

d. Fluid strength and volume vary from body to body or even from right side to left side. Continue injection until the hand has cleared and distribution is evident. Manipulate the arm, flexing at the elbow and the wrist, to assist distribution along with intermittent drainage. It may also be necessary to place digital pressure on the cephalic vein to increase distribution by blocking the loss of fluid from the superficial drainage route.

e. If fluid is not flowing into the hand, try the following: lower the hand while injecting, massage by pushing very firmly along the arterial route (axillary, brachial, radial, and ulnar arteries), increase injection pressure (using pulsation if available), and use intermittent drainage. Finally, the radial and the ulnar arteries can be raised and injected. If fluid still does not enter the fingers, treat by hypodermic injection of preservative fluid.

8. Inject the head:

a. Raise the right and the left common carotid arteries (**Fig. 17–6**). If the common carotid has been cut by the pathologist, try to find the external carotid. The common carotid bifurcates at the level of the superior border of the thyroid cartilage. This point is quite high in the neck. If the artery can be located, insert a small arterial tube. Clamp it in place with a hemostat.

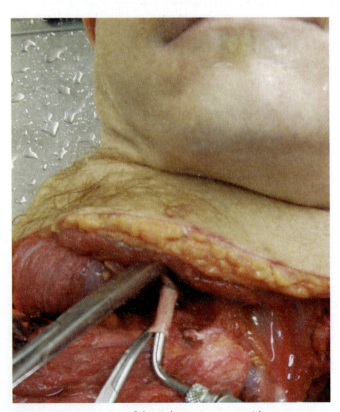

**Figure 17–6.** Injection of the right common carotid artery.

*Option 1.* Inject the left side of the head first. Certain arteries must be clamped for leakage if the **left common carotid** artery is injected. The **left internal carotid** is located inside the cranial cavity just lateral to the sella turcica of the sphenoid bone. Clamp this vessel after arterial injection has begun. In this way, filling of the vascular system supplied by the common carotid artery can be observed. This will not be necessary if the cranial cavity was not autopsied. The **superior thyroid artery** is located in the neck; this branch of external carotid artery leaks if the neck organs have been removed.

Inject the right side of the head. Arteries to be clamped are the **right internal carotid**, found lateral to the sella turcica in the cranial cavity when the cranial cavity has been autopsied, and the **right superior thyroid**, found in the neck if the neck organs have been removed.

The left is injected first so that a certain amount of fluid flows to the right side via anastomosis (cross connection). It also gives the embalmer a chance to observe the effects of the fluid and the dyes on the left side. If there is any problem, the arterial solution can be changed before the right side is injected. This method also prevents overinjection of the right side of the face.

*Option 2.* Once tubes are in place in the right and the left common carotid arteries, attach them to a Y tube. Inject both right and left sides at the same time. Clamp all arteries, such as internal carotids and superior thyroids or any other major leaking arteries, with hemostats.

*Option 3.* When no cranial autopsy has been performed but the major cavities have been autopsied, inject the left and the right sides of the head. If each side of the head is separately injected, clamp the carotid artery not being injected to encourage distribution and prevent arterial solution loss. Since a cranial autopsy was not performed, collateral circulation will occur through the Circle of Willis. Where there is an anastomosis of vessels, the arterial solution will pass from one side of the face to the opposite side. An alternative injection technique is to inject right and left sides of the head simultaneously using a Y-tube.

b. *Enucleation.* If the eyes have been enucleated, loosely pack the eye orbits with cotton saturated with autopsy gel. Close and pose the lids. A light coating of massage cream can be placed on the surrounding facial tissues. Slightly increase the strength of the arterial solution. Inject using a low rate of flow and low pressure. If leakage occurs from the corner of the closed eyelid, allow the fluid to escape. If the leakage is stopped by tightly packing the base of the orbit, it increases the possibility of the eyelids swelling during injection. After arterial injection, the cotton will be removed and the eyes will be restored.

c. If the inner ear has been removed, tightly pack the area of the temporal bone from which the tissues were removed with cotton saturated with autopsy gel. If this area leaks profusely during injection, apply a hemostat to the leaking vessels.

d. *Tongue removed.* Many medicolegal autopsies remove the neck organs, the floor of the mouth, and the tongue (glossectomy). Distribution of the embalming solution to the facial tissues will be interrupted due to the severance of a sufficient number of small arteries. It is difficult to clamp these leaking vessels during arterial injection with hemostats. First, close the mouth and pose the lips. A light coating of massage cream can be placed on the tissues of the buccal cavity and lips. Insert cotton saturated with cavity fluid or autopsy gel through the neck. Tightly pack the cotton into the floor of the mouth. This puts pressure on the severed arteries and limits leakage of the arterial solution. The arterial solution can be slightly increased in strength when this condition exists. Dye should be added to the arterial mixture so evidence of arterial fluid in the facial tissues can be easily observed. The cotton inlay can remain in place and need not be removed after arterial injection.

e. Observe the parotid, sublingual, and submaxillary glands for swelling. Use of a stronger solution and pulsation, a slower rate flow, and reduced pressure during the injection helps to limit swelling of these glands. If swelling occurs, apply digital pressure against the glands. These glands can also be pierced from under the skin with a scalpel, which, together with digital pressure, helps to reduce swelling. If the swelling is too pronounced, the glands may have to be excised from under the skin by going up through the neck.

## SUPPLEMENTAL HYPODERMIC INJECTION

The incisions made by the pathologist and extent of vessel removal may cause only a portion of the trunk to receive arterial solution. The embalmer can preserve areas of the trunk that did not receive fluid by using hypodermic embalming. Preservative solution is injected by trocar or hypovalve trocar attached to the embalming machine (**Fig. 17–7**). Arterial solution or cavity fluid may be used for hypodermic injection.

It is important that all tissues be channeled: the trunk walls (anterior, lateral, and posterior), with special emphasis on injection of the buttocks, breasts, shoulder, and neck regions. After channeling the tissues, inject the arterial solution, the solution will follow and fill the channels. Surface embalming can also be practiced.

1. A scalpel is used to cut the intercostal muscles between the ribs in the thoracic area. Coat this area with autopsy gel

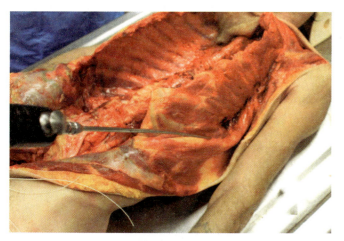

**Figure 17–7.** Supplemental injection of the trunk walls using a hypovalve trocar.

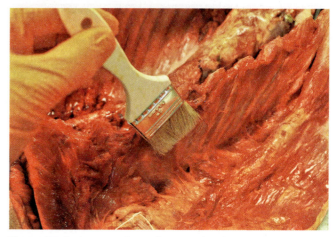

**Figure 17–8.** Intercostal muscles coated with preservative autopsy gel.

using a wide-bristled brush (**Fig. 17–8**). Autopsy gels penetrate rapidly. A high viscosity formulation allows the gel to cling to the lateral tissues.

2. The trunk walls can be dissected further from the rib cage and coated with autopsy gel. Internal compresses can also be saturated with cavity fluid and placed between the tissues and the rib cage.
3. All inside surfaces of the cavities can be coated with autopsy gel.
4. The cavities can be lined with cotton, paper toweling, or sheeting and saturated with cavity fluid before the viscera bag is placed into the cavities. Autopsy compounds can also be used. This is done before viscera are replaced directly into the cavities or the viscera bag is replaced.
5. Care should be taken to pack the pelvic cavity, so there is no leakage from the rectum.
6. When the neck organs have been removed, brush the internal surface of the neck with autopsy gel before cotton is inserted. Cotton is used for contouring the neck. Saturate the cotton with preservative fluid. This is necessary because circulation to the skin of the neck is interrupted when the neck organs are removed.

## TREATMENT OF THE VISCERA

Return the viscera bag to the abdominal and the thoracic cavities. Move the viscera within the bag until contents are positioned uniformly in the cavities. Incise hollow organs to release any gases. Add cavity fluid to the bag. Coat the sternum (breastplate) on both sides with autopsy gel and preservative powder. The sternum can also be wrapped in cotton sheeting and saturated with cavity fluid (**Fig. 17–9**). Replace and align the sternum with the rib cage.

Alternatively, viscera may be soaked in cavity fluid several hours before being returned directly to the cavities, with or without the viscera bag. Cover the replaced viscera with an absorbent hardening compound before suturing the autopsied trunk incisions. If thick cotton is used to fill the cavities, cover the breastplate and exposed cotton with webbed cotton. Thick cotton has a tendency to get caught in the needle during suturing and is pulled through the needle holes.

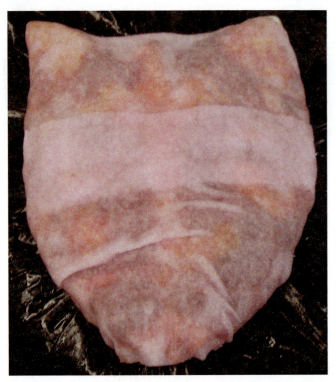

**Figure 17-9.** Sternum wrapped with saturated cotton.

## CLOSURE OF THE CAVITIES

Bring all three tissue flaps together and secure them at the central point with gathering forceps. Place individual bridge sutures every few inches along each of the separate incisions to align the tissue margins for suturing. A combination of temporary sutures and forceps can also be used (**Fig. 17-10**).

Begin to suture using a double-curved postmortem needle and linen suture cord. Linen suture cord is much stronger than cotton suture cord. When pulling the cord to tighten the stitches, pull on the thread, not on the needle. The thread may weaken or break from repeatedly rubbing against the eye of the needle.

Start the suture for the abdominal cavity at the level of the pubic symphysis. Begin the suture by tying the ligature in place or tying a knot on the end of the suture. The baseball suture is recommended for closure. This suture is tight and leakproof when properly executed. Ligature should not be visible upon completion of the baseball suture. When ligature is visible, it is too loose. Pull sutures tightly after every two or three stitches. The opposing folds of skin should overlap slightly, forming an impervious seal and concealing the actual ligature. Single- or double-cord cotton suture thread may be used. A single strand of linen thread may be sufficient. When the hole made by the suture needle appears large, double the thread to fill the void.

Every 4 or 5 inches, pass the needle through both sides of the incision to lock down the previous suture. This technique prevents slipping or unraveling and releases tension on the suture thread. Repeat this technique throughout the suturing process. If the suture thread should break when a lock down has not been practiced, pull enough thread to tie a knot in the end and begin suturing with a new length of thread. Another approach is to suture from the opposite direction and tie the two ends together when they meet.

As the suture reaches a bridging stitch or gathering forceps, remove the temporary stitch or instrument and continue. Upon reaching the xiphoid process, continue the suture up one branch of the Y-incision toward the shoulder and end the suturing at that point. Apply incision seal powder as you suture to prevent leakage. The area closest to the shoulder is the most dependent area and most likely to leak. Begin another suture from the xiphoid process to the opposite shoulder.

The skin of bodies with wasting diseases is difficult to suture because it tears easily. A widely spaced inversion (worm) suture may be necessary to close the incisions.

If trapped air is present in the thoracic area after suturing, insert the trocar through the abdominal wall just beneath the skin surface to remove. This method will flatten the thoracic area for a natural appearance.

## PREPARING THE CRANIAL CAVITY

Following arterial embalming of the head, various practices may be used to prepare the cranial vault, replace and secure the calvarium, and complete the suturing of the scalp. In the following process, calvarium clamps are not addressed but may be used to effectively secure the calvarium in place. The internal surfaces of the cranium are treated with absorbent, drying, and preservative products prior to closure.

1. Remove the absorbent material placed following cranial autopsy (**Fig. 17-11A**).
2. Aspirate or sponge any remaining liquids (**Fig. 17-11B**).
3. Brush the walls of the cranial vault with autopsy gel.
4. Place incision seal powder followed by cotton into the foramen magnum. Add absorbent compound (**Fig. 17-11C**).
5. Pack the entire vault tightly with cotton (**Fig. 17-11D**).
6. Brush glue on the margins of the calvarium and the margins of the skull (**Fig. 17-11E**).
7. Replace and align the calvarium (**Fig. 17-11F**).
8. Suture through the temporalis muscles.
9. Apply mortuary putty along the seam where the bone of the skull meets the calvarium. Continue with a coating of putty over the entire calvarium.

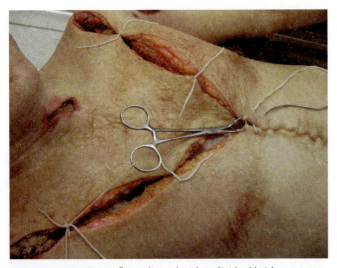

**Figure 17-10.** Tissue flaps aligned with individual bridge sutures and gathering forceps.

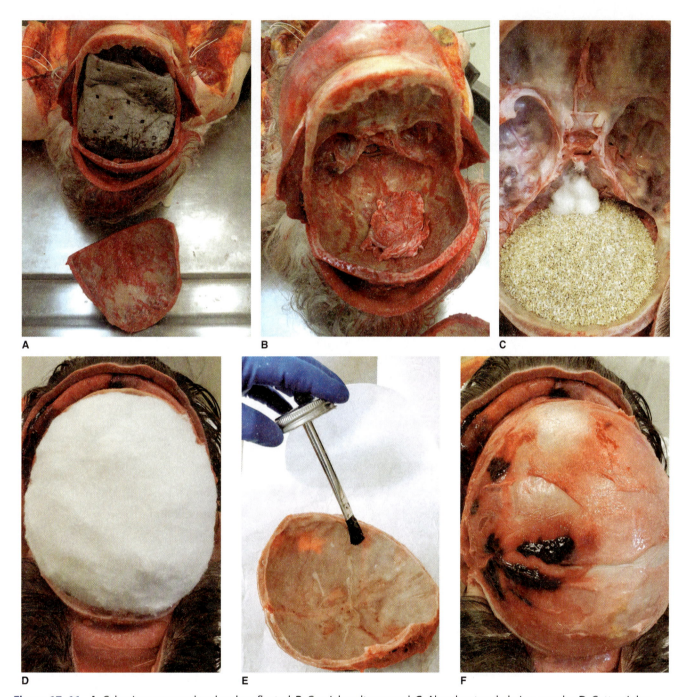

**Figure 17–11.** **A.** Calvarium removed and scalp reflected. **B.** Cranial vault exposed. **C.** Absorbent embalming powder. **D.** Cotton inlay. **E.** Glue applied to margins of calvarium. **F.** Calvarium replaced.

10. Reflect the scalp to its original position, fully covering the calvarium. The scalp will adhere to the mortuary putty and hold the calvarium in place.

## Suturing the Cranial Cavity

Prior to suturing, wet the hair and apply hair conditioner. Use a comb to direct the hair away from the incision. Elastic hair bands or barrettes can be used to hold longer hair out of the way. Trim the hair with barber shears closely to and along the margins of the incision (**Fig. 17–12A**). This method ensures a clean suture closure by preventing the needle from pulling individual hairs through each suture (**Fig. 17–12B**). The hairline meets after the suture is completed; combing the hair will hide the incision entirely (**Fig. 17–12C**).

Begin sutures on the right side of the head (viewing side) and complete them on the left side. This direction of suturing ensures that any puckering that may occur from the slipping of the scalp tissues will occur on the left side. Using a double-curved needle, tie the first suture into place behind the right ear. Avoid knots as they have a tendency to pull through the scalp tissues. Single- or double-linen suture cord can be used.

The inversion (worm) suture is made entirely on the surface of the scalp (**Fig. 17–12D**). At completion, the line of closure is flat, tight, and leakproof. Suture thread is not visible

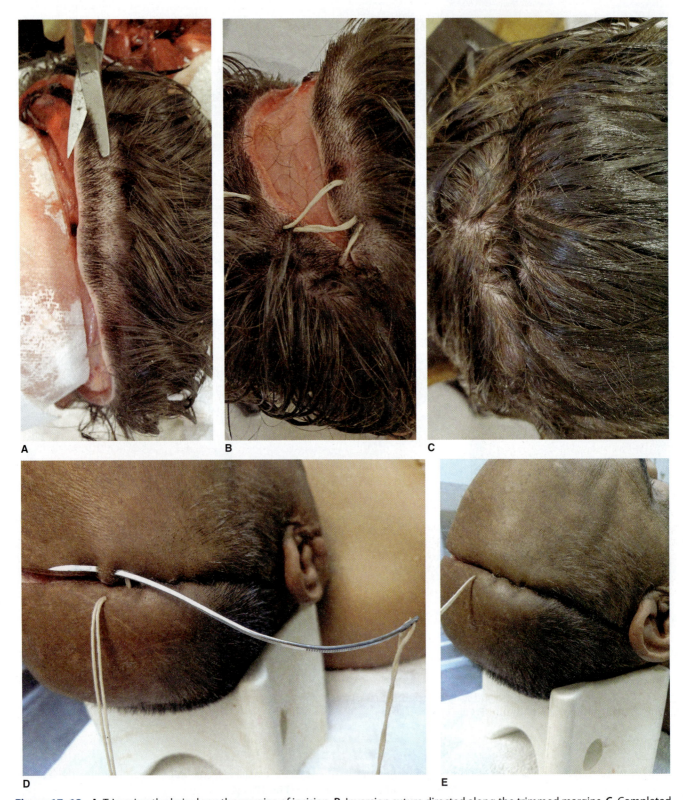

**Figure 17–12.** **A.** Trimming the hair along the margins of incision. **B.** Inversion suture directed along the trimmed margins. **C.** Completed closure with hairline restored. **D.** Inversion suture on scalp without hair. **E.** Completed inversion suture.

(Fig. 17–12E). The inversion suture is ideal when the scalp does not have hair. The incision is easily concealed with cosmetics and/or waxes.

The baseball suture is also used for cranial autopsy closure. A greater incidence of tissue damage exists during suturing with the baseball stitch. As the thread is pulled tightly with each pass of the needle, the marginal tissues may tear. Baseball sutures will produce a visible tissue ridge after completion. This suture is not ideal on a head without hair or when the autopsy incision is made nearer to the forehead; it is not as easily concealed as the inversion suture.

Super adhesive glue is an alternative to sutures for scalp closure. This method is advantageous for the preparation of infants and for tissues that may be easily torn during suturing.

Super adhesive glue is also beneficial to repair extraneous scalpel marks caused during cranial autopsy.

## FINAL PROCEDURES

After suturing the cranium, wash the hair to remove blood, mortuary putty, and loose hair. Dry the towel. Bathe and dry the entire body. Cover sutures with glue and strips of cotton (**Fig. 17–13**). Dress the body in a plastic garment, such as a unionall. Place embalming powder into the garment to control condensation, minor leakages, and odors.

## OUTLINE FOR TREATMENT OF PARTIAL AUTOPSIES

The order for treatment of all autopsied cases is determined by the judgment of the professional embalmer and based upon factors and individual conditions discovered during embalming analysis.

### Death from Pulmonary Embolism

When autopsy reveals a pulmonary embolism, the pathologist may trace the origin of the blood clot. Exploratory incisions are often made along the medial and posterior areas of the lower legs. The incisions can be packed with cotton inlays and saturated with chemicals while the body is embalmed. Remove the inlays, replace with dry cotton and apply mortuary putty during suturing. Incision seal powder will spill from the posterior incisions. A baseball suture is recommended for the length of these incisions. Cover completed incisions with glue and cotton. Plastic stockings are advised when incisions are on the dependent areas of the legs.

### Death from Overdose

Postmortem examination may involve tissue excision of keloid scars (fibrous tissue) formed from repeated use of hypodermic needles in the same tissue area. The size of sample tissue removed may prevent suturing of the area. Cover the area with a saturated chemical compress during embalming. Force dry the tissue with a hairdryer and cover with glue and cotton. Use a plastic garment over the area.

### Partial Autopsy—Cranial Only

The cranial cavity is opened, examined, and the brain is removed during cranial autopsy. Arterial embalming of both the trunk and head can be accomplished by several methods.

#### Method 1

Raise the right and the left common carotid arteries. Insert arterial tubes into both arteries directed toward the head. Also, insert an additional arterial tube into the right common carotid directed toward the trunk. Ligate, or clamp the lower portion of the left common carotid. Insert a drainage instrument into the right internal jugular vein.

Inject the trunk and extremities first. Clamp the right and the left vertebral arteries inside the cranium to prevent loss of arterial solution. The vertebral arteries are branches of the subclavian arteries. Inject upward through both the left and the right carotids to embalm the head; maintain closure of the vertebral arteries to retain solution in the facial tissues.

#### Method 2

Raise only the right common carotid artery for injection and the right internal jugular vein for drainage. Insert one arterial tube toward the head and a second arterial tube toward the trunk. Insert a drainage instrument into the right internal jugular vein. Inject the trunk and extremities first. Clamp the right and left vertebral arteries to prevent solution loss. Clamp the left internal carotid artery to stop solution from entering the head. Inject the right side of the head. Maintain closure of the vertebral arteries to retain solution in the facial tissues.

#### Method 3

Raise the right femoral artery and vein. Insert one arterial tube directed toward the head and the second directed toward the foot. Inject toward the right foot first. Inject toward the head. Clamp the right and left internal carotid arteries and the right and the left vertebral arteries.

### Partial Autopsy—Thoracic Cavity Only

One or more organs may be removed during postmortem examination of the contents of the thoracic cavity.

#### Method 1

Locate the terminal portion of the thoracic aorta on the vertebral column at the central posterior portion of the diaphragm. Insert a large arterial tube into the aorta. Either clamp the arterial tube in place with an arterial hemostat or, ligate the tube in place. Inject downward through the arterial tube. This embalms the abdominal walls, abdominal contents, and lower extremities. Leakage may occur from the right and the left

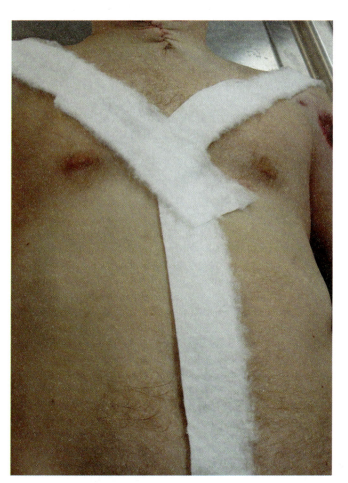

**Figure 17–13.** Trunk sutures covered with glue and cotton.

inferior or superior epigastric arteries. Clamp any leaking vessels to prevent solution loss.

### Method 2
Raise the right femoral artery and insert an arterial tube directed toward the abdomen. Also, insert a tube downward to inject the right leg. Inject the right leg first. Next, inject upward to embalm the left leg, the abdominal contents, and the trunk. Ligate by tying or clamping the thoracic aorta when fluid is observed flowing from this artery into the thoracic cavity.

After arterial injection, check for preservation of the thoracic walls, the back, and the shoulders. If the preservation is inadequate, treat these areas by hypodermic injection. The thoracic cavity can be brushed with autopsy gel and filled with absorbent material. Saturate the cavity before closure with a baseball suture. Complete cavity aspiration is accomplished externally from the standard trocar entry site.

## Partial Autopsy—Abdominal Cavity Only
One or more organs may be removed during postmortem examination of the contents of the abdominal cavity.

### Method 1
To inject the thorax, the upper extremities, and the head, locate the abdominal aorta as it passes through the diaphragm. The aorta can be located at the level of the vertebral column in the central posterior position of the diaphragm. Clamp or ligate an arterial tube into the aorta. Upward injection will embalm the thorax and its contents, the arms, and the head.

### Method 2
Raise the right common carotid artery. Insert a tube upward for the right side of the head. Insert a tube downward. Inject downward toward the trunk; the arms, the thorax, and the left side of the head will receive arterial solution. When leakage is noted from the aorta, clamp or ligate the aorta in the abdominal cavity. After the downward injection, inject the right side of the head.

Check the abdominal walls, the buttocks, and the back for fluid distribution. The location of the pathologist's incision may create leakage from the superior epigastric arteries during injection. Hypodermic injection of solution can be used to preserve the abdominal walls and buttocks. Injection of the male genitalia may also be necessary. The direct injection of both internal iliac arteries will provide good distribution of arterial solution to the buttocks, the genitalia, and the upper thighs. The walls of the cavity can be brushed with autopsy gel and the abdominal cavity filled with absorbent material. The material can be saturated with cavity chemical or other preservative chemical before suturing.

Suture the abdominal incisions using a baseball suture. After final washing and drying of the body glue may be applied to seal the incisions. Aspiration and cavity fluid injection of the thorax can be effective either through the diaphragm or by inserting the trocar through the rib cage. If aspiration and injection are to be done through the external rib cage wall, this treatment can be done before or after the autopsied cavity has been closed by suturing.

# RESTORATIVE TREATMENTS FOR FACIAL TRAUMA
Restoration of the deceased to a natural appearance is one of the primary functions of embalming. Restorative treatments begin in the pre-embalming period and continue throughout embalming. The majority of restorative work is routinely accomplished in the post-embalming period.

The following outline suggests the order of preparation for autopsied bodies that have sustained facial trauma. Two criteria must be met for effect tissue restoration; the tissues of the body must be (1) firm and (2) dry.

In addition to the presence of trauma, other postmortem conditions must be considered. Complete autopsy requires sectional embalming; six injection sites are used to deliver arterial solution to the various regions of the body. Sectional injection allows the embalmer to use different fluids and solution strengths for each area. Facial trauma will necessitate a strong arterial solution to control swelling, dry, and firm tissues. A moderate-strength solution may be desired for the extremities (arms and legs).

1. Sanitize and position the body.
2. Assess the damage to all body areas.
3. Begin with injection of the legs; then inject the arms.
4. Prepare the head and face:
   a. Open the cranial cavity and inspect for bone damage. Inspect the scalp for lacerations or abrasions.
   b. Inspect superficial tissues of the face for punctures, lacerations, abrasions, and hematomas. Debride loose skin to expose undamaged tissues. Excise dehydrated margins of lacerated tissues with a razor or scalpel to expose undamaged tissues.
   c. Apply digital pressure to the surface of the face to inspect for fractures of the mandible, maxillae, and nasal bones, and for the presence of subcutaneous emphysema.
   d. Perform mouth closure. Select a method to align the jaw bones if fractured. Suturing or the needle injector may be required. Temporarily glue the lips to maintain natural closure.
   e. Close the eyes using cotton or eye caps. The lids may be glued prior to injection.
   f. Fill depressed fractures with mortuary putty (mastic compound).
   g. Align lacerated tissues. Temporary bridge sutures using dental floss or super adhesive glue can be used. After embalming, remove the temporary sutures, align the tissues, and apply glue.
   h. Prepare a strong arterial solution using a high-index fluid (30-index and above). Add dye to the arterial solution.
5. Inject the left side of the face first using the instant tissue fixation method. Pulse the solution repeatedly until the tissues firm; stop if swelling begins. Repeat for injection of the right side.

A great volume of solution may leak from damaged tissue areas; leakage will actually reduce tissue swelling.

## CONCEPTS FOR STUDY

Define the following terminology:
- Complete autopsy
- Forensic (medicolegal) autopsy
- Medical (hospital) autopsy
- Partial autopsy
- Viscera
- Y-incision

1. List several types of death that routinely result in forensic autopsy.
2. Recall five reasons forensic autopsies are performed.
3. Relate three functions performed during complete autopsy.
4. State several best practices for autopsy embalming.
5. Outline the treatments for both complete and partial autopsies.
6. Describe one method of arterial injection for cranial only autopsy.
7. Name two sutures commonly used for closure of the scalp after cranial autopsy.
8. Repeat one method for embalming after partial autopsy of the abdominal cavity.
9. Describe preservation demand in autopsied bodies that have undergone mortuary refrigeration.
10. Explain the process of debriding loose skin from the facial areas prior to restoration.

## FIGURE CREDIT

Figures 17–2, 17–7, 17–8 are used with permission of Kevin Drobish. Figures 17–3, 17–4, 17–5, 17–6, 17–9, 17–10, 17–11A-F, 17–12A-E, 17–13 are used with permission of Sharon L. Gee-Mascarello.

## BIBLIOGRAPHY

Altman LK. Sharp drop in autopsies stirs fears that quality of care may also fall. *New York Times*, July 21, 1988.

Altman LK. Diagnosis and the autopsies are found to differ greatly. *New York Times*, October 14, 1998.

DiMaio V, DiMaio D. *Forensic Pathology*, 2nd ed. Boca Raton, FL: CRC Press, 2001.

Ninker R. Ethics goes beyond self-interest. *The Director* 1997; 7:18.

Slocum RE. *Pre-embalming Considerations*. Boston, MA: Dodge Chemical Co.

CHAPTER 18

# Preparation of Organ and Tissue Donors

## CHAPTER OVERVIEW
- Organ and Tissue Donation Defined
- Federal Legislation and Regulations Relating to Donation
- The Donation and Consent Process
- Impact of Donation
- The Moment of Silence
- Recovery and Preparation of Organ, Tissue, and Eye Donors
- Recent Advancements in Surgical Transplants

## ORGAN AND TISSUE DONATION DEFINED

Organ and tissue donation is the process of surgically removing an organ or tissue from one person (*the donor*) and placing it into another person (*the recipient*). The donor may be a **living donor** or a **deceased donor**. An organ is defined as any part of the body exercising a specific function, such as respiration, secretion, and digestion. Commonly transplanted organs include the heart, lungs, liver, kidneys, pancreas, and intestines. Tissue is defined as a collection of similar cells that function together as a unit. Commonly transplanted tissues include the eyes (sclera and corneas), blood vessels, cartilage, skin (partial and full thickness), bone, pericardium, and soft tissues.

Organ and tissue donation usually follows a sudden and unexpected death. The donation and transplantation process involves a complex series of events. Numerous medical professionals and donation and transplant specialists collaborate to accomplish a wide variety of tasks under strict time constraints. Funeral service professionals are key participants as they help families to navigate the donation process and explore options for honoring the donor's life.

## FEDERAL LEGISLATION AND REGULATIONS RELATING TO DONATION

The enactment of federal legislation ensures that equitable distribution of donated organs and tissues proceeds in a fair and efficient manner. The National Organ Procurement and Transplantation Network (OPTN) is established as a national computer registry for the purpose of matching donor organs to waiting recipients. The OPTN is managed by the United Network for Organ Sharing (UNOS). The UNOS cooperates with Organ Procurement Organizations (OPOs) throughout the country to place organs at the local, regional, and national level. Tissue donation is regulated by the U.S. Food and Drug Administration (FDA). There are numerous federal regulations impacting hospital deaths and how hospitals must work with OPOs. Most are contained within the **Conditions of Participation for Hospitals** (*482.45 Condition of Participation Interpretive Guidelines: Organ, Tissue & Eye Procurement*): U.S. Department of Health & Human Services (DHHS) and Centers for Medicare & Medicaid Services (CMS).

## THE DONATION AND CONSENT PROCESS

1. Hospitals must report all deaths to the OPO in a timely manner. This allows the OPO to screen all hospital deaths for the potential for organ, tissue, and eye donation. Timeliness is defined by the hospital; however, CMS recognizes that notification to the OPO within 1 hour is ideal for preserving the opportunity for donation; within 1 hour of clinical triggers being met on vented patients to refer potential organ donors; and within 1 hour of cardiac death to refer potential tissue donors, Nonhospital deaths are typically reported by medical examiners or coroners. Guidance and regulations for referrals of nonhospital deaths vary from state to state.
    a. An individual who is brain dead is on a ventilator and has a beating heart is a potential organ donor: heart, lungs, liver, kidneys, pancreas, and intestine.
    b. An individual that was never on a ventilator, and has no cardiac or respiratory activity is a potential donor for tissues only: eyes/corneas, blood vessels, cartilage, skin, bone, pericardium, and soft tissues.
2. Upon notification of the death or imminent death, the OPO or recovery organization assesses the potential donor's

suitability. The medical evaluation of a potential donor includes a detailed health history and physical assessment.

3. The donor registry is checked to determine if the decedent is a registered donor. The Revised Uniform Anatomical Gift Act (UAGA) is adopted in all 50 states to allow any person 18 years or older, upon their death, to donate their organs and/or tissues for medical purposes. Prior to death, the individual signs a document authorizing the gift; this is known as *first person consent* and is legally binding. If the donor is registered, the recovery organization works with the family to honor their loved one's gift. The UAGA represents a departure from centuries of common-law precedent, which held that a body, immediately after death, became the property of the next-of-kin.

4. When a decedent is not a registered donor and does not have another document of gift, the next-of-kin or authorizing party must consent to donation. The OPO explains the donation process and presents donation options to enable the family to make this decision on behalf of their loved one.

5. With donation consent received and transplant suitability established after comprehensive evaluation, the donor organs and tissues are surgically recovered.

6. The donor organs and tissues recovered are matched to potential recipients and sent to institutions for transplant or preservation.

7. The deceased donor is released to a funeral home for final disposition, as directed by the donor's next-of-kin or legally authorized representative.

## IMPACT OF DONATION

Organ, tissue, and eye donation can pose unique challenges for funeral professionals. The nature and scope of the recovery can impact the embalmer's preparation methods. To maximize the benefit to the greatest number of recipients, every effort is made to recover multiple organs from a single donor. Recovery specialists are sensitive to the role the embalmer plays in providing the type of donor care requested, including open casket presentations. If a specific donation creates an unusual challenge, most recovery organizations have an appointed liaison to address concerns and facilitate acceptable resolution.

OPOs across the country are forming work groups to collaborate with funeral directors and embalmers. These groups produce best practices guides and host educational seminars and forums for their memberships. OPO's are increasingly visible at funeral service conventions. Opening dialogues strengthens appreciation for each entity's role and sustains the allied professional relationship.

Professionals working together to honor the gift of donation and in support of the donor family can yield productive healing. Recent studies regarding the attitudes of donor families demonstrate that when the entire donation process, including funeral arrangements and services, is handled with care and sensitivity, donor families can achieve immediate and long-term benefits. Knowing that some good has resulted from the death can be comforting. For virtually all, the donation of self is the ultimate gift and affirms their loved one's fundamental humanity and generosity.

## THE MOMENT OF SILENCE

Teams of recovery specialists affirm the sanctity of the gift by offering a moment of silence at the beginning of every procurement. Many embalmers have co-opted this gesture to honor the donor in their own preparation rooms.

## RECOVERY AND PREPARATION OF ORGAN DONORS

Several types of surgical incisions are used to access the internal anatomy for organ recovery. The full median sternotomy is a complete midline incision from the xiphoid process to the pubic bone (**Fig. 18–1**). The midline incision is versatile and allows access to most organs. U- and V-incisions resemble their respective letters of the alphabet (**Fig. 18–2**). The tissue flap created by the incision is reflected to allow the specialist full access to the cavities during organ recovery (**Fig. 18–3**). The recovered heart from this donor is placed in normal saline and sent to the processor for further dissection to produce transplantable heart valve grafts (**Fig. 18–4**).

The preparation of organ donors is similar in many ways to embalming the complete trunk autopsy. The incisions for organ recovery bear similarity to the standard Y-incision used for trunk autopsy. Both provide internal access to the vessels for arterial embalming. Supplemental treatments such as hypodermic and surface embalming are routine. And each requires restoration of the cavities and control of any residual leakage after embalming. Delay between death and embalming in both cases

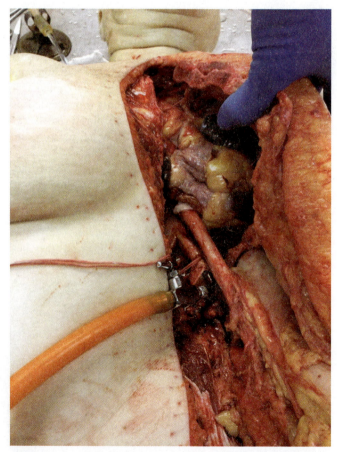

**Figure 18–1.** Midline incision. Injection of abdominal aorta in multiple organ donor. The heart was not recovered.

CHAPTER 18 • Preparation of Organ and Tissue Donors 265

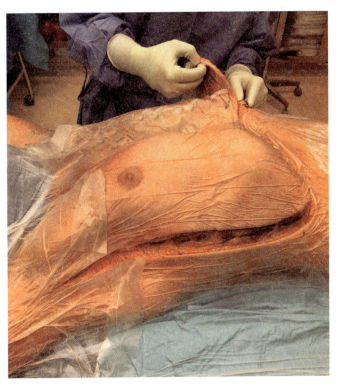

Figure 18-2. U-incision for recovery of costal cartilage, pericardium, and heart for valve grafts.

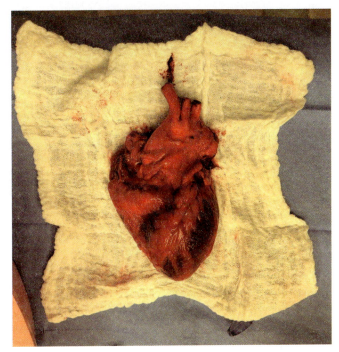

Figure 18-4. Recovered heart for valve grafts.

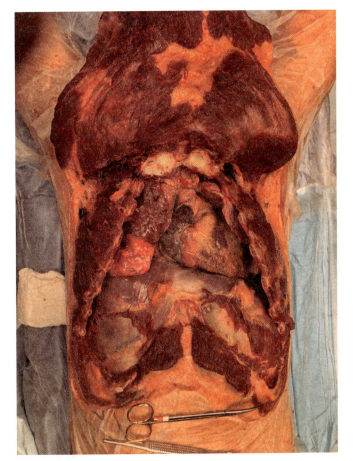

Figure 18-3. Skin reflected to expose thoracic organs: heart, lungs, and diaphragm are intact.

necessitates a higher index, concentrated embalming solution. Tracer dye is used to indicate which areas are not receiving adequate solution. Thorough blood drainage can be expected in both cases (the organ donor is administered a blood-thinning agent presurgically while much of the blood is absent following autopsy).

The embalming process begins with removing temporary sutures binding the incision at the recovery site. Internal access allows the embalmer to evaluate the scope of the recovery and determine which organs have been recovered. This information is documented on Embalming and Decedent Care Report. Suitable vessels are next identified for embalming the donor. Long suture ties are routinely placed on major vessels by the recovery specialist and left in place to benefit the embalmer.

Unlike the complete trunk autopsy, some organs and internal structures may remain intact in the donor. Complete assessment of the remaining anatomy is crucial to successful embalming. The following vessels are suggested. The remaining length of each artery will determine the optimal point for insertion of the arterial tube.

- Inject the left and right subclavian arteries to embalm the arms and shoulders.
- Inject the left and right common carotid arteries to embalm the head.
  - If the abdominal aorta is intact or the brachiocephalic artery (at the level of the aortic arch), either vessel can be used to inject the right side of the head, right shoulder, and arm simultaneously.
- Inject the left and right common iliac artery when intact, or both external and internal iliac arteries, to embalm the legs.
  - If the abdominal aorta is intact, this vessel may be used to embalm the trunk walls and legs simultaneously.
- The vena cava is ideal for blood drainage. Companion veins can also be opened for blood drainage. Blood and fluid

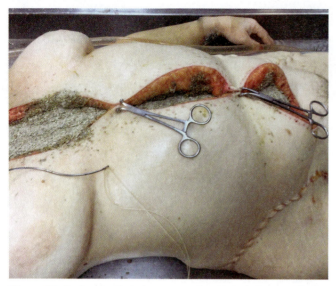

**Figure 18–5.** Post-embalming restoration. Embalming powders added and midline incision aligned and secured with gathering forceps prior to suturing.

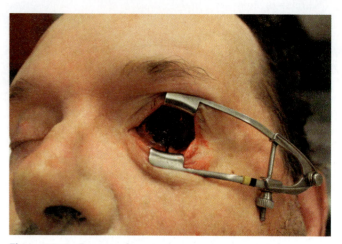

**Figure 18–6.** Eye speculum.

discharge should be aspirated regularly to reduce fumes and maintain clear visibility.

- External incisions may be necessary to locate arteries nearest to insufficiently embalmed distal areas such as the arms and hands (axillary, brachial, radial, ulnar) and the legs and feet (femoral, popliteal, anterior and posterior tibial, dorsalis pedis).

After arterial injection is complete, the use of hypodermic injection and surface embalming (compresses and/or inlays) is recommended for optimal preservation. Cavity aspiration and injection of cavity fluid may be completed after suturing. Multiple organ recovery may warrant the placement of drying, hardening, and preservative compounds into the body cavities prior to suturing (**Fig. 18–5**). The baseball suture can be intermittently locked along lengthy runs. This can prevent the incision from opening should the suture cord fail. Cover the closure with incision seal and cotton. Dress the donor in a plastic garment, such as a coverall or shirt-jacket to fully cover the recovery area. Add an absorbent powder to the garment to address condensation or minor residual leakage.

# RECOVERY AND PREPARATION OF TISSUE DONORS—EYES

## Recovery of Eyes for Corneal and Scleral Transplant

The cornea is the clear, dome-shaped tissue covering the front of the eye; often called the *lens*. The sclera is the white portion of the eye. The entire eye may be recovered for research and education on conditions such as glaucoma, macular degeneration, and diabetic retinopathy, but only the sclera and cornea can be transplanted. The cornea by itself may be recovered, or the entire eye globe is recovered. The full recovery is called eye **enucleation**. The corneal transplant is the world's oldest human transplant procedure; the first transplant was performed in 1905. Today, corneas are the most frequently transplanted tissues. For patients with corneal abrasions or clouding, or with rare keratoconus, a condition causing a cone-shaped cornea, transplant has a 90% success rate of restored vision. The sclera of the eye is used to implant glaucoma filters and in eyelid reconstruction. The sclera is also used in ocular implantation to wrap the recipient's prosthetic eye. The muscles are then attached to the donor sclera to allow the artificial eye to move with the companion eye.

To facilitate recovery of eyes, the facial area is sterilely draped. The head of the donor is kept elevated during the entire process to decrease blood pooling behind the eyes and to reduce periorbital swelling and bruising. The recovery specialist uses an instrument called a *speculum* to fully open the lids (**Fig. 18–6**). After the cornea or globe is recovered, the specialist fills the orbital cavity with cotton, inserts an eye cap, and gently closes the lid in preparation for transportation to the funeral home.

### Embalming Best Practices for Eye Donors

Apply a thin layer of massage cream or lanolin spray, using a soft brush or fingertips, to the tissues surrounding the eye. This serves as a barrier to prevent drying of facial tissues caused by excess embalming solutions draining from the eye orbit.

- Remove the eye cap and cotton packing from the orbit using spring forceps. Avoid overstretching the eyelids, which could damage the soft tissues (**Fig. 18–7**).
- Replace cotton saturated with preservative gel in the same manner. Loosely fill the orbital cavity to encourage some

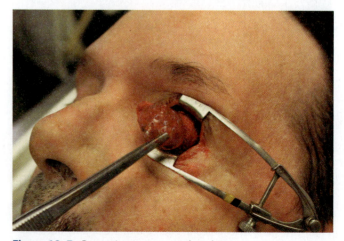

**Figure 18–7.** Removing eye cap and packing.

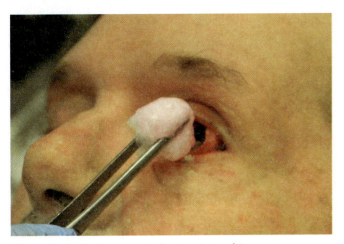

Figure 18-8. Placing saturated cotton into orbit.

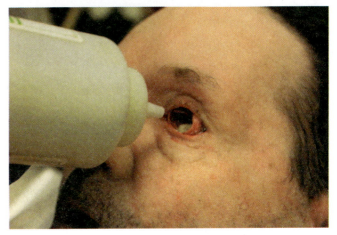

Figure 18-10. Placing incision seal powder into orbit.

leakage of embalming solution to prevent swelling of the eyelids and orbital tissues (**Fig. 18-8**).
- Insert an eye cap over the cotton to recreate the natural appearance of the closed eye (**Fig. 18-9**).
- Complete the arterial embalming (see sections **Fluid Selection** and **Arterial Injection Methods**).
- Remove eye cap and saturated cotton following arterial embalming.
- Dry and cauterize the orbital cavity.
- Embed a trocar button into the base of the orbit.
- Gently exercise the lid from beneath to increase flexibility for proper closure.
  - Select a rounded tip instrument to avoid damaging the fragile tissues.
- Place incision seal powder into the base of the orbit (**Fig. 18-10**).
- Fill the cavity with mastic compound or tightly packed cotton.
- Insert an eye cap (**Fig. 18-11**).
- Establish proper eye closure (**Fig. 18-12**).
  - Upper lid represents 2/3 and lower lid 1/3 of closed eye.
  - Center of eye is highest prominence. Check profile height by resting a flat instrument from eyebrow to cheek.
- Secure line of closure with an adhesive cream or glue.

- Apply a thin coating of lanolin spray to the eyelids and surrounding tissues to prevent dehydration and lid separation.
- Maintain head elevation (**Fig. 18-13**).

A 10-step illustration is provided for embalming and restoration of the eye donor (**Fig. 18-14**).

### Fluid Selection

Select a medium- to high-index arterial chemical to create a moderate to strong solution strength (2–4%). Fluid choice should meet preservative demands and also achieve tissue pliability to maintain natural facial contour. A co-injection fluid is recommended to replace some of the added water, maintain the overall solution strength, and reduce overall harshness of the formulation. Pre-injection and humectant fluids may not be suitable to achieve the necessary drying and firming of eye tissues.

### Arterial Injection Methods

#### Restricted Cervical Injection

Among the numerous benefits of restricted cervical injection (RCI) is the ability to restrict the volume of embalming solution reaching the head and eye tissues. This can alleviate swelling around the eyes during injection of the trunk and extremities. Note that RCI is incompatible with autopsy and multiple organ recovery.

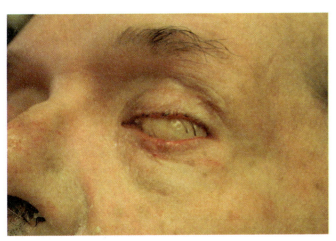

Figure 18-9. Placing new eye cap prior to embalming.

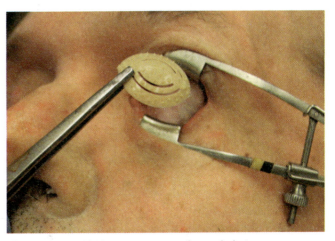

Figure 18-11. Placing new eye cap after embalming.

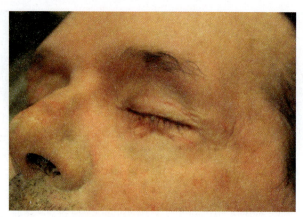

**Figure 18–12.** Closed eye.

- Inject the right common carotid artery toward the trunk and extremities.
  - Allow embalming solution to drain freely from the recovery site.
  - Lower injection pressure and/or rate of flow if eye tissues begin to distend.
  - Evaluate the trunk and extremities for sufficient distribution of solution.

Perform sectional embalming of the extremities, as needed, before injection toward the head. Solution can still reach the eye tissues when embalming from additional sites.

- Inject toward the head.
  - Inject the left side of the face using the left common carotid artery.
    - Allow embalming solution to drain freely from the recovery site.
    - Lower injection pressure and/or rate of flow if eye tissues begin to distend.
  - Inject the right, viewing side of the face, using the right common carotid artery.
    - Allow embalming solution to drain freely from the recovery site.
    - Lower the pressure and/or rate of flow if eye tissues begin to distend.
- Evaluate both eyes for symmetry; minor re-injection of one or both arteries may be necessary to achieve this.

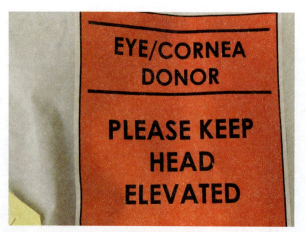

**Figure 18–13.** Eye donor notification label.

### Instant Tissue Fixation

Instant tissue fixation (ITF) is a high-pressure injection method designed to maximize preservation and minimize swelling. ITF is compatible with injection toward the head to prevent eye distension. Co-injection is supplemented in place of water to make a high-strength waterless (no added water) solution. A minimal volume is injected in a burst-rest pattern. The vessel is expanded quickly during the burst phase, creating intravascular pressure; the solution diffuses slowly during the rest phase.

### Corrective Treatments for Eye Distension

#### Surface Compresses

The weight from a wet cotton compress applied overtop the orbital cavity can alleviate swelling during and after injection. The cotton must remain fully saturated with water for optimal effectiveness.

### Surface Embalming

A chemical compress saturated with a gel or liquid cauterant, or cavity fluid, can also be effective in drying and reducing swollen eye tissues.

### Operative Aids: Tissue Channeling and Tissue Reducing Spatula

Channeling the affected tissues with a hypodermic needle and gently applying periorbital pressure can relieve the swollen tissues of accumulated fluids. Avoid over manipulation of the eyelids to prevent minor tearing; surface discoloration marks may appear later where fragile tissues have been damaged. Severe distension may require the use of a tissue-reducing spatula. Also called an *electric* or *heat spatula*. This electric-powered device resembling a hair curling iron reduces tissue moisture by direct application of the heated tip to the affected area. The threaded attachment tips come in a variety of shapes and sizes.

## RECOVERY AND PREPARATION OF TISSUE DONORS—SKIN

### Recovery of Split-Thickness and Full-Thickness Skin

Partial or split-thickness skin recovery is achieved using a surgical instrument called a dermatome. The dermatome removes very thin layers of skin approximately 10–20/1000 of an inch thick and approximately 4 inches wide. These layers resemble the tissue paper-like skin overlying a blister. In patients who have suffered extensive burns, split-thickness skin serves as a human bandage to decrease the potential for infection, help the body to maintain temperature and decrease fluid loss. Split-thickness skin may be recovered from both the anterior and posterior sides of the body. Full-thickness skin grafts are recovered by the free-hand method. Recovery sites include, but are not limited to, the abdomen (**Fig. 18–15**), back, and thighs (**Fig. 18–16**). Both the dermal and adipose layers are recovered down to the muscle layer. Full-thickness skin retains more of the patient's skin characteristics, including color, texture, and

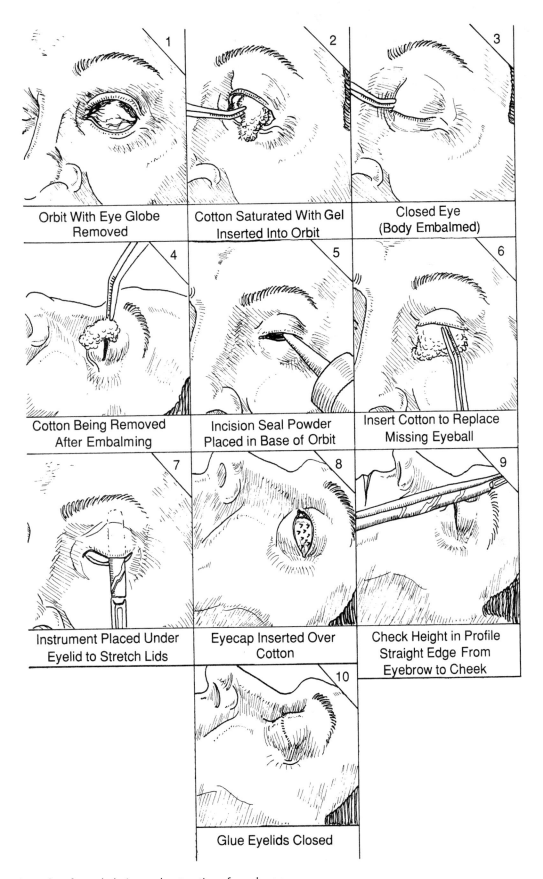

**Figure 18–14.** Procedure for embalming and restoration of eye donor.

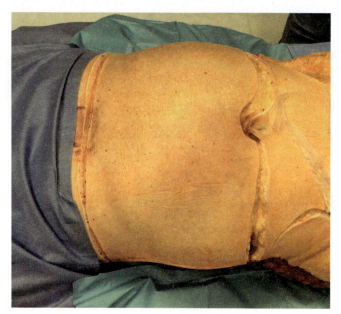

**Figure 18–15.** Surgical margins shown for recovery of full-thickness abdominal skin.

thickness. For this reason, full-thickness grafts provide better outcomes for facial, joint, and hand wounds. In addition, the benefit of full-thickness transplants in children is the likelihood that the skin will grow along with the child. Large sections of full-thickness skin are needed for structural support in the repair of large abdominal hernias and to fill soft tissue defects caused by extensive trauma or invasive cancer surgery.

To facilitate full-thickness back skin recovery, the donor is placed in the prone position (flat and face downward). The recovery site is shaved and disinfected with a series of preoperative skin solutions (**Fig. 18–17**). Surgical draping exposes only the skin that is intended for recovery (**Fig. 18–18**). According to need, the specialist may recover only to the level of the adipose or continue to the muscle layer (**Fig. 18–19**). Postrecovery the donor is bathed and placed upon a large absorbent pad inside of the body bag. Many OPO's provide a supportive care product kit to benefit the embalmer. Supportive care kits usually contain an additional absorbent pad, topical preservative gel, and plastic garment such as a unionall.

Preparation of the tissue donor presents the embalmer with three main objectives: (1) Pre-embalming inspection, drying, and treatment of the tissue recovery areas; (2) clearing of any facial discolorations during embalming that may have been caused while the donor was in a prone position during the recovery; and (3) post-embalming control of any demonstrable leakage from the recovered areas.

### Embalming Best Practices for Tissue Donors

Two persons are recommended for transfer to and from the embalming table and to roll the donor during inspection and treatment of tissues recovered from posterior areas.

- Place plastic sheeting on the embalming table and position an absorbent pad in the center of the plastic.
- Transfer the donor to the embalming table.
- Roll the donor to one side and treat the recovery site with a phenol-based liquid or gel (**Fig. 18–20**).
- Lower the donor onto the pad. Adjust the pad placement to ensure contact with the recovery site.
- Proceed with arterial embalming. Select a higher index arterial fluid and mix in a moderate to strong concentrated solution (hypertonic solution of 2% and above) for desired drying of tissues.
- During injection, some embalming solution will weep from the dependent site onto the pad. Allow the pad to remain in place throughout the cavity embalming process.
- Roll the donor, remove the pad and plastic sheeting, and inspect for untreated or under embalmed areas.
- Hypodermically treat insufficiently preserved areas.
- Apply a coating of preservative gel over the treated tissues.
  - Raise the donor with body bridges to allow air current to pass beneath or position the donor tilted slightly to one side using body blocks.
  - Allow several hours, or overnight, for tissues to dry.
  - An auxiliary fan or hair dryer directed toward the treated tissues can speed air drying.

Once the tissues are dried:

- Prepare a dressing table by draping plastic sheeting to extend over the sides of the table.
- Place another absorbent pad, or thick cotton, on top of the plastic.
- Transfer the donor to the dressing table.
- Roll the donor to one side and liberally apply an absorbent preservative compound to the pad.
  - Adjust the pad to make full contact as the donor is lowered.
- Pull the plastic sheeting up and around the donor and secure with mortuary tape.
- Dress the donor in a plastic garment that fully covers the area of tissue recovery.
  - Add an absorbent powder to the garment to address condensation or minor residual leakage.

## RECOVERY AND PREPARATION OF TISSUE DONORS—BONE

### Recovery of Bone, Connective Tissue, and Vessels

Lengthy incisions are made to procure bone in both the upper and lower extremities (**Fig. 18–21**). Bone, along with attached cartilage and muscle may be recovered as a whole or *en bloc*. The en bloc surgical procedure is used to preserve continuity

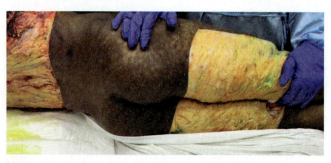

**Figure 18–16.** Recovery of full-thickness skin from back and thighs.

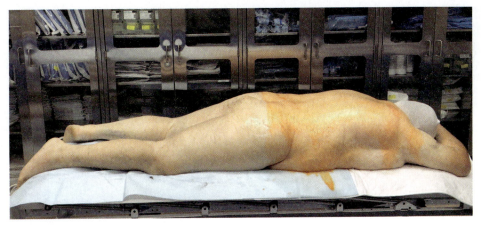

**Figure 18–17.** Preoperative preparation for back skin recovery.

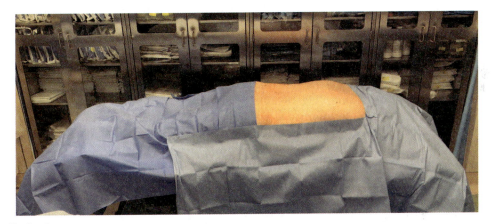

**Figure 18–18.** Sterile draping.

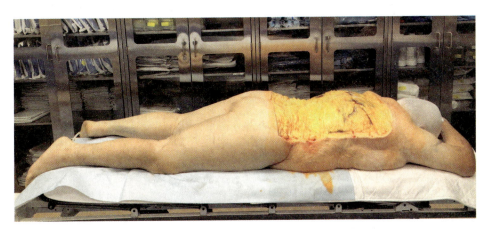

**Figure 18–19.** Post tissue recovery.

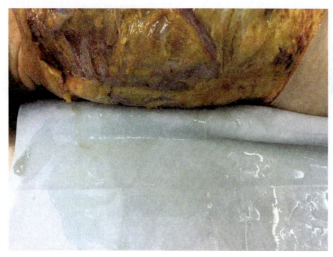

**Figure 18-20.** Absorbent pad with preservative gel.

with adjacent tissues and vessels for better outcomes. Following recovery, a prosthetic device replaces the bone and provides form to the donor limb. Transplanted bone has life-enhancing applications; amputations can be prevented, pain and nerve damage reduced, and mobility restored for its recipients. Some examples of donated bone tissue include humerus, femur, tibia, fibula, iliac crest, acetabulum, rib, radius, and ulna (**Fig. 18-22**). A single rib used in mandible repair can restore normal facial appearance. Connective tissues can restore mobility for independence in activities of daily living. Some examples of connective tissues include patellar tendon, Achilles tendon, cartilage, fascia lata, and rotator cuff. Donated saphenous veins restore circulation to the lower extremities impaired by peripheral vascular disease (**Fig. 18-23**). Femoral vessels are often used as superficial dialysis shunts in patients requiring chronic treatment.

## Embalming Best Practices for Long Bone Donors

Long bone recovery is time and labor-intensive for both the procurement team and the embalmer. The extent of the donation will influence the embalming plan. When neither autopsy

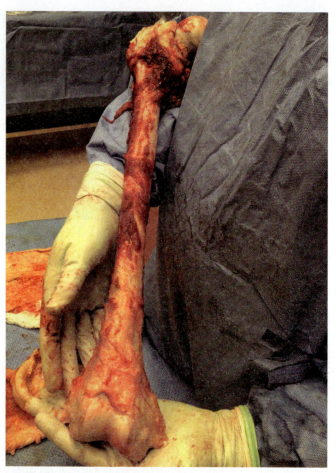

**Figure 18-22.** Recovered femur.

nor organ recovery has occurred, standard embalming injection sites can be used.
- Prior to arterial injection, remove all sutures, open incision sites, and remove the prostheses.
- Evaluate the recovery site for vascular disruption, noting any accessible and/or ligated vessels.
- Drain any residual body fluids before packing the limb with cotton.

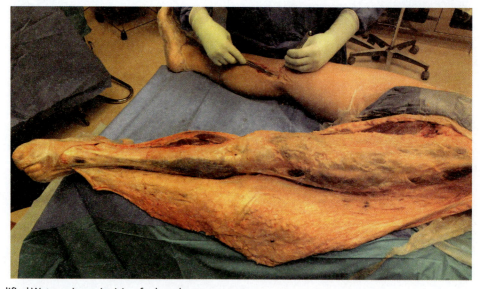

**Figure 18-21.** Modified Watson-Jones incision for long bone recovery.

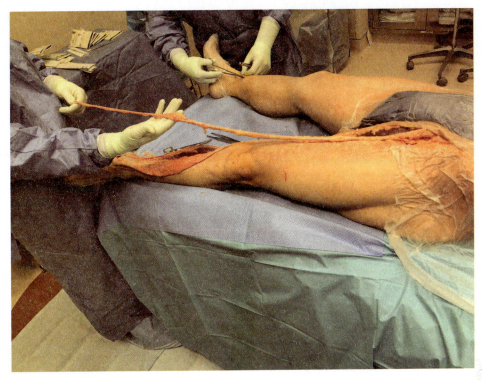

**Figure 18–23.** Saphenous vein recovery.

- Saturate the cotton with a phenol cauterant, cover to reduce fumes, and proceed with injection.
  - Embalming solution will further saturate the cotton as it exits from the vessels incised during recovery.
  - Allow the inlays to remain in place throughout cavity embalming.
- Remove inlays and assess tissue preservation.
  - Hands not affected by recovery can be injected at this time utilizing the radial or ulnar arteries.
  - Identify and clamp any leaking vessels to build intravascular pressure and prevent loss of excessive embalming solution.
- Supplemental hypodermic embalming is indicated for all tissues in the recovery area.
  - Feet not affected by recovery are best embalmed hypodermically.
- Coat tissues with cauterant gel for supplemental surface embalming.
- Replace the prostheses. Secure in place with sutures if needed.
- Apply drying, hardening, and preservative compounds.
- Tightly pack the extremity with cotton to create natural form.
- Align the tissue flaps with multiple bridge sutures or gathering forceps (**Fig. 18–24**).
- Close the recovery site, throwing tight sutures and intermittently locking them along lengthy incisions. Locking sutures prevent the incision from opening should the suture cord fail.
- Cover the closure with incision seal and cotton or an absorbent pad (**Fig. 18–25**).
- Dress the donor in a plastic garment, such as a capri or stockings.

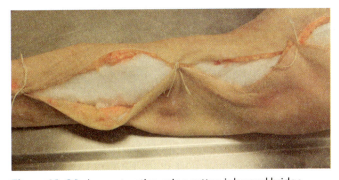

**Figure 18–24.** Leg restoration using cotton inlay and bridge sutures.

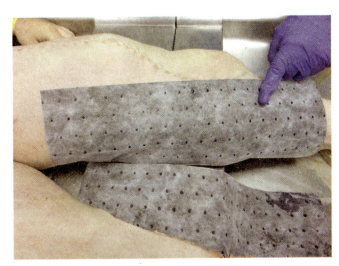

**Figure 18–25.** Absorbent pads.

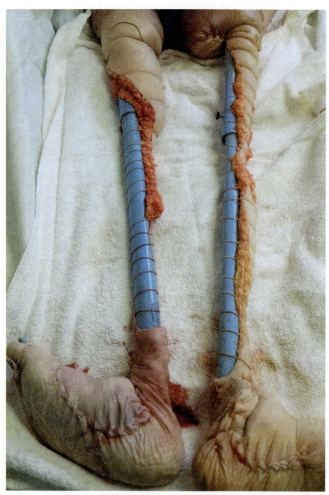

**Figure 18–26.** Full-thickness skin and long bone recovery.

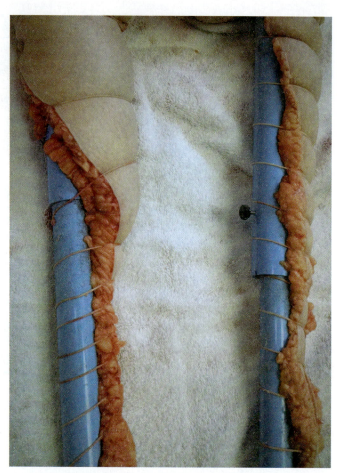

**Figure 18–27.** Prostheses secured to the remaining length of full-thickness skin for structural integrity of the anatomy.

- Add an absorbent powder to the garment to address condensation or minor residual leakage.

Full-thickness skin and long bone recovery of the legs might be viewed as the most dramatic of all multiple tissue recoveries. A thin length of tissue is left intact deliberately, connecting torso to feet to maintain the integrity and the height of the donor (**Fig. 18–26**). The prostheses and tissue are secured together for anatomical and structural integrity (**Fig. 18–27**). Hypodermic and surface embalming techniques are efficient preservation methods for these donors.

## RECENT ADVANCEMENTS IN SURGICAL TRANSPLANTS

Rapid advancements in medical technology continue to change the donation landscape. In late 2020, the first successful face and bilateral hand transplant took place in the United States. This is an example of a vascular composite allograft (VCA); the transplantation of multiple structures that can include skin, bone, muscles, blood vessels, nerves, and connective tissue. Unlike internal organs, face and hands are also matched for size, skin color, gender, and age range. In this case, both hands to the mid-forearm and full facial tissues were recovered from a single donor and received by a single recipient. The 23-hour surgery involved a team of more than 140 health care professionals, led by Eduardo D. Rodriguez, MD, DDS at NYU Langone Health.

Only a few dozen hand transplants and half as many face transplants have ever been attempted in the United States. Worldwide, the only other two combined face and hand transplants were both unsuccessful.

New life-saving and life-enhancing surgeries provide transformative benefits for their recipients. Embalmers can anticipate an ever-increasing number of preparations of organ and tissue donors. The groundbreaking transplant mentioned, utilized state-of-the-art technology. Photographs of the donor's face and arms produced printable three-dimensional (3D) replicas that helped to ease the family's tragic loss while also honoring end-of-life rituals.

## CONCEPTS FOR STUDY

1. Compare similarities between the preparation of an autopsied case and an organ donor.
2. Define vascular composite allograft.
3. List several benefits for recovering multiple organs and tissues from a single donor.
4. Describe the best practices for embalming an eye donor.
5. Describe the best practices for embalming a full-thickness skin donor.
6. Describe the best practices for embalming a long bone donor.
7. Evaluate the benefits of using higher index concentrated solutions to embalm donors.
8. Indicate the benefits of both instant tissue fixation and restricted cervical injection.
9. Explain the role of the funeral professional in the donation process.

## FIGURE CREDIT

Figures 18–1, 18–5, 18–20, 18–25 are used with permission of Duff Chamberlain.
Figures 18–2, 18–3, 18–4, 18–15, 18–17, 18–18, 18–19, 18–21, 18–22, 18–23 are used with permission of Gift of Life Michigan (photographer: Curpri Sanders).
Figures 18–6, 18–7, 18–8, 18–9, 18–10, 18–11, 18–12, 18–16, 18–24 are used with permission of Kevin Drobish.
Figures 18–13, 18–26, 18–27 are used with permission of Sharon L. Gee-Mascarello.

## BIBLIOGRAPHY

American Association of Tissue Banks (AATB)—general information from the web page.

The Dodge Company, booklet—*Best Practice: Preparation of Human Remains Following Tissue Procurement, Practices and Procedures for the Embalmer*, 2019.

Donate Life America—from the web page—*Understand Organ, Eye and Tissue Donation.*

Gift of Life Michigan (GOLM) and Eversight. booklet—*Eye, Organ and Tissue Donation Best Practices.*

Musculoskeletal Transplant Foundation (MTF) booklet—*After the Gift: A Guide to organ and tissue donation for funeral directors*, 2007. And, resource binder—*Embalmer Friendly Recovery Techniques: Keys to Good Recovery Team/Embalmer Relations*, 2011.

# CHAPTER 19

# Delayed Embalming

## CHAPTER OVERVIEW

- Preparation During the Stages of Rigor Mortis
- Preparation Following Mortuary Refrigeration
- Preparation During the Stages of Decomposition
- Advanced Decomposition Protocol

Postmortem changes begin at the moment of death. Embalming can substantially delay the organic decomposition processes that occur naturally after death. Lengthy intervals between death and embalming can exacerbate these postmortem changes. Even refrigerated mortuary shelter does not stop the progression of decomposition entirely. Optimal embalming outcomes with the fewest complications are achieved when embalming is performed within a short time interval following death. In addition to time, intrinsic and extrinsic factors influence the rate of decomposition; a spectrum of factors can speed or slow postmortem changes. Embalming considerations in this chapter include those commonly encountered when there is a delay between death and body preparation:

- Bodies embalmed during the stages of rigor mortis.
- Bodies that have been cooled by mortuary refrigeration.
- Bodies showing early signs of decomposition.
- Bodies in advance stages of decomposition.

Numerous factors are considered during the pre-embalming analysis; a listing of postmortem conditions appears on the Embalming and Decedent Care Report.

1. Conditions present in the body; intrinsic factors such as protein and moisture levels.
2. Cause and manner of death, including underlying conditions.
3. Evidence of conditions related to disease or trauma.
4. Medical therapies, surgeries, medications.
5. Postmortem physical and chemical changes.
6. Time interval between preparation and disposition; and between preparation and final disposition.

Postmortem chemical and physical changes do not occur simultaneously throughout the body. Time delays between death and preparation present three common embalming challenges: nonuniform distribution of embalming solution, tissues that easily swell, and an increased preservative demand.

1. **Nonuniform distribution.** The embalmer can anticipate challenges in achieving uniform distribution of the injected arterial solution. This can be caused by any of the following: the presence of rigor mortis, increased postmortem coagula, increased viscosity of arterial and venous blood, and the breakdown of the capillary network. This results in some areas receiving too much solution and other body areas receiving too little or no arterial solution at all.
2. **Tissues easily swell.** Tissue swelling can occur anywhere; especially in the unsupported tissues of the neck and eyelids, and the facial glands: parotid, submandibular, and submaxillary glands. Bodies dead for long periods of time do not assimilate the arterial solution well.
3. **Increased preservative demand.** The longer decomposition processes can continue, the greater the preservation need. The breakdown of body proteins increases the sites available for attachment of embalming preservative. Decomposition continues until the process is chemically arrested. Time delay between death and embalming allows for the breakdown of body proteins (**Fig. 19-1**). Even in cooler temperatures, decomposition slows but does not stop.

Preservative absorption by tissue proteins is usually greatest immediately after injection. Most bodies exhibit some degree of firming during the injection process. One reason for this early fixation is that the concentration of preservative (fixative) is greatest when the arterial solution is first introduced into the tissues. If a sufficient amount of preservative has been injected, complete firming of the body will occur several hours to a day later. Degree of decomposition, tissue pH, and temperature and concentration of arterial solution all play a role in determining the speed and degree of fixation. Cool temperature slows these reactions; alkaline pH above 7.4 slows fixation; and decomposed proteins will demand more concentrated preservative.

This increased preservative need is brought about by the breakdown of tissues. As circulation is impaired in most of these bodies, distribution challenges can be anticipated. As these bodies are all subject to distension, use of a minimum amount of a stronger arterial solution best establishes good preservation and minimizes tissue distension. Stronger (hypertonic) arterial solutions help to minimize swelling of the tissues.

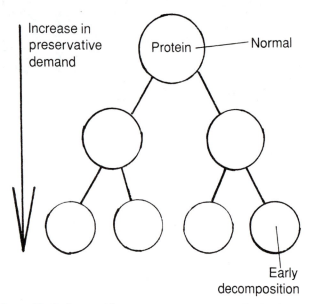

**Figure 19–1.** Demand for preservatives is increased in bodies as protein breaks down.

## MECHANICAL, MANUAL, AND OPERATIVE AIDS

Achieving adequate distribution of the preservative solution with a minimum of tissue swelling is desired. **Manual aids:** lowering hands below the table; squeezing the sides of the fingers and the nailbeds; bending, rotating, and flexing of limbs; and massaging the dependent areas help to distribute the arterial solution. **Mechanical aids:** drainage instruments, injection pressure, pulsation, rate of flow adjustments, and diameter of the arterial tube help to control the speed and volume of embalming solution.

When localized swelling of unsupported tissues such as the eyelids or neck occurs, **operative aids:** invasive treatments such as channeling, wicking, incising, and excising tissues are used for correction. Manual aids can also correct minor swelling: elevation of the affected area, chemical compresses to dry the wet tissues, water compresses, and pneumatic collars.

## GENERAL EMBALMING TREATMENTS INJECTION PROTOCOL

> **EMBALMING OF A BODY INVOLVES FOUR STEPS**
> 1. Observation of the body
> 2. Evaluation of the conditions present
> 3. Implementation of an injection and drainage plan
> 4. Observation of the results achieved

Throughout the process of arterial injection, the embalmer asks the following questions to evaluate the degree of preservation:
1. Which body areas are receiving arterial solution and which are not?
2. What can be done to stimulate arterial solution into body areas where the arterial solution is not being distributed?
3. Is there sufficient arterial solution volume in all body areas?

For underembalmed areas, the embalmer has three choices: (1) arterial injection, (2) hypodermic embalming, and (3) surface embalming.

Restricted cervical or six-point injection are the optimal choices for delayed embalming. One-point injection is not recommended; the volume of solution entering the head is difficult to control when a single injection site is employed.

### Restricted Cervical Injection

First, inject the trunk and limb areas. **Be certain that the arterial tubes directed toward the head remain open during injection of the trunk.** Arterial solution that has reached the face and head by collateral routes will exit from the arterial tubes to prevent overinjection of the head. Inject the head last; left side then right side. If purge develops during trunk injection, the RCI method allows the features to be set and the body to be aspirated **before** the head is injected.

### Six-Point Injection

Raise all six arteries; both left and right common carotid, axillary, and femoral vessels. In order, from left to right, inject the legs, the arms, the trunk, and the head. If purge develops, the body can be aspirated and the features set before the head is injected. Drainage can be taken from each accompanying vein as well as the right internal jugular vein.

### Autopsied Remains

If the body has been autopsied, the six-point or multisite injection is standard. Drainage occurs passively into the cavities.

> **FACTORS DETERMINED BY THE EMBALMING ANALYSIS**
> 1. Vessels for injection and drainage
> 2. Method of mouth closure
> 3. Strength of the embalming solution
> 4. Volume of the embalming solution
> 5. Injection pressure
> 6. Injection rate of flow
> 
> *Note:* These factors will vary by the individual body and can vary in different areas of the same body.

### Arterial Solution Strength and Volume

A moderate to strong well-coordinated arterial solution is needed when decomposition is evident and when the body is in the active stage of rigor. 30-index and above arterial fluids are recommended. Special-purpose fluids are also recommended for difficult cases. Co-injection fluids work synergistically with the arterial fluid to produce optimal results. The first half-gallon injected can be less strong to clear blood discolorations. Hypertonic solutions, 2.0% strength and higher can follow. Waterless solutions may be used effectively. Additional dye indicates distribution, or not, of arterial solution. Dye helps to prevent graying of embalmed tissues. For extreme cases, the **instant tissue fixation** method is recommended to minimize tissue swelling and provide maximum preservation. The total volume of solution depends on body mass as well as the intrinsic and extrinsic factors considered during analysis. The effectiveness of arterial solution distribution influences the volume injected as well.

## Pressure and Rate of Flow

When there has been a lengthy delay between death and embalming, inject solution *slowly*. Slower injection helps to prevent coagula in the arterial system from moving into and blocking the smaller distal arteries. Rapid injection can cause intestinal distension, which creates internal pressure upon the contents of the stomach and results in purge.

During sectional injection of the arms and legs in the autopsied body, higher pressures and faster rates of flow may be needed to establish distribution. Tissue distension can be controlled easily. The pulsation setting on the embalming machine is effective in distributing fluid to the extremities; higher pressures can be used with pulsation. A pulsed flow can be created manually by turning the rate of flow valve on and off, turning the stopcock valve on and off, and by bending and unbending the delivery hose to start and stop the delivery of fluid.

## PREPARATION OF BODIES IN RIGOR MORTIS

Rigor mortis is the postmortem stiffening of muscles. Embalming a body in the intense state of **rigor mortis** is challenging. Particularly when well-developed musculature is observed. These bodies develop intense rigor mortis. Fully established rigor is difficult to relieve when large amounts of muscle protein are affected. Rigor is more easily relieved in bodies with underdeveloped musculature and those with low protein content. **Cachexia** is an example of a wasting disease that reduces muscle protein.

Rigor mortis affects all muscles in the body, some more noticeably than others. Rigor begins when the body cannot replenish adenosine triphosphate (ATP). Any activity that reduces ATP prior to death will speed the onset of rigor. Rigor rapidly occurs in bodies with elevated temperatures such as when physical exertion or exercise preceded death. In sudden death, rigor can occur in the form of cadaveric spasms. Rigor mortis is recognized within the first 2–4 hours following death. Within 6–12 hours, it is fully established. Rigor passes in approximately 36 hours following death. The adage, "the sooner the onset, the sooner the passage" holds truth. Depending on cause of death, environmental temperature, and activity prior to death, the rigor can occur sooner or be delayed. It is easy to see how easily this postmortem change varies from body to body. The passage of rigor is indicative of the start of the decomposition cycle.

Rigor comprises three general stages: (1) primary flaccidity, the period in which the rigor develops and is hardly noticeable, (2) the active period of rigor, and (3) secondary flaccidity, in which the rigor has passed from the body. The most challenges are encountered when the body is to be embalmed while in intense rigor.

**Table 19-1** summarizes the preservative demand of the muscle tissues during the stages of rigor.

Preservative demand during primary flaccidity, the period before the onset of rigor, is related to the postmortem conditions observed during the embalming analysis; rigor is not a factor. Bodies embalmed during and after rigor mortis have a higher preservative demand. A body in an active state of rigor absorbs very little preservative; higher strengths and volumes of solution are necessary to compensate for the poor absorption. Once rigor passes, indicated by secondary flaccidity, the demand for preservative increases greatly. Saturate the tissues with a well-coordinated solution of sufficient strength to meet the preservative demands of the body when rigor has passed. Otherwise, the tissues will soften as decomposition progresses.

**TABLE 19–1. Preservative Demand of the Muscle Tissues During Rigor**

| | | |
|---|---|---|
| Pre-rigor | Great absorption of preservative | The protein centers to which preservative attaches and cross-links the proteins are readily available. Tissue pH is slightly alkaline and fluids work best in this pH range. |
| Active rigor | Little absorption of preservative | The protein centers to which preservative attaches are engaged in maintaining the state of rigor mortis; vessel lumens are reduced so distribution is decreased. Muscle protein is contracted so fluid does not penetrate the muscle fibers well. The acidic pH retards the absorption of preservative. |
| Post-rigor | Great preservative demand | Proteins have disorganized (or broken) and many centers are available for preservative attachment. The alkaline pH increases preservative absorption; nitrogenous wastes increase the need for preservative. |

### Challenges Associated with Embalming

#### Bodies in Rigor

Rigor may be relieved by physical manipulation of the muscle tissues and joints of the extremities. Firmly massaging, rotating, flexing, and bending the joints help to relieve the rigor condition. **Once relieved, the condition does not recur**. In persons with a well-developed musculature, it may be very difficult to relieve rigor in the firmly abducted arms. The following challenges may also be encountered in the preparation of the body in active and intense rigor:

- Positioning challenges are expected.
- Features may be difficult to set when the jaw is firmly fixed. Opening and packing the throat may not be possible.
- Distribution of fluid may be poor due to extravascular pressure upon arteries; narrowed lumens result from contraction of muscle cells in the arterial walls.
- Drainage may be poor due to extravascular pressure upon the small veins.
- Tissues easily swell; solution follows the path of least resistance.
- The pH of the tissues is not ideal for fluid reactions.
- Tissues may not firm well after the passage of rigor due to poor absorption during rigor and lack of sufficient volume of arterial solution injected.
- Tissue firmness caused by rigor can be a false sign of tissue fixation by the preservative.

#### Other Considerations for Bodies in Rigor Mortis

During active rigor, the pH of the tissues is slightly acidic. It has been found that the preservative protein reaction occurs most readily at slightly basic pH, about the same as that of normal, healthy tissues (7.38–7.4). Also, pH values will not be the same in the various muscles. Where rigor has passed from the muscles, autolysis and hydrolysis have proceeded to a point where protein has decomposed and the pH has become increasingly alkaline (basic).

Increase of tissue pH into the alkaline range after rigor mortis has passed, indicates that the muscle proteins have begun to break down or decompose. There are now additional sites for reaction with preservative. During rigor, there are few sites for the reaction of preservative and proteins. A body embalmed during rigor should be saturated with sufficient preservative, so that it will be available later as the state of rigor passes. Rigor and varying pH challenge uniform preservation of the body.

> **BODIES IN RIGOR MORTIS**
> Degree of rigor varies within different muscle groups.
> Tissue pH varies throughout the body.
> Lack of uniform solution distribution.
> Preservative demand varies in the different tissues.

As the absorption of preservative results in firming, there is a relationship between the rate of preservative absorption by tissues and the rate of firming. This is why bodies embalmed prior to the onset of rigor rapidly firm; preservative is rapidly absorbed and rapidly attaches to the proteins. During rigor, the proteins are "locked" together, and it is difficult for the preservative to attach to the proteins. As a result, there is little absorption of preservative by muscles in the active state of rigor mortis. Most of the firming that occurs during injection is caused by the swelling of the tissues. If a mild or a weak arterial solution is used, underembalmed tissues will later soften. After the passage of rigor, demand for preservative increases greatly.

In addition to selecting strong embalming fluids, a high strength solution includes the addition of co-injection fluids. The supplemental co-injection fluid adjusts tissue pH, buffers the arterial fluids, and promotes uniform distribution and diffusion of the preservative. Co-injections modify the harshness of the arterial fluid for better absorption. The strength of the solution is not altered by the addition of co-injection.

Preservative Absorption and Firming

| | | |
|---|---|---|
| Pre-rigor | Good absorption | Firming is good |
| Active rigor | Poor absorption | Firming is due to tissue swelling |
| Post-rigor | Good absorption | Firming is difficult to achieve |

Tissue firmness cannot be relied on as an exclusive measure of preservation; firmness may only indicate muscle-stiffening caused by the rigor. As rigor is relieved through bending, flexing, and rotating the limbs, capillary beds can become damaged and cause tissue swelling. Distended tissues that feel firm to the touch could be mistaken for tissues that are embalmed.

## Feature Setting of the Mouth

Massage of the soft tissues at the temporomandibular joint and the temporalis muscles can be effective in relieving rigor that has firmly set the jaw. Press the chin firmly upward with the palm of the hand to exercise the joint. A slight parting of the teeth will allow placement of packing material into the throat using long forceps. When the mouth can be fully opened for sanitation and packing, use a suture closure or needle injector to align and secure the jaw.

### Body Positioning

Firmly rotate, bend, flex, and massage the joints and muscles of the neck, arms, and legs. Rigor in the neck is relieved by moving the head back and forth and rotating side to side. Relieve rigor in the arms by rotating the joints of the shoulders, elbows, and wrists, and bending and flexing the fingers. Grasp all fingers together and gently straighten them. To relieve rigor in the legs, exercise the hip joint and bend and flex the knee joint. Rotate feet side to side.

### Arterial Injection

Restricted cervical or a six-point injection may be needed to thoroughly embalm bodies during rigor mortis. The right internal jugular vein is the most suitable drainage site. If a six-point injection is used in addition to the right internal jugular, drainage can also be taken from accompanying veins. Clear blood discolorations first by injecting a milder solution (such as 1.5%) then meet preservative demands by increasing the solution strength (above 2%). Dye and co-injection fluid can be added to the solution. The extra dye serves as a tracer and prevents tissue graying. In the embalming of these bodies, blood drainage is often minimal and formaldehyde gray can easily develop hours after embalming. The co-injection fluid assists in fluid penetration and adjustment of tissue pH. The dye merely indicates that surface tissues have received fluid; dye cannot indicate effect on the deeper tissues.

Inject slowly. During arterial injection, continue massage and manipulation of the limbs to encourage distribution. When drainage is established, the injection speed can be slightly increased to encourage better distribution. If a six-point injection is used, higher pressure and rate of flow can be used for direct injection of the limbs. Pulsation assists in distribution of the solution. This technique may prove effective for injection of an autopsied body in intense rigor mortis. Waterless embalming uses a minimum volume of a very strong solution to reduce tissue swelling and achieve overall preservation.

## PREPARATION OF REFRIGERATED BODIES

Short-term mortuary refrigeration is necessary to suspend naturally occurring postmortem changes. Most bodies transferred from medical or forensic institutions have undergone refrigeration for some length of time. While cool temperatures slow the cycle of decomposition, refrigeration does not halt the process entirely. Numerous decomposition changes are often evident in bodies refrigerated for lengthy intervals (**Fig. 19–2**).

The embalmer can overcome many challenges presented by decomposition. Thorough embalming, coupled with feature restoration and cosmetic application can produce acceptable results (**Fig. 19–3**).

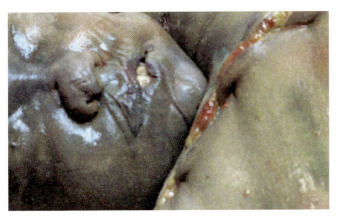

**Figure 19-2.** Decomposition evident in autopsied body following long-term mortuary refrigeration.

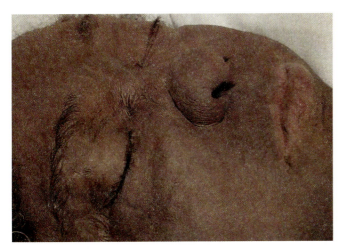

**Figure 19-3.** Restoration of decomposed body for viewing.

Some advantages of short-term refrigeration include (1) slows the progression of rigor mortis, (2) slows decomposition, and (3) maintains blood in a liquid state. Long-term refrigeration can present a number of challenges for the embalmer.

Prior to the routine use of body bags, tissue dehydration was a common condition. When bodies were wrapped in cotton sheets and refrigerated, surface dehydration occurred readily. Lips, eyes, and fingertips were noticeably affected by moisture loss. Plastic body pouches prevent excessive dehydration, but do not completely stop moisture from leaving the tissues. Instead, the plastic enclosure traps body heat and moisture. As the core temperature of the body cools, condensation forms within the bag. Desquamation, discolorations, and gas accumulation in the body cavities are accelerated by trapped heat and moisture in the pouch. Both types of body coverings present disadvantages over time.

There is usually a slight elevation of body temperature after death (postmortem caloricity) because metabolism continues until the oxygen surplus is exhausted. As the blood no longer circulates, the heat produced by the catabolic phase of metabolism is trapped in the body, causing the temperature to increase. Heat speeds the cycles of rigor mortis and decomposition. The greenish discoloration outlining the abdomen is a common indicator of decomposition. Autolysis and bacterial activity continue during refrigeration, faster while the body is still warm; slower as the tissues gradually cool. **Figure 19-4** illustrates some of the challenges associated with refrigeration.

Disadvantageous of long-term mortuary refrigeration using plastic body pouches:

- Increased capillary permeability.
- Rupture of capillaries during arterial injection.
- Tissue structure breakdown (result of autolysis and bacterial enzymes).
- Increased coagula in the vascular system; increased blood viscosity.

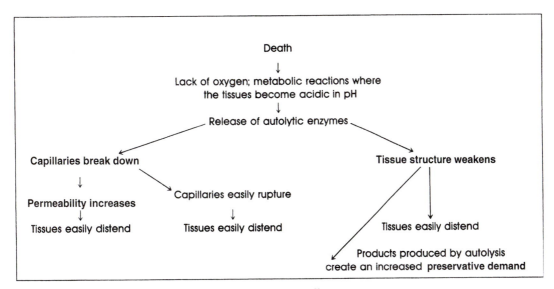

**Figure 19-4.** Challenges associated with refrigeration: time–temperature effects.

- Gravitation of blood and body liquids into the dependent body tissues; skeletal edema.
- Intense livor mortis.
- Rapid hemolysis; postmortem extravascular stain.
- Decomposition changes: discolorations, gas accumulation, purge, skin slip.
- Rapid distension of abdominal organs during injection, resulting in stomach and/or lung purge.
- Refrigerated tissues can be easily mistaken for embalmed tissues; firm to the touch and the hemolysis of red blood cells create a cosmetic effect.

Blood gravitates to dependent areas. Blood thinners and cooling of the body both contribute to the hypostasis of the blood. In refrigerated bodies, livor mortis can be intense. Postmortem stain can rapidly occur and petechiae and purpura (Tardieu spots) are common. As the body cools, hemolysis easily occurs, causing the blood cells to rupture and release **heme** into the tissues. Heme is the deep red, iron-containing component of blood. This results in **postmortem staining**. Extravascular blood discolorations cannot be removed by arterial injection and blood drainage. When elevation of the head is not maintained, discolorations can affect facial tissues. Some bleaching is possible with the use of a strong arterial solution, a bleaching co-injection fluid, and surface compresses of bleaching agents. Postmortem stain and the Tardieu spots can be lightened but *not* removed. Blood will also thicken as moisture leaves the body. Gravitation of tissue fluids forces the liquid portion of the blood into the dry tissues, causing postmortem edema, especially in the dependent tissues.

If the body has been refrigerated for a long period and wrapped in cloth sheeting, dehydration will be an issue. The amount of moisture in the dependent tissues increases because of hypostasis of the blood and tissue fluids into these areas. The upper areas of the body may be darkened from dehydration, including the lips, eyelids, fingers, and base of the nose. The cheeks and forehead may also exhibit dehydration. Airbrushing and application of opaque cosmetics can conceal discolorations. Surface dehydration creates a loss of moisture from the blood vascular system. Coagula in the vascular system will impede distribution of the arterial solution.

Rigor usually passes 36–72 hours after death. During refrigeration, the cycle of rigor slows. Rigor may still be present at the time of embalming. Decomposition breaks the rigor cycle but is also slowed by cool temperatures.

### Arterial Preparation

Swelling is always a concern when embalming is delayed (**Fig. 19–5**). Distension of the hollow abdominal viscera is caused by trapped heat and gas accumulation. Visceral swelling can create sufficient pressure on the stomach to cause purge. The presence of rigor mortis and the increased moisture content in the dependent tissues increase the preservative demand. Arterial injection of the trunk areas should be **slow** using a strong, well-coordinated arterial solution with added tracer dye. Distribution may be difficult to achieve and drainage may be limited. The amount of fluid and volume of solution is determined during pre-embalming analysis and adjusted during arterial injection based upon observable results.

If the head has been excessively elevated during extended refrigeration, the tissues of the face can become dehydrated. This is caused by the gravitation of interstitial fluids from the facial tissues. Application of massage cream to the lips, eyelids, and face reduces dehydration of these areas. Eyes can appear sunken from the effects of moisture loss in the orbital tissues. Tissue builder injected hypodermically into the tissues behind the globe of the eye will improve appearance. This treatment is done after arterial injection. Direct injection of the eye globe may cause leakage of the vitreous; eye collapse can occur hours later if the needle entry site is not sealed. Super adhesive glue can be applied to the needle entry site as the needle is withdrawn. The addition of humectant co-injection to the arterial solution can add moisture to facial tissues. RCI is recommended for separate injection of the face from the trunk. The trunk and limbs can receive a solution different than the solution used to inject the head.

Drainage may be difficult to establish because of increased blood viscosity and coagula; the right internal jugular vein would be the best choice for the primary drainage site. Multiple injection sites should be used for arms and legs not receiving sufficient arterial solution. Injection should be slow to prevent abdominal distension and to keep arterial coagula from moving and blocking smaller arteries.

Dependent areas of the trunk, buttocks, and shoulders that do not receive sufficient fluid are treated by thorough hypodermic injection. Cavity fluid can be injected using either a small gauge or infant-size trocar. Unembalmed tissues are sources of bacterial activity.

### Cavity Embalming

When restricted cervical injection is used, the cavities can be aspirated before the features are set, and the head and the facial

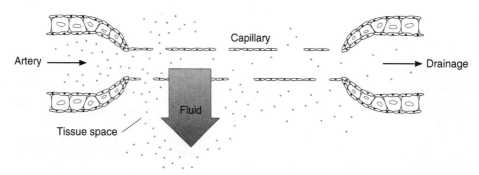

**Figure 19–5.** Refrigerated bodies and bodies in which decomposition has begun easily swell because of capillary breakdown and increased capillary permeability.

tissues are embalmed. If purge develops during embalming of trunk areas, aspirating **before** setting of the features eliminates the need to reopen the mouth and remove **purge**. Cavity embalming should be thorough. A total of 32–48 ounces of concentrated cavity fluid is suggested in accordance with embalming analysis. Re-aspiration is always advised. If gases escape when the trocar button is removed for re-aspiration, the abdomen appears distended, or the large surface veins of the neck appear distended, the cavities should be re-injected with concentrated cavity fluid after re-aspiration.

### Final Treatments

The hair and body should be washed at the completion of the preparation and thoroughly dried. Allow the body to reach room temperature prior to cosmetic application. Condensation on cold tissues impacts the adherence of cosmetics. Apply a light coating of massage cream to prevent surface dehydration. Hypodermic injection of tissue builder enhances the contour of sunken and dry features.

### Frozen Tissues

Sub-temperature refrigeration units used for extremely long storage will actually freeze body tissues. Medical examiners may use this type of refrigeration to completely stop decomposition of unidentified remains. Ice crystals form in frozen tissues and will damage capillaries as the body is handled during transfer and embalming. Damaged capillaries cause tissue swelling during arterial injection. Manipulate the body as little as possible. Allow the body to warm gradually to room temperature. Avoid the use of warm water to thaw tissues; desquamation will be accelerated.

Expect minimal blood drainage from frozen bodies. Inject arterial solution slowly to prevent capillary rupture and exacerbate swelling. Waterless solutions should be considered. Additional fluid dyes trace distribution of the preservative solution. Sectional embalming is anticipated along with supplemental hypodermic and surface treatments.

## PREPARATION OF BODIES THAT SHOW SIGNS OF DECOMPOSITION

After the passage of rigor mortis, noticeable signs of decomposition begin to be observed. Some of the factors that speed the onset of decomposition include elevated environmental heat, elevated and retained body heat, high moisture content within the body, and translocation of intestinal bacteria.

### Color Changes

#### Trunk Areas

One of the first external signs of decomposition is a green discoloration in the lower right quadrant of the abdomen. As decomposition advances, the outline of the large intestine can be observed (**Fig. 19-6**). Hydrogen sulfide produced in the colon after death reacts with end products of hemoglobin breakdown to produce the green discoloration. In time, it will spread throughout the anterior abdominal and thoracic walls, as far as the neck and chin.

#### Vascular Changes

Early decomposition color changes visibly affect the small veins. Blood in the superficial vessels decomposes; the hemoglobin

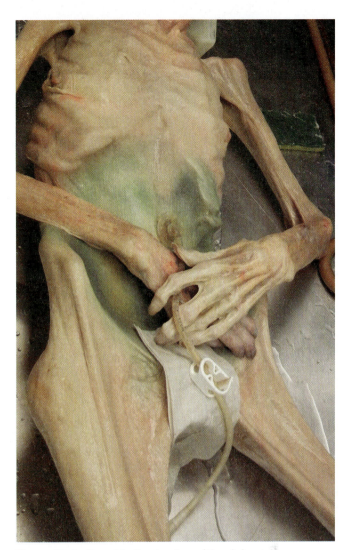

**Figure 19-6.** Greenish discoloration of the abdomen.

combines with hydrogen sulfide to produce greenish-black discolorations. Vessels take on a spider-web appearance. This extravascular discoloration is called "marbling."

#### Livor Mortis and Stain

Livor mortis is completely established in the dependent tissues. Livor is intravascular and will favorably clear during arterial injection. Extravascular postmortem stains do not clear. Stain develops as a result of hemolysis; heme passes from the capillaries into the tissue spaces. Stain can be lessened by bleaching; bleaching agents are arterially and hypodermically injected or applied as a surface compress. Petechia and purpura called *Tardieu spots* are extravascular discolorations that do not clear by arterial injection.

#### Dehydration

Prolonged exposure to air currents draws moisture from the tissues. Common areas that exhibit dehydration are the lips, eyelids, and fingertips. Dehydrated tissues will shrink and become wrinkled. Extreme dehydration causes the tissues to harden, a condition known as **desiccation**.

### Odors

Cadaverine and putrescine are commonly associated with the odor of human decomposition. During life, putrescine is associated with the smell of bad breath. Eight gases are identified as the primary contributors to the *smell of death*:

- Indole: odor of mothballs
- Skatole: odor of feces
- Putrescine: odor of rotting fish
- Cadaverine: odor of rotting fish
- Dimethyl disulfide: odor of foul garlic
- Dimethyl trisulfide: odor of foul garlic
- Hydrogen sulfide: odor of rotting eggs
- Methanethiol: odor of rotten cabbage

Foul amines and mercaptans combine with ammonia and hydrogen sulfide to produce odors of decomposition. Embalming converts the amines, mercaptans, and hydrogen sulfide to odorless compounds. Formaldehyde converts ammonia to odorless hexamethylene. Strong odors can be reduced by bathing the surface of the body with a solution prepared by mixing 2 pints of hydrogen peroxide with one-half cup of baking soda and adding a tablespoon of liquid soap. This solution is left on the skin surface for several minutes before rinsing and drying.

*Clostridium perfringens* is an anaerobic bacterium. In some bodies, its postmortem activity can create intense gas accompanied by a very foul odor.

### Purges

If gases have developed in the abdominal cavity and products of partial digestion were present in the stomach at the time of death, purge can be expected. Ruptured capillaries and congested lung passageways may also create a lung purge. Abdominal pressures may also cause purging from the rectum through the anal orifice.

### Gases

In some bodies, especially those in which bacterial activity increased after death, the tissues and cavities may contain gases. Conditions favoring gas formation are heat and humidity; those hindering formation are cold and dry environments. Gas can cause bloating and swelling of the body, protrusion of the tongue and eyes, and distension of the male genitalia. Distension of the abdominal cavity can create lung, stomach, and anal purges (**Fig. 19–7**).

### Desquamation (Skin Slip)

The autolytic changes that begin immediately after death weaken the superficial layer of the skin. Gases can easily move into the weakened superficial tissues, resulting in blisters and separation, or slipping of the skin layers.

### Chemical Changes

Although not visible, important postmortem chemical changes occur in the tissues. Autolytic and proteolytic decomposition of the body proteins result in numerous nitrogenous products. These products neutralize formaldehyde and greatly increase the preservative demand of the body. Their presence also shifts the body pH to alkaline (basic). Embalming solutions react best with proteins under slightly alkaline pH conditions.

### Embalming Protocol

During the **pre-embalming analysis,** observe: (1) general conditions of the body, (2) immediate cause and manner of the

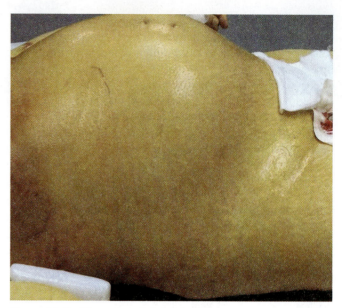

**Figure 19–7.** Distension of abdominal cavity.

death, (3) disease processes, (4) effects of drugs and medications, (5) postmortem changes, and (6) postmortem conditions such as time between death and disposition. The postmortem changes and conditions present are the most important factors in determining the embalming techniques to be used.

The protocols for embalming the bodies discussed in this chapter are similar, because all of these bodies have undergone a delay between death and preparation and all have a high preservative demand. Some of the complications encountered during embalming of the body with early signs of decomposition follow:

- Fluid distribution is poor because coagula are present in the arterial system.
- Drainage is poor because blood elements have decomposed.
- Tissues easily swell because capillaries have broken down or are easily torn by the pressure of the fluid; tissue structure has been weakened by autolytic and putrefactive changes.
- Ammonia and nitrogenous products in the tissues greatly increase the preservative demand.
- Little or no firming is exhibited because of protein breakdown.

Select maximum index fluids (36-index or higher) to mix a hypertonic solution. Supplemental chemicals enhance the effectiveness of the arterial solution. The goal is to deliver a minimum volume with maximum preservation. Avoid pre-injection fluid, which may waterlog and distend tissues. Use additional dye to trace distribution of solution. Dye only indicates the presence of fluid in the surface tissues and is not evidence of deeper embalming solution diffusion.

Two injection methods are recommended for injection, **six-point injection** and **restricted cervical injection**. Drainage can be taken from each accompanying vein or exclusively from the right internal jugular vein. Little or no drainage can be expected from these bodies. With both protocols, the head is injected last. Collateral circulation delivers preservative to all areas of the body regardless of the direction of injection; the face receives solution while other regions are directly injected.

Facial tissues would likely become oversaturated if injected first.

If the abdomen is distended tightly with gas prior to arterial injection, introduce a trocar into the abdominal cavity to relieve this pressure. The trocar should be kept just beneath the anterior wall.

The trunk should be injected at a very slow rate of flow to prevent swelling of the abdominal viscera and purge. Limbs can be injected slowly at first, and then at a higher pressure and faster rate of flow to secure distribution. Pulsation is recommended. If desired, each extremity can also be injected by the instant tissue fixation and waterless embalming methods.

If sectional arterial embalming has produced unsatisfactory results, sectional hypodermic injection will be necessary. Undiluted arterial fluid may be injected by machine through a hypovalve or infant trocar. To inject the arms, insert the trocar into the area of the bend of the elbow; from this point, the upper as well as the distal portion of the arm and possibly the palm of the hand can be reached. An alternative point of entry can be at the upper anterior portion of the arm—from this point, the upper portion of the arm can be reached, shoulder, back of the neck, and upper pectoral regions of the chest. To inject the legs, insert the trocar on the medial side of the leg either above or below the knee; from this point, fluid can be injected as far as the buttocks and as far as the foot. An alternative point of entry is the base of the foot. From this point of entry, fluid could be injected as far as the knee. The trunk walls can be injected from points of entry on the lateral walls of the trunk at approximately the level of the midaxillary line. It may be necessary to insert the hypovalve trocar or infant trocar into the upper shoulder area to inject the posterior portions of the back, shoulder, and neck. All of these points of entry can be closed with trocar buttons or a purse-string suture. Glue can be applied over the trocar button or suture to ensure against leakage. Fingers and the foot can be separately injected with a hypodermic syringe and a small-gauge needle. The use of super adhesive helps to ensure against leakage from each point where the needle is inserted.

These bodies need to be re-aspirated several hours after embalming. Reinjection is strongly advised, especially if any gases are evident during the re-aspiration. If desquamation is present, the loose skin should be removed at the beginning of embalming. Surface compresses can be applied to help dry these areas. Air drying also helps to dry the raw skin after the compresses have been removed.

Plastic garments with embalming powder should be used. Preservative powder produces some surface preservation and helps to control odors.

## Treatment of the Features

In preparing a body in which decomposition is evident, the embalmer may wish to vary the technique used to set features. When restricted cervical injection is selected, the mouth can be closed after arterial injection. As the lips and areas around the mouth may swell, it may be easier to obtain a proper closure after injection.

The embalmer should evaluate the preservation of tissues surrounding the mouth. It may be necessary to place cotton in the mouth and saturate it with concentrated cavity fluid to help ensure preservation. Dehydration should not be a concern. The lips can be secured with super adhesive glue.

Eyes can also be closed after arterial injection when restricted cervical injection is used. In this way, the embalmer has an opportunity to observe if the eyelids have received sufficient fluid. If the lids appear underembalmed, cotton can be used for closure. This cotton can be saturated with concentrated cavity fluid to help ensure preservation of the lids. Several hours later, the cotton packs can be removed or remain in place. Eyelids, especially if underembalmed, should be handled very gently to avoid skin slip. A super adhesive glue is effective for eye closure. Dehydration is not a concern in the preparation of these bodies.

Areas of the face that have not received sufficient arterial solution can be reached by hypodermic injection from inside the mouth (buccal cavity). Cavity fluid should be used to treat these areas. Do not dilute the cavity fluid; use the concentrated fluid. Make all injections from inside the mouth, because cavity fluid, unlike tissue builder, has a tendency to leak from the tissues. Any leakage will remain in the closed mouth. The sides of the nose can be reached, as well as the cheeks and the lower eyelids, from inside the mouth. A 17- to 22-gauge needle is ideal for hypodermic treatments.

In bodies dead for a long period, the submaxillary, sublingual, and parotid glands tend to swell during injection. If this happens, apply very firm digital pressure to these areas immediately after arterial injection. If the swelling is not reduced, make a semilunar flap incision at the base of the neck. Use the hypodermic or infant-sized trocar as an operative aid to lance the glandular tissue several times and apply digital pressure. If this treatment is unsuccessful, another operative correction, excision of the swollen tissues, may be necessary.

In bodies exhibiting decomposition, the tongue often protrudes and appears grossly swollen. The protruding tongue can be covered with folded cotton or cloth, and firm pressure applied to push the tongue back into the mouth; perform this treatment prior to arterial injection. Excision of the protruding tongue is the last option for consideration. Excision may be considered mutilation; permission should be secured from the authorizing agent prior to this procedure.

### Advanced Decomposition Protocol

Severe conditions may prevent acceptable restoration for viewing. The primary purpose of postmortem treatment for severely decomposed bodies is to control odor and slow the progress of decomposition until final disposition. Some level of preparation of the body should be attempted. Best practices include donning a respirator (when medically approved) and operating the ventilation system for the maximum of room air changes.

Confirm identity. Photograph all original identification bracelets or tags (place the photo in the decedent file); leave the physical tags with the body. Prepare two external identification tags to affix once the bag is closed. Remove, document, and secure any personal effects prior to final treatments. Reopening the body bag poses a high risk of chemical exposure. Proceed with treatments after donning the appropriate personal protective equipment.

Arterial injection can be effective for preservation purposes only. The arteries are one of the last structures in the body to decompose. Some level of distribution is expected.

Intense swelling of tissues and body cavities is also anticipated during injection. Special-purpose fluids are available for arterial injection. Drainage is not expected.

Aspiration of the cavity may not be necessary. Cavity injection can be effective for preservation purposes. Inject a large volume of cavity fluid to ensure internal drying of the viscera and to control odors and leakage.

The extremities and trunk walls can be treated by hypodermic injection. Treat body surfaces with a liberal application of autopsy gel followed by preservative and drying powders. The powders will adhere to the gel. Wrap the body in a blanket or several sheets before transferring to a heavy-duty body bag. Decomposing tissue is difficult to handle. Prior to zippering the bag, saturate the blanket or sheets with cavity fluid or a phenol solution. Apply glue along the zipper and cover with strips of cotton to prevent escape of odor and leakage. A second body pouch may be necessary. Affix another identification tag when a second pouch is used.

## CONCEPTS FOR STUDY

Define the following terminology:

- Excision
- Manual aids
- Mechanical aids
- Operative aids
- Primary flaccidity
- Rigor mortis
- Secondary flaccidity

1. List three challenges common with delay between death and embalming.
2. Recall the embalming time period when preservative absorption by body proteins is greatest.
3. Name the four steps in the embalming process.
4. Give examples of each: manual aids, mechanical aids, operative aids.
5. List three questions the embalmer asks throughout the arterial injection process to evaluate the degree of preservation.
6. Repeat the three methods of embalming.
7. How is the muscle rigidity, caused by the condition of rigor mortis, relieved? Once relieved, will rigor return to the muscles?
8. Review several advantages for postmortem cooling by mortuary refrigeration.
9. Review several disadvantages of cooling a body in a body bag. Review disadvantages of cotton sheeting as a body covering.
10. State eight gases associated with the odors of human decomposition.
11. Discuss which areas of the face may be reached with hypodermic injection from within the buccal cavity.
12. Relate the principal reasons for performing some type of postmortem treatment for severely decomposed bodies.

## FIGURE CREDIT

Figures 19–2, 19–3, 19–6, 19–7 are used with permission of Sharon L. Gee-Mascarello.

## BIBLIOGRAPHY

American Board of Funeral Service, *Course Content Syllabus*, 2016.

Boehringer PR. *Controlled Embalming of the Head*. Westport, CT: ESCO Tech Notes, February–March, 1969: No. 57.

DiMaio VJ, DiMaio D. *Forensic Pathology*, 2nd ed. Boca Raton, FL: CRC Press, 2001.

Dorn JM, Hopkins BM. *Thanatochemistry*, 3rd ed. Upper Saddle River, NJ: Prentice Hall, 2010.

Jones H. A chemist looks at embalming challenges. *Casket and Sunnyside* May 1968.

Pervier NC. *A Textbook of Chemistry for Embalming*. Minneapolis, MN: University of Minnesota, 1961.

Sanders CR. Refrigeration (Parts 1-2-3). *Dodge Magazine* March/April/May 1987.

Sawyer D. Treatment of refrigerated bodies. *Dodge Magazine* June/July/August 1989.

Slocum RE. *Pre-embalming Considerations*. Boston, MA: Dodge Chemical Co., 1945.

Strub CG. Why bodies decay. *Casket and Sunnyside* February–March 1959.

Weber DL. *Autopsy Pathology Procedure and Protocol*. Springfield, IL: Charles C. Thomas, 1973:69–70.

CHAPTER 20

# Discolorations

**CHAPTER OVERVIEW**
- Blood Discolorations
- Pathological Discolorations
- Pharmaceutical and Surface Discolorations
- Post-embalming and Decomposition Discolorations
- Conditions Related to Discolorations

A main objective of embalming is to create an acceptable appearance of the body. Discolorations on visible surfaces of the body challenge this objective. Concentration is customarily focused on features that will be viewed: face, neck, hands, and arms of the deceased. Other areas of the body may also be visible. Consideration is given to clothing choices: cultural and religious custom may require ceremonial dress or shrouding; less formal attire is common for infants and children. Geographical climate considerations can also influence skin exposure. Regardless of norms that influence body presentation and viewing, the expectation is for complete body-wide embalming treatment to take place. Discolorations on the nonexposed areas may not necessitate the level of restoration reserved for the face; however, the need to treat the underlying cause of the discoloration cannot be understated. Achieving an acceptable appearance of the body depends primarily on the overall success of tissue preservation. Firm and dry tissues are the foundation for acceptable restorative treatments.

The term **discoloration** holds two definitions; each of the meanings is addressed by the embalmer. First, *to discolor* means that *color is removed or lost*. Natural or lost skin color is restored during arterial injection with cosmetic coloring agents called *active dyes*. After embalming, external cosmetic products are applied. Second, *to discolor* means *to change color*. These types of discolorations are defined in embalming as *any abnormal color appearing in or on the dead human body*. Unnatural discolorations typically accelerate after death until some form of treatment is applied.

Discolorations can be **localized** as in a black-eye or **generalized**, affecting entire areas such as livor mortis, dehydration, and jaundice. Concealing a discoloration may produce satisfactory appearance; addressing the cause of the discoloration produces satisfactory embalming.

## GENERAL SKIN COLOR

Skin covers the entire body surface and is the body's largest organ. Skin is also defined as the cutaneous layer of tissue forming the natural outer covering of the body. Skin consists of two distinct layers: the superficial **epidermis** and the deeper **dermis** or **dermal layer**.

Skin color is a combination of hemoglobin, melanin, and carotene. Hemoglobin is a protein present within the red blood cells and exhibits a bright red color. Melanin is a pigment. Melanin occurs in various shades, from yellow and red to brown and black. Melanocytes are primarily responsible for skin color. Melanocytes are present in all people in the same relative number. Melanin color and melanocyte activity varies among individuals and ethnicities. Heredity and exposure to light also influence the degree of pigmentation in the skin. Carotene is an acquired yellow-orange pigment. Melanin and carotene are cellular elements, which remain in the skin after death. Hemoglobin and oxyhemoglobin are blood elements, which undergo color and positional changes after death. The red blood cells, containing the hemoglobin, no longer receive a fresh supply of oxygen which diminishes their bright red color. Blood also gravitates from the nondependent areas of the body into the dependent vessels, a process called *postmortem hypostasis*. The deceased body is often described as having a **death pallor** or a paleness to the skin. In effect, the blood coloring is lost.

## DISCOLORED AREAS

Deceased bodies ordinarily present with some level of discoloration. Changes in the natural complexion of the skin are observed during the pre-embalming analysis. At this time, the choice of embalming techniques, selection of chemicals, and post-embalming restoration is also addressed. The ability to identify classifications and probable causes of discolorations and to differentiate between discolorations that **can** and **cannot** be reduced during arterial injection and drainage is fundamentally important.

### Classification of Discolorations According to Cause

There are six classifications of cause-related discolorations.
1. Blood discolorations.
2. Drug and therapeutic discolorations (pharmaceutical agents).
3. Pathological discolorations.

4. Surface discoloring agent discolorations.
5. Reactions to embalming chemicals on the body.
6. Decomposition changes.

One *type* of discoloration can belong in more than one *classification*. For example, ecchymosis is a type of intravascular blood discoloration. Ecchymosis can be classified as a blood discoloration when caused by trauma, a pathological discoloration when it results from disease, and a therapeutic discoloration when caused by a drug. Jaundice can be classified as both a therapeutic discoloration and a pathological discoloration.

### Classification of Discolorations According to Time of Occurrence

Antemortem discolorations appear before death. The fact that they remain after death does not change their classification. Postmortem discolorations appear *only* after death and are always classified as postmortem discolorations.

1. Antemortem
   a. Blood discolorations
   b. Drug and therapeutic discolorations
   c. Pathological discolorations
   d. Surface discoloring agent discolorations

2. Postmortem
   a. Blood discolorations
   b. Surface discoloring agent discolorations
   c. Reactions to embalming chemicals on the body
   d. Decomposition discolorations

### Classification by Location

Blood discolorations are also classified as intravascular, within the circulatory system, or extravascular, outside of the circulatory system. Intravascular blood discolorations, both antemortem and postmortem, are readily cleared through venous drainage during embalming. Extravascular discolorations may be lightened during embalming, but will not clear completely because they exist outside of the vascular system.

### Blood Discolorations

Blood discolorations result from changes in blood composition, content, and location (**Table 20–1**).

1. Antemortem blood discolorations
   a. Intravascular
      (1) Hypostasis of blood (blue–black discoloration).

| TABLE 20–1. Embalming Considerations and Blood Discolorations | | | | | | | |
|---|---|---|---|---|---|---|---|
| Antemortem Hypostasis | Postmortem Hypostasis | Time | Livor Mortis | Time | Postmortem Stain | Time | Formaldehyde Gray |
| Occurs prior to death or during the agonal period | Begins at death | | Seen as soon as blood fills superficial vessels; begins approximately 20 min after death; depends on postmortem/antemortem hypostasis | | Normally occurs approximately 6 h after death; rate varies with the cause of death and the blood chemistry | | Occurs after embalming |
| *Intravascular* | *Intravascular* | | *Intravascular* | | *Extravascular* | | *Intravascular or Extravascular* |
| Movement of blood to dependent tissues | Movement of blood to dependent tissues | | Postmortem blood discoloration as a result of postmortem/antemortem hypostasis | | Postmortem blood discoloration as a result of hemolysis | | Embalming discoloration |
| Antemortem physical change | Postmortem physical change Speed depends on blood viscosity | | Postmortem physical change Color varies with blood volume and viscosity and the amount of O2 in blood | | Postmortem chemical change May occur prior to, during, or after arterial injection | | – Seen after arterial injection |
| Antemortem – – – | Postmortem – – Arterial injection stops progress Speeded by cooling of body, low blood viscosity | | Postmortem Clears when pressed on Removed by blood drainage Arterial injection (mild) clears with drainage Speeded by cooling, blood "thinners," low blood viscosity, CO deaths | | Postmortem Does not clear when pressed on Not removed by blood drainage Strong solutions bleach and "set" livor as stain Speeded by cooling, rapid red blood cell hemolysis, CO deaths | | Postmortem Seen as a gray stain Methemoglobin (HCHO and blood) – Speeded by poor drainage, small amount of arterial fluid Vascular system not well cleared of blood |

(2) Result of carbon monoxide (CO) poisoning (cherry-red coloring).
(3) Capillary congestion (hypostatic, active, or passive).
d. Extravascular
  (1) Ecchymosis: a large bruise caused by escape of the blood into the tissues.
  (2) Purpura: flat, medium-sized hemorrhage beneath the skin surface.
  (3) Petechia: small pinpoint skin hemorrhages.
  (4) Hematoma: swollen blood-filled area within the skin.
2. Postmortem blood discolorations
  a. Intravascular
    (2) Livor mortis.
  c. Extravascular
    (1) Postmortem stain.
    (2) Tardieu spots.

## Intravascular Blood Discolorations

Intravascular blood discolorations occur within the circulatory system and are effectively cleared through sufficient blood drainage during arterial injection. Intravascular blood discolorations include antemortem hypostasis of blood into dependent tissues, cyanosis, results of carbon monoxide (CO) poisoning, capillary congestion, and livor mortis.

Livor mortis, a postmortem **physical** change, is an intravascular blood discoloration caused by the gravitation of blood into the dependent capillaries. Livor mortis is first observed approximately 20–30 minutes after death and is well established by the sixth hour. Mortuary refrigeration and drugs such as blood thinners speed the onset and increase the intensity of livor mortis. If the discolored area is pressed upon and the area clears, this indicates that the discoloration is intravascular. Livor mortis can be gravitated. This is the reason for elevating the head above the heart during embalming; livor mortis is pulled by gravitational force, which serves to clear the discolored facial tissues (**Fig. 20–1**). If the decedent were lying flat, blood from the heart could gravitate toward the face, resulting in discoloration of the face.

Elevation of the head and the shoulders should be consistently maintained throughout embalming and the memorial event, until final disposition. When facial discolorations do not clear during preliminary bathing of the body, this might indicate the presence of clotted material in the vessels; usually the right atrium of the heart or the right or left internal jugular veins. These are the same vessels recommended for clearing facial discolorations. Direct access to the right atrium of the heart allows coagula to be manually removed with angular spring forceps.

Pre-injection fluids assist in clearing blood discolorations such as livor mortis. Use continuous, **concurrent drainage** and inject a sufficient volume of solution until the discoloration clears. When pre-injection fluid is unavailable, a mild arterial solution may be substituted. The use of a mild, **hypotonic** arterial solution prevents the conversion of livor mortis to stain. Subsequent injections of arterial solutions can be stronger, **hypertonic** to meet preservative demand. Reaction-controlled arterial fluids are formulated to distribute and diffuse before the chemical reaction with cellular proteins occurs. Reaction-controlled arterial fluids effectively clear livor mortis without causing stain, despite their astringent composition. Manual tissue massage and raising and flexing the limbs will increase solution flow toward the discolored tissues and drain the blood away from the area. During embalming analysis, observe the nail beds for livor mortis. Clearing of livor mortis during embalming indicates that arterial solution is reaching the hands. Summary of livor mortis:

1. Postmortem physical change.
2. Appears in dependent tissues.
3. Speeded by refrigeration and blood thinners, CO deaths, low blood viscosity, and large blood volume.
4. Intravascular condition.
5. May be cleared by arterial injection and blood drainage.
6. May be gravitated and massaged from a body region.
7. Color varies from light to dark dependent on blood volume and viscosity.
8. When pushed on (or palpated), tissues clear.
9. Pre-injection or mild arterial solutions are recommended as primary solutions to clear the discoloration. Follow with stronger subsequent solutions to meet preservative demand.

Discolorations from deaths by carbon monoxide (CO) poisoning are antemortem and intravascular and should be readily cleared with blood drainage. However, delay between death and preparation is expected. CO poisoning deaths are routinely investigated by the coroner or the medical examiner. Intravascular discolorations become extravascular discolorations following lengthy time delays. Hemolysis also creates postmortem stain; extravascular blood discolorations do not clear during arterial injection. The addition of an active dye to the arterial solution will trace the distribution of the arterial fluid and provide the embalmer a visual inspection of body areas not receiving adequate solution. The dye will also prevent the condition known as **formaldehyde gray**. When formaldehyde reacts with excess blood, the tissues will turn gray. Dye counterstains the gray tissues and is available in numerous tint colors to match various complexion shades.

## Extravascular Blood Discolorations

Extravascular blood discolorations do not respond well to clearing during arterial injection and blood drainage because they exist outside of the vascular system. Some extravascular discolorations may be slightly lessened in appearance but most are not substantially cleared. Examples of these discolorations are ecchymosis,

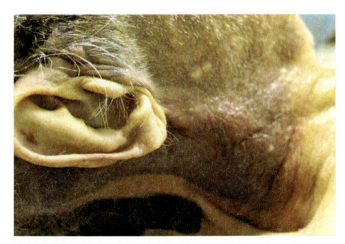

**Figure 20–1.** Livor mortis clearing from the face and settling in the tissues of the neck.

purpura, petechia, hematoma, and postmortem stain. Injection of a stronger arterial solution assists in bleaching some of these discolorations. Both livor mortis and postmortem stain can be present in the same dependent area. The livor might be flushed from the vascular system but the stain remains. Pre-injection, co-injection, or "special arterial" fluids cannot completely remove these extravascular discolorations. Formaldehyde gray can result.

Ecchymosis, purpura, and petechia are all extravascular. They are types of blood discolorations, but can be classified as both pathological and drug discolorations; caused by disease as well as therapeutic agents. Treatment for extravascular discolorations routinely involves all three types of embalming: arterial, hypodermic, and surface.

Tardieu spots are pinpoint petechial hemorrhages visible in the areas of advanced livor mortis (**Fig. 20-2**). The pinpoint hemorrhages are due to capillary rupture. This is an extravascular condition and the dark spots cannot be removed by arterial injection and blood drainage.

Ecchymoses are very large discolorations. Purpura and petechiae are smaller discolorations, and very frequently, simple arterial embalming satisfactorily bleaches and preserves them. Ecchymoses are of concern when they occur in a visible area such as on the face, the neck, the arms, and on the back of the hands. If the ecchymosis was caused by an intravenous needle puncture, one of three scenarios can be anticipated: (1) Arterial solution will perfuse the area, there will be little distension, and the area will be sufficiently preserved. (2) The area will distend dramatically. (3) The area will not receive arterial solution; ecchymosis is now treated by supplemental methods: hypodermic or surface embalming, or both.

### Post-Embalming Hypodermic Treatment

Two types of chemicals can be used: a concentrated phenol cautery or a cavity fluid containing phenol. A concentrated solution acts quickly to cauterize, dry, and preserve tissues. Steps for hypodermic treatment using the channeling method:

1. If the ecchymosis is on the back of the hand, insert a hypodermic needle between the webbing of the fingers.
2. Repeatedly direct the needle through the discolored tissues *prior* to injecting any of the solution from the syringe. This creates pathways, or *channels* within the tissues; the channels will readily accept the injected solution.
3. Inject the solution and apply digital pressure to the area to uniformly distribute the chemical throughout the discolored tissues.
4. Injected chemical may leak from the points of entry between fingers. Digital pressure and elevation of the area is suggested.
5. Allow the chemical to saturate the discolored tissues for 15–20 minutes. Eliminate as much of the chemical as possible by squeezing the fluid through the needle entry sites.
6. Dry and seal all needle sites with a drop of super adhesive glue.

### Surface Embalming

In addition to formaldehyde and phenol solutions, a variety of cream and gel preservatives are available. Surface treatments can be applied before, during, or after arterial injection.

1. Brush the surface of the ecchymosis with a preservative cream or an autopsy gel. Or, saturate cotton with a preservative chemical to create a compress of undiluted cavity fluid or a bleaching chemical and apply the cotton pack to the ecchymosis.
2. Cover the compress with plastic to decrease chemical odor and prevent evaporation of the chemical.
3. Allow sufficient time for chemicals to penetrate and preserve discolored tissues. Phenol-based solutions bleach rapidly. Other products may require additional time.
4. Remove surface compresses, rinse the area with water, and dry the tissues.
5. Apply a surface adhesive to the affected area.

### Ecchymosis or Hematoma of the Eye

Ecchymosis or hematoma of the eye, commonly known as a *black eye* (**Fig. 20-3**) is effectively treated by arterial injection of both the left and the right common carotid arteries. A stronger solution can be employed and the embalmer can directly control the amount of solution entering the head. Using the stronger solution, a smaller volume can be used in the event that the eye begins to distend. Avoid pre-injection and mild solution strengths; swelling will be exacerbated by hypotonic solutions.

Use cotton to close the eyes. Place a few drops of cavity fluid on the cotton. Place the cotton beneath the eyelid. This acts as a compress to preserve and bleach the discoloration. This

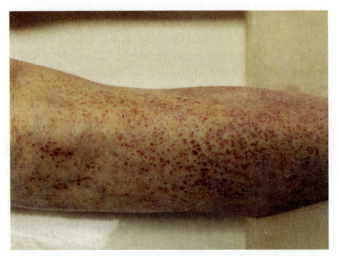

**Figure 20-2.** Pinpoint petechial hemorrhages known as tardieu spots.

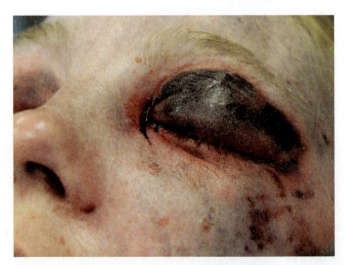

**Figure 20-3.** Ecchymosis or hematoma of the left eye.

method is also good for routine embalming when the eyelids have not received sufficient preservation.

Another approach is to inject the tissues around the eyes and the lids with a phenol cautery chemical prior to arterial injection. Allow 15–20 minutes for the chemical to cauterize the tissues; then proceed with the arterial injection. This method cauterizes the tissues and prevents arterial solution flow into the area. A post-embalming operative correction may be needed to directly incise, puncture, or channel the swollen discolored eyelids. The procedure is applied to the underside of the lids. Pressure upon the lid removes extravasated blood and accumulated serum. Facial tissues should be coated with massage cream or lanolin spray to protect against surface dehydration caused by contact with strong chemicals.

### Postmortem Stain

Postmortem stain, a postmortem **chemical** change, is an extravascular blood discoloration caused by the hemolysis of red blood cells. Stain usually indicates a period of time has elapsed between death and embalming. Heme is the pigmented portion of the hemoglobin molecule responsible for postmortem stain. Heme passes through the capillaries and into the tissue spaces. Postmortem stain can occur in combination with livor mortis in the same tissue regions. When pressed upon, or palpated, the stain will not gravitate. During arterial injection, stain may lighten but will not entirely clear.

Distribution of arterial solution may be inhibited in areas of postmortem stain. Tissue swelling after lengthy postmortem intervals is common. Moderate to strong, well-coordinated solutions minimize distension. Co-injection is an ideal supplemental fluid to enhance the efficiency of the arterial solution; coordinating better distribution and diffusion. Active dye can be added to the solution to trace distribution and counterstain formaldehyde gray discolorations.

Factors for consideration when evaluating postmortem stain:
1. Lengthy postmortem intervals are probable.
2. Caused by hemolysis.
3. Extravascular discoloration.
4. Discoloration does not clear when pressed upon.
5. Not removed by arterial injection and blood drainage.

## Pharmaceutical Discolorations

Antemortem discolorations can result from the long-term administration of pharmaceutical and chemotherapeutic agents. There are many discolorations under this classification; some are specific to a particular agent. All drugs affect the organs, particularly the vascular, renal, and hepatic systems. The skin is also affected; capillaries are fragile and bruising occurs easily. The disruption of normal liver and kidney function creates elevated levels of bilirubin in the blood. Diseases affecting the kidneys (renal) and liver (hepatic) can lead to organ failure and cause a condition called *jaundice*. The classic indication of jaundice is the yellowish discoloration of the skin and sclera of the eye.

## Pathological Discolorations

Some examples of pathological discolorations include:
1. Gangrene
    a. Wet gangrene: caused by the venous obstruction; infected tissues appear bright reddish to black.
    b. Dry gangrene: caused by arterial insufficiency; appear dull reddish to black
    c. Gangrene commonly occurs in the distal limbs, feet, and fingertips.
2. Jaundice: renal failure
3. Specific diseases
    a. Addison disease: adrenal gland impairment; darkening of the skin
    b. Leukemia: blood cancer, skin hemorrhages
    c. Meningitis: Contagious—oral and respiratory spread; bacterial or viral inflammation of the meninges; reddish-purple rash of petechia and purpura
    d. Tumors: unregulated cell growth, benign or malignant; local discolorations
    e. Lupus (Systemic lupus erythematosus): autoimmune disorder; chronic inflammation; malar "butterfly rash" over bridge of nose and cheeks

### Jaundice

There are three types of jaundice: prehepatic, hepatocellular, and posthepatic. Posthepatic jaundice causes obstruction of biliary drainage; bilirubin that is not excreted by the kidneys results in hyperbilirubinemia. Elevated levels of bilirubin present as a yellowish discoloration in the skin and in the **sclera**, the white portion of the eye. This condition is known as *conjunctival icterus* (**Fig. 20–4**). Some causes of jaundice include alcoholic liver disease, cirrhosis, carcinoma, heredity and autoimmune disorders, iatrogenic drug therapies, and viral hepatitis.

During embalming, the discoloration of the skin can change from shades of yellow to intense green; the *yellow*

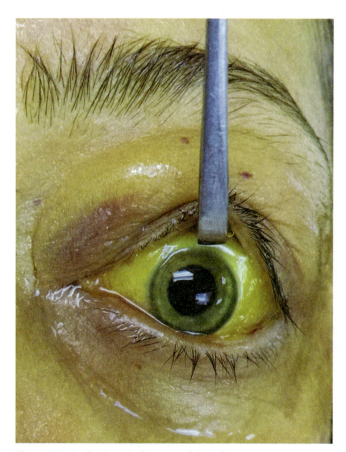

**Figure 20–4.** Conjunctival icterus of the left eye.

bilirubin converts to the *green* biliverdin. This chemical reaction is caused by the presence of a strongly acidic environment. Formaldehyde is a strong reducing agent. The conversion of bilirubin to biliverdin is a chemical oxidation reaction. Chemist Leandro Rendon, former Director of Research and Development for The Champion Company issued this narrative about the actual cause of this conversion:

*When aldehydes react with proteins, one of the chemical reactions that occur is said to be that of release of hydrogen ions which, of course, results in a low pH (acid) that is acid in nature. A given amount of formaldehyde or aldehyde can unite with a given amount of protein to form a given aldehyde condensation resin (fixed protein). Once the proteins have received the necessary amount of aldehyde to form these condensation resins, any excess aldehyde tends to become more acid in character and, therefore, causes oxidation changes. From another point of view, aldehydes, in combining with protein or amino acid, increase the local acidity in the tissues by the release of proton. The hydrogen ($H_1$) ions which produce the acid condition result from the chemical reaction between aldehyde and protein. This acid medium, in turn, results in oxidation changes. The yellow (bilirubin) is converted to green (biliverdin).* **It is not the formaldehyde** *which causes the oxidation (formaldehyde is a reducing agent). It is the chemical reaction (oxidation) as a result of the presence of the acid.*

**Preservation takes precedence over the cosmetic clearing of jaundice discolorations.** Confronting the potential to change a mild yellow discoloration to a deep green discoloration during arterial injection often gives the embalmer pause. A common error is to focus entirely on the discoloration rather than consider the sum of postmortem conditions present. Edema, emaciation, and decomposition may also be present and necessitate varied treatments. Consideration of the totality of postmortem conditions is fundamental. Discolorations that remain after embalming are customarily concealed by cosmetic application.

**Restricted cervical** injection is recommended so that varied fluids and solution strengths can be used for separate injection of the trunk and face. This method focuses on meeting the preservative demand of the trunk tissues first. A large volume of a strong well-coordinated solution with an active dye will counterstain the discoloration, regardless of its intensity. And nitrogenous waste products will be arrested by the strength of the solution. In the next phase of injection, the focus is shifted to the discoloration in the face. A specialty fluid is selected to clear the discoloration. Once the discoloration is cleared, a moderate strength can be injected to meet preservative demand.

Ascites caused by jaundice is a source of tissue discoloration. Edematous fluids in the abdomen can be removed prior to arterial embalming by trocar aspiration (**Fig. 20–5**).

**Method 1: Jaundice Fluid.** Specialty jaundice fluids are formulated to be very low in formaldehyde, or contain no formaldehyde. They are high in dye content. Glutaraldehyde is substituted in some formulations. Jaundice fluids may not be strong preservatives; once the discoloration is cleared, a stronger preservative solution can be injected.

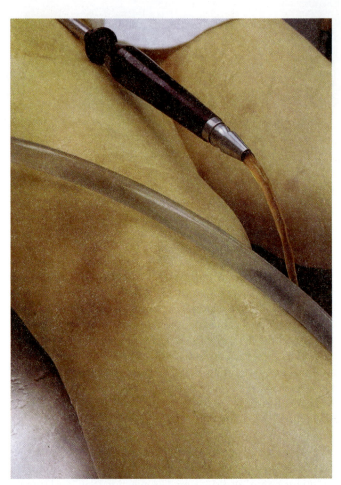

**Figure 20–5.** Aspiration of edema and jaundice discoloration prior to embalming.

**Method 2: Pre-injection.** Pre-injection fluid clears the vascular system prior to preservative embalming. Intravascular discolorations clear with the blood drainage. Dye can be added to the pre-injection solution to counterstain the discoloration.

**Method 3: Mild Arterial Solution.** Mild arterial fluid solutions can substitute for a pre-injection. Dye can be added to the solution for counterstaining discolorations. After the primary injection, the strength of the solution can be increased to meet preservative demand.

**Method 4: Nonformaldehyde Fluid.** Nonformaldehyde-based fluids function as preinjections.

**Method 5: Bleaching Co-injection Solution.** Co-injection bleaching fluids are added to the arterial embalming solution. Dye can also be added.

**Method 6: Cavity Fluid.** The bleaching properties of cavity fluid lighten the discoloration. A lower index fluid is recommended. Dye can be added. Cavity fluid may be too harsh for arterial embalming. The warranty on the embalming machine may be voided when phenol, a common ingredient in cavity fluids, is used.

### Nephritis

A sign of chronic renal failure is the sallow yellow color or bronzing of the skin resulting from urochrome in the tissues. This antemortem pathological discoloration takes on the appearance of mild jaundice. Urea in the blood vascular system and in the tissues is converted to ammonia. Ammonia neutralizes formaldehyde. Treatment of renal failure requires strong arterial solutions to establish firming and counteract the ammonia present.

### *Diabetes*

Uncontrolled diabetes mellitus can lead to renal failure. Poor peripheral circulation is common with diabetes. Gangrene in the distal extremities is another complication. A strong arterial solution with the addition of co-injection fluid increases distribution and diffusion. An active dye added to the solution indicates areas receiving distribution.

## Surface Discoloring Agents

Surface discoloring occurs antemortem or postmortem. Examples include blood, betadine, adhesive tape residue, gentian violet, paint, mercurochrome, and tobacco stains. Most of these can easily be removed with soap and water or with a solvent.

Surface discolorations should be removed prior to arterial injection. The pores of the skin are easier to clean at this time. During arterial injection, as the tissues firm and contour, pores are reduced in size. Removal of surface matter allows evaluation of tracer dye during injection. Removing blood, dirt, and grease from the fingers prior to embalming allows the embalmer to observe the presence of livor mortis in the nail beds and its subsequent clearing.

Mechanical and chemical methods can be used to remove surface discoloring material. Mechanical means include the use of abraded scrubbing pads, soft cloths, gauze, and brushes. Warm water and antiseptic soap can be used along with these mechanical aids. Chemical solvents can be used to remove specific discolorations that do not respond well to mechanical scrubbing. Blood is the most common surface discoloration and is easily removed with *cold* water and soap. The gentle friction of a scrubbing pad will remove dried blood.

## Discolorations Related to Embalming Chemicals

Postmortem discolorations can react with embalming chemicals; they can intensify or change color. Examples include razor burns, dehydration of tissues, formaldehyde burn, formaldehyde gray, flushing, conversion of yellow to green jaundice, and postmortem bruising and contusions.

### *Dehydration*

Dehydration is a drying of the skin. The classic colors of this discoloration are yellow, brown, and black. Dehydration can be caused internally by (1) injection of too much arterial solution, (2) use of an arterial solution that is too strong, and (3) continuous or concurrent drainage. It can also be caused externally by the passage of air over the body. Dehydration can also be the result of loss of the superficial layer of skin (e.g., abrasion) or the drying of cut edges of skin (e.g., laceration). Dehydrated tissues cannot be bleached and will progressively darken. The application of opaque cosmetics conceals this discoloration. The embalmer must be able to distinguish this darkening of the tissues from a similar darkening caused by decomposition. Dehydrated skin areas are generally very hard to touch, whereas a skin area that has decomposed is generally very soft and the use of light digital pressure can cause desquamation, or skin-slip.

Dehydration of the fingers should be mentioned. If strong chemicals were employed (or an edema-reducing chemical), the fingertips may have wrinkled and darkened because of dehydration. An application of massage cream or mineral oil over the fingers and the hands will help to reduce further dehydration. To correct this condition, tissue builder can be injected into each finger after embalming. Another area of the hand that frequently darkens as a result of dehydration brought about by the embalming is the tissue between the thumb and the index finger. Again, filling out this area with some tissue builder after arterial injection will minimize the discoloration. The arterial solution may also draw moisture from the lips. Wrinkling and separation of the mucous membranes can occur. Tissue builder (after arterial injection) can be injected from the corners (sulcus) to contour the lips and restore natural fullness.

Addition of a humectant co-injection fluid to the arterial solution adds and retains moisture in the tissues. Excessive use of humectants can work in the reverse and cause dehydration. Restricted drainage (intermittent or alternate) retains tissue moisture.

### *Yellow to Green Jaundice*

The conversion of bilirubin (yellow) to biliverdin (green) is an oxidation reaction. One theory is that formaldehyde, being a strong reducing agent, is only indirect to the cause of this reaction. Strong formaldehyde solutions create an excess of formaldehyde in the tissues. The excess formaldehyde gradually converts to acid. The acidic condition in the tissues, it is thought, converts the yellow jaundice to green jaundice. Oxygen from the air plays a role in this conversion. Coating the face and the hands with massage cream can help to prevent the oxygen contact with the tissues. The most important point is the **preservation** of the body. This is more important than clearing the discoloration. Counterstaining with an active dye is effective. If this fails to cover the jaundice condition, an opaque cosmetic treatment will be necessary.

### *Embalmer's (Formaldehyde) Gray*

Graying of the tissues results when blood removal during venous drainage is inadequate. The remaining blood mixes with the preservation fluids in the tissues and produces a putty-gray discoloration. This condition can be avoided by the injection of a large volume of arterial solution accompanied by thorough drainage and thorough aspiration of the heart. It is also important the head and the shoulders of the embalmed body are kept elevated. This elevation prevents blood present in the heart after embalming from moving into the facial and neck tissues.

### *Flushing*

Flushing is seen in those body areas into which the embalmer has been able to distribute arterial solution but has been unable to obtain good drainage of blood. Take as an example the body in which the femoral artery is used for injection and the accompanying femoral vein for drainage. If drainage is poor because of clotting in the right atrium of the heart or in one of the internal jugular veins or because of abdominal pressures, arterial solution will quite often flow into the facial tissues. Blood, however, will not be able to rapidly drain from these tissues. The facial tissues and the neck take on a cyanotic appearance.

Establishing drainage from another point such as the right internal jugular vein will clear this problem. If there is edema of the pleural sacs, often seen with pneumonia, drainage from the jugular will help to remove blood from the facial tissues and the neck. Flushing can result from leaving the drainage closed too long when using intermittent or alternate drainage. The establishment of drainage should clear the problem.

### Razor Abrasion (Razor Burn)

A razor "burn" abrasion is a cut of the skin during the shaving of the dead human body. Air drying alone turns these areas dark brown. With razor burn, application of a light layer of massage cream during embalming helps to prevent the nicked area from dehydrating and browning. If cream cosmetics are to be used and a small layer of wax is placed over the area, the discoloration should not darken or be noticed. The darkening may also be considered an advantage, because it indicates that the areas have dried, and an opaque cosmetic can be used to cover the discoloration. Dried tissues accept cosmetics and, when necessary, wax very well. The embalmer can promote the drying of these areas by using a hair dryer for few minutes. This ensures that there will be no further leakage and establishes a good surface for cosmetics.

### Postmortem Bruising

Postmortem bruising is rare; it occurs if sufficient pressure is applied to tissues to damage the capillaries. This condition is particularly noted in persons who have been on blood thinners and in elderly people whose skin is thin. When an eye enucleation has been incorrectly performed—if the eye speculum used to keep the lids open has crushed capillaries in the lids, blood will escape into the eyelids. The discoloration resembles an ecchymosis or "black eye." It will possibly further discolor and swell during the injection of the head. When present, restricted cervical injection is advised. Use a preservative solution that is a little stronger than that normally used so only a minimum of solution needs to be injected to ensure preservation. Avoid pre-injection treatment of the head and facial tissues in these bodies. Injection using a lower pressure and slower rate of flow will help to control swelling. Post-embalming treatments include: hypodermic injection of a phenol solution may help preserve and reduce the distension or surface compresses of a phenol solution or other preservatives such as cavity fluid or the autopsy gels may also be used to reduce any distension, bleach the discoloration, and ensure preservation.

Confluent hemorrhage into the eyelids is also seen when death occurs due to head trauma. This is caused by fracturing of the orbital plates. Almost all gunshot wounds to the head will exhibit some amount of hemorrhage into the eyelids. Restricted cervical injection is recommended to control swelling along with those recommendations suggested in the previous paragraph.

### Formaldehyde Burn

In bodies dead for long periods of time some of the capillaries in the skin may have broken. When a large volume of a strong formaldehyde solution circulates through such localized skin areas—fluid can escape directly into the tissues. This can create a raised rash-like appearance. Often this is seen near the injection site and is possibly caused by excessive collateral circulation through the tissues. In a few hours the raised skin areas will decrease. The tissues generally feel very firm to the touch and depending on dyes in the fluid the area can remain discolored.

### Decomposition Discolorations

Decomposition color changes are postmortem discolorations brought about by the action of bacterial and/or autolytic enzymes on the body tissues as a result of decomposition. These colors may be yellow, green, or blue-black to black. Examples are progressive skin color changes and "marbling" of the veins on the skin surface.

Decomposition is evidenced by five signs: odor, desquamation, gas, purge, and color changes. The first external sign of decomposition is a color change, usually a green discoloration of the right inguinal or iliac area of the abdomen. This green discoloration enlarges over a period and outlines on the abdominal wall, the ascending, transverse, and descending colon. The green then proceeds upward over the chest area into the tissues of the neck and the face. A color change is also evidenced throughout the skeletal tissues. Generally, the color changes from yellow to green to blue-black to black. In addition, the blood in the veins begins to break down. This discoloration progresses from the red of the postmortem stain to a black, and follows the course of the particular vein. The pattern resembles a "spider web" and the veins are described as being marbled (**Fig. 20–6**).

Both the general progression of color changes resulting from decomposition and the marbling of the veins are discolorations that can be bleached with external compresses such as phenol solutions, cavity fluid, or autopsy gel. These discolorations can be lightened but not to normal skin color. Post-embalming hypodermic treatment can also be used to lessen the discolorations and to help ensure preservation.

## CONDITIONS RELATED TO DISCOLORATIONS*

*Conditions discussed relating to discolorations and lesions pertain to those conditions located on the face and/or the hands of the deceased or other areas of the body that will be viewed.*

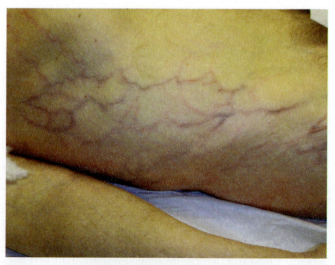

**Figure 20–6.** Marbling pattern of the veins in the torso.

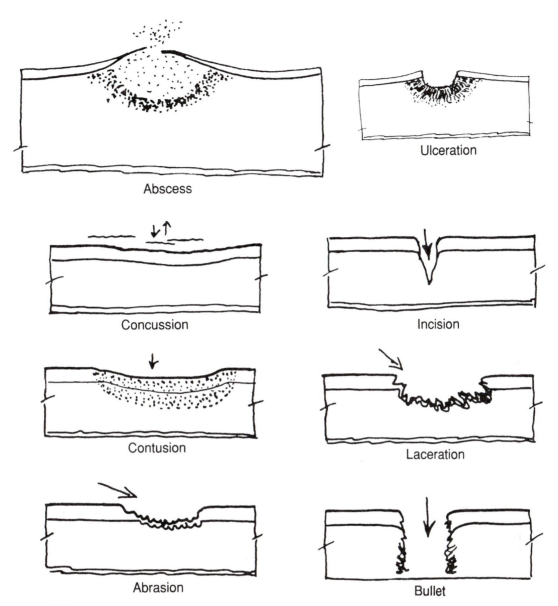

**Figure 20–7.** Types of skin trauma.

A discoloration is simply any abnormal color appearing in and on the dead human body. The discolorations already described involved color changes and possibly some swellings. There were no breaks or tears in the skin surface with the exception of the razor abrasion. In the following conditions, a discoloration is present but, in addition, there is some form of disruption of the skin surface (**Fig. 20–7**). The emphasis is not so much on the pathological origins of these conditions, but rather on the treatment of these conditions from an embalming standpoint.

A **skin lesion** is any **traumatic** or **pathological** change in the structure of the skin (**Fig. 20–8**).

The objective of the embalmer is to properly sanitize skin lesions, clean them of debris, remove skin that cannot be used in the restorative treatment, and secure adequate preservation and drying of the tissues. There are four categories of skin lesions: (1) unbroken skin, (2) scaling skin, (3) broken skin, and (4) pustular or ulcerative lesions.

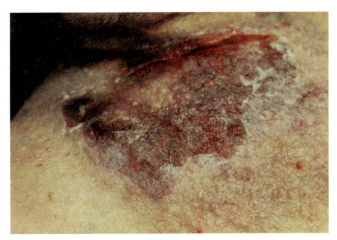

**Figure 20–8.** Pathological skin lesion.

Treat all broken, eruptive, pustular, scaling, and ulcerated tissues as potentially infectious. Exanthema is a skin eruption or rash manifested by certain diseases, common examples include chickenpox, measles, and scarlet fever. Use a search engine to identify unknown conditions; compare photos and review descriptions of those conditions. Wear the appropriate personal protective equipment (PPE) and thoroughly disinfect skin areas prior to treatment.

### Unbroken But Discolored Skin

Skin may remain unbroken but discolored for a variety of pathological and traumatic cases, for example, allergic reaction, inflammation, trauma, and tumors. Generally, a discoloration will result from an increase in blood flow into the tissues of the affected area and some swelling. If this area is to be viewed (face, neck, or hands), a strong arterial solution can be used to help decrease further swelling or surface compresses can be used to help bleach the area and possibly reduce some of the distension. A phenol solution can be injected beneath the skin after arterial injection to preserve, bleach, and reduce the swelling.

### Scaling Skin

Dry skin and large amounts of medications can result in extensive scaling of the skin on the face and the hands. Some of the skin breaks away, as in the healing of sunburn. The embalmer must make certain that as much of the loose skin as possible is removed. This is necessary for a good cosmetic treatment on the affected area. Methods of removal include shaving the loose skin with a razor; firmly wiping with a solvent (e.g., hydrocarbon solvents such as dry hair washes); and cleaning the area using an abrasive and massage cream.

If there is any question as to preservation, brush autopsy gel over the affected area for several hours or apply compresses of a surface preservative. The gels work well because they can be evenly applied and are not harsh bleaching agents. Surface compresses or gels should always be covered with plastic to reduce fumes.

### Broken Skin

Three types of broken skin are discussed: abrasions, blisters, and skin-slip.

An **abrasion** is defined as an antemortem injury resulting from friction of the skin against a firm object resulting in the removal of the epidermis. When raw skin is exposed to the air, it dries and darkens. An abrasion must be fully dry before restorative treatments. During embalming, the surrounding tissues can be protected with massage cream. **Do not apply massage cream to the abrasion.** Instead, allow the fluid to flow through the broken skin. After embalming use a hair dryer to force-dry the tissues. The tissues will darken and become firm and dry; ready for restorative treatment. If there is a preservation issue and fluid did not reach the abraded tissue, a surface compress of phenol cautery or cavity fluid will help promote preservation and drying of the tissues. When tissue is dehydrated, it cannot be bleached.

**Blisters** are elevations of the epidermis containing a watery liquid. When blisters are present on an area of the face, dry them with preservative gel. Lip blisters can be drained and cauterized. Mortuary wax and cosmetics will restore natural lip contour and appearance.

Blisters are characteristic of second-degree burns. In most second-degree burns, the blisters are opened and drained as part of medical treatment. When present on the face, these lesions should be debrided of loose skin with a sharp razor. A stronger-than-average solution should be used to embalm the affected area. Then the lesions could be force-dried with a hairdryer, or treated with phenol solution.

#### *Treatment for Blisters*
1. Lance and drain.
2. Debride loose skin.
3. Cauterize.
4. Dry.

### Desquamation (Skin Slip)

Desquamation, more commonly called *skin-slip*, is the separation of the superficial layer of skin (epidermis) from the deeper dermal layer. Desquamation can be a sign of early decomposition. The embalmer's goal is to achieve good preservation and ensure that denuded areas are dry. Remove all loose skin prior to arterial injection. Friction created by using a soft pad will gently remove **denuded** skin. Denuded skin is the bare skin exposed when the epidermis is lost. For larger desquamated areas, use a scalpel to incise at the point where the loose skin remains attached to unaffected skin. For exposed areas with desquamation, the following protocol is recommended:

1. Apply a topical disinfectant.
2. Open and drain fluid-filled blebs or blisters.
3. Remove all loose skin.
4. Apply surface compresses of cavity fluid or phenol solution to the raw tissue or brush with autopsy gel.
5. Sectional embalming may be necessary. Use a strong arterial solution.
6. Check preservation. Compresses can be continued or hypodermic treatment instituted with cavity fluid or phenol solution.
7. Allow time for these chemicals to take effect.
8. Clean away all preservative chemicals with a solvent or water.
9. Dry the area with a hair dryer to ensure no further leakage.

If desquamation is present on the eyelids or in the vicinity of the eye orbit, cotton can be used to close the eye. Saturate the cotton with a few drops of cavity fluid. This will serve as an additional internal compress to help establish good preservation. Leave it in place and use cosmetics over the affected skin areas when dried.

Desquamation in unexposed body areas can be treated in the following manner:

1. Apply a topical disinfectant.
2. Open and drain fluid-filled blebs or blisters.
3. Remove all loose skin.
4. Embalm the body with a strong, well-coordinated arterial solution.
5. Apply a cavity or phenol compress to the raw tissue or brush with an autopsy gel.
6. Check for preservation. If not complete, hypodermically treat the area with cavity fluid.

7. Brush again with autopsy gel, cover with embalming powder, or do both.
8. Cover the area with absorbent cotton.
9. Use plastic garments over the affected area.

## Pustular and Ulcerative Lesions

Examples of pustular or ulcerative lesions are ulcerations, pustules, herpes fever blisters, boils, carbuncles, and furuncles. These lesions are pustular and contain dead tissue. Treat these lesions in the following manner:

1. Disinfect the surface of the lesion.
2. Open and drain or remove any material in the lesion; clean the lesion and coat with autopsy gel or compress with cotton saturated with cavity fluid or a phenol cautery solution.
3. Embalm the body.
4. Check for preservation. Hypodermic treatment with a preservative or surface compress may be necessary.
5. Dry the area with a solvent and force-dry with a hair dryer.

## Decubitus Ulcers (Bedsores)

Because of their size and the fact that most occur on body areas that are not visible, decubitus ulcers bear special mention. These lesions are the result of a constant inadequate blood supply to the tissues overlying a bony part of the body, against which prolonged pressure has been applied. These ulcerations can be very large and are most frequently seen over the sacrum, heels, ankles, and buttocks. In addition, bacterial infections occur at these locations. Not only does the skin break and drain, but an odor is emitted because of the infection, commonly a staph infection.

Routine treatment of these ulcerations (when present on body areas that are not visible) can be summarized:

1. Disinfect the surface. Remove all bandages and apply a droplet spray.
2. Temporarily pack the area to reduce odors and to promote surface preservation.
   a. Autopsy gel can be brushed onto the ulceration.
   b. A cavity or phenol-saturated compress can be placed over the ulcer.
3. Embalm the body.
4. Hypodermically inject cavity fluid (via infant trocar) into all the areas surrounding the ulceration.
5. Apply new surface compresses of cavity fluid or autopsy gel to the ulceration.
6. Clothe the body in plastic garments (stockings, pants, coveralls, etc.). If plastic garments are unavailable, use an adult incontinence brief as a substitute.
7. Spread embalming powder within the plastic garments to control odors.

## Conditions Related to Discolorations—Unnatural

**Preservation is the most important objective.** Discolorations can be concealed with cosmetics. Airbrushing cosmetics is ideal for severe discolorations. Deaths from unexpected and unnatural causes are investigated by legal authority, coroner, or a medical examiner. Autopsy, or postmortem examination commonly follows. Delay between death and embalming is expected. Mortuary refrigeration is routine (**Table 20-2**). With time delays, circulation and preservation challenges

| TABLE 20-2. Unnatural Conditions Related to Discolorations | |
|---|---|
| Burns | First degree—redness of the skin<br>Second degree—blistering and redness<br>Third degree—charred tissue |
| CO poisoning | Bright red color to the blood<br>Low blood viscosity, intense livor<br>Rapid postmortem staining |
| Drowning | Low blood viscosity, intense livor<br>Head faced downward, livor and stain<br>Possible abrasions and bruising |
| Electrocution | Point of contact, burn marks can be present |
| Exsanguination | Little livor mortis, paleness to skin surfaces |
| Gunshot wounds | Eyelids can show ecchymosis, swelling of eye area when injury is to face or head |
| Hanging | Intensive livor in facial tissues; some capillary rupture showing petechial discolorations; no blood present in facial tissues |
| Mutilation | Loss of blood—little livor mortis Ecchymosis and bruising at affected areas |
| Poisons | Variable—from generalized conditions such as jaundice and cyanosis to localized discolorations such as caustic burns and petechiae |
| Refrigeration | Low blood viscosity, intense livor<br>Postmortem stain speeded<br>Dehydration of mucous membranes and skin surface after long exposure to cold air |

can be expected. The use of a strong preservative arterial solution is usually indicated. Restricted cervical injection is suggested when the body is not autopsied. Sectional, or six-point injection is expected for autopsied bodies.

### Death by Hanging and Strangulation

Hanging and strangulation deaths cause closure of the carotid arteries and jugular veins causing cerebral hypoxia. Death by hanging can create extensive blood discolorations. Tardieu spots and pinpoint petechial hemorrhages occur as a result of localized blood congestion. Discolorations appear on the face. The eyes may bulge and the tongue may protrude. Postmortem stain can be expected.

Cyanosis is caused by asphyxia. Many cyanotic and blood discolorations in the facial tissues clear after the pressure has been relieved from the neck. Autopsy is expected. During the autopsy as vessels are cut, blood drains from the facial tissues. Restricted cervical injection is recommended. The strength of the solution is determined through analysis of body conditions. A moderate to strong 2.0–2.5% well-coordinated arterial solution is typical when autopsy is the only remarkable condition present.

Ligature markings on the neck may appear as abraded tissues; exposure to air causes abraded tissues to discolor, dry, and firm. Thin ligatures, such as wire can deeply cut the tissues in the neck.

### Burned Bodies

Burns may be caused by numerous sources: heat (thermal burns), electrical current, radioactive agents, and chemical agents. Extensive burns cause bacterial infections, inadequate

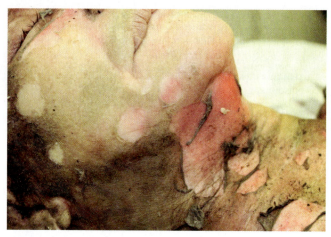

**Figure 20–9.** Second-degree burns to the face and neck.

blood supply to peripheral areas, and kidney failure (resulting in waste accumulation in the blood and tissue fluids). Both the local effect of the burn and its systemic effects are considered by the embalmer.

Burns have four classifications:

- **First-degree:** Superficial; affects the epidermal layer only. The skin surface appears red.
- **Second-degree:** Deep; affects the posterior dermal layer (**Fig. 20–9**). Skin blisters may develop. *Bullae* are blisters beneath and within the epidermis.
- **Third-degree:** Full-thickness; destruction of both the epidermal and dermal layers. The tissues are black, brown, white, or yellow; may appear charred. Hair follicles and glandular inclusions are destroyed (**Fig. 20–10**).
- **Fourth-degree:** Most severe. Destroys all skin layers and underlying tissues; possibly involves muscle and bone. Nerve endings are destroyed.

Burns may affect large regions of the body. Odor may be noticeable. Brushing these areas with an autopsy preservative gel ensures preservation and reduces odor. To prevent leakage and again, to control odors, a **unionall** garment is recommended. This plastic garment covers the entire body, except the face and the hands. Ample embalming powder should be spread within the garment, especially to cover the burned areas. The autopsy gel may be left in place. The embalming powder adheres to the gel.

The need to achieve preservation cannot be overemphasized in the preparation of burned bodies. Many of these bodies should be embalmed with a waterless solution using a high-index arterial fluid. These bodies have a very high preservative demand. Circulation may be very difficult to establish. Very strong or waterless arterial solutions are needed to prepare these bodies. Dye is added to trace the distribution of solution. Multipoint injection, if the body has not been autopsied, is routine. Suturing of incisions may be challenging in areas of burned tissue; the inversion suture (worm) may be more successful than the baseball suture.

Treatment to contain leakage and control odor is necessary even when the body will not be viewed, nor present at the memorial event. The zipper of the body pouch can be glued and sealed with cotton. The use of a second pouch may be necessary.

### Electrocution

Electrocution is related to discoloration because a burn is evident. Direct contact with an electrical source produces a local burn. The area where the electrical current exits may appear as a burn, more commonly the skin is broken at the exit site and the deep tissues are damaged. Rigor mortis can occur rapidly in death by electrocution. Routine autopsy protocol is followed when applicable. Damaged tissues are treated to halt leakage. Embalming gels and powders are applied. The affected area is covered with cotton, wrapped in plastic sheeting, or placed into a plastic garment.

### Carbon Monoxide Poisoning (CO)

The primary concern for discolorations associated with deaths from CO poisoning is the classic "cherry-red" coloring of the tissues (**Fig. 20–11**). The bright color is due to carboxyhemoglobin, a component of blood. Low blood viscosity is anticipated; with little to no clots. Distribution of the embalming solution and favorable blood drainage is expected.

The bright reddish color is found in the dependent areas of the body where blood gravitates after death. If the facial tissues and the neck are dependent, intense livor and staining can be expected in these tissues. Areas of the body where livor mortis is not present, appear normal. Blood trapped in the superficial anterior tissues can be falsely observed as dye from the embalming solution.

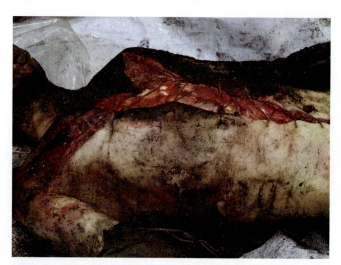

**Figure 20–10.** Third-degree burns to the entire body.

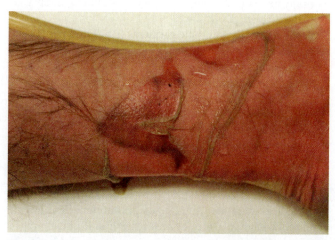

**Figure 20–11.** "Cherry-red" discoloration due to carbon monoxide poisoning. Skin slip is also evident.

Carbon monoxide poisoning discoloration is classified as an antemortem, intravascular blood discoloration. It should clear during arterial injection and subsequent blood drainage. Lengthy postmortem intervals can lead to hemolysis and postmortem staining.

Solution strength is based on the embalming analysis. Delay and refrigeration necessitate use of a stronger-than-average solution. Extra dye should be used to indicate solution distribution and diffusion. Once circulation is established, the solution strength can be increased.

With regard to the selection of vessels, if there are no major challenges or delays, any vessel is appropriate. Where there has been a delay, pathological challenges, and so on, the ideal vessels are the common carotid artery and the internal jugular vein. If the embalmer feels that large volumes of solution are needed, restricted cervical injection is recommended.

### Drownings

Death by drowning is caused by asphyxia; water blocks the airway. The most noticeable discoloration presented with drowning deaths is intense livor mortis, petechia, and possibly cyanosis (from asphyxia). Livor mortis can be maintained due to the cool temperature of the water, similar to mortuary refrigeration. Blood viscosity will be low. Excessive postmortem gas in the cavities will eventually bring the body to the water surface; trapped gases cause the body to float face down. Livor and other postmortem discolorations will appear intense in the facial areas.

Each case must be evaluated on an individual basis. Extrinsic factors such as water temperature, quality and speed of water current, presence of aquatic life, and underwater debris are important postmortem considerations. Intrinsic factors are considered for every embalming case. Preparation can be delayed when the body is unrecovered for days, weeks, or even months. Lengthy time in the water does not necessarily prevent viewing. However, bodies recovered within just a few days can exhibit severe decomposition that may hinder viewing.

Purge is very common. Pack the throat with liberal amounts of cotton after embalming. The packing material can be a combination of chemically saturated and dry layers. Selection of vessels should be based on the condition of the body. If the embalmer has any doubts, use of the common carotid artery and the internal jugular vein is recommended. The ideal is restricted cervical injection. The strength of the fluid depends on the extent of decomposition, the size of the body, pathological complications, and other factors in the case analysis. Aspiration should be thorough, followed with injection of a minimum of two to three bottles of cavity fluid. These bodies should be reaspirated, and if gases are evident or the viscera do not appear firm, reinject cavity fluid.

### Gunshot Wounds

**Face and Head.** Each body is considered on an individual basis. The scope of trauma varies considerably.

Common factors of deaths by firearm:
- Autopsy is expected
- Eyelids and surrounding eye tissues discolored (ecchymosis)
- Eyelids and surrounding tissues swollen
- Torn or bruised tissues easily swell during arterial injection
- Fractures of the facial and cranial bones

If the bullet passed into the cranial vault, did not exit, and there is not an autopsy, arterial fluid leakage into the cranium is probable. If sufficient arterial fluid fills the cranial cavity, sufficient pressure can be created to create brain or fluid purge. Frequently these purges are seen from the nose or the ear if surrounding bones are fractured. Purge may also exit at the site of the bullet entry or exit. The embalmer needs to make a thorough examination of the face and the skull to determine where there is bone and tissue damage. Pre-embalming local treatments include:

- Clean and disinfect the face, cranium, and cranial hair.
- Pack entry and exit points with cotton saturated with a phenol-cautery chemical to dry and firm surrounding tissues.
- Protect unaffected skin by a light application of massage cream.
- Align fractured bones to achieve a normal contour to the head or the face.
- Temporary bridge sutures or super adhesive glue may be needed to align torn tissues.
- Apply compresses of bleaching or cavity chemical over discolored and/or swollen facial areas, for example, eyelids and skin of the forehead.

Injecting the head with a strong, well-coordinated, arterial solution or a waterless arterial solution accomplishes the following:

- Good preservation.
- Firm and dry tissues for restorative treatments.
- Control and reduction of swollen tissues.
- Bleaching of discolored tissues.

Sectional embalming is used for injection of the autopsied body. **Restricted cervical** injection is recommended for the unautopsied body. Restricted cervical injection gives the embalmer the greatest control over fluid entering the face and the head—solution strength, pressure, and rate of flow is controlled.

**Instant tissue fixation** is an ideal method of injection for this type of body. Strong solution, under high pressure is injected in a burst-suppression pattern. A minimum volume of preservative creates maximum firming without tissue swelling.

After arterial embalming is completed, a phenol cautery chemical (or cavity fluid) can be injected using a hypodermic syringe and needle into the discolored or distended tissues. This solution should be injected from a hidden point of entry for these chemicals can leak. It may be necessary to aspirate the cranial cavity of the unautopsied body. Undiluted cavity fluid should be injected into the cranial cavity. Aspiration and injection can be performed through the point of entry or exit of the bullet or through the nose, passing the instruments through the ethmoid foramen of the cribriform plate of the ethmoid bone.

Post-embalming if the eyelids are distended, a phenol-reducing and bleaching agent can be hypodermically injected using "hidden points of entry." It is possible for this solution to leak out of the hypodermic needle punctures; the hidden points provide a location where leakage is least likely to be seen. The following points of entry are suggested:

1. Lower eyelid and surrounding tissues
   a. Inside the mouth
   b. Inside the nostril

c. Behind the ear
   d. In the hairline
2. Upper eyelid and surrounding tissues
   a. In the hairline of the eyebrow
   b. In the hairline of the cranial hair

Let the phenol solution remain undisturbed for 20–30 minutes; then apply pressure to decrease swelling. Remove excess liquids through the needle punctures.

Surface compresses (of cavity fluid or a surface bleaching compound) may be applied as weight to reduce the eye distension as well as to preserve and bleach tissues. Cotton may be used to close the eyelids; saturated with cavity fluid and then the lids glued.

If eyelids are grossly distended, surgical reduction may be necessary. First achieve good preservation of the eyelids. The globe of the eye, or *eyeball* can be collapsed by aspiration. The eyelids should be reflected and the tissue excised from beneath the eyelids.

### Poisoning

A variety of discolorations are associated with poisoning deaths. Some poisons act in a very short time. Others have a cumulative effect on the body. The latter poisons may affect the liver, which, in turn, leads to jaundice. Some poisons induce shock; the blood is drawn into the large veins and the body exhibits very little livor mortis.

A large number of poisons act on the nervous and muscular systems. Respiration becomes difficult and the tissues become cyanotic. Other poisons are corrosive and will burn areas that they contact. Ingested corrosive agents destroy tissues of the gastrointestinal tract, causing the rupture of veins and arteries in these organs. Some poisons cause petechiae on the skin surface. Others bring about anaphylactic shock, causing the skin to redden and swell. Cyanide produces a bright pink color similar to CO poisoning.

Most of these bodies are autopsied. Dyes can be used to counterstain discolorations. Preservation should be the first concern. Areas burned by corrosive poisons need to be cleaned and dried before restorative treatment begins.

### Mutilations and Blunt Force Trauma

The conditions caused by the various types of mutilation and blunt force trauma could fill an entire book. Tissues can be crushed, lacerated, punctured, and abraded, and so on. If injuries are to the face, the area affected can easily swell during arterial injection.

These bodies should not be embalmed by the "one-point" method of arterial embalming. Most require multipoint arterial embalming. In addition, some amount of hypodermic and surface embalming is necessary to achieve adequate preservation of the body.

Discolorations usually manifest as ecchymoses, both antemortem and postmortem. Autopsy is expected.

In mutilated tissue areas, severed arteries stand open, making them relatively easy to locate. These vessels can be used for the injection of embalming solution. Drainage need not be a concern as many of these bodies have sustained major blood loss; postmortem drainage will be minimal. Strong arterial solutions should be used. Such cases constitute an excellent example of the type of body for which special purpose high-index fluids can be used. Use dyes to trace arterial solution distribution.

### Exsanguination

Exsanguination is the excessive blood loss to the point of death. The blood loss is not always external, as in massive hemorrhage. It can be internal, for example, rupture of a blood vessel. Blood loss can also occur without vascular damage or rupture, as evidenced in the condition of shock. Shock is a sudden loss of blood flow; blood does not leave the vessels.

Exsanguination deaths are characterized by a lack of color in the tissues. Whether blood is lost externally, internally, minor livor mortis is evident. In cases of shock, the blood tends to congeal in the large veins and drainage may be difficult to establish. The largest vein possible should be selected; the right internal jugular vein leads directly into the right atrium of the heart.

In injecting the bodies that have sustained a large blood loss, a slightly stronger arterial solution should be used, for there is likely to be a loss of arterial solution depending on the cause of blood loss. Additional dye should be added to the arterial solution to trace the distribution of arterial solution.

When necessary, sectional arterial embalming should be employed. If an artery such as the aorta has ruptured, the trunk walls will require supplemental hypodermic embalming. A small gauge trocar is used to deliver arterial solution into these tissues. Several points are used to introduce the trocar into the trunk. Emphasis is given to the dependent tissues of the buttocks, nape of the neck, and the shoulders.

Two postmortem conditions, which are not causes of death, can create discolorations, so are included here: bodies refrigerated prior to embalming and mold.

### Refrigerated Bodies

Intense livor mortis can be expected in bodies that undergo mortuary refrigeration shortly after death. The cooling process helps to keep the blood liquid. When the body has been cooled 6–12 hours prior to preparation, the dependent tissues can turn a variety of dark hues from red to blue-black. It is important to elevate the head and the shoulders of to prevent intense livor mortis in the tissues of the neck and the face.

Hemolysis is also accelerated by cool temperatures. Hemolysis causes the blood vessels to rupture, producing postmortem stain (**Fig. 20–12**). Blood trapped in the tissues

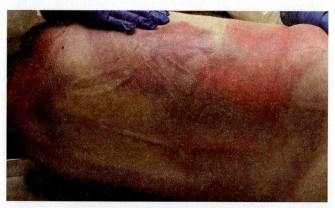

**Figure 20–12.** Postmortem stain.

appear red or pink. The capillaries are porous and postmortem stain can be expected when cooling exceeds 12 hours. Discolorations caused by hemolysis can be mistaken for embalming fluid dye.

When mortuary refrigeration continues for several days, expect surface dehydration of the tissues. The lips, fingertips, and other features that have a thin skin covering will shrink and darken after extended refrigeration. Cotton sheeting used as a body covering increases surface dehydration; cool air circulates freely. Plastic body bags decrease dehydration, but increase moisture. Condensation forms inside the pouch from trapped body heat.

### Mold

The growth of mold on the surface of the body occurs after lengthy refrigeration. Darkness and moisture encourage mold growth. Cold molds also grow on the body surface in refrigeration. Molds will grow on both the unembalmed and the embalmed body. When the embalmed body is to be stored for several weeks, air should be allowed to circulate around the body. The exposed tissues (face and hands) can be sprayed with a surface mold preventative. Mold can be scraped from tissues and the area swabbed with a solution of 1% phenol and 1% creosote. Or, a mixture of equal parts methyl alcohol and acetic acid. Cosmetic treatment will be necessary.

## CONCEPTS FOR STUDY

Define the following terminology:

- Abrasion blisters
- Bilirubin
- Biliverdin
- Carbon monoxide poisoning
- Carotene
- Counterstaining method
- Death pallor
- Desquamation
- Discoloration
- Ecchymosis
- Embalmer's gray
- Exsanguination
- First degree burn
- Hematoma
- Jaundice
- Livor mortis
- Melanin
- Pathological discolorations
- Petechia
- Postmortem stain
- Purpura
- Razor abrasion
- Second degree burn
- Skin lesion
- Surface discoloration agents
- Tardieu spots
- Therapeutic discolorations
- Third degree burn

1. Recall two different meanings of "to discolor."
2. Describe the role of melanocytes in determining skin pigmentation.
3. List methods and fluids that can be used to clear livor mortis.
4. Give an example of an arterial injection method used to treat a hematoma of the eye.
5. Explain the cause of postmortem stain.
6. Discuss several types of fluid used to embalm a jaundiced body.
7. What is the condition known as embalmer's gray and how is it treated after embalming?
8. Defend the importance of dry, well-preserved tissues for the purpose of restoration.
9. List the classifications of burns and explain the effect on tissues in each stage.
10. Relate the cause of the classic cherry-red discoloration common in deaths by carbon monoxide poisoning?

## FIGURE CREDIT

Figures 20–1, 20–2, 20–3, 20–6, 20–8 are used with permission of Kevin Drobish.

Figures 20–4, 20–5, 20–9, 20–10, 20–11, 20–12 are used with permission of Sharon L. Gee-Mascarello.

## BIBLIOGRAPHY

Adams J. Embalming the jaundice case—Part IV. *Dodge Magazine*, January-February 1995.

American Board of Funeral Service, *Course Content Syllabus*, 2016.

Bedino JH. Waterless embalming—an investigation. *Champion Expanding Encyclopedia no. 656*, 1993:619–620.

DiMaio VJ, DiMaio D. *Forensic Pathology*, 2nd ed. Boca Raton, FL: CRC Press, 2001.

Dorn JM, Hopkins BM. *Thanatochemistry*, 3rd ed. Upper Saddle River, NJ: Prentice-Hall, 2010.

Kazmier H. *Essentials of Systemic Pathology*. Dubuque, IA: Kendell-Hunt Publishing Co., 1976.

Knight B. *Simpson's Forensic Medicine*, 11th ed. London: Arnold, Hodder Headline Group, 1997.

Mayer JS. *Color and Cosmetics*, 3rd ed. Dallas: Professional Training Schools, Inc., 1986.

Mayer JS. *Restorative Art*, 6th ed. Bergenfield, NJ: Paula Publishing Co., 1974.

New Jersey State Funeral Directors Assn. "Putting Alternative Preservations to the Test." In *The Forum*, Vol. 76, No. 3, Wall, NJ: New Jersey State Funeral Directors Assn., January 2010.

# CHAPTER 21

# Moisture Considerations

## CHAPTER OVERVIEW
- Maintaining Moisture Balance after Embalming
- Dehydration Causes and Treatment
- Causes, Classifications, and Treatments of Edema
- Renal Failure
- Fatal Burns

There are three main objectives in the embalming process: temporary preservation, sanitation of body tissues, and restoration of the deceased to create an acceptable appearance. Water and moisture play an important role in achieving each of these objectives. Areas customarily viewed, the face, neck, arms, and hands should present a natural appearance. Dehydrated tissues, visible discolorations, and features swollen with edema are unacceptable. The control of moisture is a primary concern for the embalmer. Establishment and maintenance of proper moisture balance prevents extreme conditions associated with dehydration and edema. Good tissue moisture begins during arterial embalming and is supplemented with various embalming treatments, and continues with proper post-embalming care.

Three conditions characterize the various tissues of the dead human body with regard to moisture: normal tissue moisture, dehydration, and excess tissue fluid accumulation (edema). Dehydration and edema can be caused by disease processes, drug therapies, surgical procedures, and long-term mortuary refrigeration. Moisture extremes can be localized or generalized within the body. It is possible for all three tissue conditions to be present within the same body. An example is the patient who dies following open heart surgery for aortic repair. The face can be severely swollen with edema, while the rest of the body is unaffected.

Embalming analysis and professional judgment determines the selection of embalming fluids and the techniques used for arterial injection. Body moisture plays a significant role in these decisions. The following factors are considered during the analysis:
- Type of arterial fluid (index, firming action, etc.)
- Dilution of the arterial fluid
- Volume of arterial solution to inject
- Use of co-injection or humectant fluid
- Vessels used for injection and drainage
- Injection and drainage techniques to increase, maintain, or remove moisture
- Pressure and speed (rate of flow) of arterial injection
- Other techniques and fluids that add or remove moisture

## NORMAL BODY MOISTURE

Ideal body water percentage for males is 50–65% and for females is 45–60%. Edema is said to be established when there is a 10% increase in total body water.

After death, several factors bring about dehydration. Mortuary refrigeration is a leading cause of postmortem loss of moisture. Dry, cool, or warm air moving across the body promotes dehydration. Between death and embalming, the blood and the tissue fluids begin to gravitate into dependent body regions, increasing the moisture levels in the dependent tissues but reducing the moisture in the elevated body areas.

The embalming process itself can either add or greatly reduce moisture. The primary ingredient in almost all embalming fluids is formaldehyde, and formaldehyde dries tissues. During arterial injection, the skin becomes dry to the touch. The lips, the fingers, and the area between the thumb and the index have a tendency to rapidly dehydrate; wrinkling of these body areas is easily evidenced if the arterial embalming produces dehydration (**Fig. 21–1**). This dehydrating effect can often be seen even before arterial injection is completed. The embalmer must see that a good moisture balance is established or maintained (**Fig. 21–2**). The well-embalmed body should not show signs of wrinkled, dark dehydrated tissue during the funeral. **Thoroughly embalmed tissues dehydrate LESS than under-embalmed tissues.** Changes in the appearance of the body during the interval between embalming and final disposition should be minimal. Continued care of the deceased on a periodic basis ensures the body remains stable.

An article published many years ago by Philip Boehringer in **ESCO Review** cited some interesting relationships dealing with the loss of moisture from the dead human body:

If a pint of water weighs approximately 1 pound, consider the following: If the embalmer injects 3 gallons of arterial solution, 24 pounds of liquid is injected.

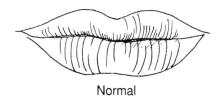

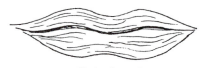

**Figure 21-1.** Dehydration causes horizontal wrinkles to form on the lips. Lips with good moisture content have vertical lines.

The following liquid losses were estimated:

1½ gallons of drainage = 12 pounds of moisture lost; 1 quart of liquid aspirated = 2 pounds of moisture lost. Up to 3 pints can be lost per day by dehydration; funerals average 3 days = 9 total pounds of moisture lost.

Only one pound of moisture remains (or was added) by the preceding example. No dehydration should have occurred during viewing. It is important that the embalmer maintain proper moisture in the tissues. The process of embalming should **add** moisture to the body to retain natural appearance. This is one of the reasons why so much water is used to dilute arterial fluid. The following techniques can help to maintain a good balance of moisture in the body:

1. Avoid the use of astringent or hypertonic arterial solutions unless case analysis indicates strong solutions. Consider dilution recommendations available in the product catalog or on the company website. Hypotonic solutions distribute better, and diffusion and retention rates are increased. A mild primary solution strength of 1.75% can assist in retaining moisture to the tissues as long as subsequent injections meet preservative demands.
2. Avoid the use of concurrent or continuous drainage after surface discolorations have cleared. Intermittent or alternate drainage helps to distribute and diffuse the arterial solution. These methods also help the body to retain arterial solution.
3. Avoid rapid arterial injection and drainage. A slower injection rate reduces short-circuiting of fluids. Gradual injection rates allow the solution to distribute, diffuse, and be retained in the tissues. Less tissue fluid is withdrawn from the tissues to exit as drainage. For best results, the final portion of arterial solution is injected against closed drainage to allow the solution ample time to diffuse into the tissues.
4. Delay cavity aspiration for a brief time, 20–30 minutes, to promote deeper diffusion of arterial solution into the tissues.
5. Use a body pouch during mortuary refrigeration to prevent the surrounding air from dehydrating the surface tissues.
6. Strong alkaline or acid fluids can alter the reaction between protein and preservative. Formaldehyde has a drying effect on the tissues. Acid or rapid-acting arterial fluids often produce very firm and dry tissues. Avoid old and outdated fluids. These fluids cause the tissues to dehydrate rapidly.
7. Disinfectants should not dry and bleach the surface tissues.
8. Use of absorbent cotton to set features can cause tissues to dehydrate. Nonabsorbent cotton can be used as a substitute for absorbent varieties.
9. Fumes from the injection of cavity fluids into the neck area can dehydrate the mouth and the nose. These areas can be packed tightly so fumes cannot enter.
10. Short-circuiting of arterial solution causes dehydration of the areas in which the solution is circulating. Distribution is uneven, and the short-circuiting regions are very firm and dry.
11. Warm water solutions increase fluid reaction. Cool solutions slow the formaldehyde reaction allowing better distribution and diffusion of the arterial solution throughout the entire body.
12. After embalming, maintain coverage of the body to prevent circulating air from dehydrating the surface. Application of cream cosmetics and massage cream to the surface tissues helps to reduce moisture loss to the atmosphere.
13. If there is to be a long delay between embalming and viewing of the body **do not** excessively elevate the head during storage of the body; elevation will cause gravitation of liquids from the facial tissues resulting in dehydrated features.
14. Tissue building of the cheeks, lips, temples, fingertips, etc. after embalming prevents dehydration of these areas.
15. A light coating of massage cream applied to face, neck, and hands during and following embalming will help to prevent dehydration of these tissues.

# PREPARATION OF THE DEHYDRATED BODY

## Antemortem Dehydration

A number of disease processes can result in a loss of fluid from the body cells and tissues: hemorrhage, febrile diseases, kidney diseases, diabetes, some cancers and localized neoplasms, and some first- and second-degree burns. Decades ago, tuberculosis and acquired immunodeficiency syndrome (AIDS) were classic examples of illnesses that produced severe emaciation and dehydration. Dehydration may also be caused by excessive vomiting & diarrhea, drugs that increase urine excretion

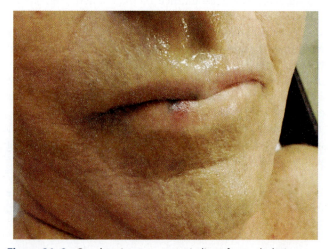

**Figure 21-2.** Good moisture content in lips after embalming.

(diuretics), and decreased water intake. Medical care incorporates hydrating therapies to lessen body dehydration.

### Postmortem Dehydration—Pre-Embalming

Dehydration following death is classified as a postmortem physical change. Mortuary refrigeration and hypostasis remove moisture from the upper, nondependent areas of the body such as the face and the neck. The dry, cool air draws moisture gradually from the tissues into the surrounding air. This is an example of surface evaporation. Short-term mortuary refrigeration also maintains the blood in a fluid state; this is advantageous for copious blood drainage during embalming.

Dehydration causes the viscosity of the blood to increase. Postmortem emboli in the arteries prevent good arterial solution distribution; coagula in the veins hinder drainage. Direct exposure to forced air heating and air conditioning currents also rapidly dehydrate tissues.

The skin of a dehydrated body appears dry and can also be flaky (**Table 21–1**). Loose skin, if not removed from facial areas will interfere with cosmetic application. Massage cream can be applied liberally, allowed to remain several minutes, then gently wiped away. The remainder of loose skin is removed with a mildly abrasive pad, saturated with solvent. Several applications may be necessary. Rinse solvent from the skin thoroughly as this product will also dehydrate tissues. Reapply massage cream as a moisture barrier.

### Desiccation

Dehydrated bodies decompose slowly because water is necessary for decomposition. In the absence of water or moisture, extreme dehydration occurs. This is called **desiccation**. Desiccation is a form of preservation insofar as water is withdrawn to such a degree that enzymatic cellular destruction is fully arrested. Moisture cannot be restored to desiccated tissues. Areas of thin tissue, such as the ears, nose, lips, and eyelids, become desiccated after long-term refrigerated or frozen storage. Desiccated lips appear black, severely wrinkled, and shrunken. Desiccated fingertips are commonly observed; the skin becomes parchment-like and turns a yellowish brown. Minor areas of desiccation may be removed and restored using restorative treatments. Arterial injection or hypodermic injection is ineffective. Widespread facial desiccation can severely impact viewability.

## LOCAL DEHYDRATION CHALLENGES

Dehydration is associated with several situations where the epidermis layer of the skin has been removed. When the epidermis is removed and the area is allowed to dry or force-dried, the affected area will turn dark brown in color and appear quite firm to the touch. Examples frequently encountered: **abrasion**, **razor burn** (**abrasion**), nicking of the face during shaving of the body, **skin-slip**, where the dermis has dried, **epidermis removed** for transplant. This type of discoloration does not respond to bleaching by preservative surface compresses. Opaque cosmetic treatment is necessary when this occurs in a visible body area.

The drying of the tissues in the preceding examples is actually desired by the embalmer, for the skin surface is now sealed and there is no leakage from these areas. Opaque cosmetics or waxes can be applied over these dried areas. To speed the drying of abraded tissues, following arterial injection, a hair dryer can be used. Massage cream should not be applied to these areas, because it slows the drying of tissues.

## ARTERIAL EMBALMING CHALLENGES

Dehydration occurring during the antemortem, agonal, and postmortem periods prior to arterial embalming can result in a thickening of the blood. Satisfactory blood removal is essential to establish uniform distribution and even diffusion of arterial solution. Drainage may be difficult to establish in these bodies. Thickened blood in the arterial system can prevent arterial solution from reaching the smaller arteries, or block solution distribution entirely.

Blood should be drained from the largest vein; the right internal jugular vein. Arterial injection from the right common carotid artery or restricted cervical injection pushes arterial coagula toward the legs. A secondary injection point may be necessary, and if this is not successful, hypodermic and surface treatment of the legs can be used to establish preservation.

Injection from the femoral or external iliac arteries, when clots are present, may force arterial clots into the carotid arteries and affect distribution to the face. Slow injection will minimize arterial coagula from being dislodged and blocking smaller arteries.

| TABLE 21–1. Problems Associated with Dehydration | |
|---|---|
| Darkened skin | Corrected by cosmetic application; use fluid dyes to ensure fluid distribution to all body areas |
| "Flaking" or peeling of skin, especially in facial areas | Apply massage cream and then clean with a solvent to remove all loose skin; mortuary cream cosmetics further reduce skin drying |
| Firm feel to the skin | Skin feels embalmed; additional dye helps to trace the distribution of fluid |
| Desiccated lips, eyelids, or fingertips | May need correction with restorative waxes; tissue building; opaque cosmetics needed to hide discolorations |
| Thickened blood | May be diluted with a pre-injection fluid; use right internal jugular as drainage point; inject from the carotids to push arterial coagula toward the lower extremities |
| Dehydration created by the embalmer; wrinkled lips, fingertips; facial areas | Use correct dilutions for arterial and humectant fluids; areas may be filled out with tissue builder after embalming |
| Dehydration of large facial area from embalming and passage of air over body | Use massage cream on exposed areas prior to cosmetic application; if skin is discolored, opaque cosmetics will be needed; cream cosmetics further reduce dehydration; fingertips and facial areas may also be treated with tissue builder to reduce dehydration |

## TREATMENTS THAT MINIMIZE OR PREVENT POST-EMBALMING DEHYDRATION

Dehydration occurs to some extent in all embalmed bodies; the process of embalming removes a great amount of tissue moisture through blood drainage. And, formaldehyde is inherently dehydrating. The following are treatments for adding and maintaining moisture:

1. Use a moderate arterial solution with an overall strength of 2.0% or above. Many fluids are reaction-controlled and do not release the preservative ingredients until they come into contact with body cells. Many arterial fluids contain antidehydrants in their formulations. Larger volumes of a mild solution can also be used to add tissue moisture and secure preservation.
2. Very slow injection of the arterial solution will help to fill the vascular system without causing arterial emboli to block small arterial branches.
3. Use a co-injection fluid with the arterial solution. The co-injection fluid helps to reduce the astringency of the arterial solution and also adds moisture to the tissues. It is recommended that equal amounts of co-injection and preservative arterial fluids be used.
4. Use a humectant co-injection fluid along with the arterial solution. These fluids are designed to maintain or add body moisture. Excessive use of humectants will have the opposite effect and instead will cause tissues to dehydrate.
5. Inject large volumes of fluid to replenish the lost moisture.
6. Intermittent or alternate drainage can be used to help the tissues retain the arterial solution and also to reduce short-circuiting of fluids to achieve more uniform embalming. This type of drainage also helps the arterial solution to penetrate the deeper body tissues (**Fig. 21–3**).
7. Apply massage cream, stone oil, or lanolin spray to exposed skin surfaces of the face and the hands to act as a barrier to retard moisture loss. Applications are done during and immediately after arterial injection. Repeated applications may be needed if tissue drying is noticed.
8. Avoid excessive massage of the hands, neck, and face. Massage is practiced to encourage fluid to reach these areas, but excessive massage will instead, remove fluid from these areas.
9. Do not expose bodies to direct air currents. Maintain body coverings. Forced air heating and air conditioning currents quickly dehydrate exposed areas of the body.

## EDEMA

**Edema is defined as the abnormal collection of fluid in tissue spaces, serous cavities, or both.** Interstitial or tissue fluids enter and leave the bloodstream (in a similar manner to embalming fluids) through the walls and the pores of the capillaries, the small vessels connecting the smallest arteries (arterioles), and through the smallest veins (venules). If more fluid leaves the blood vascular system and enters the tissues than is absorbed from the tissues into the blood, the tissues become saturated and swell. Edema may be localized in a specific area or generalized throughout the body. Localized edema is generally named for the region affected. Generalized, body-wide edema is called **anasarca**. Edema is a frequent condition encountered by embalmers (**Table 21–2**).

Abnormal accumulations of fluid (edema) can be found:
1. within the individual cells—*Intracellular*.
2. within the spaces between the cells—*Intercellular*.
3. within the body cavities.

Edema can be **localized,** for example, when surgery has involved the heart or repair of the aorta. Following these surgeries, the head and the face can be severely swollen with fluid, while the body trunk and the limbs display no trace of edema. Anasarca or generalized edema is present in all tissues. A number of diseases and conditions can cause generalized edema: diseases that affect cardiac function and result in increased venous pressures, diseases that affect the renal system, increased permeability of the capillary walls, inflammation, and allergic reactions. In addition, long-term use of drugs can damage such vital organs as the liver and kidneys and the circulatory system. Failure of these organs or systems can lead to edema. Some drugs also act upon cell membranes, causing the cells to retain or take up moisture which creates a condition of edema within the cell. This is commonly seen in long-term corticosteroid use. Edema can be present in one or more body cavities without edema present in the skeletal tissues. Likewise, edema can be demonstrated in the skeletal tissues and not present in the body cavities.

The following diseases and conditions are often associated with edema:

- Alcoholism
- Burns
- Cirrhosis of the liver
- Carbon monoxide poisoning
- Congestive heart failure
- Allergic or inflammatory reactions
- Extended drug therapy

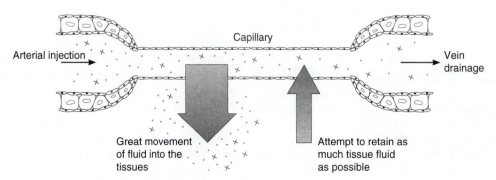

**Figure 21–3.** Hypotonic arterial solutions help the tissues retain moisture.

### TABLE 21-2. Summary of Edema

| Edema | Definition | Challenges | Treatment |
|---|---|---|---|
| Solid | Edema within body cells | Swollen tissues; difficult preservation | Must be excised for reduction |
| Pitting | Edema in tissue spaces, between the cells | Distension; fluid dilution; leakage; difficult preservation | Strong arterial solutions; co-injection fluids |
| Anasarca | Generalized edema in all body tissues | Leakage; distension; arterial fluid dilution | May be gravitated; use strong arterial solutions; may be punctured and drained; use plastic garments to protect from leakage |
| Edema of face | Edema in facial tissues | Swollen tissues, eyelids, and tongue | Strong arterial solutions; hypodermic and surface embalming; plastic garments; gravitation; puncture and drain |
| Edema of hands | Edema in tissues of the backs of the hands | Swollen tissues; possible leakage from intravenous punctures; wrinkles after removal | Restricted cervical injection; strong coordinated arterial solutions; possible use of salt solutions or high-index solutions to reduce swelling; elevate head; channel with trocar neck area for drainage into thorax; surface weights for eyes and lips; surface and hypodermic embalming to ensure preservation with cavity fluid |
| Edema of legs | Edema in thighs and lower legs | Dilution of arterial fluid; leakage | Sectional injection from axillary artery; surface packs with cavity fluid to ensure preservation; bleach any discolorations; elevate to gravitate edema into arm |
| Pulmonary edema | Edema in the alveoli of the lungs | Purge | Sectional injection of legs from femoral or external iliac artery; use of strong arterial solutions; use of salt solutions or dehydrating solutions to remove edema; hypodermic injection with undiluted cavity fluid; surface treatment using autopsy gel; plastic stockings containing embalming powder and autopsy gel; elevate to gravitate edema into abdominal cavity; puncture and drain |
| Hydrothorax | Edema in the thoracic cavity | Purge; dilution of cavity fluid; pressure can cause venous congestion of neck and face; facial distension | Aspiration and injection of lungs |
| Ascites | Edema of abdominal cavity | Pressure can cause purge of stomach contents; anal purge; dilution of cavity fluid | Aspiration; injection of cavity fluid; careful draining prior to arterial injection |
| Hydropericardium | Edema of pericardial cavity | Dilution of cavity fluid pressure could cause drainage challenges | Aspiration and injection of undiluted cavity fluid; pre-embalming draining via trocar or drainage tube; re-aspiration and re-injection |
| Hydrocele | Edema of scrotum | Leakage; dilution of arterial fluid; distension; challenges in dressing | Aspiration and injection of undiluted cavity fluid |
| Hydrocephalus | Edema of cranial cavity | Purge in infant | Channel with trocar to drain into abdominal cavity; inject via trocar undiluted cavity fluid; surface coating with autopsy gel; use of plastic garments and embalming powder |
| | | | Drain in infant via ethmoid foramen; inject cavity fluid via ethmoid foramen |

- Steroid therapy
- Renal failure
- Trauma
- Lymphatic obstruction
- Venous obstruction
- Phlebitis
- Malnutrition
- Hepatic failure and/or obstruction
- Surgical and transplant procedures

## CLASSIFICATION OF EDEMA BY LOCATION

### Cellular (Solid) Edema

Cellular, or solid edema occurs when an abnormal amount of interstitial fluid passes into, and is retained by the cell (intracellular). The tissues are swollen and firm to the touch. Solid edema does *not* respond to embalming treatments. When facial tissues are affected, excision of the deep tissues after completion of arterial treatment is an optional restorative method.

### Intercellular (Pitting) Edema

Pitting or intercellular edema occurs when fluids accumulate between the cells of the body. Digital pressure applied to the edematous area causes an indentation, or *pit* to remain in the tissues. Pitting edema responds well to embalming treatments. It can be drained from the tissues into the circulatory system and removed along with the blood drainage. This edema may be localized as is frequently seen in bodies dead from cardiac diseases where only the legs are distended, and pulmonary edema (edema of the alveolar spaces in the lung tissue). Or, it may be generalized as is frequently encountered after death from liver or renal failure. Generalized edema is referred to as anasarca.

### Edema of the Body Cavities

**Ascites** is edema of the abdominal (or peritoneal) cavity; the edema is found within the cavity and surrounds the abdominal viscera. **Hydrothorax** is edema of the pleural cavity; it may involve one or both pleural cavities. **Hydrocephalus** is edema of the cranial cavity, and **hydropericardium** is edema of the pericardial sac surrounding the heart. **Hydrocele** is an accumulation of serous fluid in the sac-like cavity in the tunica vaginalis testis of the male scrotum.

*Edema of the cavities (ascites) does not mix with, or dilute the arterial solution. Ascites* **will** *dilute the cavity fluid.*

## EMBALMING CHALLENGES CREATED BY EDEMA

Generalized edema presents a number of challenges for the embalmer. The tissues in which edema is present are swollen. When this involves the face and the hands, measures must be taken to reduce the distortion. Edema of the skeletal tissues has a tendency to gravitate into the dependent body areas, during life as well as after death.

In the bedridden patient, the edema is found largely in the dependent areas such as the back, the buttocks, the shoulders, and the backs of the legs. After death, this edema in the dependent tissues can in time lead to the passage of this fluid through the skin. This exit of fluid from the body can dampen the clothing of the deceased and the casket bedding, unless precautions are taken (e.g., use plastic garments and absorbent powders to trap and hold the fluids).

Bodies with large amounts of edema also exhibit leakage from intravenous punctures and small openings such as those made with hypodermic needles. Any surgical or embalming incisions are possible sites of leakage. Another major concern with edema is that the excess moisture in the tissues will hasten the decomposition cycle. A good, moist environment for bacterial growth is provided. Autolytic and hydrolytic enzymes will have an ample source of water for their role in decomposition. A secondary dilution of the embalming fluid is created by this excess fluid.

## EMBALMING CHALLENGES CREATED BY ANASARCA

1. Affected tissues are swollen with fluid.
2. When edema gravitates or moves from a region, the skin can wrinkle and appear distorted.
3. Fluid can leak from intravenous or invasive punctures through the skin surface by gravitation, through hypodermic needle punctures, through surgical incisions, and through incisions made for embalming purposes.
4. Arterial fluid is diluted (secondary dilution).
5. Decomposition is speeded.
6. The possibility of separation of the skin layers (skin-slip) is increased.

When the face is affected by edema, the embalmer must first determine whether **solid** or **pitting** edema is involved. This can be done by gently applying digital pressure to the swollen tissues. Solid edema **cannot** be indented by pressure from the fingers. With solid edema, the extra fluids are located within the individual cells of the tissues. This type of edema is seen in allergic reactions and as the result of certain drug therapies, such as the extended use of corticosteroid drugs. Solid edema cannot be removed by arterial or mechanical means. It would not be wise to attempt to reduce the swelling by surgical removal of subcutaneous tissues after arterial embalming. Uniformity of the tissue reduction and leakage would be major concerns. Solid edema, especially of the facial tissues, is not as frequently encountered as pitting edema.

In pitting edema, the fluid is in the interstitial spaces (between the cells). **Pitting edema can be gravitated**. Merely elevating the head helps to drain some of the fluid from the tissue spaces. Elevation of the head and the shoulders, during and following arterial injection, can drain a considerable volume of edematous fluids from the facial tissues. Passing the trocar through the tissues of the neck, while aspirating, will provide channels through which these fluids can pass from the face into the thorax. A sufficient amount must be given for this drainage to occur.

## ARTERIAL TREATMENT FOR GENERALIZED EDEMA

Anasarca or generalized edema presents a number of challenges for the embalmer. Foremost is the increased rate of decomposition resulting from the presence of excess body moisture. Water is necessary for the cycle of decomposition. Excess moisture causes secondary dilution of the arterial fluid, reducing the ability of the embalming solution to dry, sanitize, and preserve tissues. Edema can seep through the skin and skin blebs can form at edematous sites and rupture, releasing fluids. Soiling of clothing or casket interior fabrics can result.

The objectives of the embalmer are to (1) inject an arterial solution of sufficient strength and volume to counteract the secondary dilution that occurs in the edematous tissues, (2) remove as much of the edema from the tissues as possible, and (3) establish tissue drying and satisfactory preservation.

The underlying cause of the edema is helpful in determining the embalming treatment. For example, generalized edema could be the result of renal failure. In addition to the edema, renal failure creates a buildup of nitrogenous wastes in the tissues. The nitrogenous wastes can neutralize the preservative solution, rendering it ineffective. The use of strong astringent solutions should be used to overcome neutralization. Edema also coexists with nitrogenous wastes in deaths from second-degree burns and exacerbated when death occurs after an extended period.

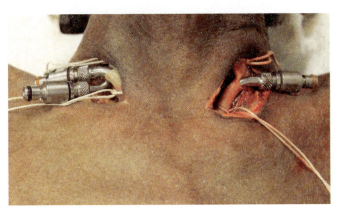

**Figure 21-4.** Restricted cervical injection to reduce generalized edema and to prevent facial dehydration.

Edema affects all body types, even emaciated bodies. One primary concern is to achieve preservation and to dry the tissues. Overdehydration of the face and the features is best avoided by raising both common carotid arteries for restricted cervical injection method (**Fig. 21-4**). Inject the trunk first with a hypertonic solution followed by separate injection of the head using a less astringent solution.

Liver cancers, generalized edema, and jaundice are comorbidities. Primary importance is the preservation and drying of the tissues. The jaundice discoloration is secondary. RCI with a waterless solution is recommended. A jaundice fluid is selected to embalm the head, and large volumes of strong arterial solution are used for the trunk.

Supplemental hypodermic injection of concentrated (hypertonic) arterial solution can be used to treat areas receiving insufficient arterial solution. The hypovalve trocar can be used for the injection. The trocar entry site is easily closed with a trocar button. Application of super adhesive around the trocar button prevents leakage. Plastic garments are recommended.

When edema affects the head and the facial tissues, the features may become severely distended and the tongue can protrude (**Fig. 21-5**). Digital pressure on the dependent portions of the scalp can also reveal the presence of pitting edema. Elevation of the head and the shoulders is necessary. Hypertonic arterial solutions draw edema from the tissues into the circulatory system (**Fig. 21-6**). The edematous fluids are removed along with blood drainage.

In addition to employing a hypertonic arterial solution for the injection of the head, the embalmer can use the channeling method during cavity embalming. From within the cavities, the trocar is directed into the affected tissues; fluids will drain from the face, scalp, and neck into the thoracic cavities for aspiration. Massage of the facial tissues toward the neck and chest gravitates excess fluids.

In severe cases when edema remains after arterial injection and cavity treatment, the body can be transferred and secured to the mortuary cot for additional treatment. The cot is fully lowered and only the head end of the cot is raised. Allow several hours to encourage edema to gravitate from the head and neck. Transfer the body back to the embalming table for reaspiration.

Swollen tissues around the eyes can be treated by channeling with a hypodermic needle from beneath the eyelids. Firm digital pressure upon the lids will gravitate the edema. Cotton saturated with phenol or cavity fluid can be placed into an eye cap to dry edematous eyelids and ensure preservation.

If areas of the face appear to lack adequate arterial solution, surface compresses of undiluted cavity fluid or preservative gels can be applied and remain in place several hours. Facial areas can also be preserved hypodermically. Consider the points of needle entry as the edema may leak from these points. Hypodermic injection from within the oral cavity is recommended. When the head has been autopsied, a long hypodermic needle can be introduced from within the margins of the cranial incision. In the majority of bodies with generalized edema, the embalmer can expect copious (abundant) drainage and good fluid distribution. Preservative demand is met by injection of a moderate to strong arterial solution.

### Injection Site

In the body with generalized edema, it is recommended that restricted cervical injection be employed. This allows saturation of the trunk tissues without overly injected the head. Separate injection of the head follows after the trunk has been embalmed. Facial features may be set after the trunk has been embalmed and after cavity aspiration.

### Drainage Site

The center of blood drainage is the right atrium of the heart. If the right internal jugular vein is used for drainage, instruments can be inserted directly into the right atrium and the head and neck drained from this site. Or, drain from both right and the left internal jugular veins when preparing a body with severe facial edema. Continuous drainage encourages removal of edematous fluids from the body.

### Rate of Flow (speed of delivery)

Begin at a slow rate of flow. Once distribution is established, increase the rate of flow to ensure good distribution to distal body areas.

### Interrupted Injection

It is very important when removing edematous fluids from the tissue spaces to allow the injected embalming fluid time to bring about osmotic exchange; wherein the edematous fluids move into the capillaries and the preservatives move from the

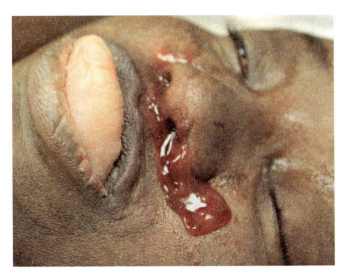

**Figure 21-5.** Protruding tongue caused by severe facial edema.

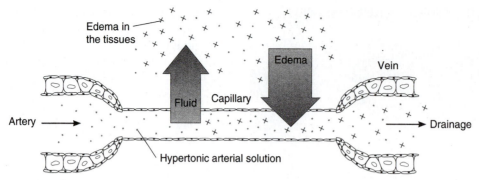

**Figure 21-6.** Hypertonic arterial solutions and arterial solutions containing large colloid molecules help to draw the edema from the tissues into the circulatory system.

capillaries into the tissue spaces. Best practice is to periodically stop injection to allow these physical exchanges to occur. Massage and squeeze the limbs from their distal portion toward the heart to encourage drainage of the edematous fluids from the veins into the blood drainage. Elevation of the arms and the legs also encourages the edematous fluids to move into the large veins. The injection of additional arterial solution after a rest period helps to force edematous fluid out of the vascular system into the drainage.

## Arterial Solutions

The following examples are offered for consideration in the treatment of generalized edema. Embalming analysis and professional judgment determine the selection of embalming fluids and strengths of arterial solutions.

## LOCAL TREATMENTS FOR EDEMA

### General Techniques

1. Sectional arterial injection
2. Direct hypodermic injection
3. Elevation and gravitation
4. Channeling and wicking
5. Lancing and draining
6. Plastic protective garments and absorbent powders

### Legs

When only the legs are affected by edema, raise the femoral vessels and separately inject the legs. If the edema is severe, after arterial injection use the trocar to pierce the upper thighs beneath the inguinal ligaments while embalming the cavities. Elevate the legs and, if desired, wrap them with an elastic bandage beginning at the foot and moving up the leg. This pushes some of the edema into the pelvic cavity from which it can later be aspirated. The legs should be elevated several hours to make this treatment effective.

The legs can also be injected with cavity fluid or a high-index arterial fluid using an infant or hypovalve trocar. This is done **after** the arterial injection of the legs. The fluid is placed in the injection machine, and the delivery tube is attached to an infant trocar. The inside of the calf is a good point of entry. From this point, the lower leg and thigh can be reached. Saturate the leg with the fluid and close the entry point with a trocar button. The leg can also be coated with autopsy gel and placed into a plastic stocking. Embalming powder can also be placed inside the stocking. The powder and the gel assist in the preservation of the leg. When edema is more extensive and affects the hips and the buttocks, plastic coveralls or pants should also be used. When shoulders and trunk walls are affected in addition to the legs and arms, a plastic unionall is recommended to fully cover these areas.

**Tissue blebs** can accompany severe edema (**Fig. 21-7**). The bleb contains edematous fluid that has seeped from the deeper tissues into the superficial layer. Lance the bleb and cauterize the moist tissues with phenol or cavity fluid. Apply surface chemical compresses and wrap the affected area (**Fig. 21-8**).

**Lymphedema**, or lymphatic obstruction is a long-term condition caused by the collection of excess fluid in tissues. The obstruction prevents lymph fluid from draining from the area; fluid buildup leads to swelling and hardened tissues. Tissues become necrotic in the advanced stages of the condition. This condition commonly affects the limbs. Post-embalming treatment includes hypodermic injection of the affected area and surface chemical compresses (**Figs. 21-9** and **21-10**). Plastic garments are recommended.

### Arms

When only the arms and the hands are affected with edema, the arm can be separately injected after the body has been embalmed. The hand and the arm can be elevated to gravitate some of the edema into the upper arm. Wrinkling of the back of the hand now becomes a problem.

If distal areas such as the fingers become badly wrinkled, a small amount of tissue builder can be injected into each finger.

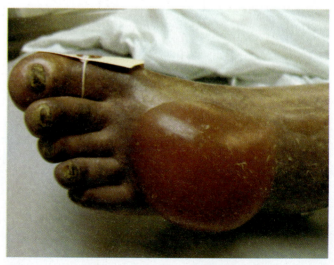

**Figure 21-7.** Edema of the foot accompanied by tissue bleb.

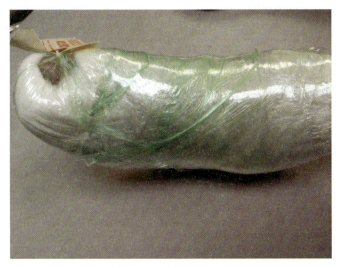

**Figure 21–8.** Tissue bleb treated.

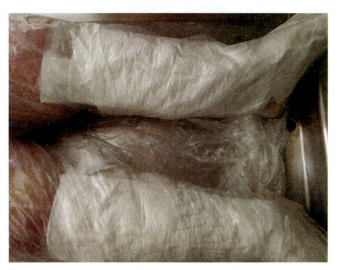

**Figure 21–10.** Surface embalming treatment for lymphedema.

Some wrinkling may be removed by the injection of tissue builder; good points of needle entry would be between the fingers. If there are intravenous or needle punctures on the back of the hand, the embalmer can remove a considerable amount of edema through these openings by squeezing and then sealing the openings with a drop or two of super adhesive.

If only the elbow area is swollen with edema, it may be unwise to lance and drain the edema after embalming, UNLESS a sufficient amount of time is available for the fluids to drain and the tissues would be strong enough to be sewn closed. Wicking the edema is possible—time permitting. Cavity fluid can be injected into the elbow area by use of an infant or hypovalve trocar. The trocar can be inserted through a high point in the upper arm. The opening can be securely closed with a trocar button.

### Edema of the Trunk

After death, edematous fluid gravitates to the dependent areas. Sectional arterial injection of the trunk is not possible. When edema is present in the dependent trunk areas (e.g., shoulders, buttocks, lateral walls), direct hypodermic injection will serve best to increase the preservation of these regions. An infant or hypovalve trocar can be inserted into the lateral walls on each side of the body. The point of entry can be along the midaxillary line in the soft tissues inferior to the rib cage. From this point of entry, the trocar should be able to reach as far up as the axilla and also as far down as the buttocks. Cavity fluid or very concentrated arterial solution can be injected through the embalming machine. This added embalming measure, of course, is done after arterial injection of the body. Coveralls or a unionall can be placed on the body, and a liberal amount of preservative powder can be sprinkled into the plastic garment. Eventually this edema will pass through the skin of the back and the dependent trunk walls. This exit of fluid can occur even before the disposition of the body. It is essential to protect the clothing and the interior of the casket by use of the plastic garments.

### Ascites (Edema of the Abdominal Cavity)

Ascites can exist undetected until the embalmer begins to aspirate the cavity, or it can noticeably distend the abdominal cavity. The edematous fluid is located within the cavity and around the visceral organs. Ascites is unaffected by arterial fluid treatment or blood drainage. Ascites will not dilute arterial fluid, because the arterial solution and the edema in the abdominal cavity do not come into contact. **Ascites will dilute cavity fluid.** When ascites is present and the abdomen is very tense prior to arterial embalming, the pressure in the abdominal cavity may be sufficient to interfere with arterial distribution and blood drainage. The pressure and fluid should be removed prior to arterial injection (**Fig. 21–11**).

Several techniques can be used to relieve the pressure caused by ascites:

1. Using a scalpel, make a small opening in the abdominal cavity and insert a drain tube or a trocar from which the point has been removed. Make this incision in the inguinal or the hypogastric area of the abdominal wall. At this lower point, more liquid can be removed from the cavity. Attach the aspirating hose to the drainage tube or trocar for removal of the edematous fluids directly into the drainage or collection system.
2. Insert a trocar keeping the point just under the anterior abdominal wall. Pierce the transverse colon to release gases. Attach the aspirating hose to the trocar.

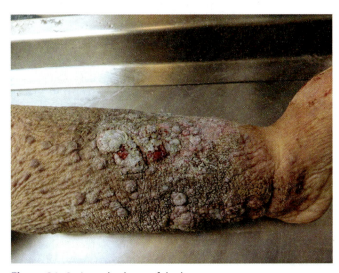

**Figure 21–9.** Lymphedema of the leg.

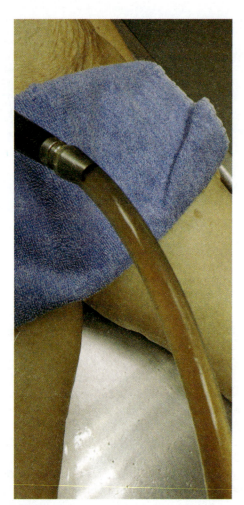

**Figure 21–11.** Aspiration of ascites; edema of the abdominal cavity.

head and the arms. Aspiration should immediately follow arterial injection. Very often distension of the neck will diminish and any swelling that may have occurred in the facial tissues will be reduced.

### Hydrocele

In the male, the scrotum can become distended with edematous fluid (**Fig. 21–12**). Insufficient arterial solution reaches the tissues of the scrotum, which can be a site for decomposition. This condition is treated during aspiration and injection of the body cavities, after arterial injection. During aspiration pass the trocar over the pubic symphysis and pubic bone and enter both sides of the scrotum. Place a towel around the scrotum and apply pressure. This forces the edematous fluid through the channels that have been made with the trocar and into the pelvic cavity. The scrotal sac is filled with undiluted cavity fluid to ensure preservation. Care should be taken not to puncture the scrotum with the trocar. If the scrotum is punctured, use the wicking method to remove as much fluid as possible (**Fig. 21–13**).

**Wicking** is a post-embalming process to remove edema from body regions. A scalpel is used to create one or several small openings in a dependent area of the edematous tissue. Long lengths of dry cotton serve as wicks to draw the edema from the area. Wicks are inserted directly into the area using forceps

When the distension of the abdomen is not severe enough to restrict the flow of arterial solution or interfere with blood drainage, the ascites can be removed during cavity aspiration. Reaspiration is recommended.

### Hydrothorax

In hydrothorax, edema is present in the pleural cavity, the space between the wall of the thoracic cavity and the lung. This condition is not easy to recognize because the rib cage cannot expand like the abdomen when edema is present. This condition can be expected in deaths from heart disease or pneumonia. Distension of the neck is common. Both the face and the neck can exhibit intense livor mortis after death. Aspiration after embalming removes the fluid. Direct the trocar into the posterior portions of the thorax, where the fluid has gravitated. Often large volumes of fluid can be aspirated from the thorax when this condition is present.

If it is necessary to relieve some of this pressure prior to or during arterial injection, a trocar can be introduced from the standard point of trocar entry and guided along the lateral wall of the abdomen into the thoracic cavity. This provides a drainage outlet for the fluid, but does not rupture any large arteries or veins. When hydrothorax is suspected, use the common carotid artery for injection and drain from the right internal jugular vein. This is the best location from which to drain the

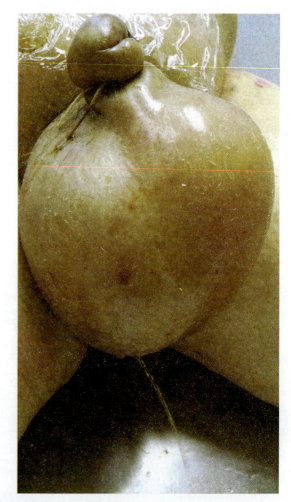

**Figure 21–12.** Hydrocele; edema of the scrotum, prior to treatment.

# CHAPTER 21 • Moisture Considerations

plunger of the syringe. Several ounces of undiluted cavity fluid or phenol solution can be injected in the same manner as the fluid was aspirated. The nostrils should be tightly packed with cotton to prevent leakage.

## SPECIAL CONDITIONS

### Fatal Burns

When an individual initially survives a burn trauma, edema will occur, especially in second-degree burns. Blistering of the skin is characteristic of second-degree burns. It is unlikely the embalmer will see the blistering phase of tissue repair. The blisters have been lanced during medical intervention. Death commonly results from renal failure. Preservation is the primary objective and demand for preservative is high. Restricted cervical injection of hypertonic or waterless solutions is recommended. Fluid dye can be added to the arterial solution to trace distribution. Areas not reached by the arterial solution are treated by hypodermic injection of cavity fluid or a very strong arterial solution.

Denuded skin surfaces can be thoroughly dried after embalming by allowing air exposure and by force-drying with a hair dryer. Select a suitable plastic garment that covers all affected areas. Coat the affected surfaces of the body with autopsy gel and liberally apply embalming powder. Place embalming powder into the garment as well.

### Renal Failure

Renal failure, acidosis, and anemia may not be recognized during Pre-embalming analysis. Conversations with next-of-kin or review of documents from the releasing institution may yield information about cause of death, or the presence of underlying conditions. Kidney dialysis indicates a potential for renal failure. Pungent and persistent odors of ammonia or urine can indicate renal failure. Uremic pruritus is a chronic itching of the skin affecting up to 50% of patients with advanced and end-stage renal failure. Also called chronic kidney disease-associated pruritus (CKD-ap).

Kidney disease and renal failure do not occur in a vacuum; simultaneous disease processes called *comorbidities* can occur. The proximity of the kidney to the liver, for example, means both organs can be affected by jaundice; a common complication of liver disease. Chronic renal failure accumulates toxic wastes (urea, uric acid, ammonia, and creatine) in the blood and the tissues of the body. Retention of waste products in the tissues causes acidosis. The presence of urochrome turns the skin to yellow or brown in tone. Loss of natural complexion color is referred to as sallow. Anemia, gastric ulcerations, and gastrointestinal bleeding are common. Over time, a decrease in cardiac function can lead to congestive heart failure and pulmonary edema.

Bodies with renal failure rapidly decompose. Special purpose high-index fluids are recommended to address the following embalming concerns: (1) edema further dilutes the arterial solution, (2) waste products in the bloodstream and the tissues neutralize the formaldehyde, and (3) altered proteins inhibit tissue firming.

The primary objective is thorough preservation. Restricted cervical injection is recommended. Dye can be added to the

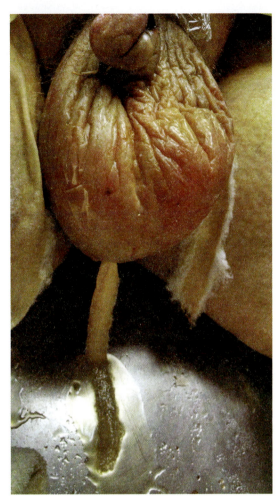

**Figure 21–13.** Reduction of hydrocele using the wicking method.

or a hemostat. The opposite end of the wick extends into the side drain of the embalming table. Numerous wicks can overlap to create additional length. The capillary action of the wick will draw the edema from the tissues over time. Manual pressure placed on the edematous area can increase and speed the drainage of the edema. Allow passive drainage to continue for several hours. The opening can be closed with a trocar button or a reverse suture and sealed with a surface adhesive. Plastic pants or an adult incontinence brief is recommended.

### Hydrocephalus

Hydrocephalus is an abnormal accumulation of cerebrospinal fluids in the ventricles of the brain. This condition can happen at any age; more commonly infants and adults over sixty. Causes include: bacterial meningitis, lesions, tumors, stroke, or other traumatic brain injury. Infant hydrocephalus is usually congenital (present from birth). The head presents as severely distended. Infants may survive after birth and live many years with this condition.

In adults and unautopsied infants, it is necessary to drain some of this fluid. Rapid decomposition of the brain and fluids of the cranial cavity can occur. After embalming, drainage is established using a long hypodermic needle and syringe. Pass the needle through the nostril and direct it through the anterior portion of the cribriform plate of the ethmoid bone. The fluid is aspirated from the cranial cavity by drawing back on the arterial solution to trace the distribution of fluid and counterstain the sallow appearance.

Cavity treatment in renal failure cases is vital to remove nitrogenous waste and inactivate bacteria. Thorough cavity aspiration followed by injection of a large volume of cavity fluid halts bacterial proliferation and gas formation. Re-aspiration and re-injection of cavity fluid is a best practice. Areas not receiving adequate arterial solution should be sectionally injected. If necessary, undiluted cavity fluid can be injected hypodermically, or compresses of undiluted cavity fluid or autopsy gel can be applied to the surface to ensure preservation.

## CONCEPTS FOR STUDY

Define the following terminology:

- Acidosis
- Anasarca
- Ascites
- Channeling
- Dehydration
- Desiccation
- Edema
- Hydrocele
- Hydrocephalus
- Hydropericardium
- Hydrothorax
- Intercellular edema
- Intracellular edema
- Pulmonary edema
- Renal failure
- Uremic pruritus
- Wicking

1. List antemortem and postmortem conditions that cause dehydration.
2. Apply techniques for maintaining proper moisture balance in the embalmed body.
3. Explain the process of channeling and wicking edematous tissues.
4. Review the impact of ascites upon arterial fluid and cavity fluid.
5. Defend the selection of restricted cervical injection for treatment of edema isolated to the trunk; not affecting the head or facial features.
6. Recall numerous embalming concerns presented with renal failure.

## FIGURE CREDIT

Figures 21–2, 21–4, 21–5 are used with permission of Kevin Drobish. Figures 21–7, 21–8, 21–9, 21–10, 21–11, 21–12, 21–13 are used with permission of Sharon L. Gee-Mascarello.

## BIBLIOGRAPHY

American Board of Funeral Service, *Course Content Syllabus,* 2016.

Elkins J. Major body elevation as a technique for the reduction of swelling in the face and hands of embalmed bodies. In: *Champion Expanding Encyclopedia,* No. 554. Springfield, OH: Champion Chemical Co., 1985.

Ennis JS. *Embalming and Renal Failure: A Silent Danger for Embalmers.* 2018

Henson RW. Controlling the moisture content of the tissues. *Professional Embalmer*, November 1940.

Henson RW. Controlling the moisture content of the tissues. *Professional Embalmer*, October 1940.

*Regulating the Moisture Content of Tissues.* Wilmette, IL: Hizone Supplements; 1938:11.

Sheldon H. *Boyd's Introduction to the Study of Disease*, 10th ed. Philadelphia: Lea & Febiger, 1988.

Shor MM. Can magnesium sulfate be safely used to rid body of fluid in lower extremities? *Casket and Sunnyside*, July 1965.

Sturb CG. Distribution and diffusion. *Funeral Directors Journal*, May 1939.

Venes D. *Taber's Cyclopedic Medical Dictionary,* 19th ed. Philadelphia: F.A. Davis, 2001.

# CHAPTER 22

# Vascular Considerations

## CHAPTER OVERVIEW
- Pathological Conditions
- Vascular Diseases
- Arterial and Venous Coagula
- Intravascular and Extravascular Resistance

Arterial embalming utilizes the entire blood vascular system to distribute embalming solution throughout the body. Arteries carry the embalming solution to the capillaries. At the capillary level, some of the solution will move into the interstitial spaces and make contact with cells and cellular proteins. The solution remaining in the vascular system moves into the veins and forces the blood present to be eliminated in the form of drainage. Damage to the vessels within the system hinders the embalming process. Natural degenerative changes in the circulatory system are common with aging. Pathological and traumatic conditions can also cause damage. When damage occurs to any of the vessel layers, the opening, or lumen can narrow or become fully obstructed. Both arteries and veins have three layers (**Fig. 22-1**):

- *Tunica intima.* The inner lining of endothelial cells, which continue to form the walls of the capillaries and then the inner walls of the veins and arteries (this endothelial layer of cells lines the entire blood vascular system).
- *Tunica media.* The middle layer, composed of muscle cells and elastic tissue.
- *Tunica externa, or adventitia.* The outer layer, composed mostly of connective tissue.

Heart and vascular disease, along with prescribed drug therapies influence the integrity of the vascular system. Any type of intravascular condition that changes the structure of the blood vessel walls, or affects its lining, is of concern. Arteriosclerosis and arterial coagula are frequently encountered by the embalmer. **Table 22-1** lists intravascular conditions that disrupt the processes of distribution and drainage.

## ARTERIOSCLEROSIS

Arteriosclerosis is a pathological condition causing the arterial walls to thicken, harden, and lose elasticity. Diet, exercise, heredity, and stress are precipitating factors. This condition affects all age categories. Arteriosclerosis is more commonly noted in the femoral arteries than the common carotid arteries. The severity of the condition determines whether the artery is viable for injection (**Fig. 22-2**).

- *Type 1.* The intimal wall of the artery is thickened; the lumen is well defined. Use of a standard size arterial tube and unrestricted injection is expected.
- *Type 2.* Vessel walls are thickened and/or hardened; lumen size is reduced and off center. A smaller gauge arterial tube is recommended for injection.
- *Type 3.* The lumen is completely occluded and the artery cannot be used for injection. Collateral circulation can circumvent a blockage and continue to circulate blood beyond the area of occlusion. As the severity of the condition increases, a process called **canalization** creates tiny pathways or canals within the vessel to allow the passage of blood. Canalization may be visible in vessels affected by Type 3 arteriosclerosis.

In comparison to other arteries, the common carotid artery less frequently exhibits arteriosclerosis and is a good choice when vascular problems are anticipated (**Fig. 22-3**). Begin injection at low pressure and slow rate of flow; increase as solution distribution is evidenced. When distribution is mediocre, the strength of the arterial solution can be increased. A stronger solution supports sufficient preservation when a large volume cannot be distributed. Multisite injection allows for higher pressures and pulsation to establish local distribution. Once circulation is established, the pressure and the rate of flow can be reduced.

Co-injection chemicals aid in both fluid distribution and diffusion. Dye is added to indicate which tissues have, and have not received solution. Firm massage helps to move the solution to the affected area. Lowering the hands or feet below the sides of the table increases distribution by gravity.

When the femoral vessel is sclerosed, avoid forcing the arterial tube into the artery. Damage to the intimal layer can cause the lining to slough (shed) and block the lumen. Choose an area of the artery to incise that is not thickened by fatty deposits, or **atheroma.** The vessel wall is weakened in this area and can easily rupture. Make the incision in an unaffected portion

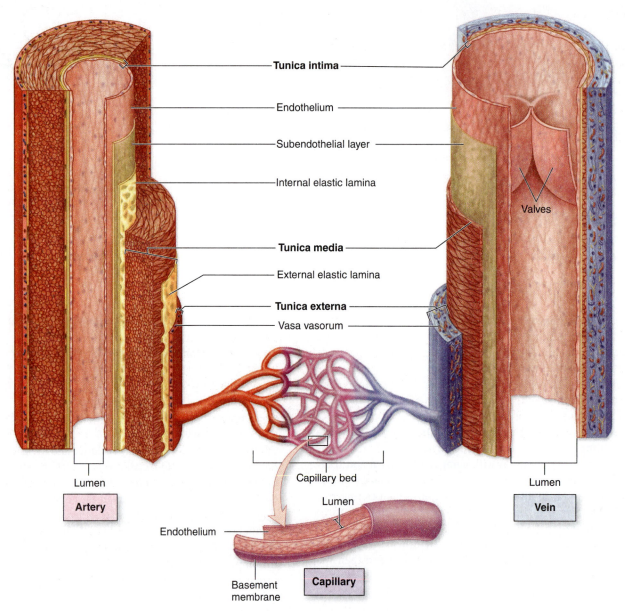

**Figure 22–1.** Comparison of blood vessels. (Used with permission from McKinley M et al. *Human Anatomy*. 5th ed. New York: McGraw Hill, 2017, Fig. 23.1.)

of the artery. Sclerotic arteries are less flexible and may not tolerate being stretched and raised from the incision. Secure arterial tubes in place with an arterial hemostat or thick cotton ligature. Thin linen ligatures may tear the vessel.

## AORTIC ANEURYSM

Ruptured abdominal aortic aneurysm can significantly impair arterial solution distribution. Restricted cervical injection is a recommended best practice. A single-site injection is improbable after severe aortic rupture. Extreme facial edema and sclerotic femoral arteries can be anticipated. Use a strong arterial solution with additional dye to trace distribution. Inject slowly. Continue to inject if drainage is established. If no drainage appears and the abdomen immediately swells, stop the injection. This indicates a loss of embalming solution from the ruptured aorta into the thoracic and abdominal cavities. Begin multipoint injection to sectionally embalm each of the body areas. The trunk walls may require supplemental injection using a hypodermic or infant trocar.

## VALVULAR HEART DISEASES

Disease or malformation may prevent the aorta from being the center of arterial solution circulation according to Murray M. Shor in his article, "Damage to Aorta May Bring Embalming Problems"

*Because of the position of the aortic semilunar valve, embalmers generally consider the aorta as the center of arterial fluid circulation. In most cases, this seems to be true. In the absence of damage to the circulatory system or the heart, it is only after the aorta is filled with fluid that its*

## TABLE 22-1. Conditions Resulting from Intravascular Disease Processes

| Vascular Condition or Injury | Description | Embalming Concern |
|---|---|---|
| Advanced decomposition | Breakdown of the body tissues | Arteries are one of the last "organs" to decompose. Some circulation may be possible. Expect a large number of intravascular clots. Distribution is very poor. Capillary decomposition causes rapid swelling of the tissues. |
| Aneurysm | Localized dilation of an artery | If aneurysm ruptures, fluid cannot distribute. |
| Arteriosclerosis | Hardening of the arteries | Vessel may not be suitable as an injection site. Narrowed arteries may easily trap arterial coagula. |
| Arteritis | Inflammation of an artery | Artery may narrow, resulting in poor distribution of arterial solution. Artery may also weaken and rupture from pressure of injection. |
| Asphyxiation | Insufficient oxygen supply | Right side of heart is congested (poor drainage). Purging can result as blood flows back into lungs instead of draining. Tissue is cyanotic. Intense livor mortis is present in neck and facial tissues. Blood may remain liquid. Capillary permeability is increased. Swelling could easily occur. |
| Atheroma, atherosclerosis | Patchy or nodular thickening of the intima of an artery | Flow of arterial solution may be restricted or occluded. Arterial coagula may be easily trapped during injection. Vessel is poor injection site. |
| Burns | Local or general damage to tissue from heat | Capillaries constrict resulting in extensive coagulation. Distribution of arterial solution may be reduced. Large burns can result in kidney failure, with retention of nitrogenous wastes, thus increasing the preservative demand of the tissues. |
| Cerebrovascular accident | "Stroke" caused by a clot or the rupture of a small artery in the brain. | Vasoconstriction may occur on one side of the body, reducing the distribution of arterial solution. |
| Clots or coagula | Antemortem or postmortem clumping of blood elements | Arterial clots can block or reduce fluid flow to a body region, and may not be removed through drainage. Venous clots may often be removed; if clots are unmovable, swelling and discoloration can result. |
| Congestive heart failure | Decreased heart function | Venous congestion and clotting and cyanosis occur. Legs and feet are edematous. Capillary permeability increases. Tissues can easily swell. |
| Corrosive poisons | Toxic and corrosive chemicals | If poisons are swallowed, purge can usually be expected. Corrosive action may destroy blood vessels causing loss of solution or blood into the gastrointestinal tract. |
| Diabetes | An endocrine disease affecting the control of blood glucose levels | Poor peripheral circulation can reduce solution distribution. Gangrenous areas require surface and/or hypodermic embalming treatments. Dehydration frequently occurs. Breakdown of protein results in poor firming of tissues. |
| Emboli | Detached blood clot | Blockage of a small artery interrupts solution distribution. Venous emboli can block drainage. |
| Esophageal varices | Swollen, tortuous veins caused by a stagnation of blood and generally seen in the superficial veins | Drainage may be difficult to establish. Rupture and massive purge may occur. |
| Extracerebral clot (stroke) | A clot, usually in the carotid artery, that stops blood supply to the brain | The clot can occlude the artery, making it impossible for arterial solution to flow to one side of the face. Blockage may occlude the carotid so it cannot be used as an injection site. Resulting stroke may cause vasoconstriction on one side of the body, reducing arterial solution distribution. |
| Febrile disease | A disease or condition accompanied by an elevation of body temperature | Decomposition may be speeded. Dehydration is possible. Blood coagulates and causes congestion. Distribution and drainage may be hard to establish. |
| Freezing (postmortem) | Cooling of the body to the point where ice crystals form in body tissues | Small vessels and tissues easily swell on injection of solution. |
| Gangrene (dry) | Poor arterial circulation into an area of the body, causing death of body cells | Distribution of arterial solution into the affected area is impossible to establish. Surface and hypodermic treatment is needed. |

(Continued)

## TABLE 22-1. Conditions Resulting from Intravascular Disease Processes (Continued)

| Vascular Condition or Injury | Description | Embalming Concern |
|---|---|---|
| Gangrene (moist) | Occlusion of veins draining a body area that becomes the site of bacterial infection | Very strong fluid must be injected into the general area arterially. The affected necrotic tissues require hypodermic and surface treatments. |
| Gunshot wounds | Entry of a foreign missile into the body | Arterial system may rupture. Multisite injection may be needed. Conditions vary depending on location of wound. Blood loss may result in very little drainage. Bodies are usually autopsied. |
| Hanging | Asphyxiation resulting from exertion of pressure against the large vessels of the neck | Livor mortis is intense or absent in facial tissues. Vessels may be damaged or severed. Restricted cervical injection and jugular drainage are recommended. |
| Hemorrhage | Loss of blood caused by a break in the vascular system | Blood volume may be quite low so there is little drainage. Livor mortis may be minimal. If hemorrhage is the result of a ruptured artery, arterial solution may be lost to body cavities. Multisite injection may be necessary. If a vein has ruptured, much of the drainage may collect in the body cavity where the hemorrhage occurred. If the stomach or esophageal veins are affected, stomach purge can be expected. |
| Ischemia | Lack of blood supply to an area, frequently resulting in tissue necrosis | Arterial solution cannot reach the affected tissues. Hypodermic and surface embalming treatments are needed. |
| Leukemia | Cancer of the tissues that form white blood cells | Purpura is observed over the thorax, arms, and abdomen. Edema may be present. Circulation of arterial solution and drainage may be difficult to establish. |
| Mutilation | Traumatic tissue injuries | Several arteries may result in difficulty in establishing distribution. Multipoint injections may be needed. |
| Phlebitis | Inflammation of a vein | Edema may be present in the area. Blood does not easily drain from the area and discolorations may result. |
| Pneumonia | Acute inflammation of the lung | Broken lung capillaries can result in lung purge. Fever speeds the onset of rigor and decomposition. Congestion may lead to hydrothorax. Distension of the neck can easily occur. Body should be aspirated immediately after arterial injection. |
| Shock | Sudden vital depression, reduced blood return to the heart | Vasodilation may be present, which can cause swelling. In other types of shock, capillaries constrict and blood congestion occurs in the large veins, making drainage difficult to establish. Capillary congestion may interfere with the distribution and diffusion of arterial solution. |
| Syphilis | Venereal disease caused by the spirochete *Treponema pallidum* | Aneurysms may occur in arteries. Rupture can make distribution of arterial solution impossible. |
| Thrombosis | Blood clots attached to the inner wall of a blood vessel | Arterial solution distribution may be difficult. If occurring in a vein, drainage may be hard to establish from the affected tissues. |
| Tuberculosis | Infection of the lungs by *Mycobacterium tuberculosis* that may spread to other organs (e.g., bone, brain, kidney) | When the lungs are affected, cavitation may result; this causes small vessels and capillaries to rupture. There may be a great loss of arterial solution through purging. Purge can be expected. Untreated dehydration and emaciation may be observed. |
| Tumor | Benign or malignant growth of cells | Pressure may be exerted on the outside of an artery or a vein. Distribution to and drainage from an area may be difficult to establish. |
| Vasoconstriction | Narrowing of a blood vessel | When arteries are affected, as in a "stroke," it may be difficult to supply sufficient arterial solution to the affected side of the body. Multipoint injection may be necessary. |

branches can be expected to receive fluid under any appreciable pressure.

Were it not for the position and construction of the aortic valve, fluid would pass from the ascending portion of the aorta into the left ventricle. Under those conditions, the aorta would not be considered the center of embalming fluid circulation. If because of disease or malformation of the aortic semilunar valve fluid did pass into the left ventricle and was confined there by the proper functioning of the mitral valve, the problem would be merely academic. It is when other heart valves are impaired concurrently that embalming problems are created.

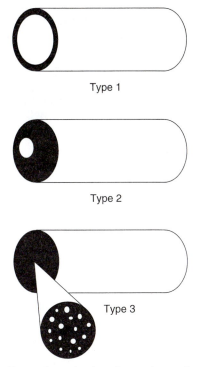

**Figure 22-2.** Types of arteriosclerosis seen in arteries used for arterial injection.

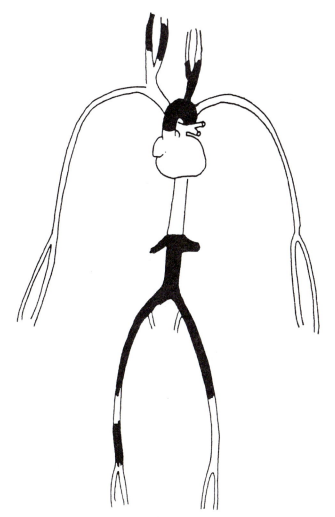

**Figure 22-3.** Common sites of arteriosclerosis. The common carotid arteries are least commonly affected by arteriosclerosis. (*Used with permission of HE Kazmier.*)

## Anatomy of the Heart

The functioning valves are the **left atrioventricular or mitral** (which allows blood to pass from the left atrium to the left ventricle); the **right atrioventricular or tricuspid** (which opens from the right atrium into the right ventricle); the **pulmonary semilunar**, a tricuspid valve (which opens to allow blood to flow from the right ventricle into the lungs via the pulmonary artery); and the **aortic semilunar**, a tricuspid valve (that opens into the aorta from the left ventricle).

During life, heart valves can be affected by congenital malformation, bacterial damage, and the same degenerative diseases that affect arteries. The circulation of blood during life and the distribution of preservative during embalming are substantially altered by disease conditions.

When the mitral and the aortic semilunar valves are damaged, embalming solution (injected under pressure) moves from the aorta into the left ventricle, and then into the left atrium. The left atrium receives the pulmonary veins from the lungs. The pulmonary veins do not have valves, so the embalming solution in the atrium (under pressure) passes back into the capillaries of the lung. The result is the purge of embalming solution from the lungs.

## Lung Purge Caused During Embalming

During embalming, the pulmonary capillaries also receive fluid from the bronchial arteries (from the descending thoracic aorta). When the two fluid masses meet (the first from the bronchial arteries and the second from the pulmonary veins), the collective volume and pressure creates a lung purge. The contents of the hollow portions of the lungs are virtually squeezed through the trachea.

## CONGESTIVE HEART FAILURE

When congestive heart failure is the primary cause of death, these complications are commonly noted:

1. Blood is congested in the right side of the heart.
2. The neck veins are engorged with blood.
3. Facial tissues are discolored due to blood congestion.
4. Lips, ears, and fingertips appear cyanotic (bluish-purplish discoloration due to a lack of oxygenated blood).
5. Generalized pitting edema, ascites, and edema of the legs and feet may be present.
6. Blood may be more viscous due to an increase in red blood cells (polycythemia).
7. Salt is retained in the body fluids.

Selection of the right common carotid and right internal jugular vein or, restricted cervical injection is recommended. Both methods support thorough blood drainage from the head and the right atrium of the heart. The first gallon of arterial solution is prepared as a mild solution to clear blood congestion and discolorations. When edema is present, subsequent solutions are mixed stronger to meet the preservative demands of the tissues. Severe ascites and intestinal gases create pressure upon the inferior vena cava that can prevent adequate drainage from the lower portions of the body. Edematous fluids can be drained using a trocar or drain tube. Incise the skin at the point of entry with a scalpel; this allows insertion of the trocar with minimal effort. Insert the instrument into the ventral portion of the abdominal cavity to prevent puncturing any of the major trunk vessels.

Lower the arms over the table at the onset of arterial injection to promote capillary expansion; this helps to clear discolorations from the hands and fingers. Massage facial tissues to clear discolorations. Drain from both the right and left internal jugular veins when extensive discoloration of the face is present. Use continuous drainage until congestion has cleared. Pressure and rate of flow may be increased as the embalming progresses; the pressure and the rate of flow should be sufficient to move arterial solution through the entire body.

The liver may be enlarged and its functions decreased. This should improve drainage, as the level of clotting factor in the blood will be low.

Pulmonary edema is often observed in cases of congestive heart failure, lung purge is anticipated. Coat the facial tissues with massage cream and allow purge to continue during the embalming process. Perform thorough cavity treatment and pack the nasal cavity with cotton after embalming. In the presence of anasarca, or generalized edema, good distribution and drainage is anticipated. However, ascites dilutes cavity fluid. Reaspiration and reinjection of the cavities may be indicated.

Distension in the neck tissues can be removed during cavity aspiration. Direct the tip of the trocar into the neck and channel the tissues.

## VASODILATION AND VASOCONSTRICTION

The dye used to trace the distribution of arterial solution can indicate that one side of the body has received a large amount of solution and the other side a small amount. This difference is often evident down the midline of the body. This unequal distribution of arterial solution is evident in death from cerebrovascular accident, or stroke. Vasoconstriction occurred on one side of the body while vasodilation, in an effort to supply more oxygen to the tissues, occurred on the opposite side of the body. Multisite injection may be necessary with injection of a sufficient quantity of solution to remedy the discoloration.

## BLOOD VESSEL CLOTS

Internal changes within an artery or a vein causes the lumen to narrow or collapse, creating resistance within the vessel. This is called **intravascular resistance.** Intravascular resistance restricts flow within the vessel. Blockages caused by clot formation are commonly encountered during embalming.

### Arterial Coagula

At death, some blood remains in the arteries, especially in the large aorta. During the postmortem period, this blood can congeal. Injection of the arterial solution may loosen and push coagula into the smaller arteries. When the common carotid is used as the primary injection site, arterial coagula are moved into the iliac and femoral arteries. The femoral arteries can be injected at higher pressures to clear coagula and embalm the legs. Supplemental hypodermic and surface embalming enhance the areas that do not receive sufficient arterial solution.

When the femoral artery is used as the primary injection point, coagula can be moved into the common carotid arteries and prevent arterial solution from reaching the facial tissues

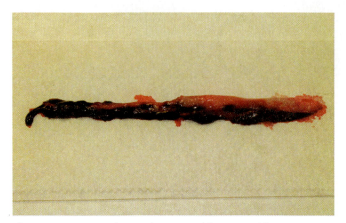

**Figure 22–4.** Arterial coagula removed from carotid artery.

(**Fig. 22–4**). Arterial coagula can also block the left subclavian artery. Raise and inject the axillary or brachial artery to embalm the lower arm and hand.

### Venous Coagula

Small venous blood clots are readily cleared during blood drainage from the right internal jugular vein. Heavier clots lodged in the right atrium can be reached with angular spring forceps for manual removal (**Fig. 22–5**). Coagulum that cannot be

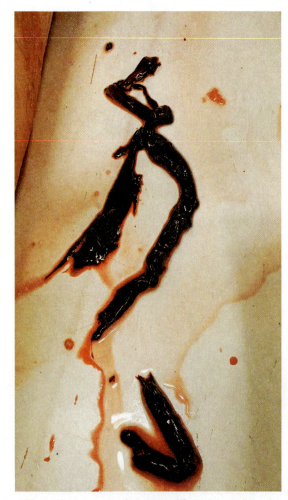

**Figure 22–5.** Venous coagula removed from internal jugular vein.

removed can lead to tissue distension and discoloration. Massaging from distal points toward the heart promotes thorough blood drainage. Intermittent drainage also helps to increase venous pressure and loosen coagula from the veins. Multisite injection and drainage may be warranted. When this condition is encountered in a localized area, use a stronger arterial solution to ensure that a minimum amount of arterial fluid delivers the maximum preservative.

## DIABETES

Arteriosclerosis, cardiovascular disease, hyperlipidemia, obesity, and poor peripheral circulation are common comorbidities with diabetes. Proper fluid selection and thorough distribution are primary embalming concerns. The presence of increased bacterial and mycotic infections requires strong arterial solutions. To assist in establishing distribution and clearing of blood discolorations, the first gallon of arterial solution can be milder than subsequent injections. Use of a co-injection fluid assists in clearing discolorations. Restricted cervical injection is suggested along with a moderate to high pressure to distribute the solution. Massaging the extremities and using intermittent drainage also facilitates fluid distribution. High pressure and pulsation promote flow to the peripheral tissues (fingers, toes, ears, nose, and lips). Bluish discoloration in the fingertips can be manually cleared by squeezing the nailbeds and forcing the discoloration to be removed through blood drainage (**Fig. 22–6**). Dye can be added to trace the distribution of solution in the tissues.

Abnormal pH values may prevent embalmed tissues from adequately firming. A moderate to strong solution strength accompanied by a co-injection fluid and dye should meet the preservative demands, despite lack of tissue firming.

Restricted cervical injection and drainage from the right internal jugular vein ensures thorough tissue saturation. A large volume of solution can be injected without concern of swelling the features of the face. Large volumes also promote better fluid diffusion.

Cavity embalming must be thorough to arrest mycotic infections that may be present in the lungs. Arterial solution does not treat the visceral organs. Abscesses, necrosis, and gangrene

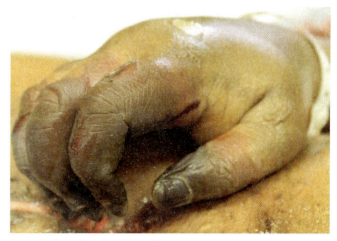

**Figure 22–7.** Fingers affected by gangrene.

of the pancreas and the liver are treated by a sufficient amount of cavity fluid. Cavity fluid is injected into each major body cavity: thoracic, abdominal, and pelvic for a recommended total volume of 32–48 ounces. Based on embalming analysis, additional volumes may be necessary.

Decubitus ulcers are topically disinfected. Marginal tissues are injected hypodermically with cavity fluid or a phenol cautery solution. Surface compresses are applied to the necrotic surface tissues. When the compress is to remain in place, an adult incontinence brief is helpful. Plastic pants are recommended to protect clothing and contain odors.

Gangrene may also be present in distal tissues such as the fingers and the toes (**Figs. 22–7** and **22–8**). These areas will not receive arterial solution when the body is arterially injected. Cavity fluid or phenol cautery can be hypodermically injected into these areas. The surface of the feet affected by gangrene can be coated with autopsy gel or cavity fluid compresses. Plastic stockings protect clothing and contain odors.

## EXTRAVASCULAR RESISTANCE

External pressure upon an artery or a vein causes the lumen to narrow or collapse, creating resistance within the vessel. This is called **extravascular resistance.** Extravascular resistance restricts

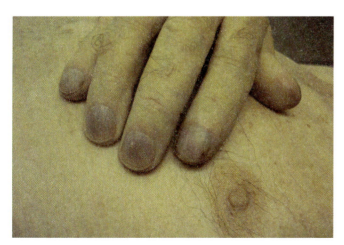

**Figure 22–6.** Bluish fingertips can be cleared by squeezing the nailbeds.

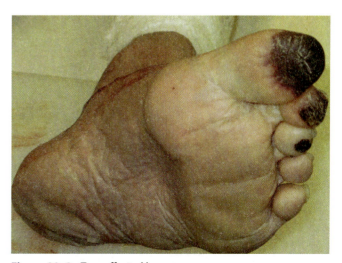

**Figure 22–8.** Toes affected by gangrene.

flow within the vessel. Sources of extravascular resistance and suggestions on how to overcome resistances are listed here:

- *Rigor mortis.* Relieve as much rigor as possible prior to arterial injection.
- *Ascites.* Drain the fluid in the abdomen prior to, or during arterial injection.
- *Gas in the cavities.* Release gases in the abdomen prior to, or during arterial injection.
- *Bandages.* Remove tight bandages prior to injection.
- *Contact pressure.* Massage the affected areas.
- *Tumors.* Excise when necessary; permission is required.
- *Swollen lymph nodes.* Treat with sectional injection.
- *Hydrothorax.* Drainage of the pleural cavities may be impractical prior to embalming.
- *Visceral weight.* Utilize injection and drainage points above and below the heart.

Multipoint injection is recommended when extravascular resistance is present. Higher embalming pressures improve distribution. Moderate to strong well-coordinated arterial solutions are effective when distribution is limited. A method for preventing blood discolorations involves pausing injection and allowing drainage to continue before injecting again. Alternate drainage is practiced as a sequence: inject-pause, drain-pause, repeat. Tissue massage also promotes optimal fluid distribution and blood drainage.

## CONCEPTS FOR STUDY

Define the following terminology:

- Aneurysm
- Arteriosclerosis—Type 1, Type 2, Type 3
- Arteritis
- Asphyxiation
- Atheroma
- Canalization
- Cerebrovascular accident
- Congestive heart failure
- Corrosive poisons
- Diabetes
- Dry gangrene
- Emboli
- Esophageal varices
- Extracerebral clot
- Extravascular resistance
- Febrile disease
- Hemorrhage
- Ischemia
- Leukemia
- Moist gangrene
- Phlebitis
- Pneumonia
- Shock
- Syphilis
- Thrombosis
- Tuberculosis
- Tumor
- Tunica externa
- Tunica intima
- Tunica media
- Vasoconstriction
- Vasodilation

1. Define the types of arteriosclerosis and present embalming complications caused by this condition.
2. Describe embalming considerations for ruptured aortic aneurysm.
3. Recall how arterial injection can cause embalming solution lung purge.
4. State seven complications anticipated with congestive heart failure.
5. Discuss treatment of ascites prior to, or during arterial injection.
6. Relate a manual treatment for clearing bluish discolorations from the fingertips.
7. Describe treatment for decubitus ulcers.
8. Give several reasons for the use of plastic garments.
9. Name nine causes of extravascular resistance.
10. Illustrate interrupted injection as a method to prevent blood discolorations.

## FIGURE CREDIT

Figures 22–4, 22–5, 22–6, 22–7 are used with permission of Kevin Drobish.
Figure 22–8 is used with permission of Sharon L. Gee-Mascarello.

## BIBLIOGRAPHY

American Board of Funeral Service, *Course Content Syllabus*, 2016.
Day DD, Poston G. Embalming the diabetic case. In: *Champion Expanding Encyclopedia*, No. 560. Springfield, OH: Champion Chemical Co., 1985: 2254–2257.
Mulvihill ML. *Human Diseases: A Systemic Approach*, 2nd ed. Norwalk, CT: Appleton & Lange, 1987.
Sheldon H. *Boyd's Introduction to the Study of Disease*, 9th ed. Philadelphia, PA: Lea & Febiger, 1984.
Shor MM. Damage to aorta may bring embalming problems. In: *Casket and Sunnyside*, June 1960.

CHAPTER 23

# Effect of Drugs on the Embalming Process

## CHAPTER OVERVIEW
- Impact of Drug Therapy Upon Embalming
- Preservative Demand
- Chemotherapeutic Agents
- Radioactive Isotopes
- Oral Diabetic Drugs
- Opioid Use

## THE CHEMISTRY OF PROTEINS

The chemistry of embalming is essentially the chemistry of proteins. Proteins are responsible for the structure, function, and regulation of the body's tissues and organs. During embalming, proteinaceous materials within the dead human body must be rendered chemically inert. Proteinaceous materials are those that contain protein. Essentially, this means that decomposition is halted or suspended for a time that exceeds the memorial event or until the time of final disposition.

Proteins are labile (easily altered or broken down) substances that break down rapidly even without bacterial action. **Proteolytic enzymes** are specialized enzymes that break down protein. Enzymes are endowed with a physicochemical structure that allows catalytic activity; they can speed up decomposition reactions. Even if a cadaver were completely sterile (free from bacteria and microbes), the proteolytic enzymes in the cells and tissues of that body would still be fully active and capable of causing the breakdown of tissue proteins.

The preservation objective of embalming is to render the proteins resistant to attack by catalytic enzymes. There are two ways to do this: (1) The proteins can be treated so that they are no longer susceptible to the action of proteolytic enzymes. (2) The enzymes can be changed or inactivated so that they cannot exert catalytic action on proteins. Embalming chemicals are formulated to do both. To illustrate how preservation is achieved in a hypothetical decedent, a brief mathematical formula is helpful.

> **AVERAGE BODY PROTEIN**
> Body weight is 150 pounds, or 65.3 kg
> The 150 pound body is comprised of 10.7 kg, or 10,700 g of protein
>
> **Preservative (Formaldehyde) Demand**
> 100 g of soluble protein requires 4.4 g of formaldehyde for preservation
>
> **Formula Calculations**
> Divide protein (10,700) by soluble protein (100) and multiply by preservative needed (4.4)
> 10,700 ÷ 100 x 4.4 = 470.8 g of formaldehyde needed
>
> **Solution Needed**
> One 16-ounce bottle of a 30-index arterial fluid contains 142.08 g of formaldehyde
> Preservative demand is 470.80 g of formaldehyde
> 470,80 ÷ 142.08 = 3.31
> 3.31 bottles of a 30-index fluid needed to embalm a 150-pound body
> Or, approximately 53 ounces of arterial fluid

## THE CHEMOTHERAPY CASE

Many chemotherapeutic agents are nephrotoxic and can decrease kidney function. Since the kidneys are the main organs responsible for elimination of nitrogenous wastes, waste materials such as ammonia, urea, and uric acid are retained in the tissues. There is no better way to neutralize formaldehyde than to react it with ammonia, and this is exactly what happens in the body. If there has been a buildup of nitrogenous waste materials as a result of chemotherapy-induced kidney dysfunction, a moderate arterial solution will not be sufficient. A large proportion of the formaldehyde in the embalming solution will be neutralized when it encounters the nitrogenous wastes in the body. The remainder is insufficient to preserve the tissues, and the body begins to undergo postmortem putrefactive changes. Strong solution strengths are recommended.

Customarily, arterial embalming fluids are packaged in 16-ounce concentrates. Arterial fluids are diluted with water and other supplemental fluids to create the arterial embalming solution for injection into the body. An embalming fluid containing 30% formaldehyde supplies 142 g of formaldehyde per bottle. To embalm a body containing 10.7 kg of protein, 470 g of formaldehyde is needed, that is, a minimum of three bottles of arterial embalming fluid. Double this amount may be necessary when therapeutic drug therapies were administered. (See Selected Readings: The Mathematics of Embalming Chemistry: Part I. A Critical Evaluation of "One Bottle" Embalming Chemical Claims.)

One axiom could be universally applicable to all drugs that enter the body, regardless of the method of delivery: cellular and tissue changes occur. Drug-induced changes may be relatively minor. Postmortem, a minor skin discoloration will respond favorably to cosmetic treatment. Intense complications, such as acute jaundice can saturate the body tissues with uremic wastes. The fixative action of the preservative chemical during arterial embalming will be impaired.

Chemotherapeutic agents exert numerous effects: impairment of organs and systems within the body: decreased kidney, liver, and lung function; changes in the circulatory system (heart and blood vessels); and changes of the skin. Drugs can decrease permeability of the cell membrane, making it difficult for embalming solution to enter the cell and denature cellular proteins. Hair follicles are commonly affected; hair loss (alopecia) is a common side effect of chemotherapy (**Fig. 23–1**).

The **liver** is the main detoxification center, every drug eventually enters the hepatic circulation. While in the liver, the drug may be changed to an innocuous form by hepatic enzymes or the drug may cause profound changes in the liver itself. When the liver is damaged, the embalmer may encounter a jaundiced body.

All drugs ultimately pass through the kidneys. Kidney damage leads to renal insufficiency and the resulting buildup of nitrogenous wastes in body tissues. Saturated with urea, uric acid, ammonia, creatinine, and other wastes, the tissues become spongy and difficult to preserve. In such cases, preservation treatment must be modified.

Drugs also change the biochemical constituents of the blood and can damage the blood vessels. The circulatory system may become blocked as a result of extensive clot formation, lysis of the blood cells, or extensive damage to the walls of the arteries and veins.

The effects on the **skin** are closely associated with the changes in the circulatory system. Widespread areas of discoloration caused during hemolysis: hemorrhages, ecchymosis, and purpura are frequent discolorations of the skin (**Fig. 23–2**).

## IMPACT OF DRUG THERAPY UPON EMBALMING

Embalming preservation challenges do not result from direct reaction between the drug and the preservative. The drug causes physiological changes in the body. The physiological conditions present in the body create the embalming challenges. For example, a drug that causes nephrotoxic changes enhances the accumulation of nitrogenous waste products in the body. These waste products, which result indirectly from the physiological effect of the drug, are responsible for the inactivation or, more specifically, the neutralization of the formaldehyde:

$$4NH_3 + 6CH_2O \rightarrow (CH_2)_6N_4 + 6H_2O$$

This neutralization reaction, whereby formaldehyde is converted to hexamethylene, is probably at the root of at least 90% of the preservation challenges.

Changes in cellular membrane permeability is another effect of systemically administered drugs. It is through this membrane that everything must pass, either to enter or to leave the cell. Preservative chemicals such as formaldehyde must pass through the cell membrane to inactivate the intracellular enzymes that cause protein decomposition. When a chemotherapeutic agent reduces or destroys membrane

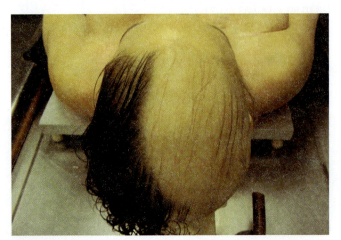

**Figure 23–1.** Hair loss and jaundice discoloration due to chemotherapy.

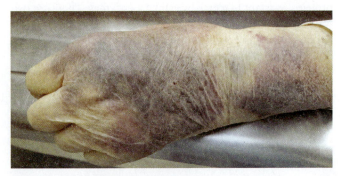

**Figure 23–2.** Ecchymosis and purpura.

permeability, preservative solutions cannot pass through. The antibiotic tetracycline is a case in point. Although most antibiotics exert their effects on bacteria, they also have an effect on the human cell. They are chelating agents and tend to lodge in the cell membrane, causing calcium to form an impenetrable layer around the cell. "Chelating" means they have an affinity for metallic ions, particularly calcium and magnesium. Antibiotics appear to act selectively on cell membranes. After they are entrenched in the membrane, they start chelating or sequestering calcium and magnesium ions. There is generally not a shortage of calcium in the body; calcium is present in all biological fluids.

Eventually, as more calcium and magnesium ions become lodged in the cell membrane, the permeability of the membrane changes. It becomes increasingly more difficult for some chemicals to enter such a cell. Because the goal of embalming is the inactivation of the intracellular enzymes present, it is essential that the preservative enter the cell. If it does not, the proteolytic enzymes inside the cell can proceed to break down the proteinaceous materials in the cell, and the tissue is subject to decomposition and lysis of its structural features.

## MULTIDRUG THERAPY

Two or more drugs may be prescribed together to treat a single disease or condition; called a multidrug approach or combination therapy. The embalming challenges resulting from synergistic combinations of drugs can be more intense than the effects caused by a single drug.

## ANTIBIOTICS

Antibiotics are the most widely used class of drugs. Antibiotics are used to treat or prevent some bacterial infections; they are not effective against viral infections. Long-term antibiotic use can cause liver damage and kidney failure. Tissues may become saturated with ammonia and nitrogen waste. Higher index arterial fluids and strong, hypertonic solutions are necessary to compensate for waste products that neutralize formaldehyde. Firming of tissues may be difficult to achieve.

## CORTICOSTEROIDS AND ANTI-INFLAMMATORY DRUGS

Cortisone and its derivatives may constitute a close second for their wide applications and common use. Corticosteroids are commonly used for chemotherapeutic cancer treatment. Anti-inflammatory drugs primarily reduce inflammation. Nonsteroidal anti-inflammatory drugs (NSAID) are pain relievers.

With regard to specific embalming problems caused by these drugs, the chief effect is blockage of the cell membrane. Corticosteroids decrease the permeability of this membrane and thereby block passage of liquids into the cell. On a gross macroscopic level, liquids are retained by the cells and tissues, resulting in an increase in cell turgor and waterlogging of tissues. Cell turgor refers to the rigidity of cells from the absorption of liquids.

The use of cortisone for the treatment of chronic diseases may result in gastrointestinal ulcerations and perforations of the gut. Prolonged use in the treatment of ulcerative colitis can result in dehydration of the body.

Corticosteroids have been shown to exert a protective effect on proteolytic enzymes. This is demonstrated by the challenge of denaturing enzymes in cortisone-treated bodies. Even if these enzymes are extracted from such cortisone-treated tissues and are obtained in an almost pure form, they are still difficult to inactivate. They retain the protective effect originally conferred by the corticosteroids. This means that more undenatured proteolytic enzymes remain in the body after embalming. Such bodies tend to decompose very rapidly after an uncomplicated embalming.

Denaturing of proteins means to destroy the characteristics of proteins. Embalming denatures proteins by cross-linking them. Undenatured proteins are those that embalming did not cross-link or destroy leaving them susceptible to decomposition.

In pharmacology, similar chemical structures elicit similar biological reactions. Progesterone, an oral contraceptive, and its derivatives have chemical structures similar to that of cortisone. Embalming reactions observed from corticosteroid therapies are similar to the reactions observed from oral contraceptive use.

Long-term use of corticosteroids suppresses immunity. Reactivation of the mycobacterium responsible for tuberculosis creates an undetectable hazard to the embalmer. Personal protective equipment (PPE) to cover the mouth and nose of the embalmer is a best practice during any type of decedent care. Sufficient room air exchanges that produce fresh air will reduce circulation of harmful airborne populations in the preparation area.

Pre-injection and co-injection types of fluids restore cell membrane permeability; the surface-active chemicals in the formulation facilitates entry of the preservative across the membrane.

## CHEMOTHERAPEUTIC AGENTS

Cancer chemotherapy agents are classified according to their chemical nature and function. Some of the common cancer chemotherapy agents include alkylating agents, plant alkaloids, antimetabolites, anthracyclines, topoisomerase inhibitors, and corticosteroids. These drugs are cytotoxic, meaning they are capable of damaging or killing cells. The basic mechanism of cytotoxic drugs is to cause immunosuppression by toxic effects to lymphocytes. *Cyto*—cell; *toxic*—poison. Cytotoxic drugs slow the growth of quickly dividing cells. They are commonly used to treat leukemias and cancers of the breast, ovary, and intestinal tract. Antimetabolite drugs are a type of cytotoxic drug. Antimetabolite drugs mimic the molecules that a cell requires for growth; the cell cannot differentiate between its own molecule and that of the mimicking version. The drug is readily received by the cell.

## SIDE EFFECTS OF CHEMOTHERAPEUTIC AGENTS

The antemortem side effects of chemotherapeutic drug therapies can influence the postmortem conditions present in the dead body. Common side effects include diarrhea and vomiting, loss of appetite, loss of hair, skin rashes and dry, cracked skin, inflammation of the mouth and lips, and higher levels of liver enzymes. Related postmortem conditions may include body and tissue dehydration, severe weight loss, hair loss, abdominal fluid retention, yellowish discolorations of the skin, and swollen features (Table 23–1).

## RADIOACTIVE ISOTOPES AND THEIR EFFECTS

Radioactive materials are also used for cancer therapy. Medical institutions provide some form of warning indicating exposure to radiation. A warning sticker might also be affixed to the body bag. The release paperwork should include contact information for the Radiation Safety Officer. The institution is not permitted to release the body until the level of radioactivity has dropped below 30 millicuries for unautopsied bodies; 5 millicuries or below for autopsied remains.

Three precautions are followed for embalming a body treated or exposed to radiation: **protection**, **time of exposure**, **and distance from the body**. Best practice for PPE selection includes the addition of heavy rubber gloves worn over standard surgical gloves, a heavy rubber apron, and all other applicable equipment. Universal Precautions protocol is strictly followed.

Task-sharing is an effective method to reduce time of exposure and distance of exposure. During preparation, embalmers work in pairs and alternate embalming tasks. For example, one embalmer sets features and steps back while the second embalmer raises vessels. This method is followed throughout the procedure. Having instruments ready and fluids mixed, as soon as the body is observed, reduces the time spent in preparation. Avoid raising a vessel where tissues have been seeded with a radioactive isotope for cancer treatment. Common implant areas include the upper chest and neck tissues. Selection of the femoral vessels for embalming is indicated in this case.

For every 3 feet of distance from the body, exposure is reduced substantially. When not performing a procedure, one embalmer should remain at a distance from the body. Maintain a constant flow of water onto the embalming table, beneath the body. Positioning devices and body bridges support the body and allow water to flow freely.

Terminal disinfection best practices:
- Flush all instruments with running water before submerging in cold chemical sterilant.
- Dispose of soiled paper toweling, cotton, suture material, hospital gowns, and the like, in the approved biohazard waste container.
- Washable gowns, towels, and clothing are readily laundered in-house or placed in a laundry bag for the service provider.
- Document the decedent's exposure to radiation on the Embalming and Decedent Care Report.
- Triage all exposure incidents and report for medical attention. Consult the Radiation Safety Officer at the releasing institution.

## OPIOID USE

Opioids are controlled-substances used primarily in medicine for pain relief or anesthesia. Fentanyl is a commonly prescribed synthetic opioid similar to morphine; yet 50–100 times more potent. It is medically administered as an injection, a transdermal patch, or as an oral lozenge.

Direct skin contact with Fentanyl poses a risk to the embalmer. PPE is required. Patches should not be manually removed by gloved hands as gloves have pores that will expand with time and use. Transmission of the narcotic through the pores in the glove is possible. Safe removal of transdermal Fentanyl patches requires instrument usage and proper disposal; the biohazard sharps container is ideal (Fig. 23–3A-C).

**TABLE 23–1. Side Effects of Chemotherapeutic Agents[a]**

| Drug | Problem |
|---|---|
| Antibiotics (penicillins, synthetic penicillins, aminoglycosides, tetracyclines) | Cotton-like circulatory blockages (fungal overgrowth); jaundice; bleeding into skin; poor penetration |
| Corticosteroids (cortisone) | Cell membranes less permeable; retention of fluids; mild to severe waterlogging of tissues; "protects" proteolysis enzymes, resulting in more rapid breakdown of body proteins |
| Cancer chemotherapy (antimetabolites, cytotoxic agents, radioisotopes) | Emaciation and dehydration; extensive purpura; jaundice; low protein (because of anorexia and vomiting); perforation of gut; brittleness of bone; nitrogenous waste retention |
| Tranquilizers (phenothiazines) | Dehydration; weight loss and emaciation; low protein; kidney dysfunction and retention of nitrogenous waste products |
| Stimulants (amphetamines, cocaine) | Weight loss; emaciation; low protein; mucous membranes bleed easily; other problems as for tranquilizers |
| Sedatives (barbiturates, meprobamate) | Emaciation; dehydration; low protein; difficult to firm |
| Oral antidiabetic agents (tolbutamide) | Muscle atrophy; mild to severe jaundice; some emaciation and edema |
| Circulatory drugs (antihypertensives, anticlotting agents) | Blood clots; impairment of circulation; poor distribution of fluids; purpura; urine retention and spongy nitrogenous waste-filled tissues |

[a]Table has been adapted and summarized from many published works. It is neither complete nor exhaustive. It is designed to point out categories of chemotherapeutic agents in use now. It is hoped that this table will stimulate both the student of embalming and the licensed professional to read about the latest developments in journals and trade magazines. As new chemical agents are introduced so frequently by the medical profession, it is impossible to publish up-to-the-minute tables. Keeping up with the literature is of the utmost importance.

PPE is advised to be worn during the transfer of the deceased. Fentanyl "dust" can adhere to clothing and mortuary cot fabrics. Remove contaminated PPE, launder transfer sheets, and clean all transfer equipment.

## ORAL DRUGS FOR TREATMENT OF DIABETES

Drugs that treat diabetes can induce changes in the voluntary muscles (site of glycogen storage and breakdown) and the liver (main glycogen storage organ of the body). Continuous use of oral diabetic agents has been linked with circulatory problems, which can cause poor distribution of the arterial solutions. Acidosis sometimes occurs as a result of the altered carbohydrate metabolism and leads to the formation of high concentrations of lactic acid in muscle tissue. Such bodies firm very rapidly unless an alkaline co-injection is used in combination with the arterial embalming fluid.

## DILUTION OF CHEMOTHERAPEUTIC AGENTS WITHIN THE BLOODSTREAM

Once absorbed into the bloodstream, a drug is rapidly diluted. An average body contains about 6 L, or 2.1 pints of blood. This entire volume of blood circulates once per minute and comes into contact with an additional 35 L of liquid. Most oral dosages are measured in milligrams. Once the drug is absorbed into the bloodstream, it becomes diluted to the point where it becomes insignificant to the embalming process. The direct chemical reaction between the drug and the embalming preservative is negligible.

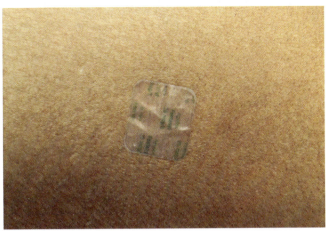

A

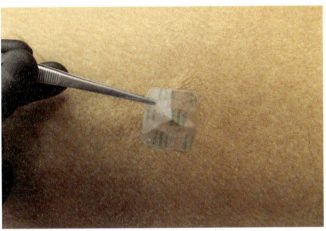

B

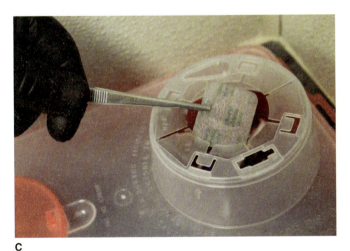

C

**Figure 23–3** **A.** Transdermal Fentanyl patch. **B.** Removal of Fentanyl patch by forceps. **C.** Disposal of Fentanyl patch in biohazard sharps container.

When a drug is taken beyond the time period prescribed, in amounts larger than the prescribed dosage, or without a prescription, it is termed drug abuse. Fentanyl is the drug most commonly attributed to overdose deaths in the United States. Opioid usage produces a state of euphoria in the user. Fentanyl has numerous routes of transmission, including ingestion by pill or powder form, transdermal absorption, and mucous membrane absorption by eye drops or nasal sprays.

> ### CONCEPTS FOR STUDY
> 
> Define the following terminology:
> - Chemotherapy
> - Cytotoxic drugs
> - Millicurie
> - Nephrotoxic
> - Opioids
> - Proteolytic enzymes
> - Radioactive isotopes
> 
> 1. List three functions of the proteins in the body.
> 2. Relate several postmortem conditions related to chemotherapeutic agents.
> 3. Explain the method of task-sharing as it relates to preparation of bodies treated by radiation.
> 4. Describe the procedure for safely removing and disposing of narcotic transdermal patches.
> 5. Recall how oral drugs taken for diabetes can influence tissue firming during embalming.
> 6. Express the process of drug dilution once the drug enters the bloodstream.
> 7. What effects do nitrogenous waste products have upon formaldehyde?

## FIGURE CREDIT

Figures 23–1, 23–3A-C are used with permission of Kevin Drobish.
Figure 23–2 is used with permission of Sharon L. Gee-Mascarello.

## BIBLIOGRAPHY

American Board of Funeral Service, *Course Content Syllabus,* 2016.

American Cancer Society, *Evolution of Cancer Treatments: Chemotherapy.* Retrieved January 11, 2020 from www.cancer.org/cancer/cancer-basics/history-of-cancer.html.

Brozek J. *Body Composition.* New York, NY: New York Academy of Sciences, 1963.

Dorn J, Hopkins B. *Thanatochemistry*, 3rd ed. Upper Saddle River, NJ: Prentice-Hall, 2010.

Fredrick JF. An alpha-glucan phosphorylase which requires adenosine-5-phosphate as coenzyme. *Phyto-chemistry* 1963;2:413–415.

Fredrick JF. *Embalming Problems Caused by Chemotherapeutic Agents.* Boston, MA: Dodge Institute for Advanced Studies, 1968.

Gomori G. Microtechnical demonstration of phosphatase enzymes in tissue sections. *Proceedings of Society for Experimental Biology and Medicine* 1939;42:23–26.

Goodman L, Gilman A, eds. *The Pharmacological Basis of Therapeutics,* 4th ed. New York, NY: Macmillan, 1970.

Goth A. *Medical Pharmacology,* 6th ed. St. Louis, MO: C.V. Mosby, 1972.

Julian RM. *A Primer of Drug Action.* San Francisco, CA: Freeman, 1975.

Long YG. *Neuropharmacology and Behavior.* San Francisco, CA: Freeman, 1972.

Merck, Sharpe, & Dohme. *Merck Index*, 10th ed. Rahway, NJ: Merck & Co., 1983.

*Physician's Desk Reference (PDR).* Oradale, NJ: Medical Economics, 1984, No. 38.

Windholz M, Budavari S. In: *Merck Index*, 10th ed. Rahway, NJ: Merck & Co., 1983.

Yessell ES, Braude MC. *Interaction of Drugs of Abuse.* New York, NY: New York Academy of Sciences, 1976.

# CHAPTER 24

# Selected Conditions

### CHAPTER OVERVIEW
- Types of Gases and Purges
- Facial Trauma
- Alcoholism
- Renal Failure
- Obesity
- Mycotic Infections

## PURGE

**Purge** is defined as the postmortem evacuation of any substance from any external orifice of the body as a result of pressure. This condition can occur prior to, during, and after embalming (**Fig. 24–1A–B**). Purge is generally described by its source: stomach, lung, brain, anal, or embalming solution. Purge occurring during the arterial injection is often the result of excessive injection pressure and rapid rate of flow. Embalming solution forced into the lungs may exit as purge from the oral and nasal cavities.

The pressure responsible for the purge can develop in several ways:

1. **Gas**—Gas in the abdominal cavity or in the hollow intestinal tract can create sufficient pressure on the stomach to force the contents of the stomach through the mouth or the nose. This abdominal pressure can also push on the diaphragm with sufficient force to cause the contents of the lungs to purge through the mouth or the nose. Gas can originate from early decomposition or from partial digestion of foods or may be true tissue gas formed by *Clostridium perfringens.*

2. **Visceral Expansion**—When bodies have been dead for several hours and arterial solution is injected too fast, the hollow visceral organs (intestinal tract) tend to expand. The abdomen is a closed cavity, this expansion creates sufficient pressure to push on the stomach walls and create a stomach purge. The expansion also pushes on the diaphragm and squeezes on the lungs, possibly resulting in lung purge.

3. **Arterial Solution**
   a. Injection of arterial solution at a faster rate of flow, especially in bodies dead for long periods, causes expansion of the viscera.
   b. If an area of the stomach, the upper bowel, or the lung is ulcerated, the arterial solution can leak through the ulcerated vessels, fill the stomach, the esophagus, or the lung tissue, and the trachea, and develop into a purge.
   c. If esophageal varices break, sufficient blood and arterial solution can exit to create purge.
   d. Gastrointestinal bleeding accompanies a variety of diseases and the long-term use of many drugs. If a sufficient amount of arterial solution and blood leak from these tissues during injection, anal purge results.
   e. Purge can occur when leakage of arterial solution from an aneurysm in the thoracic or abdominal cavity develops sufficient pressure to push on the lungs or the stomach.
   f. Sufficient injection pressure can cause leakage from recent surgical incisions. The arterial solution lost to the stomach or the abdominal cavity builds up enough pressure to create purge.

4. **Ascites and Hydrothorax**—When edema fills the thoracic or abdominal cavity prior to death, a great amount of pressure builds up and on injection of arterial solution forces purge.

---

**CONDITIONS PREDISPOSING TO PURGE**
Decomposition
Long delay between death and embalming
Drowning or asphyxia
Recent abdominal, thoracic, or cranial surgery
Tissue gas
Hydrothorax or ascites
Peritonitis or bloodstream infections
Esophageal varices, ulcerations of the gastrointestinal tract, or internal hemorrhages
Warm environment which speeds decomposition

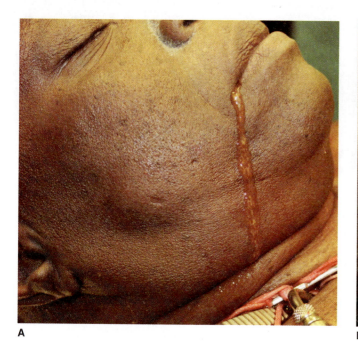 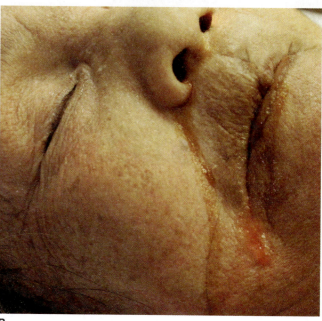

Figure 24–1. **A.** Embalming solution purge during arterial injection. **B.** Lung and stomach purge post-embalming.

## Protecting Skin Areas from Purge

When purge occurs prior to or during arterial injection from the nose or the mouth, the surrounding tissues of the face should be protected by an application of massage cream. Stomach purge contains hydrochloric acid and can desiccate and discolor the skin. If arterial fluid is contained in the purge material, the dye from the fluid can stain the skin. Cover the facial tissues and the neck area with the massage cream. Only a light coating is needed. Be certain that the inside of the lips is covered as well as the base of the nose. Tightly packing with cotton or webbed cotton the throat, the nostrils, the ears, and the anus prior to embalming should greatly reduce the possibility of a purge during or after embalming.

## General Pre-Embalming and Embalming Treatments

When the abdomen is tightly distended from gas or edema (ascites) prior to embalming, a trocar should be introduced into the upper (ventral) area of the cavity. Piercing the transverse colon can help to relieve gas pressure. The stomach can also be punctured, as it can contain a large quantity of liquid. If ascites is present, removing some of the edema from the abdominal cavity will relieve the pressure. To drain ascites, insert a trocar or make a puncture in the lower left inguinal area of the abdomen (just above the inguinal ligament). Insert either a trocar or a drain tube to which a drainage hose is attached. From this location a portion of the liquid should gravitate from the cavity. By keeping the trocar (or drain tube) just under the abdominal wall (ventral), there should be no piercing of any large blood vessels.

## Time Period Treatments

Two factors are necessary for purge to occur. First, there must be a substance to purge, such as stomach contents, blood, arterial fluid, and respiratory tract contents. Second, there must be pressure on an organ such as the stomach, the rectum, or the lung to evacuate the material.

## Pre-Embalming Purge

### Stomach or Lung Purge

Pre-embalming purge generally consists of the stomach contents (**Table 24–1**). If esophageal varices have ruptured or if a stomach ulcer has eroded a blood vessel, blood can also be expected in the purge. As the stomach contains acid, this purge usually is brown. Stomach purge is often described as coffee grounds, by its appearance. Removal of this material at the beginning of embalming decreases the possibility of a post-embalming purge. A nasal tube aspirator can be used to remove purge from the throat and the nasal passages. Disinfect the oral cavity and the nose and tightly pack the passage with cotton. Or, allow the purge to continue during embalming and make a final setting of the features after embalming. When restricted cervical injection is used, the body can purge during injection. After arterial injection, the body can be aspirated, nasal and throat passages can be tightly packed, the features can be set, and the head can be separately embalmed. Any purge on the face before or during embalming can create cosmetic problems. Protect facial tissues with massage cream. Coat the lips on the inside as well as the outside.

### Anal Purge

Pre-embalming anal purge material should be forced from the body by applying firm pressure to the lower abdomen; flush material with running water. Use controlled water pressure to avoid splattering material. Allow purge to continue during embalming. Fecal matter is difficult to aspirate from the body. The anal orifice can be tightly packed with cotton saturated with cavity fluid or a phenol cauterant solution **after** cavity treatment. During final bathing, turn the body on its side to clean beneath the body and clean the embalming table. Protect the clothing of the deceased from soiling by use of plastic garments, such as pants or capri garment. Add embalming powder to garments to control any odors.

| TABLE 24–1. Postmortem Purge |||||
| Source | Orifice | Description | Contents | Time |
| --- | --- | --- | --- | --- |
| Stomach | Mouth/nose | Liquid/semisolid<br>"Coffee grounds" appearance<br>Foul odor<br>Acid pH | Stomach contents<br>Blood<br>Arterial solution | Pre-embalming<br>Embalming<br>Post-embalming |
| Lung | Mouth/nose | Frothy<br>Blood remains red<br>Little odor | Respiratory tract liquids<br>Residual air from lungs<br>Blood<br>Arterial solution | Pre-embalming<br>Embalming<br>Post-embalming |
| Esophageal varices | Mouth/nose | Bloody liquid | Blood<br>Arterial solution | Pre-embalming<br>Embalming<br>Post-embalming |
| Brain | Fracture in skull<br>Nose<br>Fractured ethmoid<br>Fractured ear<br>Temporal bone<br>Surgical opening | White semisolid | Brain tissue<br>Blood<br>Arterial solution | Pre-embalming<br>Embalming<br>Post-embalming |
| Anus | Anal orifice | Semisolid/liquid | Fecal matter<br>Blood<br>Arterial solution | Pre-embalming<br>Embalming<br>Post-embalming |
| Embalming solution | Mouth/nose | Color of arterial solution injected | Arterial solution | Embalming |
| Cavity fluid | Mouth/nose<br>Anal orifice | Color of cavity fluid<br>Blood present is brown in color | Cavity fluid | Post-embalming |

### *Brain Purge*

Pre-embalming brain purge results from a fracture of the skull, a surgical procedure in the cranial cavity, or a trauma such as a bullet penetrating the bone of the skull. It is possible for gas (a type of purge) to build up in the cranium and travel along the nerve routes to distend such tissues as the eyelids. Numerous foramina (opening or hole, especially in bone) in the eye orbit communicate with the cranial cavity. Brain purge from the nose is rare and is usually the result of a fracture of the cribriform plate in the floor of the anterior cranial cavity. The ear can also be the site of brain purge, usually as a result of a fracture of the temporal bone. It is best to let these purges continue during the embalming procedure.

### Embalming Purge

During arterial injection, the injected solution can expand the viscera. Pressure on the stomach or diaphragm can result in expulsion of the contents of the stomach and/or the respiratory tract. Also, during arterial injection, arterial solution can be lost to the respiratory tract, the stomach, or the esophagus as a result of ruptured capillaries, small arteries, or veins. Ulcerated or cancerous tissues easily rupture because of the pressure of the solution being injected.

Tuberculosis of the lungs, cancer, pneumonia, and bacterial infections of the lung can cause fluid loss through weakened capillaries. A second cause of lung purge during embalming is congestion in the right atrium of the heart, which easily occurs if disease has involved the valves of the heart. Assume that drainage is being taken from the right femoral vein but has been very difficult to establish. Blood continues to push into the right atrium but cannot be drained away. The pressure builds to the point where the blood flows into the right ventricle and into the pulmonary arteries, squeezing the lung tissues and forcing a purge. Rupture of small veins can also produce a bloody lung purge.

During embalming purge may simply be composed of the contents of the stomach, lung, or rectum or, as already explained, arterial solution. As a large amount of arterial solution is lost in the drainage and possibly as purge, be certain that a sufficient volume of arterial solution is injected to replace these losses. It is not always necessary to turn off the machine and begin a multipoint injection when purge contains arterial solution. When arterial solution is present in purge during arterial injection and **drainage is occurring**, inject a sufficient volume to satisfy the preservative demands of the body. When arterial solution is present in purge during arterial injection and **drainage has stopped,** a major fluid loss is occurring and distribution is not taking place. Evaluate the body and use sectional arterial injection where needed.

Rarely does anal purge contain arterial solution; however, long-term use of some drugs can cause gastrointestinal bleeding; rectal and colon cancers can erode tissues; and ulcerative colitis can destroy vessels. These conditions make possible a loss of arterial solution as well as blood drainage into the colon and the rectum. If a sufficient amount of blood or arterial solution accumulates in the lower bowel, purge containing arterial solution can exit from the anal orifice.

It is usually during arterial injection that brain purge occurs. As already stated, for brain purge to occur, an opening must be present in the skull as a result of fracture, surgery, or trauma. Arterial solution escapes through small leaking arteries within the cranium, building up pressure that forces blood, arterial solution, and tissues of the brain through the openings.

## Post-Embalming Purge

Purge that occurs prior to or during arterial injection can easily be controlled by the embalmer. Post-embalming purge is a concern to the embalmer. After cavity embalming, purge should be minimal. Many times, purge from the mouth, the nose, or the anal orifice after cavity embalming is simply cavity fluid that has been injected into passages of these orifices. Tightly repack the nostrils with cotton and replace moist cotton in the mouth with dry cotton.

Re-aspirate prior to dressing whenever possible. If there appears to be a buildup of gas in the abdominal cavity, consider re-injection. Treat post-embalming anal purge by forcing as much of the purge material from the body as possible. Then pack the rectum with the cotton saturated with a phenol solution, autopsy gel, or cavity fluid. Clothe the body in plastic pants or coveralls as added protection.

A purge that occurs from the mouth or the nose after the body has been dressed and casketed may be temporarily stopped by removing the trocar button and passing a trocar through the viscera to relieve the pressure that has accumulated. The body should be re-aspirated and reinjected.

## Prevention of Post-Embalming Purge

1. Thoroughly aspirate the body cavities. Inject sufficient cavity fluid based on body mass and embalming analysis into the abdominal, thoracic, and pelvic cavities.
2. Inject additional cavity fluid into obese bodies, bodies with ascites, bodies that have recently undergone abdominal surgery, and bodies which evidence decomposition.
3. If the abdominal trunk or buttock walls do not appear to have received sufficient fluid, hypodermically inject these areas with cavity fluids. Gases can form in unembalmed tissues and gradually move into the body cavities.
4. Re-aspirate, especially those bodies that exhibit abdominal gas. This gas is easily detected when the trocar button is removed.
5. Re-aspirate all the bodies that have been shipped from another funeral home.
6. Pack the throat and the nose with cotton. Nonabsorbent cotton should be used, because absorbent cotton may act as a wick to draw cavity fluid into the throat or the upper nasal passages. Apply massage cream or autopsy gel to the nonabsorbent cotton before it is inserted into the nostrils or the throat.
7. Remove moist cotton if purge has occurred during embalming. Be certain that the mouth is completely dried.
8. When purge has been expelled from the skull as a result of fracture, decomposition, or surgical procedure (brain purge), the cranial cavity can be aspirated by passing an infant trocar or large hypodermic needle through the surgical opening, the body fracture, or the cribriform plate. To aspirate through the cribriform plate, insert the needle through the nostril. Direct the needle toward the anterior portion of the cranial cavity. The brain can be injected with a small amount of cavity fluid using a long hypodermic needle and a syringe.
9. Incise the trachea and the esophagus from inside the incision used to raise the carotid artery. Pack with cotton.
10. Re-aspirate and re-inject as necessary prior to dressing.

## GASES

Five types of gases may be found in the tissues of the dead human body: (1) subcutaneous emphysema, (2) air from the embalming apparatus, (3) gas gangrene, (4) tissue gas, and (5) decomposition gas (Table 24–2).

In the dead human body, gases move to the superior body areas when the body is in the supine position (lying flat on the back). When the head is elevated, gases can move into the unsupported tissues of the neck and the face. The **source** of the gas can be in the **dependent** body areas. Gas can be detected in several ways in the body. It distends weak unsupported tissues such as the eyelids and the tissues surrounding the eye orbit, the temples, the neck, and the backs of the hands. In a firmly embalmed body, distension of veins is a possible sign that gas has formed. Pushing on the tissues where the gas is present may elicit a crackling sound that is both heard and felt. This is called **crepitation.** The area under the skin feels as if it is filled with cellophane.

### Types of Gases Found in Tissues

#### Subcutaneous Emphysema

The most frequently encountered gas condition is caused by antemortem subcutaneous emphysema, brought about by a puncture or a tear in the pleural sac or the lung tissue. As the living individual gasps for air, the air escapes from the injury site into the tissues. Subcutaneous emphysema can follow a compound fracture of a rib, tracheostomy, lung surgery, or other injury to the pleural sac. During life-saving cardiopulmonary resuscitation (CPR) injury to the lung tissue can happen inadvertently and cause subcutaneous emphysema.

This condition is *not* caused by a microbe and does not continue to intensify after death. The gas, however, moves from the dependent areas to the upper body areas such as the neck and the face. No odor accompanies this condition; skin-slip or blebs do not form on the skin surface. In the male, the scrotum can distend to several times its normal size. It is best to remove the gas from the tissues *after* the body is embalmed.

## COMMON CONDITIONS CAUSING ANTEMORTEM SUBCUTANEOUS EMPHYSEMA

- Rib fractures that puncture the pleura or a lung
- Puncture wounds of the thorax
- Thoracic surgical procedures
- CPR compression causing a fractured rib or sternum to puncture a lung or pleura
- Tracheostomy surgery

| TABLE 24–2. Gases That Cause Distension | | | |
|---|---|---|---|
| Type | Source | Characteristics | Treatment |
| Subcutaneous emphysema | Puncture of lung or pleural sac; seen after CPR; puncture wounds to thorax; rib fractures; tracheostomy | No odor; no skin-slip; no blebs; gas can reach distal points, even toes; can create intense swelling; rises to highest body areas | Gas escape through incisions; establishment of good arterial preservation; channeling of tissues after arterial injection to release gases |
| "True" tissue gas | Anaerobic bacteria (gas gangrene), C. perfringens | Very strong odor of decomposition; skin-slip; skin blebs; increase in intensity and amount of gas; possible transfer of spore-forming bacterium via cutting instruments to other bodies | Special "tissue gas" arterial solutions; localized hypodermic injection of cavity fluid; channeling of tissues to release gases |
| Gas gangrene | Anaerobic bacteria, C. perfringens | Foul odor, infection | Strong arterial solutions; local hypodermic injection of cavity chemical |
| Decomposition | Bacterial breakdown of body tissues; autolytic breakdown of body tissues | Possible odor; skin-slip in time; color changes; purging | Arterial injection of sufficient amount of the appropriate strong chemical; hypodermic and surface treatments; channeling to release gases |
| Air from embalming apparatus | Air injected by embalming machine (air pressure machines and hand pumps are in limited use today) | First evidence in eyelids; no odors; no skin-slip; amount depends on injection time | If distension is present, channeling after arterial injection to release gases |

## Gas Gangrene

Gas gangrene is a fatal disease caused by contamination of a wound infection by a toxin-producing, spore-forming, anaerobic bacterium. This bacterium can be found in soil and the intestinal tract of humans and animals. *C. perfringens* is the most common of the *Clostridium* bacteria responsible for this condition. The organisms grow in the tissue of the wound, especially muscle, releasing exotoxins and fermenting muscle sugars with such vigor that the pressure build up by the accumulated gas tears the tissues apart.

The gas causes swelling and death of tissues locally. The exotoxins break down red blood cells in the bloodstream and, thereby, damage various organs throughout the body. The bacteria enter the blood just before death (the incubation period is 1–5 days). Because of the destructive action of the exotoxins and the enzymes produced, tissue involvement and spread are very rapid. Gas gangrene usually occurs after severe trauma, especially farm or automobile accidents and close-range shotgun discharges, where the wound may be contaminated with filth, manure, or surface soil. Gas gangrene is particularly likely after compound fractures; the bone splinters provide foreign bodies that enhance the infection as well as permit entrance of embedded debris or dirt.

The gangrenous process begins at the margins of the wound. The skin, dark red at first, turns green and then black, and there is considerable swelling that extends rapidly over the body. The tissues are filled with gas, sometimes to the point of bursting. The affected tissue decomposes, blisters and skin-slip form on the surface, and there is no line of demarcation. A very foul odor permeates the surroundings.

Gas causes the tissue to crackle when touched. The danger involved, as an embalming complication, lies in the fact that if death occurs shortly after injury, the gas gangrene may not be visible; it may be totally internal. If embalming treatment is not sufficient to control the spread of the organisms or their by-products, the symptoms of gas gangrene may show up several hours after embalming. In addition, if the postmortem examination is delayed, internal spread will be extensive and could create disastrous post-embalming complications.

## Tissue Gas

Tissue gas is caused primarily by *C. perfringens*. It may begin prior to death as gas gangrene. After death, the condition may result from the contamination of tissues by the gas bacillus, which has translocated from the intestinal tract. Contaminated hypodermic needles have also been known to transfer *C. perfringens* to the tissues of the extremities. Contaminated autopsy instruments have spread this condition from one body to another. This condition may also be spread when embalming instruments (cutting instruments, i.e., scalpels, scissors, trocar, suture needles) are not thoroughly disinfected. These organisms are very resistant to most disinfectants. Thus, the condition can occur after the body has been embalmed if all the tissues of the body and the visceral organs have not been adequately sanitized and preserved.

The gas is ordinarily formed more rapidly and with greater intensity in the dependent tissues and the organs. These areas are frequently congested with blood and later poorly saturated with arterial solution and, therefore, provide an ideal medium for bacterial growth. Lighter than the liquids displaced, the gas rises to the highest receptive parts of the body. In addition, the gas is larger in volume than the liquid it displaces, and thus tears and distends the tissues.

Distension is usually greatest in soft tissue areas such as the eyelids, the neck, and the scrotum of the male. The gas spreads rather rapidly through the tissue, causing blebs to form on the surface. As the condition progresses, the blebs grow and burst, releasing the gas and putrefactive fluids and causing skin-slip.

## CONDITIONS PREDISPOSING TO TISSUE GAS

- Recent abdominal surgery
- Presence of gangrene at the time of death
- Intestinal ulcerations or perforations
- Contaminated skin wounds or punctures
- Intestinal obstruction or hemorrhage
- Unsatisfactory embalming
- Contact with contaminated instruments

### Decomposition

In the dead human body two factors are responsible for decomposition: bacterial enzymes and autolytic enzymes. Gases are formed that accumulate in the visceral organs, body cavities, and the skeletal tissues. These gases are responsible for the odor of decomposition. As the gases accumulate in the body cavities, sufficient pressure is produced to cause purge. The gases produced by decomposition are not often as intense as tissue gas or gas gangrene. Likewise, decomposition cannot be spread from body to body by contaminated instruments. The generation of gas ceases when the tissues are properly embalmed. Gases can be removed by cavity aspiration and post-embalming channeling of the tissues.

### Embalming Protocol

#### Subcutaneous Emphysema

Because subcutaneous emphysema does not involve microbes, treatment involves merely removal of the gas from the tissues. There are no foul odors, blebbing, or skin-slip with this condition. During arterial injection, some of the gas in the tissues may relocate, especially into higher body regions such as the neck and the facial tissues.

Restricted cervical injection should be used for the arterial injection. Fluid strength should be based on the postmortem and pathological conditions. A slightly stronger solution should be used to embalm the head; if gas should relocate into the head after embalming (if the tissues are firm), sufficient resistance will be exerted to prevent distension. In restricted cervical injection, two incisions are made at the base of the neck. These incisions provide an exit for the gas in the tissues. The incisions can also be used as points from which to channel the neck so air can be pushed from the facial tissues.

#### Decomposition Gas, Gas Gangrene, and True Tissue Gas

Decomposition gas, gas gangrene, and true tissue gas all have a bacterial origin. It is very important to saturate the tissues of the body with a very strong arterial solution. Restricted cervical injection should be used so large quantities of sufficient-strength arterial solution can be injected into the trunk. Chemicals specifically made for the treatment of decomposing bodies and tissue gas should be used, for example, special-purpose arterial fluids, co-injection chemicals, and cavity fluids that can be injected arterially.

If the gas appears to have originated in an extremity, sectional arterial embalming should be done. If the condition is well advanced, 100% chemical should be injected into the localized area. A co-injection chemical can be added for each ounce of the arterial chemical. High pressure may be needed to inject the solution into the affected area. Often tissue gas is not noticeable at the time of death. As the organism responsible is anaerobic, after death the human body becomes an ideal medium.

Gases can form very rapidly after death. These postmortem changes can be devastating enough that a viewing of the body would be impossible. It is imperative that the preparation be started as soon after death as possible. If the gas source is an extremity or an area such as the buttocks, a **barrier** can be made by hypodermic injection of undiluted cavity fluid in addition to sectional embalming.

### Clinical Example

The source of the tissue gas appears to be a gangrenous condition of the left foot. The lower portion of the leg has turned a deep purple-black. The leg is swollen and gas can be felt beneath the tissues. A high-index special-purpose arterial fluid and six-point injection is selected. Drainage is taken from the right internal jugular vein.

Following arterial injection of the body, the left femoral artery is raised and the left leg injected. Pulsation and high pressure are used to distribute the solution. Next, the leg is hypodermically treated using a trocar introduced from the medial side of the middle of the thigh. Cavity fluid is injected throughout the area above the knee and into the deep tissues of the lower leg. A barrier has now been formed with cavity fluid in an attempt to contain the *C. perfringens* and prevent it from migrating to other body areas. The femoral incision can remain open several hours, providing an exit for the gas to escape.

Cavity treatment should be very thorough. Gas rises to the anterior portions of the viscera and the cavity. Carefully aspirate the cavity, including the walls, to provide exits for the gas if it can be felt in the trunk walls. Inject cavity fluid based on body mass and embalming analysis. The trocar entry site can remain open to allow the escape of gases. The site can be closed following re-aspiration and re-injection of the cavities.

Tissue gas can also form in bodies that have not been thoroughly embalmed. *C. perfringens* is a normal inhabitant of the gastrointestinal tract and can rapidly translocate to other body areas after death.

### Removal of Gas from Tissues

Regardless of the source of the gas, the method of removing it is the same. There is only one effective way to remove gas from the distended tissues and that is to lance and channel the tissues and release the gas. Arterial injection and subsequent blood drainage may remove gases in the circulatory system, but do little to remove gas trapped in the subcutaneous tissue. The incision made to raise any vessels is an escape route for gas from the body.

Remember that in bodies with true tissue gas, release of the gas from the tissues does not stop its generation. The microbe causing the gas must be killed. Although gas accumulates in the superficial body tissues, the source of the gas may be located in a distal extremity or in the dependent tissues.

### Trunk Tissues

Gases in trunk tissues can be removed by trocar after arterial injection. During aspiration of the cavity, the trocar is channeled through the thoracic and the abdominal walls. If the scrotum is affected, it too can be channeled by passing the trocar over the pubic bone.

### Neck and Face

After arterial embalming, the trocar can be used to channel the neck to remove gas. Insert the trocar into the abdominal wall, after making certain that the trocar can reach the neck tissues. Pass the trocar beneath the rib cage and under the clavicle to reach the neck. The trocar can also be inserted into the neck by passing under the clavicle. Make a large half-moon incision at the base of the neck lateral from the center of the right clavicle to a point lateral from the center of the left clavicle. Reflect this flap and, with an infant trocar or scalpel, channel the neck tissue. Squeeze the neck tissues. Force the gas toward the openings. The half-moon incision can also be used for restricted cervical injection. If restricted cervical injection is used, this incision prevents more gases from entering the neck and the facial tissues. If possible, leave these incisions open several hours or until the body is to be dressed and casketed.

### Eyelids and Orbital Areas

The eyelids are loose unsupported tissues, gas easily distends the lids. After embalming, the eyelids can be opened and slightly everted (turned inside out). Using a large suture needle, make punctures along the undersurface of the lids. Deep channels can also be made from this location to the surrounding orbital areas. By digital pressure move the gases from the most distal areas toward the punctures. A bistoury knife or large hypodermic needle can also be inserted from within the hairline of the temple area to remove gases in the orbital area and the temple. Cotton should be used for eye closure. It absorbs the small amount of liquid that may seep from the punctures. It may be best not to seal these punctures, for they are an escape route for any further gas that may accumulate in the orbital area. In the autopsied body, after arterial injection, the orbital area can be channeled by carefully reflecting the scalp. A bistoury blade or scalpel can be used to dissect into the orbital areas. All of this can be done from beneath the skin surface through the tissues exposed by the cranial autopsy.

### Facial Tissues

Gases present in the cheeks and the facial tissues can be removed after arterial injection and cavity embalming. Aspiration of the thoracic cavity and channeling of the neck tissues may help to remove some of the gases present in the facial tissues. From inside of the mouth direct a bistoury knife, scalpel, or hypodermic needle deep into the tissues of the face (to the level of the facial bones) to make channels for the gases to escape. Digital pressure forces the gases from the tissues. Apply pressure at the distal points of the face and move gases to the insertion points made by the instrument. Any liquid leakage will drain into the mouth and the throat areas and may be aspirated. In the autopsied body, reflect the scalp and use a dissecting instrument or large hypodermic needle to make channels into the facial tissues to release accumulated gases.

### Instrument Disinfection

Tissue gas and gas gangrene involve a spore-forming bacillus, *C. perfringens,* which can easily be passed from one body to another via contaminated instruments. Great care should be taken in the disinfection of cutting instruments and suture needles. Wash instruments in cool running water using a good disinfectant soap. Then, soak them in a very strong disinfectant solution for several hours. Be certain that the disinfectants used in the preparation room are active (most disinfectants have a specific shelf life) following use, place disposable scalpel blades in an approved biohazard sharps container. Care should be given to the disinfection of the trocar and the suture needles.

## BODIES WITH FACIAL TRAUMA

In the preparation of bodies with facial trauma, the embalmer's goal is maximum tissue preservation with a minimum amount of swelling. If good preservation can be established, the restorative and cosmetic procedures will be easier to perform and will provide satisfactory results.

Traumatic injuries vary greatly; however, blunt force facial trauma can be classified into two categories: injuries in which the skin is broken (abrasion, laceration) (**Fig. 24–2**) and injuries in which the skin is not broken (contusion, hematoma).

| Skin | Broken Skin |
|---|---|
| Depressed fractures | Abrasion |
| Swollen tissues (hematoma) | Laceration |
| Ecchymosis | Incision |
| Simple fracture | Compound fracture |
| Contusion | |

Traumatic injuries also vary with respect to their location on the head. A laceration of the cheek may be simple to restore; however, a lacerated upper eyelid may involve swelling and

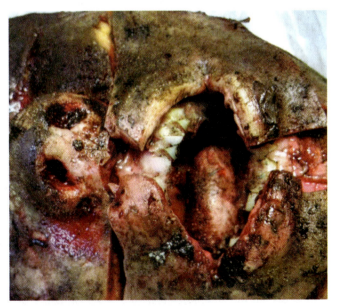

**Figure 24–2.** Blunt force facial trauma.

discoloration, as well as torn skin, resulting in a much more serious problem for the embalmer to restore.

It is not within the scope of this text to detail the restorative treatments for each type of facial trauma and describe how treatment varies with location. It is the intent of this text to give a general outline of embalming protocol for traumatic facial injuries. Most of these injuries involve delay, for there usually is an inquiry by the coroner or the medical examiner. Quite frequently, when an autopsy is performed, refrigeration may precede or follow the postmortem examination. This discussion is concerned only with preparation of the head. If the body has been autopsied, the head is separately embalmed by injecting first the left common carotid artery and then the right common carotid. In the unautopsied body, restricted cervical injection can be used (right and left common carotid arteries are raised at the beginning of the embalming). Insert two arterial tubes into the right common carotid, one directed toward the trunk of the body and the other directed toward the right side of the head. Open the left common carotid artery, tie off the lower portion of the artery, and insert one tube into the artery directed toward the left side of the head. Leave both arterial tubes directed toward the head **open**. Inject the trunk first, then the left side of the head, and, finally, the right side. Drainage can be taken from the right internal jugular vein. Drainage may also be taken from both the right and the left internal jugular veins.

### General Considerations

Run cool water over the facial areas and hair to remove debris and blood. If glass is present in the wounds, irrigate the area with water. Use forceps instead of fingers to remove glass.

Align fractures. Incisions may have to be made prior to embalming to properly align simple and depressed fractures. Next, align lacerated or incised skin areas. Use super adhesive glue or individual bridge sutures. Remove (debride) loose skin. Apply surface preservative and bleaching compresses. Compresses of cavity fluid or phenol bleach, preserve, and dry the tissues. Phenol solutions work rapidly. Protect unaffected tissue from harsh chemicals by applying a thin layer of massage cream to prevent dehydration. Instant Tissue Fixation is recommended. Use a waterless arterial solution. Example of a waterless solution:

- 16 ounces of 30 index (or higher) arterial fluid
- 16 ounces of co-injection fluid
- 4 ounces of water conditioner
- Arterial fluid dye
- No added water

## RENAL FAILURE

It has been estimated that six times more preservative chemical is needed to preserve tissues of bodies dead from the complications of renal failure. Evaluate each case by performing a thorough pre-embalming analysis. The following signs can indicate renal failure.

- Sallow color to the skin as a result of urochrome buildup.
- Uremic pruritus (chronic itching of the skin).
- Increase in the amount of urea, uric acid, ammonia, and creatine (urea and ammonia can be detected by their odor).
- Acidosis.
- Edema (retention of sodium by the kidneys leads to increased retention of water).
- Anemia.
- Gastrointestinal bleeding (blood in the gastrointestinal tract and purging).

Renal failure may be only a contributory cause of death; comorbidities such as diabetes and hypertension contribute to kidney failure. Comorbidity is the simultaneous presence of two, or more, chronic diseases or conditions within an individual.

The importance of this disease to the embalmer lies in the fact that these bodies rapidly decompose. The acidity of the tissues leads to rupture of lysosomes, which contain the autolytic hydroenzymes that begin the decomposition cycle. The edema present provides the moisture needed for the hydrolytic enzymes to act, the blood in the intestinal tract provides an excellent medium for the growth of putrefactive microorganisms, and the abundant ammonia in the tissues readily neutralizes formaldehyde.

### Embalming Protocol

Preparation of the body affected by renal failure calls for the use of strong arterial solutions. High-index fluid is advised. Nitrogenous wastes neutralize formaldehyde so preservative demand is high. Pre-injection fluid may not always be advised because tissues can easily swell, especially when circulation is expected to be impaired. Once circulation is established, arterial solution strength can be increased. Use dye to indicate the distribution of arterial solution. To inject strong solutions without adversely affecting the facial tissues, restricted cervical injection is advised. A large volume of strong arterial solution can be injected into the trunk followed by a more moderate solution strength to embalm the facial tissues.

When edema is also present, inject a sufficient volume of fluid to dry tissues and meet preservative demands. Inadequate embalming will result in soft tissues, skin blebs, desquamation (skin-slip), and other signs of decomposition. Dependent tissues will contact the embalming table and cause pressure points that may not receive sufficient arterial solution. Dependent areas are usually higher in moisture content; putrefactive bacteria flourish in moist conditions. Supplemental hypodermic injection is advised to ensure thorough preservation.

Thoroughly aspirate the cavities immediately after arterial injection. Gastrointestinal ulcerations can create purge during embalming; blood and arterial solution may be present in the contents aspirated from the abdominal cavity. Inject concentrated cavity fluid as indicated by the embalming analysis. Re-aspiration and re-injection are considerations. Plastic garments can be used to contain minor leakage and odors. Add preservative-deodorant powder to the garment.

## ALCOHOLISM

Prior to embalming, if ascites is present and the abdomen is fully distended, drain the serous fluid with a trocar. Keep the point of the trocar just beneath the surface of the anterior abdominal wall to prevent puncturing the aortic vessels.

Jaundice discolorations may be present as a result of liver failure. **Preservation takes precedence over presentation**. Add dye to counterstain jaundice. Liver failure can also cause edema in the skeletal tissues or the cavities (ascites, hydrothorax). In addition, hepatic failure depletes the blood of clotting factors; therefore, good drainage can be expected if the body is prepared within a reasonable time after death. Both the common carotid artery and the femoral artery are good primary injection sites; however, if skeletal edema is extensive and a large volume of strong arterial solution must be injected, restricted cervical injection is recommended. Injection should proceed at a moderate rate of flow so the tissues can assimilate the arterial solution without swelling. A moderate rate of flow also helps to prevent purging and rupture of weakened esophageal veins. Due to the effects of chronic alcoholism, tissue firming may be difficult to establish. Select a moderate to hypertonic preservative arterial solution. Add sufficient arterial fluid to firm the tissues. Oral and nasal purge may develop during arterial injection. When purge is comprised mainly of embalming solution, select additional vessels for sectional injection. The continuation of injection from a single site will result in large volumes of solution loss to purge.

Ecchymoses on the back of the hands can be treated by hypodermic injection of cavity fluid or phenol cautery solution after arterial injection. Before, during, and after arterial injection, compresses of cavity fluid, autopsy gel, or phenol solution may be applied to the skin surfaces to bleach and firm areas of ecchymosis.

Cavity embalming should be thorough, and, of course, re-aspiration is recommended.

## OBESITY

Obesity is the second highest cause of preventable death in the United States, continuing to rise in every age group, ethnicity, race, and gender. Almost 40% of Americans are considered to be overweight or obese. A measure of body mass approximates that two of every five individuals carries 30% fat on their bodies. A more startling statistic shows children, ages 2–19 years, approaching levels of obesity at 19%. The Body Mass Index, or BMI is a diagnostic tool for comparing weight to height to determine overall body mass. The National Institutes of Health (NIH) now defines normal weight, overweight, and obesity according to BMI rather than the traditional height/weight charts. Overweight and obese decedents often present with comorbidities, such as heart failure and stroke. In addition to the obese condition, the related comorbidities must also be successfully managed by the embalmer. The cardiovascular effects of obesity show that hypertension is greatest in those subjects with upper body and abdominal obesity. It can be noted that weight loss, in obese subjects, creates a decline in blood pressure. The risk of coronary heart disease (CHD) in obese and overweight person can be compounded by comorbidities such as, but not limited to hypertension, diabetes, and dyslipidemia (unhealthy levels of one or more lipids in the blood). Dyslipidemia may cause a build-up of fat in the muscles of the heart called *myocardial steatosis*. When arteriosclerosis is present, this condition can interfere with good arterial solution distribution to peripheral body areas and possible general uniform distribution of the embalming solution.

Prior to embalming, place body bridges beneath the decedent. Position the body on the bridges maintaining three levels of height: the head is highest, then the chest, and the abdomen is lowest. Raise the chin and tilt the head back to minimize fullness in the neck, for easier raising of the vessels, and to prevent purge. Position hands at the sides and keep elbows as close to the body as possible. Use numerous positioning devices to achieve acceptable positioning.

Restricted cervical injection affords the use of the largest arteries. Consider using quick-connect arterial tubes. The common carotid arteries are superficial compared to the femoral arteries. The right internal jugular vein is closest to the center of venous drainage, making it an ideal drainage site. Angular spring forceps or a jugular drain tube can be inserted directly into the right atrium. If varicose veins are present, large clots may be observed in the drainage. The internal jugular vein allows passage of these clots out of the body.

Begin arterial injection with the arms lowered over the sides of the table. Leave them in this position until the arterial solution reaches the tissues of the hands. Massaging the radial and ulnar arteries promotes the flow of fluid into the hands. Large volumes of solution may be necessary. The solution can be of moderate strength initially and increased in strength to meet preservative demands of the trunk. A higher solution strength will dry and firm the trunk tissues. Sufficient pressure should be used to overcome extravascular resistance caused by visceral weight upon the aortic vessels. Massage, manipulation of extremities, and intermittent drainage assist in fluid distribution. If the legs do not receive sufficient arterial solution, raise the external iliac artery at the level of the inguinal ligament. The vessels are more superficial near the ligament and larger than the femoral arteries.

Purge may result from abdominal weight. The contents of the stomach will exit as stomach purge. Excess adipose tissue retains heat for an extended period after death; gas formation is proliferated in the warm and moist conditions of the gastrointestinal tract. Aspirate the cavities thoroughly after embalming to eliminate gases and purge. Several aspiration sites may be necessary. The first entry point can be made 4 inches inferior to the xiphoid process in the center of the abdomen and the second entry point, just superior to the center of the right or left inguinal ligament. The first site is used to aspirate the thoracic cavity. The trocar can also be inserted through the carotid incision as a supplemental aspirating site for the thoracic cavity. The incision site is ideal for channeling to reduce swelling in the neck. Abdominal aspiration begins using the center abdominal point of entry. This is followed by insertion of the trocar into one of the lower inguinal sites. A thorough fanning of all levels of the abdomen is completed from this point. Inject 32–64 ounces of high index cavity fluid. Re-aspiration is always recommended prior to dressing and transferring to a different location.

Final bathing of the body includes areas beneath skin folds and the back of the body. Place lift straps between the body bridges and roll the decedent to one side to remove the bridges; leave the straps in place for lifting and transferring the decedent. Observe load limits on the mortuary lifting device before use. Employ additional assistance during the procedure.

# MYCOTIC INFECTIONS

Mycotic infections are fungal infections that can spread by direct contact. A fungus that invades the tissue can cause infections confined to the skin, hair, and nails. Or it can spread to the tissues, bones, and organs. Fungal infections can affect the entire body. Fungi may be saprophytic or parasitic. Parasitic fungi obtain nourishment from dead organic material. Fungal infections can affect the skin and mucous membranes in conditions such as athlete's foot (tinea pedis), jock itch (tinea cruris), oral thrush (mouth), ringworm (tinea corporis), and yeast infections (cutaneous candidiasis). Destructive parasitic fungi can produce widespread chronic mycotic lesions. Fungi can proliferate in people with weakened immune systems and those receiving prolonged chemotherapy and steroid therapy. Diseases such as diabetes mellitus, leukemia, and HIV/AIDS create susceptibility to fungal infections. Although there are many types of fungal infections, discussion is limited to those specific to embalming.

## Candidiasis (Moniliasis)

*Candida* species are commonly found in the mouth, intestinal tract, and vagina of healthy individuals. **Candida albicans** is the most common cause of candidiasis. A common form of the disease known as *thrush* affects the oral mucosa (tongue, gums, lips, and cheeks) and the pharynx and is seen most often in debilitated infants (especially premature) and children. The lesions, white patches on the mucosa, comprise an overgrowth of yeast cells and hyphae and a nonspecific acute or subacute inflammation of the underlying tissue. Similar lesions occur on the vulvovaginal mucosa, particularly in diabetic and pregnant women and women on birth control pills. The skin, especially moist skin (perineum, inframammary folds, and between the fingers), may be affected.

*Candida* may produce lesions of the nails (onychia) and around the nails (paronychia), particularly in people whose hands are always in water. Esophageal, bronchopulmonary, and widely disseminated forms of candidiasis are also observed. Invasiveness is promoted by the lowered resistance of the host, as may occur in various debilitating illnesses and with intensive antibiotic, immunosuppressive, or steroid therapy.

Oral candidiasis can occur at any age during the course of a debilitating disease. It can also occur under dentures and orthodontic appliances and can complicate other erosive mucosal diseases (pemphigus vulgaris). The moist folds at the corners of the mouth provide a friendly environment for a troublesome candidal infection. Oropharyngeal candidiasis is a common complication of immunosuppression. Mouth lesions can spread down the trachea and the esophagus and produce extensive gastrointestinal infections.

## Aspergillosis

Most species of the genus *Aspergillus* are saprophytic and nonpathogenic. Some are found as harmless invaders of the external auditory canal, nasal sinuses, and external genitalia and as secondary invaders in lung abscesses.

In involvement of the ear, the external auditory canal may be partially filled with foul moist material spotted with black granules. The lung appears to be the most common site of serious infection. Pulmonary lesions manifest as bronchopneumonia, abscesses, small infarcts (resulting from thrombosis caused by vascular invasion), or masses of Aspergillus mycelia (fungus balls) in a newly formed cavity or a preexisting inflammatory (tuberculosis) or carcinomatous cavity. Chronic granulomatous reactions to the organisms in the lungs are also possible.

A primary fatal disseminated infection is relatively uncommon. Generalized aspergillosis is more frequent as a secondary complication and tends to occur in patients with debilitating diseases and in those who have received steroid, antibiotic, or immunosuppressive therapy. Aspergillosis occurs in various tissues and organs and is characterized by abscesses, necrotic and necrotizing lesions, and sometimes chronic granulomatous inflammation.

## Phycomycosis

Phycomycosis is an infection of the lungs, the ears, the nervous system, and the intestinal tract caused by a fungus commonly encountered as a saprophyte or a contaminant. The lesions may display an intense necrotizing and suppurative inflammation process. Although this infection is commonly called *mucormycosis*, it may be caused by several members of the group Phycomycetes, including *Mucor*, *Rhizopus*, and *Absidia*. These fungi invade vessels and cause thrombosis and infarction. Phycomycosis is especially seen in patients with uncontrolled diabetes mellitus, leukemia, AIDS, and other debilitating diseases and in those receiving antibiotics, corticosteroids, chemotherapeutic agents, and irradiation. The resulting lesions are similar to those mentioned earlier.

## Histoplasmosis (Reticuloendothelial Cytomycosis)

Histoplasmosis is caused by the oval, yeast-like organism **Histoplasma capsulatum**. Histoplasmosis occurs worldwide. In the United States, *Histoplasma* is common in the central and eastern states, especially around Ohio and the Mississippi River valleys. The fungus also lives in parts of Central and South America, Africa, Asia, and Australia. Histoplasmosis is endemic in many parts of the world, particularly near large rivers and in high-humidity warm temperature regions.

Histoplasmosis is caused by breathing in microscopic fungal spores from the air as is not generally spread between individuals. It appears to be contracted from soil contaminated with fecal material of birds and bats. The lungs are the usual portal of entry of the organisms. Histoplasmosis can be classified into four forms: acute pulmonary, chronic pulmonary, acute disseminated, and chronic disseminated. The acute pulmonary form may be asymptomatic or symptomatic. The basic reaction in the lungs and the lymph nodes consists of foci of tuberculoid granulomas that tend to heal. Most cases of histoplasmosis are benign, asymptomatic pulmonary infections, with positive histoplasmin skin tests and healed calcified nodules in the lung and the peribronchial lymph nodes, often resembling the healed primary complex of tuberculosis. The symptomatic pulmonary infections may be either mild and flu-like or more severe, resembling atypical pneumonia. Positive diagnosis depends on the identification of the organisms in cultures of sputum, blood, or bone marrow or in biopsied tissue from the lymph nodes. This infection may spread throughout the body. Usually, the prognosis is good. Multiple pulmonary infiltrations, with or without hilar lymphadenopathy (involvement with the entrance to the glands), may be indicated in x-rays of the chest and, in the more prolonged cases, tend to calcify and simulate healed miliary tuberculosis. Coin lesions are removed surgically due to clinical suspicion of lung cancer.

The **chronic pulmonary** form is progressive, forming granulomatous inflammation with caseation necrosis and cavitation, and frequently is misdiagnosed as pulmonary tuberculosis, or it may occur as a secondary complication of tuberculosis. It is seen most commonly in otherwise healthy males older than 40 years. The prognosis is poor. Occasionally, either the acute primary complex or the chronic pulmonary type is disseminated, spreading through the blood to involve many organs. Involvement of the lymph system, the liver, the spleen, and the bone marrow dominate the clinical picture. The organs involved are packed with macrophages stuffed with organisms, so the histologic picture resembles that of visceral leishmaniasis. Jaundice, fever, leukopenia, and anemia lead to a condition that mimics acute miliary tuberculosis.

The **acute disseminated** form may be either benign or progressive. The acute progressive form is rapidly fatal and is usually encountered in young children or severely immunosuppressed adults. The spleen, the lymph nodes, and the liver are enlarged. There is a septic type fever with anemia and leukopenia. Bone marrow smears may reveal the organisms or granulomas. Occasionally, the organisms may be found in mononuclear cells in blood smears.

The **chronic disseminated** form may occur in the elderly and otherwise healthy individuals and may be fatal. In the more protracted form, which occurs in otherwise healthy individuals, the clinical features vary according to the organ most severely involved. For instance, involvement of the heart valves leads to endocarditis, and involvement of the adrenal glands leads to Addison's disease. Other organs that can be affected are the gastrointestinal tract, the spleen, the liver, the lymph nodes, the lungs, the bone marrow, and the meninges. In some cases, infection and ulceration of the colon, the tongue, the larynx, the pharynx, the mouth, the nose, and the lips are initial manifestations.

## Significance of Mycotic Infections to Embalming

Several other mycotic infections may be encountered but are rare. These include dermatomycosis, cryptococcosis, North American blastomycosis, and protothecosis. More than 100,000 species of fungi are known, of which approximately 100 are human pathogens. For the most part, they occur as secondary complications of other diseases. Mycotic infections are frequently encountered, especially in those with debilitating or immunosuppressive diseases and diabetes mellitus. The widespread use of immunosuppressive drugs, combined with modern medical advances that keep patients alive but debilitated, has led to a considerable increase in the incidence of fungal infections. In the modern hospital, they are one of the most important and lethal examples of opportunistic infection.

The greatest danger presented is to the embalmer and to others who work directly with the dead human bodies. Many fungal infections produce superficial lesions on the skin and the mucous membranes. As many of the fungi involved are saprophytic, they continue to multiply until they are effectively arrested. Other fungal infections involve the oral/nasal cavity, the larynx, the pharynx, the esophagus, and the lungs. These may also be saprophytic and continue to multiply in untreated or poorly embalmed dead human bodies. In all fungal infections or unidentified lesions, careful handling of the remains is essential. When moving the remains, do not compress the abdominal or thoracic cavity. Such compression causes air and fungal organisms (including spores) to be expelled into the environment. The spores may lay dormant in the environment until the conditions conducive to fungal growth arise. The spores and fungal organisms may also be inhaled by embalming personnel, establish colonies in the lungs and the throat, and cause further infections.

Bodies with superficial lesions should never be handled with bare hands. A cut or break in the skin of the hands of embalming personnel represents a portal of entry for fungal and other organisms. Should the organisms enter the bloodstream, they can spread throughout the body and cause serious infections. In addition, the embalmer's clothing may harbor fungal organisms and spores, as well as other infectious organisms, which could be spread to other persons with whom the embalmer comes into contact.

Most, if not all, fungal organisms form spores. These spores may be resistant to weak disinfecting agents. Therefore, the spores may lay dormant in an improperly cleaned and disinfected preparation room and on improperly disinfected instruments. These spores could contaminate subsequent remains embalmed in that preparation room. The greater danger, however, lies in the possibility that unsuspecting embalming personnel might inhale airborne spores or contract them through cuts or breaks in the skin. Spores may enter the ventilation system and be spread to other areas.

Personal protective equipment (PPE) is critical to prevent skin contact and breathing in of fungal spores. Clothing and bedding should be removed carefully and disposed of properly. The body should be thoroughly bathed with a proper disinfectant solution as soon as it is undressed. All superficial lesions should be treated immediately, and the mouth, the nose, and the eyes should be properly disinfected. All of these procedures must be accomplished before any embalming procedure is initiated.

Once the external disinfection has been completed, embalming procedures may be carried out as prescribed by the pre-embalming analysis. Routine arterial injection of a solution of sufficient strength and thorough cavity treatment should control internal fungal infections. Oral, nasal, vaginal, and anal cavities may be packed with disinfectant-soaked cotton as an added precaution. For autopsied bodies, careful handling of drainage is recommended.

## CONCEPTS FOR STUDY

1. Discuss the measures that can be taken to prevent post-embalming purge.
2. Discuss the difference between subcutaneous emphysema and true tissue gas.
3. Outline the embalming of a body with tissue gas isolated to the tissues of the right leg.
4. Discuss the challenges encountered in embalming a body dead from chronic alcoholism.
5. List some mycotic infections encountered by the embalmer.
6. Discuss the challenges encountered in preparation of the obese dead human body.
7. Discuss the complications encountered in embalming bodies dead from renal failure.
8. Define comorbidity and explain the embalming significance.

## BIBLIOGRAPHY

Anderson WAD, Scotti M. *Synopsis of Pathology,* 10th ed. St. Louis, MO: C.V. Mosby, 1980.

Boehringer PR. Uremic poisoning. *ESCO Rev* 1964; Second Quarter.

Boehringer PR. *Controlled Embalming of the Head.* Westport, CT: ESCO Technical Notes, 1967:57.

Grant M. Selected embalming complications and their treatment. In: *Champion Expanding Encyclopedia,* No. 573. Springfield, OH: Champion Chemical Co., 1987.

Mulvihill ML. *Human Diseases,* 2nd ed. Norwalk, CT: Appleton & Lange, 1987.

Robbins SL. *Pathology,* 6th ed. Philadelphia, PA: W.B. Saunders Co., 1999.

Sheldon H. *Boyd's Introduction to the Study of Disease,* 9th ed. Philadelphia, PA: Lea & Febiger, 1984.

Tissue gas cause and treatment. In: *Champion Expanding Encyclopedia,* No. 420. Springfield, OH: Champion Chemical Co., 1971.

Walter JB. *Pathology of Human Disease.* Philadelphia, PA: Lea & Febiger, 1989.

## FIGURE CREDIT

Figure 24–1A,B is used with permission of Kevin Drobish.

Figure 24–2 is used with permission of Sharon L. Gee-Mascarello.

CHAPTER 25

# Viewing without Embalming, Delayed Viewing, Re-embalming, and Human Remains Shipping

**CHAPTER OVERVIEW**

- Mausoleum Demolition and Disentombment Project
- Expectations of Embalming Preservation
- Preparation for Viewing Without Embalming
- Embalming for Delayed Viewing and Disposition
- Re-embalming Protocol
- Human Remains Shipping Preparations

The American Board of Funeral Service Education (ABFSE) curriculum committee revised the definition of embalming from "the preservation of the dead human body" to "the *temporary preservation* of the dead human body." Standard embalming as practiced for funeral service applications does not guarantee indefinite preservation of human remains. Embalming for funerals and final events is not the same as preparations of the dead for long-term clinical study and as museum specimens. The methods of embalming customary to funeral events provide preservation in addition to the restoration of an identifiable and acceptable appearance. Preservation methods such as alkaline hydrolysis, cryogenics, mummification, plastination, and anatomical embalming will alter appearance. In time, all organic matter will be reduced. Numerous remains of ancient Egyptian mummies have survived the ages, however any tissue that is present is severely dehydrated to the level of desiccation. Standard arterial embalming will only slow, not completely stop organic decomposition of the body. The funeral service expectation of embalming is that preservation will maintain the body in a stable form until final disposition. Standard embalming methods can potentially produce long-term preservation. Numerous intrinsic variables specific to the decedent, coupled with extrinsic conditions present within the interment and entombment environments prevent defining preservation in terms of time. Three main factors affect the degree and length of preservation:

1. Condition of the body prior to embalming.
2. Effectiveness of embalming.
3. Final disposition environment.

## Mausoleum Demolition and Disentombment Project

A unique and interesting opportunity was presented in 1996, to Professor John Pludeman, while an instructor at the Milwaukee Area Technical College. The objective of the study was to examine hundreds of disentombed bodies that had been embalmed prior to entombment. His findings are included to present evidence of long-term preservation. According to Professor Pludeman:

*"Several years ago, I managed a very unique project involving the demolition of an 85-year-old mausoleum that was in ruins. The massive project first required the disentombment of all human remains within the mausoleum. Once completed, more than 650 casketed human remains and about 350 cremated remains were re-interred in another, well-maintained cemetery. Because the mausoleum entombment records were vandalized and incomplete, every casket was*

opened to confirm occupancy and reestablish identities. By observing large numbers of embalmed human remains that had been preserved and entombed over an 85-year period, the following anecdotal information was derived about the subjects of this study.

- Between 1900 and 1960, nearly 99% of human remains were embalmed.
- In most cases, there was strong evidence of successful long-term preservation, lasting many decades.
- There was much evidence of thorough preservation through the use of adequate embalming chemicals and implementation of proper embalming methods of the day.
- In numerous cases, the deceased were very well preserved and distinctly recognizable. Facial features, hands, jewelry, and clothing remained intact.
- Some remains were completely desiccated but still recognizable while others were only skeletons. In either case, there was no odor present.
- Less than 15% (approximately 35) of all 650 disinterments were in a state of active decomposition. The majority of these cases were in sealer caskets and it appears that moisture was trapped inside the casket and could not escape, or the crypt accumulated water and it seeped into the casket.
- There was consistent evidence of extreme care given to the deceased in respectful final preparation (dressing, positioning, cosmetizing, hair dressing, etc.).
- Funeral directors achieved these admirable accomplishments without the assistance of modern embalming machines, advanced embalming chemicals, eye caps, needle wire injectors, hydroaspirators, and so on."

## Expectations of Embalming Preservation

In the United States, until the last several decades, a majority of human remains were embalmed as a matter of standard practice. Embalming was customary and an integral component of the traditional funeral. Diverse societal attitudes and cultural changes have raised questions about the value of the funeral altogether, not to mention the value of embalming and long-term preservation. As a result, the funeral director can no longer assume that embalming and preservation will be selected. The Federal Trade Commission (FTC) forbids statements that guarantee long-term embalming preservation. Frequently debated questions apply to embalming:

- What are consumer expectations of embalming?
- How long should modern embalming methods preserve human remains?
- What are the purposes and benefits of long-term preservation?
- Should the professional embalmer strive to achieve short-term or long-term preservation?
- Are the family and the public concerned about preservation beyond the funeral and final disposition?
- Are they entitled to a certain degree of preservation because they requested and paid for embalming by a professionally licensed funeral director?

Today, consumers are informed about product choices, expect variety and demand value for goods and services purchased. When faced with the decision of paying for the cost of embalming, some may question just how long embalming will preserve their loved one. If the funeral director is asked this question directly, the response may be influenced by a FTC requirement that prevents the funeral director from representing that preservation will delay the natural decomposition of human remains indefinitely.

There exists yet another consumer-related argument for long-term preservation, which involves the offering of protective funeral merchandise. Considering the many well-constructed, durable, highly protective caskets, burial vaults, crypts, and mausoleums offered to the consumer, what is it these products are protecting if long-term preservation is not possible? And will the consumer be willing to select these products if they perceive long-term preservation as unlikely?

The mausoleum demolition and disentombment project demonstrates an important principle: a thoroughly embalmed, well-preserved body is fundamental to long-term stabilization of that body. Without thorough embalming preservation, no casket, crypt, or other product can retard decomposition and protect the body in the manner that embalming can accomplish. Long-term preservation offers the assurance of a professionally prepared loved one and the peace of mind that it affords.

## VIEWING WITHOUT EMBALMING

Viewing of the body may be requested when permission to embalm is not given. Viewing the unembalmed body may also be necessary to confirm positive identification of the decedent. This is also called **identification viewing**. The following practices are suggested for preparation of the unembalmed body for viewing when a casket or other container is not selected. The same protocol may be followed for preparing a decedent for identification viewing in a casket, cremation container, or other selected container such as a combination unit for shipping.

- Inspect the human remains and document all postmortem conditions on the Embalming and Decedent Care Report.
- Do *not* remove identification tags or bracelets. Attach a new identification tag generated by the funeral home or embalming facility.
- Remove, inventory, and securely store all personal effects.
- Remove pacemakers and cardio-defibrillators (with permission when final disposition by cremation is confirmed).
- Remove medical devices affecting the facial orifices and the neck (intubation or tracheostomy tubes).
- Disinfect body surfaces, set features, and clean fingernails.
- Bathe, shampoo, and shave facial hair (with permission).
- Pack all orifices.
- Apply plastic garments as necessary.
- Dress the decedent in a hospital gown or clothing provided.
- Transfer the decedent to a dressing table or mortuary cot.
- Place the decedent's head on a pillow, comb or brush the hair.
- Drape a crisp, clean sheet and blanket similar to making a bed. The arms and hands can be positioned atop the blanket.
- Cosmetics may or may not be applied.

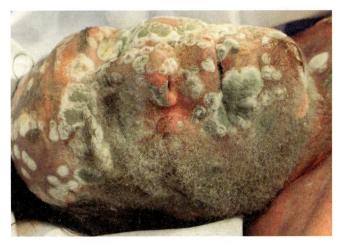

**Figure 25–1.** Mold formation after extended storage.

## DELAYED VIEWING OR FINAL DISPOSITION

All three classifications of embalming chemicals may be necessary to extend preservation for delayed viewing, delayed final disposition, and during temporary sheltering: (1) preservative embalming chemicals, (2) supplemental embalming chemicals (humectants, co- or pre-injection chemicals, dyes, tissue building products), and (3) accessory embalming chemicals (embalming powders, gels, autopsy compounds, mold inhibiting agents). The application of mold inhibiting agents prevents mold growth during extended storage (**Fig. 25–1**).

Considerations for the preparation of remains for delayed viewing and disposition:
- Multipoint injection.
- Moderate arterial solutions with humectant co-injection.
- Intermittent or restricted drainage.
- Hypodermic and surface embalming.
- Delayed aspiration and cavity treatment.
- Body bridges and positioning devices.
- Hypodermic feature and tissue treatments (cheeks, temples, lips, and fingertips).
- Apply a mold inhibiting agent to skin surfaces. Reapply at regular intervals during storage.
- Apply massage cream to the face, neck, and hands. Cover with cotton and plastic sheeting to prevent dehydration.
- Avoid excessive elevation of the head during storage.
- Perform periodic monitoring and make necessary corrections.

### Secure Sheltering of Human Remains

The deceased human body must be securely protected throughout the period of temporary sheltering. In circumstances when embalming authorization is delayed or not desired, mortuary refrigeration is recommended and is required in some states. Obtain permission for minimal care services prior to performing any treatments.

## RE-EMBALMING

Re-embalming the entire body arterially or an area of the body may be necessary when signs of decomposition appear that were not present after the initial embalming. Previously injected arteries may be re-injected and additional arteries areas can be raised for injection that are closest to the affected area. Strong or waterless solutions are recommended. Observe blood-filled veins and open them for drainage. Areas of the face that appear underembalmed can be injected hypodermically. Hidden injection points from inside the mouth and nose and at the hairline are recommended. Residual leakage from external sites can be stopped by the application of super adhesive glue. The eyelids can be treated by placing cotton beneath or overtop the eyelids and saturating the cotton with a few drops of undiluted cavity fluid. The embalmer may need to utilize all three methods for re-embalming: arterial injection, hypodermic injection, and surface embalming. Cavity re-aspiration and re-injection may also be necessary. Embalming provides temporary preservation. Lengthy intervals between embalming and final disposition and the following factors may contribute to the continuance of decomposition:

- Arterial solution strength was too weak to meet preservative demands of the tissues.
- Arterial solution was neutralized by nitrogenous waste.
- Active rigor mortis prevented adequate absorption of arterial solution.
- Arterial solution did not distribute uniformly.
- Arterial solution did not diffuse into the tissues and cells.
- Additional arterial injection sites were needed.
- Insufficient volume of arterial solution was injected.
- Inadequate blood drainage.
- Incomplete cavity aspiration.
- Insufficient volume of cavity fluid injected.
- Rigor mortis was mistaken for tissue firming.
- Blood discolorations were mistaken for arterial fluid dyes.

## HUMAN REMAINS SHIPPING

Human remains shipping is the transportation of human remains (dead human body or cremated remains) from one location to a different location. Shipping categories are based on destination: (1) intrastate—within the same state, (2) interstate—between states, and (3) international—between countries. The **Transportation Security Administration** (TSA), an agency of the U.S. Department of Homeland Security was created to improve airport security procedures following the September 11, 2001 attacks against the United States. The **Known Shipper Program** requires all funeral homes who wish to transport human remains on a passenger aircraft to register and be approved as a known shipper.

### Cremated Remains

Airline passengers are allowed to travel with cremated remains in either a checked or carry-on bag. Cremated remains may be shipped (domestic or international) through the United States Post Office by Priority Mail Express (PME).

### Shipping Human Remains (Ship-out)

Prior to providing any type of decedent care, it is advisable to contact the receiving funeral home first. Specific requests can be discussed and documented at that time. Embalming and positioning preferences vary according to geographic, cultural, religious, and other preferences. Arterial, hypodermic, and surface embalming methods should be employed to the fullest extent to alleviate post-embalming concerns during transportation. Cavity embalming should be thorough and all body orifices packed to prevent purge. Plastic garments are recommended with absorbent powders placed within. The decedent may be dressed minimally in a hospital gown or provided clothing. Massage cream may be applied to the face and hands to prevent dehydration. It is advisable to consult with the receiving funeral home regarding cosmetic application. Prepare the Embalming and Decedent Care Report and make a copy. Retain the original report and provide a copy to the receiving funeral home. Discuss any conditions or embalming concerns with the receiving funeral home prior to shipping.

### Preparation of the Casket or Shipping Container

Line the inside length of the casket or container with plastic sheeting prior to placing the decedent. Best practice is to reverse the casket pillow for shipping and elevate the head. In the shipping container, cotton can be securely packed around the head block as well as the head and neck of the decedent to prevent shifting during transportation. Position the arms according to preference. Secure the decedent in place when straps are provided to prevent shifting.

Avoid placing live floral tributes in the casket or container. Flowers can create a moist environment and soil clothing and interior fabrics. Items placed inside the casket or container should be secured in place and visible. The receiving funeral home should be alerted to the placement and provided an inventory of those items accompanying the decedent.

When closed, the casket lid or top of the container should not touch the nose or forehead. Metal caskets with locking mechanisms can be secured for shipping; leave the cap off of the locking mechanism. The cargo hold of an airplane may not be pressurized and a sealed casket may implode during transport. The cap can be secured with tape on the inside of the stationary or swing bar of the casket. Alert the receiving funeral home of the location of the cap. Casket keys are universal; supplying a key to the receiving funeral home is unnecessary.

Document the required information on the outer shipping box at the *head end*: decedent's full name and the names, addresses, and phone numbers of both the shipping and receiving funeral homes. Place all necessary documents (Burial-Transit Permit, Certificate of Death, Embalming and Decedent Care Report, etc.) in the provided document envelope. Affix the envelope to the top of the container. Do **not seal** the envelope until instructed to do so by the shipping agency; often the documentation is verified before sealing the envelope.

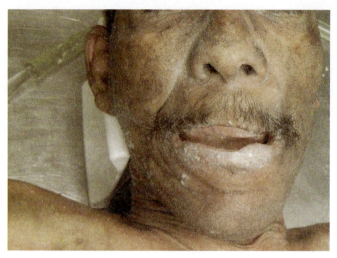

**Figure 25–2.** Mouth opened during transit.

### Shipping Regulations

Regulations and requirements related to human remains shipping vary widely and can change without notice. Best practice is to consult the most current directory published exclusively for funeral service use. For international human remains shipping, it is advised to first contact the consulate in the receiving country for specific regulations and requirements.

### Receiving Human Remains (Ship-in)

Minor adjustments are anticipated. Cavity re-aspiration is recommended for all bodies received. Facial features may have opened during transportation and require adjustment (**Fig. 25–2**). Inspect the remains thoroughly and review the Embalming and Decedent Care Report provided by the shipping funeral home. Document any custodial care treatments on the report. Provide a copy of the updated report and discuss any unanticipated concerns immediately with the shipping funeral home.

## FIGURE CREDIT

Figure 25–1 is used with permission of Kevin Drobish.
Figure 25–2 is used with permission of Sharon L. Gee-Mascarello.

## BIBLIOGRAPHY

American Board of Funeral Service Education, *Course Content Syllabus,* 2016.
Basic factors relating to the embalming process. In: *Champion Expanding Encyclopedia,* Springfield, OH: Champion Chemical Co., September 1981.
Hirst T. Diagnose your cases before you start embalming. *American Funeral Director* March 1930.
Mayer R. The secret is in its strength. *The Director* April 1992.
Peterson KD. The two-year fix: Long-term preservation for delayed viewing. *The Director* April 1992.
Sanders CR. Preventing restorative problems caused by delayed interment. *The Dodge Magazine* March/November, 1997; January, 1998.
Shor M. Condition of the body dictates the proper embalming treatment, not cause of death. *Casket and Sunnyside* November 1972.
Strub CG. Embalmed body may become "disembalmed." *Casket and Sunnyside* 1966.

# PART II

## The Origin and History of Embalming

Edward C. Johnson, Gail R. Johnson, and Melissa Johnson

This statement made in 1875 by the New York State Supreme Court remains relevant, concise, and conceptually complete today:

*The decent burial of the dead is a matter in which the public have concern. It is against the Public Health if it does not take place at all and against a proper public sentiment should it not take place with decency.*

Winston Churchill offered this timeless statement:

*Without a sense of history, no man can understand the problems of our time, the longer you can look back, the further you can look forward—the wider the span, the longer the continuity, the greater is the sense of duty in individual men and women, each contributing their brief life's work to the preservation and progress of the land in which they live, the society of which they are the servants.*

Esmond R. Long, M.D., a medical historian, said:

*Nothing gives a better perspective of the subject than an appreciation of the steps by which it has reached its present state.*

So it is with the subject of embalming. The authors of this chapter trust that this brief exposition of the origin and history of embalming will impart to the reader a sense of the tradition and technical advances achieved over nearly 5000 years that the art and science of embalming have been practiced. There is a clear indication that both tradition and new technical advances will continue to be maintained in the future.

Embalming, one of humankind's longest practiced arts, is a means of artificially preserving the dead human body.

1. **Natural means of preservation:** obtained without the deliberate intervention of humans
   a. *Freezing:* By this method, bodies are preserved for centuries in the ice and snow of glaciers or snow-capped mountains.
   b. *Dry cold:* A morgue located on the top of St. Bernard Mountain in Switzerland was so constructed to permit free admission of the elements. True mummies were produced as a result of the passage of the cold, dry air currents over the corpses.
   c. *Dry heat:* Natural mummies are produced in the extremely dry, warm areas of Egypt, south western America, and Peru.
   d. *Nature of the soil at the place of interment:* There are recorded instances of the discovery of bodies in a good state of preservation after long-term burial in a peat bog that had high tannin content or in soils strongly impregnated with salts of aluminum or copper.
2. **Artificial means of preservation:** secured by the deliberate action of humans
   a. *Simple heat:* Simple heat is the means employed to preserve bodies in the Capuchin Monastery near Palermo, on the island of Sicily. The monastery is connected to a catacomb or underground burial vault composed of four separate chambers. Treatment of the bodies consists of slow drying in an oven that is heated by a mixture of slaked lime. The desiccated bodies, quite shrunken and light in weight, are placed in upright positions along the walls of the catacombs.
   b. *Powders:* In powder methods, the body is placed on a bed of sawdust mixed with zinc sulfate or other preserving powder.
   c. *Evisceration and immersion* (used by the Egyptians and others)
   d. *Evisceration and drying* (the Guanche method)
   e. *Evisceration, local incision, and immersion* (employed in Europe, particularly in France, during the period AD 650–1830)
   f. *Simple immersion* (in alcohol, brine, or other liquid preservatives)
   g. *Arterial injection and evisceration* (used by the Hunter brothers and others)
   h. *Cavity injection and immersion* (method of Gabriel Clauderus)
   i. *Arterial injection* (mode of treatment of Gannal, Sucquet, and many others)
   j. *Arterial injection and cavity treatment* (method in daily use by all present-day embalmers; generally taught in schools and colleges of embalming today)
   k. *Artificial cold* (by a system of refrigeration to reduce the body temperature to inhibit bacterial activity; in use in most hospitals and morgues today)

## PERIODS OF EMBALMING HISTORY

Embalming originated in Egypt during the period of the first dynasty. It is estimated to have begun around 3200 BC and continued until AD 650. The motive of Egyptian embalming was religious in that preservation of the human body (intact) was a necessary requirement for resurrection, which is their religious goal. During this nearly 4000-year period of embalming practice, there obviously existed a number of variations in this technique. Egyptian embalming began to decline with the advent of Christianity, as the early Christians rejected the practice, associating embalming with various "pagan religious rites." When the Arabs conquered Egypt, they too rejected the practice of embalming.

The second period of embalming history extends from AD 650 to 1861, and its principal geographical area of practice and growth was Europe. This era is termed the *Period of the Anatomists*, as the motive was to advance the development of embalming techniques for the preservation of the dead to permit detailed anatomical dissection and study.

The third or modern period of embalming history extends from 1861 to the present day. It is during this period that embalming knowledge, which had been transferred from Europe to America during the previous period, finally reverted to its original use, principally for funeral purposes. Embalming again became available to all who requested it. Motives in this period are diverse, with sentiment probably predominant, as the average person desires to view the decedent free of evidence of the ravages of disease or injury. Public transportation is another reason to embalm, as the procedure prevents a dead body from becoming offensive during a protracted period of travel and is required by many public transport agencies.

Although the value of embalming is disputed and debated to the public health, it is most apparent that a decaying, unembalmed body is surely a health menace to those exposed to its effluvia. From earliest Egyptian times, embalmers have been closely associated with the medical profession. In fact, most embalmers in the United States were doctors of medicine until the later portion of the nineteenth century.

## EGYPTIAN PERIOD

During the early predynastic period, well before 3200 BC, the Egyptians had a very simple culture. When death occurred, the unembalmed body was placed in the fetal position (arms and legs folded), wrapped in cloth or straw mats, and placed in a shallow grave scooped out of the desert sand west of the Nile River. A few pieces of pottery and other artifacts were placed in the grave with the body, which were positioned on its side. The body was preserved by drying, and from contact with the arid, porous sand and the total absence of rainfall, or other moisture. From time to time, desert winds uncovered the bodies in their shallow graves, and cemetery guards or relatives saw that the bodies were indeed preserved (**Fig. 1**).

Then, as now, there existed members of the society who were criminals, and some devoted themselves to grave robbing. When the cemetery custodians or family survivors of such elaborate burials noted the opening and desecration of burials, they also noted and were appalled that the corpse was no longer preserved, but had begun to decay. One attempt to forestall decomposition was the enclosure of the body within a solid stone coffin cut from a single mass of stone. The body of the coffin was without seams and the cover fit tightly. These burials were subsequently plundered, and again, the custodians or relatives contemplated the remains, which, to their horror, had on many occasions completely decomposed to a skeletal status. Without a scientific knowledge of the process of putrefaction, they expressed the belief that the stone coffin ate the soft tissues. To this day, massive bronze and copper caskets are termed *sarcophagi* from the Greek *sarco* for "flesh" and *phagus* for "eater." The Egyptians, not wishing to revert to their simple method of burial in the sands, found it necessary to devise some system of preserving the human body—embalming.

It is not too difficult to understand how Egyptian embalming was first developed when it is kept in mind that Egypt has a basically warm climate. The culture was such that hunting and fishing provided some of the food requirements. Thus, a hunter or a fisherman might have a successful catch and secure more birds, fish, or game than he or his family could consume immediately. Such animals, fish, or birds could, like the human body, quickly decay and become worthless for food. The hunter, however, knew how to prepare his catch and to preserve it. He eviscerated and bled his catch and then, by one or another method such as salting, sun drying, smoking, or cooking, preserved it for future consumption. (*This procedure for the preservation of food was common knowledge and it requires little imagination to recognize the ease with which the basic food preservation process could be adapted with refinements to the preservation of the dead human body.*)

## VARIATION IN EMBALMING METHODS

The actual methods of embalming employed by the Egyptians varied from dynasty to dynasty according to the custom and the technique of the individual embalmer. History provides views of four contemporary writers on the subject who have frequently been quoted.

The earliest account is that of the Greek historian Herodotus, who lived around 484 BC:

*There are certain individuals appointed for the purpose [the embalming], and who profess the art; these persons, when any dead body is brought to them, show the bearers some wooden models of corpses; the most perfect they assert to be the representation of him whose name I take it impious to mention in this matter; they show a second, which is inferior to the first and cheaper; and a third which is cheapest of all. They then ask according to which of the models they will have the deceased prepared; having settled upon the price, the relations immediately depart, and the embalmers, remaining at home, thus proceed to perform the embalming in the most costly manner.*

In the first place, with a crooked piece of iron, they pull out the brain by the nostrils; a part of it they extract in this manner, the rest by means of pouring in certain drugs; in the next place, after making an incision in the flank with a sharp Ethiopian stone, they empty the whole of the inside; and after cleansing the cavity, and rinsing it with palm wine, scour it out with pounded aromatics. Then, having filled the belly with pure myrrh pounded, and cinnamon, and all other perfumes, frankincense excepted, they sew it up again; having so done, they "steep" the body in natrum, keeping it covered for 70 days, for it is not lawful to leave the body any longer.

When the 70 days are gone by, they first wash the corpse, and then wrap up the whole body in bandages cut out of cotton cloth, which they smear with gum, a substance the Egyptians use instead of paste. The relations, having then received back the body, get a wooden case in the shape of a man to be made; and when completed, they place the body in the inside and then, shutting it up, keep it in a sepulchral repository, where they stand it upright against the wall. The above is the most costly manner in which they prepare the dead.

For such who choose the middle mode, from a desire of avoiding expense, they prepare the body as follows: They first fill syringes with oil of cedar to inject into the belly of the

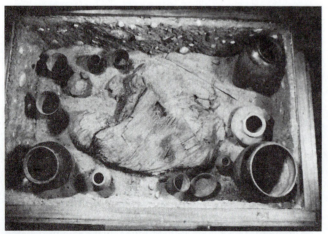

**Figure 1.** Predynastic (3200 BC) Egyptian burial site, west of the Nile. The unembalmed corpse is in the fetal position, wrapped in straw matting. (*Used with permission of the Royal Ontario Museum.*)

deceased, without making any incision, or emptying the inside, but by sending it in by the anus. This they then cork, to hinder the injection from flowing backwards, and lay the body in salt for the specified number of days, on the last of which they release what they had previously injected, and such is the strength it possesses that it brings away with it the bowels and insides in a state of dissolution; on the other hand, the natrum dissolves the flesh so that, in fact, there remains nothing but the skin and bones. When they have done this they give the body back without any further operation upon it.

The third mode of embalming, which is used for such as have but scanty means, is as follows: after washing the insides with syrmaea, they salt the body for the 70 days and return it to be taken back.

The second writer is Diodorus Siculus, who lived around 45 BC:

*When anyone among the Egyptians dies, all his relations and friends, putting dirt upon their heads, go lamenting about the city, till such time as the body shall be buried. In the mean time they abstain from baths and wine, and all kinds of delicate meats, neither do they during that time wear any costly apparel. The manner of their burials is three-fold: one very costly, a second sort less chargeable, and a third very mean. In the first, they say, there is spent a talent of silver [$1,200]; in the second, 20 minae [$300]; but in the last there is very little expense [$75]. Those who have the care of ordering the body are such as have been taught that art by their ancestors. These, showing to the kindred of the deceased a bill of each kind of burial, ask them after which manner they will have the body prepared. When they have agreed upon the matter, they deliver the body to such as are usually appointed for this office. First, he who has the name scribe marks about the flank of the left side how much is to be cut away. Then he who is called the cutter or dissector, with an Ethiopian stone, cuts away as much of the flesh as the law commands, and presently runs away as fast as he can. Those who are present pursue him, cast stones at him, curse him, thereby turning all the execrations which they imagine due to his office upon him.*

*For whosoever offers violence, wounds, or does any kind of injury to a body of the same nature with himself, they think him worthy of hatred; but those who are called embalmers are worthy of honor and respect; for they are familiar with their priests and go into the temples as holy men without any prohibition. So soon as they come to embalm the dissected body, one of them thrusts his hand through the wound into the abdomen and draws out all the viscera but the heart and kidneys, which another washes and cleanses with wine made of palms and aromatic odors.*

*Lastly having washed the body, they anoint it with oil of cedar and other things for 30 days, and afterward with myrrh, cinnamon, and other such like matters, which have not only a power to preserve it for a long time, but also give it a sweet smell; afterward they deliver it to the kindred in such manner that every member remains whole and entire, and no part of it changed. The beauty and shape of the face seems just as it was before, and may be known, even the hairs of the eyebrows and eyelids remaining as they were at first. By this method many of the Egyptians, keeping the dead bodies of their ancestors in magnificent houses, so perfectly see the true visage and countenance of those that died many ages before they themselves were born that in viewing the proportions of every one of them, and the lineaments of their faces, they take as much delight as if they were still living among them.*

The third account is given by Plutarch, who lived between AD 50 and 100:

*The belly being opened, the bowels were removed and cast into the River Nile and the body exposed to the sun. The cavities of the chest and belly were then filled with the unguents and odorous substances.*

The fourth description is by Perphry, who lived around AD 230 to 300:

*When those who have care of the dead proceed to embalm the body of any person of respectable rank, they first take out the contents of the belly and place them in a separate vessel, addressing the sun, and utter on behalf of the deceased the following prayer, which Euphantus has translated from the original language into Greek: "O thou sun, our lord, and all ye gods who are the givers of life to men, accept me, and receive me into the mansions of the eternal gods; for I have worshiped piously, while I have lived in this world, those divinities whom my parents taught me to adore. I have ever honored those parents who gave origin to my body; and of other men I have neither killed any, nor robbed them of their treasure, nor inflicted upon them any grievous evil; but if I have done anything injurious to my soul, either by eating or drinking anything unlawfully, this offense has not been committed by me, but by what is contained in this chest." This refers to the intestines in the vessel, which is then cast into the River Nile. The body is afterwards regarded as pure, the apology having been made for its offenses, and the embalmer prepares it according to the appointed rites.*

## DIFFERENCES IN TRANSLATIONS

As may be observed, there were differences in embalming methods as described by the foregoing writers. This may be, in part, due to inaccuracies in copying and translating of the original manuscripts.

Present-day translations of the *Book of the Dead*, a textbook guide for the Egyptian embalmer, do not agree on the 70-day period for the covering with natron. One of the chronologies of the most costly method states that the 1st to the 16th days were occupied with evisceration, washing, and cleansing of the body; from the 16th to the 36th days, the body was kept under natron; from the 36th to the 68th days, the spicing and bandaging took place; and from the 68th to the 70th days, the body was coffined.

## STEPS IN EGYPTIAN PREPARATION

### Step 1: Removal of the Brain

The brain was generally removed by introducing a metal hook or spoon into the nostril and by forcing it through the ethmoid bone to the brain. As much as possible was scooped out in this way.

In some mummies, the brain was not removed. A few craniums had the brain removed through the eye socket. There is one case on record in which the evacuation of the cranium was accomplished through the foramen magnum, after excision of the atlas vertebra. After the body was removed from under natron, the cranium was usually repacked with linen bandages soaked in resin or bitumen. One writer tells of removing 27 feet of 3-inch linen bandage from the cranium of a mummy. Sometimes, the cranium was filled with resin believed to have been introduced while molten with the aid of a funnel.

## Step 2: Evisceration

Many bodies were not eviscerated. The earliest incision was made vertically in the left side, extending from the lower margin of the ribs to the anterior superior spine (crest) of the ilium. This incision would measure between 5 and 6 inches in length. At a later period, the incision became oblique, extending from a point near the left anterior spine (crest) of the ilium toward the pubis. A variant incision extended vertically from the symphysis pubis toward the umbilicus. In the very late 26th dynasty (665–527 BC), some bodies were eviscerated through the anus. The incision was usually made with a flint knife called *Ethiopian stone* because of its black color. All the viscera, with the exception of the kidneys and usually the heart, were removed, washed, and immersed in palm wine or packed in natron. (*Their disposition will be referred to later.*)

## Step 3: Covering with Natron

Natron is a salt obtained from the dry lakes of the desert and is composed of chloride, carbonate, and sulfate of sodium and nitrate of potassium and sodium. Because of its corrosive action on the body, the embalmers had to affix the toes and fingernails to the body during the macerating period. This was accomplished by tying the nails on with thread or copper or gold wire. Alternatively, metal thimbles were fit over the ends of the fingers and toes for the same purpose. The body was then ready for the natron treatment. Early Egyptologists believed that the bodies were placed in a solution composed of natron dissolved in water, as described by Herodotus. Present-day authorities, in studying the original writing of Herodotus and other prime sources, detect a flaw in the translation of the text that is responsible for the misrepresentation. Present-day research, where the embalming process was recreated, indicates conclusively that only application of the concentrated dry salt over the body to some depth could dehydrate and preserve it. Experiments with different concentrations of the natron solution and immersion of specimens therein were largely unsuccessful in preventing decay.

## Step 4: Removal from Natron

At the end of the 20th day of immersion in natron, the body was washed with water and dried in the sun.

## Step 5: Wrapping and Spicing

The body was coated within and without by resin or a mixture of resin and fat. The skull was treated as in Step 1. The viscera, when removed from the body and not returned to the body, were placed in four canopic jars, the tops of which were surmounted by the images of the four children of Horus. Each jar

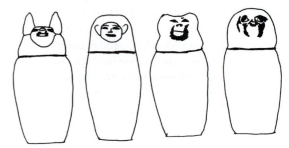

**Figure 2.** Canopic urns—containers of the viscera removed during embalming preparation and not returned to trunk of body. From left to right are the jackal's head, Duamutef (contained stomach); the human head, Imset (contained liver); the ape's head, Hapy (contained lungs); and the hawk's head, Qebeh-Snewef (contained intestines). (*Used with permission of Paula Johnson De Smet.*)

held a specific portion of the viscera. The jar topped with the human head represented Imset and contained the liver. The jar covered with the jackal's head represented Duamutef and contained the stomach. The jar topped with the ape's head represented Hapy and held the lungs. The fourth jar, surmounted by a hawk's head, represented Qebeh-Snewef and contained the intestines. No mention is made of the disposition of the spleen, pancreas, or pelvic organs (**Fig. 2**).

The canopic jars varied in size and material. They were from about 9 to 18 inches in height and 4 inches in diameter and were made of alabaster, limestone, basalt, clay, and other materials. The canopic jars were usually placed in a wooden box and kept near the body. When the viscera were placed in these jars, images in miniature of the jars were returned to the cavity, which was padded in straw, resin-soaked linen bandages, or lichen moss. On return to the body cavity, the viscera were usually wrapped in four separate parcels to which specific images were attached, as mentioned earlier. Originally, the incision was not sewn but merely had the edges drawn together. Sometimes, the edges were stuck together by resin or wax; however, there are recorded instances in the 18th, 20th, and 21st dynasties (respectively, 1700, 1250, and 1000 BC) of closure effected by sewing, which closely resembles the familiar embalmer's stitch of today. The incision was covered, whether sewn or not, by a plate of wax or metal on which the eye of Osiris (Egyptian god of the dead) was engraved.

## Ancient Restorative Art

It was during this part of the preparation in the 20th dynasty (1288–1110 BC) that a little-known process was performed. Most present-day embalmers feel that the restoration to normal of emaciated facial features of a corpse is of comparatively recent origin. On the contrary, the Egyptian embalmers performed this operation, but on a much more extensive scale. Not only were the facial features restored, but the entire bodily contours were subcutaneously padded to regain their normal shape. The methods and materials used varied.

The mouth was usually internally packed with sawdust to pad out the cheeks, while the eyelids were stuffed with linen pads. Then, working from the original abdominal incision by burrowing under the skin of the trunk in all directions, the packing material was forced into these channels. In places such as the back and arms that could not be reached from the original incision, additional local incisions were made through which to pass the padding material. In later periods, the cheeks and temples were padded with resin introduced through openings in front of the ears. This material, introduced while warm, could be molded to conform to the desired contour. The packing materials most commonly used were resin, linen bandages, mud, sand, sawdust, and butter mixed with soda. It was also during this stage of preparation that repair of bodily injuries took place. Broken limbs were splinted, and bed sores were packed with resin-soaked linen bandages and covered with thin strips of antelope hide.

There is a case of a crooked spine having been straightened. Eyes were sometimes replaced with ones of stone or, as in one instance, with small onions. The bodies that were to be gilded (covered with golden leaf) were then treated. Some were completely covered with a gold leaf; on others, only the face, fingernails, and toenails, or genitals were gilded, as there was much variation on this matter. After the complete covering of the body with a paste of resin and fat, the bandagers set to work. It is believed that there were individuals who specialized in wrapping certain parts of the body such as the fingers, arms, legs, and head. Each finger or toe was first separately swathed; then each limb. The body was first covered with a kind of tunic and the face covered with a large square bandage followed by the regular spiral bandages. Pads were placed between the bandages to aid in restoration and maintenance of the bodily contour. Lotus blossoms have been found between the layers of linen bandages. Some authorities claim that the living saved cloth all their lives to provide bandages for use as mummy wrappings. The bandages varied from 3 to 9 inches in width and up to 1200 yards in length and were inscribed at intervals with hieroglyphics indicating the identity of the enswathed person. Authorities believed that only 1 of 10 mummies was prepared by the first method. The others were prepared by the cheaper methods, as described by the earlier writers. Another means of embalming used then was simple covering of the entire body with natron or molten resin. This latter process, while preserving the body, destroyed the hair and most of the facial features, fingers, and toes.

During the last 1000 years of Egyptian embalming practice, the emphasis gradually changed from producing a well-preserved body capable of withstanding decay for all eternity to creating an increasingly elaborate external appearance of the wrapped body. Wrapping patterns became quite elaborate and cartonage and plaster were employed to present a sometimes fanciful external recreation of the deceased. During the terminal centuries of Egyptian embalming, portraits on a flat surface were painted and placed over the head area, which more faithfully resembled the dead.

### The Receptacles

The wrapped mummies were usually additionally encased and placed in boxes or coffins. An additional encasement, termed *cartonage*, was made of 20 or 30 sheets of linen cloth or papyrus saturated in resin, plaster of Paris, or gum acacia and placed over the wrapped body while wet. To ensure a tight fit, the material was drawn together in the back of the body by a kind of lacing not unlike present-day shoelacing. The cartonage, when dry, was as hard as wood and was covered with

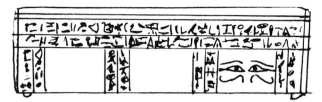

**Figure 3.** Wooden coffin. The body, placed inside, lies on its left side with the head at the end where eyes are drawn thus looking outward. (*Used with permission of Paula Johnson De Smet.*)

a thin coating of plaster, then painted with a representation of a human head and other designs. Two or more wood cases of cedar or sycamore might encase the cartonage and each other. These coffins or mummy cases were of different shape, depending on the period when they were made. The outer wooden case was, at times, rectangular in shape with a cover resembling the roof of a house. Early coffined embalmed bodies were placed within the coffins lying on their side. The exterior of the coffin contained the representation of a pair of eyes on one side near the head of the coffin (**Fig. 3**). This indicated the position of the body facing outward at this point. Coffins shaped like the human form were termed anthropoid or mummiform (**Fig. 4**). If the deceased was a member of a great family, he might be

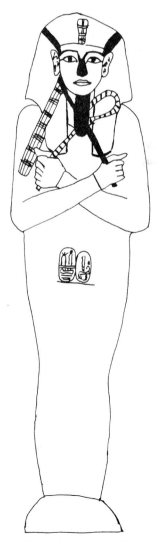

**Figure 4.** Wooden anthropoid or mummiform coffin. (*Used with permission of Paula Johnson De Smet.*)

enclosed within a stone sarcophagus, which was a stone coffin or vault fashioned of marble, limestone, granite, or slate.

Even in Egyptian times, the tombs of the dead were plundered for their valuables. Many mummy cases were broken open and the mummies themselves were damaged. The embalmers were called on to repair the damaged mummies and to rewrap and recoffin them. This may explain, in part, the so-called *faking of mummies*. In the Field Museum of Natural History in Chicago, there are numerous x-ray pictures of unopened mummy cases and unwrapped mummies. Some of these pictures show damage that may have occurred prior to or during the course of embalming. One x-ray photo of a young child displays the complete absence of the arms and bilateral fractures of the femurs at about their midpoint, with the lower broken portion entirely missing. Museum authorities advance the theory that this was done to fit the child into a smaller mummy case. Another x-ray photo reveals a wrapped mummy lacking arms and the trunk of the body. The head was connected to the legs by a board and the body has been represented by padding of straw or lichen moss.

Additional faking may be the result of a curious custom of the early middle ages of using bits of mummies as good luck pieces and as a drug for internal consumption. This demand created a brisk business for the Arabs of North Africa, and as the supply of natural mummies was difficult to maintain, the Arabs began to produce their own from the bodies of lepers and criminal dead.

Animals were also embalmed, wrapped, and coffined in a manner similar to humans. The variety of animals so treated was large and included baboons, monkeys, full-grown bulls, gazelles, goats, sheep, antelopes, crocodiles, cats, dogs, mice, rats, shrews, hawks, geese, ibis, snakes, and lizards. X-ray examination of these wrapped packages discloses an occasional falsity. Some of these false mummies are composed of straw or rags wrapped in the form of the animal they were to represent. G. Elliot Smith, in his article on "The significance of geographical distribution of practice of mummification," states that knowledge of the Egyptian method of embalming was carried westward as far as the Canary Islands. He bases his decision on the similarity of the embalming procedures carried on in these areas of the world and the knowledge that the Egyptian method preceded those in all other known parts of the world.

### Recreation of the Ancient Mummification Process

The Greek historian Herodotus wrote of the ancient mummification practice while visiting Egypt in approximately 450 BC. It was a fascinating description of the nearly 70-day process and the tools, processes, and ceremony that surrounded the preservation process.

Although this account has existed for centuries and we have seen the mummies that have been preserved through this process, there has never been a modern understanding of what takes place. In 1994, Robert Brier, an Egyptologist with the C.W. Post Campus of Long Island University, and Ronald Wade, the Director of Anatomical Services at the University of Maryland Medical School in Baltimore, Maryland, embarked on an amazing research study. They set out to recreate an authentic Egyptian mummy using the process and tools described by Herodotus. To be true to the process, they had replicas of the original tools made by a silversmith, they had a wood artisan construct an embalming table, and they visited Egypt to obtain the oils, spices, amulets, and Nile natron salt. Additionally, they had the ceramics department at C.W. Post make canopic jars to hold the internal organs.

The modern-day mummy was an elderly gentleman who donated his body to science. The body was placed on the embalming table and the process of making the mummy began with the removal of the subject's brain through the nose. Brier and Wade used the replicated "hook" to break through the ethmoid bone. The ethmoid bone is a thin bone that is located at the back of the nose and leads directly into the brain. Although the description by Herodotus suggests that the hook was used to actually remove the brain, Brier and Wade found that this was not the case. They used the hook to pulverize the brain and then turned the body over on its stomach and allowed it to drain out of the nose.

The procedure then calls for the removal of the thoracic and abdominal organs. This was done using a sharpened black stone according to Herodotus. The recreated bronze tools initially did not work because they dulled too quickly. Brier and Wade then used a stone called *obsidian* that was sharpened, and they made an incision in the left side of the abdomen to remove all the organs except the heart. The heart was considered to be the essence of the individual. The body cavities were then washed with a combination of palm wine and myrrh, whereas the brain cavity was washed with palm wine and frankincense. The body cavities were then filled with bags filled with natron. The body was then completely covered with 600 pounds of natron and placed in a room to recreate the climatic conditions that would have been found in ancient Egypt 3000 years before. The body was left for 35 days and then rubbed with oils of frankincense, myrrh, palm, lotus, and cedar. The body itself had lost over 100 pounds of water from its original weight of 160 pounds. Brier and Wade then removed tissue samples for bacterial sampling and the results were all negative for any growth. Using linen bandages and shrouds purchased in Egypt, they wrapped the body over a 6-day time period. The body was wrapped in six layers and the traditional amulet was placed directly above the heart. The mummy currently resides at the University of Maryland Anatomical Services Laboratory.

## THE PRACTICE OF BODY PRESERVATION OF VARIOUS ETHNIC GROUPS AND PLACES

### Jews

The Jews did not embalm but simply washed and shaved the body and swathed it in sheets, between the folds of which were placed spices such as myrrh and aloes. The purpose of herbs and spices was to disguise the odor of decay of the body, not to preserve it.

### Ancient Persians, Syrians, and Babylonians

Sometimes, the ancient Persians, Syrians, and Babylonians immersed their human dead in jars of honey or wax. Alexander the Great was said to have been so treated to preserve his body during the long journey from his place of death in Babylon in 323 BC (during a military campaign) to Egypt.

## Ancient Ethiopians

The ancient Ethiopians eviscerated and desiccated their dead in a manner similar to the Egyptian method. The bodily contours were restored by applying plaster over the shrunken skin. The plaster-covered corpse was then painted with lifelike colors and given a coating of clear resin-like substance believed by some authorities to be a fossil salt and by others to be a type of amber, somehow rendered fluid at the time of application.

## Canary Islands (from at least 900 BC)

In the Atlantic Ocean, about 4 degrees south of the Madeira Islands, on the northwest coast of Africa, there is a cluster of 13 islands known as the *Canary Islands*. These islands were not subdued by any European nation until the Spaniards overran them in the late fifteenth century. The original inhabitants, known as *Guanches*, are thought to have been descendants of the lost continent of Atlantis. It is believed that only prominent and influential families had the dead embalmed. The Guanches' method of embalming their dead is very similar to the Egyptian method.

The Guanche embalmers were both men and women who performed the services for their own sex. These embalmers were well paid, although their touch was considered contaminating and they lived in seclusion in remote parts of the islands. On the death of a person, the family bore the body to the embalmers and then retired. The embalmers placed the body on a stone table and an opening was made in the lower abdomen with a flint knife called a *tabona*. The intestines were withdrawn, washed, cleaned, and later returned to the body. The entire body, inside and outside, was very thoroughly saturated with salt and the intestines were returned to the body along with numerous aromatic plants and herbs.

The body, anointed with butter, powdered resin, brushwood, and pumice, was exposed to the sun, or, if the sun was not hot enough, the body was placed in a stove to dry. During the drying period, the body was maintained in an extended position; the arms of men were placed along the sides of the body, whereas women's arms were placed across the abdomen.

The embalmers maintained a constant vigil over the body during this period to prevent it from being devoured by vultures. On the 15th or 16th day, the drying process should have been complete and the relatives would claim the body and sew it in goatskins. Kings and nobles were, in addition, placed in coffins of hollowed juniper logs. All bodies were deposited in caves in the hilly regions of the islands.

In another method of preparation described, a corrosive liquid believed to be juice of the spurge or euphorbia plant was either introduced through the belly wall or poured down the throat; this was followed by the drying process described earlier. The mummies produced by these processes were called *xaxos* and the method of embalming was believed to have been introduced from Egypt about 900 BC. In T. J. Pettigrew's *History of Egyptian Mummies*, there is a description of a *xaxos* as found by a sea captain in 1764. The author points out the "flesh of the body is perfectly preserved, but it is dry, inflexible and hard as wood . . . nor is any part decayed. The body is no more shrunk than if the person had been dead only two or three days. Only the skin appears a little shriveled and of a deeply tanned, copper color." The *xaxos* were extremely light in weight, averaging about 6–9 pounds for bodies up to 5½ feet in length.

## Peru

Preservation of the body in Peru was practiced for at least a 1000 years before the Spanish conquest in the early sixteenth century. It had for its motive a religious belief in the resurrection of the body. Most authorities agree that the Peruvians had no process of embalming, but that their mummies were a product of the extremely dry climate of the region. There are reports that the Incas or ruling classes were embalmed, and because only mummies of the common people have been discovered, this report may be true. The manner in which the Inca rulers are believed to have been prepared was by evisceration. The intestines were placed in gold vases, the cavity filled with an unspecified resin, and the body coated with bitumen. The bodies were said to have been seated on their thrones, clothed in their regal robes, hands clasped on the breast, and head inclined downward. There is mention of the use of gold to plate or replace the eyes.

The usual Peruvian mummy, of which there are many specimens in the Field Museum at Chicago, was often found buried with the face toward the west, together with provisions of corn and coca contained in earthen jars. The mummies themselves were wrapped in cloth and tied with a coarse rope. The outer covering was of matting and followed a roll of cotton that, in turn, enveloped a red or varied-color wool cloth wrapped about the body. The innermost wrapping was a white cotton sheet. The corpse was found in a squatting position, knees under chin, arm over breast, with the fists touching the jaws. The hands were usually fastened together, and on most mummies, there was a rope passed three or four times around the neck. In the mouth, there was usually a small copper, silver, or gold disk. The greater part of the mummies was well preserved, but the flesh was shriveled and the features were disfigured. The hair was preserved, with the women's hair braided. Nearly all types of animals and birds have been found mummified, including parrots, dogs, cats, doves, hawks, heron, ducks, llamas, vicunas, and alpacas wrapped in the manner of human mummies.

## Ecuador

The Jivaro Indians of the Marano River region of South America had a method of preserving heads by shrinking them. Technically, this process does not come under the heading of embalming, but a brief general description of the process is of interest.

The bones of the skull were first removed through long slits in the scalp. The skin of the head, with the hair attached, was boiled in water containing astringent herbs. On completion of this process, hot stones of gradually diminishing size were inserted into the space formerly occupied by the skull bones. When the shrinking process was completed, the stones were removed and the incisions were sutured as were the mouth and eyes. The finished shrunken head is about the size of a man's fist, with the features rather clear and retaining their proper proportions. It has been stated that this same process has been applied to an entire human body with equal success, although no such specimens have been found.

### Mexico and Central America—Aztecs, Toltecs, and Mayans

On the basis of information received from Alfonso Caso, Mexico's outstanding anthropologist, there is no evidence of the employment of any artificial means of preservation of the body in the pre-Spanish era in these regions. There are accounts of finding mummies wrapped in matting and buried in the earth or in caves, but it is the opinion of Caso and others that such mummification was the result of the natural climate of the region.

### North American Indians

Although no proof exists to substantiate claims that some of the Indian tribes embalmed their dead, there are quotes from two accounts of embalming means as recounted by H. C. Yarrow in his *Study of Mortuary Customs of North American Indians* from 1880, collected from earlier publications. On page 185 of the *History of Virginia* (Beverly, 1722), this statement is found:

> The Indians are religious in preserving the corpses of their kings and rulers after death. First they neatly flay off the skin as entire as they can, slitting only the back; then they pick all the flesh off the bones as clean as possible, leaving the sinews fastened to the bones, that they may preserve the joints together. Then they dry the bones in the sun and put them into the skin again, which in the meantime has been kept from shrinking. When the bones are placed right in the skin, the attendants nicely fill up the vacuities with a very fine white sand. After this they sew up the skin again, and the body looks as if the flesh had not been removed. They take care to keep the skin from shrinking by the help of a little oil or grease, which saves it from corruption. The skin being thus prepared, they lay it in an apartment for that purpose, upon a large shelf raised above the floor. This shelf is spread with mats for the corpse to rest easy on, and screened with the same to keep it from the dust. The flesh they lay upon hurdles in the sun to dry, and when it is thoroughly dried, it is sewed up in a basket and set at the feet of the corpse, to which it belongs.

Another account appeared in Volume XIII, page 39, of *Collection of Voyages* (Pinkerton, 1812), concerning the Werowance Indians:

> Their bodies are first bowelled, then dried upon hurdles till they be very dry, and so about most of their joints and neck they hang bracelets or chains of copper, pearl and such like, as they are used to wear. Their innards they stuff with copper beads, hatchets and such trash. Then they lap them very carefully in white skins and so roll them in mats for their winding-sheets.

The Indians are known to have wrapped their dead in cloth or leather and to have suspended the bodies in a horizontal manner in trees or buried them in the earth, in caves, or in the ground covered by rocks. This may have had a religious significance, but more likely it was done to prevent vultures or animals from devouring the dead.

### Aleutian Islands and Kodiak Archipelago

It is believed that the inhabitants of the Aleutian Islands and Kodiak Archipelago practiced preservation of their dead from at least AD 1000, although the custom did not prevail on the mainland. The internal organs were removed through an incision in the pelvic region and the cavity was refilled with dry grass. The body was placed in a stream of cold running water, which was said to have removed the fatty tissues in a short time. The corpse was removed from the water and wrapped in the fetal posture, knees under the chin and arms compressed about the legs. This position was accomplished by use of force, breaking bones if necessary. In this posture, the body was sun-dried and, as a final gesture, was wrapped in animal skins and matting.

## PERIOD OF THE ANATOMISTS (AD 650–1861)

With the Arabic conquest of Egypt and the fall of the Roman Empire, European and Mediterranean civilizations declined virtually to the vanishing point. The old world of law and order as the Romans and others knew it was replaced by anarchy. Geographical areas were ruled by bands of armed men with little stability of control. The Dark Ages were to continue until the year 1000 when a gradual elimination of unstable leaders left a few more wise and capable individuals in charge of substantial geographical divisions of Europe. With a return to a more normal civilized existence came the establishment of schools and colleges in what is today Sicily, Italy, France, and England and later in Germany, Holland, Belgium, and Switzerland. The schools were, in part, the product of the Catholic Church, which throughout the Dark Ages had maintained and served as a sanctuary for work in the fields of medicine, nursing, teaching, copying of manuscripts, and establishment of orphanages and poorhouses.

The medical schools that were established used some texts originally written during the glory era of Egypt. In Alexandria, on the Mediterranean at the mouth of the Nile, there existed the greatest center for teaching that history had known. The library, before its destruction, was said to have contained more than half a million manuscripts on subjects varying from astronomy to mathematics to engineering to medicine. It was here that a famous teacher and practitioner of medicine, Claudius Galen (130–200 AD), born in Pergamum, Asia Minor, taught and wrote on the subject of anatomy. His textbook on anatomy described human anatomy principally from dissections of animals such as the pig or monkey. It must be obvious today that there are substantial differences or variations between the anatomical structure of the pig or monkey and those of the human being. Galen and others were not encouraged to dissect the human body as it was considered a mutilation and a crime under Egyptian law. Nevertheless, Galen's teachings and writings on human anatomy were to be considered as the unchallengeable authority for the next 1000 to 1200 years.

Leonardo da Vinci was the first to bring a true understanding of the human body's anatomy with his anatomical dissections and drawings. He performed more than 200 dissections and his drawings were directly from them. Nearly all previous drawings were based on animal anatomy. It has been said that he had the understanding of an anatomist. In the current era, his drawings have inspired the New York Academy of the Arts to collaborate with Drexel University College of Medicine on the first of its kind sketch classes during anatomy dissection sessions. In the 500th year of his death, we all owe Leonardo a great debt of thanks for his attention to detail and the desire to understand the human body.

With the emergence of Europe from the Dark Ages came a craving for learning that had to that time been suppressed. The medical schools lacked the authority to legally acquire dead human bodies for dissection and anatomical study until the thirteenth and early fourteenth centuries. Such authority was granted in 1242 by Frederick II, King of the Two Sicilies, and again in 1302 for the delivery of two executed criminals to the medical school at Bologna, Italy, each year for dissection. Such dissections were public affairs, often conducted in open areas or amphitheaters always during the cold months of the year because the dissection subjects were not preserved. The dissection itself was rapid, frequently confined to a 4-day period. In the actual procedure, the anatomy professor, who was seated, read from Galen's text on anatomy while pointing out (with a wand) the body structures mentioned by Galen. An assistant, a barber-surgeon, did the actual dissection as the lecture progressed. Obviously, there were frequent contradictions between Galen's description of a body part and its actual appearance as disclosed by the dissection. These most evident discrepancies encouraged the more intelligent student and medical practitioner to steal bodies from cemeteries and gallows for personal study and research. Every part of such a purloined cadaver was probed speedily for knowledge of its structure or function until it became too loathsome to conceal and had to be disposed of. In many cases, the soft tissues were thrown away and the bones boiled to secure the skeleton.

## Military Religious Campaigns

During the period from 1095 to 1291, a series of military religious campaigns mounted by the Christian nations of Europe, termed the *crusades*, were conducted to recapture the Holy Land from the Moslems. The campaigns were successful early on, but with the passing of time, the Christian occupation forces in the Holy Land became complacent and less martial and eventually were expelled from the entire conquered territory. Many prominent members of the nobility, including King Louis XIX of France, died far from home during the crusades. To allow the return to their homeland of their remains, it was necessary to develop what became a gruesome procedure, as no certain means of embalming was available during the campaigns. The procedure consisted of disemboweling and disarticulating the body, cutting off all soft tissues, and then boiling the bones until they were free of all soft tissues. The bones were then dried and wrapped within bull hides and returned to their homeland by the couriers who maintained the communication lines.

In 1300, Pope Boniface VIII issued a papal bull (a directive) that prohibited the cutting up of the dead for the purpose of transport and burial under penalty of excommunication. For a brief period, this papal bull was interpreted by some members of the medical profession as a directive to ban anatomical dissection. For example, in 1345, Vigevano stated that dissection was prohibited, and Mondino (1270–1326) said sin was involved in boiling bones. In any case, such interpretations were rare and were seldom given any regard by the majority of anatomists.

As the years passed, it became obvious that some system of preservation, even temporary, had to be contrived to permit a more careful and intensive study of body structure. Early efforts of preservation followed the ancient regimen of drying the parts, for moisture was and is the enemy of preservation. Preservation by drying of cadavers or their components was first sought by exposure to the natural heat of the sun. Later, use of controlled heat in ovens was employed to accomplish desiccation. Eventually, while probing the nature and extent of the hollow blood vessels, it was noted that warm air forced through the blood vessels removed blood and eventually dried out the tissue.

Reports of preservation attempts from the fifteenth century did not include injections of the blood vascular system. Such early injections into hollow structures of the body were made to trace the direction and continuity of blood vessels or to inflate hollow organs so as to reveal their size and shape or to make internal castings of areas under study. As early as 1326, Alessandra Giliani of Italy injected blood vessels with colored solutions that hardened; Jacobus Berengarius (1470–1550) employed a syringe and injected veins with warm water; Bartolomeo Eustaschio (1520–1574) used warm ink; Regnier De Graaf (1641–1673) invented a syringe and injected mercury; Jan Swammerdam (1637–1680) injected a waxlike material that later hardened. The great artist Leonardo Da Vinci (1452–1519), who is said to have dissected more than 30 corpses to produce hundreds of accurate anatomical illustrations, injected wax to secure castings of the ventricles of the brain and other internal areas.

## Early Instruments for Injection

Early instruments for injection were crude and usually made in two parts: a container for the injection material and some form of cannula. The cannula was often contrived from a hollow straw, feather quill, hollow metal, or glass tube that was attached by ligature to an animal bladder (stomach or intestine). The cannula was inserted into the hollow opening being studied and the bladder tied onto its free end. The bladder, in turn, was filled with a liquid and then tied to retain the bladder full. Entrance of the liquid material into the hollow area was secured by squeezing the bladder until it emptied.

As early as 1521, Berengarius wrote of using a forerunner of the modern syringe. Early syringes similar to the hypodermic syringes employed today were constructed. They were filled and then attached to a cannula in position within the opening to be injected. To refill the syringe, the operator had to detach the syringe from the cannula, refill it, and then reattach it. Bartholin (1585–1629) developed the first continuous flow syringe. It could be recharged during use without halting the injection process.

One of the best accounts of nonanatomical embalming for burial purposes is related by the Dutch physician Peter Forestus (1522–1597), who wrote about embalming. His account, in German, is contained as an appendix in the 1605 edition of Peter Offenbach's treatise on *Wound Surgery*. Forestus specifically described the embalming process and the materials used in five named cases between 1410 and 1548, two of which he personally performed:

| 1410 | Pope Alexander V of Bologna, Italy |
| 1511 | Lady Johanna of Burgundy, Holland |
| 1537 | Bishop Magoluetus of Bologna, Italy |
| 1582 | Countess of Hautekerken of The Hague, Holland |
| 1584 | Princess Auracius of Holland |

As these cases are essentially similar, only one embalming report is cited in its entirety.

Most of the above-mentioned embalmings were performed in the room of the residence where the death occurred, a practice rather commonly followed later (well into the twentieth century) in many countries including the United States.

The following is the full description of the Forestus embalming of the Countess of Hautekerken. The others listed are quite similar with some individual variations such as opening the cranium and removing the brain and making long and deep incisions in the extremities to press out the blood, then filling the incisions with the powdered mixture.

*I personally was bidden to embalm the Countess of Hautekerken, who was a daughter of a nobleman of Egmont (Holland) and who died of childbirth on January 9, 1582 at The Hague (Holland) before Johannes Heurnius (1543–1604), my good friend, and professor at Leyden in Holland was asked. Preceding all things, before the embalmment was begun, there was made the following preparation ... I took 2½ lbs. aloes; myrrh, 1½ lbs.; ordinary wermut, seven handsfull; rosemary, four hands-full; pumice, 1½ lbs.; marjoran, 4 lbs.; storacis calamata, 2 loht; the zeltlinalipta muscata, ½ loht. Mix all and reduce to a powder. Lay open the trunk of the body, remove all the viscera, afterward take such sponges which were previously immersed in cold fresh water, afterward dipped in aqua vita, and wash out the interior of the body by hand with the sponge. This having been done, fill the cavities (of the body) with a layer of cotton moistened in aqua vita; sprinkle over it a layer of the previously mentioned powders; place another layer of the moistened cotton and a layer of powder one over the other until the abdomen together with the chest is entirely full. Afterward sew the above (abdominal walls) again together. Wrap around (the body) with waxed cloth and other things. Now having heard this you understand this embalmment was performed by me, the aforementioned Heurnius and Arnold the Surgeon on January 10, 1562, in the dwelling of the wellborn Count and Countess Von Wassenaer in The Hague.*

## Ambroise Paré (1510–1590)

Born in France, Ambroise Pare was military barber-surgeon and eventually surgeon to French Kings Henri II, Francois II, and Charles IX. He was famous for rediscovery and improvement of use of ligature to control bleeding after amputations, podalic version (changing the position of an unborn infant within the uterus) to facilitate delivery, and designing of artificial limbs. Paré, like many surgeons of the period, embalmed the bodies of prominent military leaders and noblemen killed during military campaigns as well as similarly prominent civilians dying of natural causes.

In one of his books written in 1585 and entitled *Apology and Account of His Journeys into Diverse Places*, Paré described embalming a follower of the Duke of Savoy, a Monsier de Martiques, who died following a gunshot wound through the chest received in battle. The embalming was followed by coffining and transportation to the home of the deceased.

In his book, *The Works of Ambroise Pare*, translated into English and published in London in 1634, he devotes a portion of the 28th chapter, "On the Manner Howe to Embalme the Dead":

*But the body which is to be embalmed with spices for very long continuance must first of all be embowelled, keeping the heart apart, that it may be embalmed and kept as the kinsfolkes shall thinke fit. Also the braine, the scull being divided with a saw, shall be taken out. Then shall you make deepe incisions along the armes, thighes, legges, backe, loynes, and buttockes, especially where the greater veines and arteries runne, first that by this means the blood may be pressed forth, which otherwise would putrifie and give occasion and beginning to putrefaction to the rest of the body; and then that there may be space to put in the aromaticke powders; and then the whole body shall be washed over with a spunge dipped in aqua vita and strong vinegar, wherein shall be boyled wormewood, aloes, coloquintida, common salt and alume. Then these incisions, and all the passages and open places of the body and the three bellyes shall be stuffed with the following spices grossely powdered. Rx pul rosar, chamomile, balsami, menthe, anethi, salvia, lavend, rorismar, marjoran, thymi, absinthi, cyperi, calami aromat, gentiana, ireosflorent, assacederata, caryophyll, nucis moschat, cinamoni, styracis, calamita, benjoini, myrrha, aloes, santel, omnium quod sut ficit. Let the incisions be sowed up and the open spaces that nothing fall out; then forthwith let the whole body be anointed with turpentine, dissolved oyle of roses and chamomile, adding if you shall thinke it fit, some chymicall oyles of spices, and then let it be againe strewed over with the forementioned powder; then wrap it in a linnen cloath, and then in ceareclothes. Lastly, let be put in a coffin of lead, sure soudred and filled up with dry sweete hearbes. But if there be no plenty of the forementioned spices, as it usuall happens in besieged townes, the chirurgion shall be contented with the powder of quenched lime, common ashes made of oake wood.*

The procedure described by Paré was the most prevalent in use from the end of the Egyptian system to well past the discovery of arterial injection.

### Discovery of a New Technique

Anatomical dissection, nonpreservative injections, and study continued until inevitably the technique of arterial injection of some preservative substance into the blood vascular system to secure an embalmed subject was stumbled upon. Contrary to popular belief, three men, all Dutch and all friends, were involved and must be recognized for their contributions to the technique: Jan Swammerdam (1637–1680), the original inventor or discoverer; Frederick Ruysch (1638–1731), the great practitioner who refined the technique; and Stephen Blanchard (1650–1720), the person who openly published the method.

Swammerdam was educated in medicine but devoted the greatest part of his life to the study of insects and small animals. He perfected a system of injection to preserve even insects through tiny cannulas made of glass and manipulated by the aid of microscopes designed by Leeuwenhoek (the inventor of the microscope). His preservatives were said to have included various forms of alcohol, turpentine, wine, rum, spirits of wine (purer form of alcohol), and colored waxes. This injection technique was transmitted to Ruysch who applied it to human subjects, both entire bodies and portions thereof. His superb collections of anatomical specimens provided great teaching aids. His embalming of complete human remains included individuals such as British Admiral Sir William Berkley, who was killed during a sea battle off Holland in 1666, and whose body was recovered from the sea in a decomposing condition. Ruysch was requested by the Dutch government to embalm the body so that it might be returned to England for funeral and burial. It is said that the body was normal in appearance and color after his treatment.

In another episode, the Russian Czar Peter the Great, during one of his visits to western Europe, visited the medical school of Leiden, Holland, and Ruysch's home, where his museum was situated. During the visit with Ruysch, it is related that some domestic problem required Ruysch's attention and he left Czar Peter alone for a few minutes. Czar Peter began to explore the various rooms and, in opening one door, discovered an infant apparently asleep. Tiptoeing into the room he contemplated the beautiful pink child, then bent down and kissed it, only to discover by its cold exterior that it was one of Ruysch's many preparations. Czar Peter purchased one entire museum collection from Ruysch, which some historians report was lost or destroyed. The truth is that it is still on exhibit in Leningrad today. Ruysch personally never did make a full disclosure of his technique or preservative. There are many who conjecture that his preservative was alcohol, turpentine, or even arsenic.

Blanchard, an anatomist of Leiden, published a book in 1688 entitled *A New Anatomy with Concise Directions for Dissection of the Human Body with a New Method of Embalming*. Pages 281 to 287 and several diagrams of syringes and instruments constitute the appendix describing his method of embalming. He mentions the use of spirits of wine and turpentine. In one of his embalming treatments, he began by flushing out the intestinal tract by first forcing water from the mouth to the anus. Then he repeated the flushing with spirits of wine and retained it in place by corking the rectum. He opened large veins and arteries and flushed out the blood with water, then injected the preservative spirits of wine. (**This technique described in the book appears to be the earliest mention of injection of the blood vessels for the specific purpose of embalming.**)

### Gabriel Clauderus (Late Seventeenth Century)

Gabriel Clauderus, a physician from Altenburg, Germany, was a contemporary of De Bils. In 1695, he published a book, *Methodus Balsamundi Corpora Humani, Alique Majora Sine Evisceratione*, in which he described his method of embalming, which omitted evisceration. His fluid was made from 1 pound of ashes of tartar dissolved in 6 pounds of water, to which was added ½ pound of sal ammoniac. After filtration, it was ready for use and was denominated by Clauderus as his "balsamic spirit." He injected this fluid into the cavities of the body and then immersed the cadaver in the fluid for 6–8 weeks. The treatment was concluded by drying the corpse either in the sun or in a stove.

### England's Customs and Achievements

Although the British Isles are geographically grouped with Europe, they developed different customs and their scientific achievements advanced at a pace different from that in continental Europe.

Some individuals regard the Company of Barber–Surgeons of London to be the first group licensed to embalm. A brief examination of the background of this organization reveals that from about 1300 to 1540, the Company of Barbers and the Guild of Surgeons were separate entities. In 1540, they received a charter from Henry VIII consolidating these two groups under the title of the Company of Barber–Surgeons and granting them the right to anatomize four executed criminals each year. In 1565, Queen Elizabeth I granted the same privilege to the College of Physicians. In 1745, the Surgeons and Barbers ended their joint relationship and again became two separate organizations. During the Barber–Surgeons period, they were permitted to be the sole agency for embalming and for performing anatomical dissections in the city of London, although there is no record of any of the bodies for anatomy being embalmed.

This was never a well-respected or enforced monopoly. In their 200-year existence, there were fewer than 10 complaints, and in several of the cases cited in the College of Barber–Surgeons records, no fines or other punishment is noted. In several cases, no conclusion of the case appears. Most complaints were lodged against members for performing private anatomical dissections not on the premises of the College. The more influential members such as William Cheselden and John Ram simply ignored the rule and even withdrew from the organization as William Hunter did. (**The Barber–Surgeons made no progress in the development of licensing of embalmers as such, and even today in the British Isles, no license or permit is needed from any governmental agency to perform embalming and never has been so required.**)

### William Hunter, M.D.

William Hunter (1718–1783) was born in Scotland and studied medicine at the University of Glasgow and at Edinburgh. He finally settled in London where he specialized in the practice of obstetrics and taught anatomy. He became one of the great teachers of anatomy in English medical history and received many awards and appointments to honor societies, climaxed in 1764 by his appointment as Physician-Extraordinary to Queen Charlotte of England. He was the author of many brilliant treatises on medical subjects, perhaps the greatest being his *Anatomy of the Gravid Uterus*. His private collections of anatomical and pathological specimens, together with his lecture and dissecting rooms, occupied a portion of his home. All of this, plus a large sum of money, were donated to the University of Glasgow after his death.

Hunter was in the habit of delivering, at his private school at the close of the anatomical lectures, an account of the preparation of anatomical specimens and embalming of corpses. He injected the femoral artery with a solution composed of oil of turpentine, to which had been added Venice turpentine, oil of chamomile, and oil of lavender, to which had been added a portion of vermillion dye. This mixture was forced into the body until the skin exhibited a red appearance. After a few hours during which the body lay undisturbed, the thoracic and abdominal cavities were opened, the viscera were removed, and the fluid was squeezed out of them. The viscera were separately arterially injected and bathed in camphorated spirits of wine. The body was again injected from the aorta and the cavities were washed with camphorated spirits of wine. The viscera were returned to the body, intermixed with powder composed of camphor, resin, and niter, and placed in the eyes, ears, nostrils, and other cavities. The entire skin surface of the body was then rubbed with the "essential" oils of rosemary and lavender. The body was placed in a box on a bed of plaster of Paris for about 4 years. When the box was reopened, and if desiccation appeared imperfect, a bed of gypsum was added to complete the process.

One of Hunter's admonitions to his students, which is still applicable to attainment of the finest results, was to begin the embalming process within 8 hours of the death in the summer and within 24 hours in the winter.

Until the wartime aerial bombing of the Royal College of Surgeons Museum in 1941, the embalmed body of the wife of eccentric dentist Martin Van Butchell, a pupil of William Hunter, was on exhibition. There was a letter in Van Butchell's handwriting describing the embalming process. It is reproduced here verbatim:

*12-Jan.-1775: At one half past two this morning my wife died. At eight this morning the statuary took off her face in plaster. At half past two this afternoon Mr. Cruikshank injected at the crural arteries five pints of oil of turpentine mixed with Venice turpentine and vermillion.*

*15-Jan.: At nine this morning Dr. Hunter and Mr. Cruikshank began to open and embalm my wife. Her diseases were a large empyema in the left lung (which would not receive any air), accompanied with pleuropneumony and much adhesion. The right lung was also beginning to decay and had some pus in it. The spleen was hard and much contracted; the liver diseased, called rata malphigi. The stomach was very sound. The kidneys, uterus, bladder and intestines were in good order. Injected at the large arteries oil of turpentine mixed with camphored spirits, i.e., ten ounces camphor to a quart of spirits, so as to make the whole vascular system turgid; put into the belly part six pounds of rosin powder, three pounds camphor and three pounds niter powder mixed rec. spirit.*

*17-Jan.: I opened the abdomen to put in the remainder of the powders and added four pounds of rosin, three pounds niter and one pound camphor. In all there were ten pounds rosin, six pounds niter and four pounds camphor, twenty pounds of powder mixed with spirits of wine.*

*18-Jan.: Dr. Hunter and Mr. Cruikshank came at nine this morning and put my wife into the box on and in 130 pounds of Paris plaster at eighteen d. a bag. I put between the thighs three arquebusade bottles, one full of camphored spirits, very rich of the gum, containing eight ounces of oil of rosemary, and in the other two ounces of lavender.*

*19-Jan.: I closed up the joints of the box lid and glasses with Paris plaster mixed with gum water and spirits wine.*

*25-Jan.: Dr. Hunter came with Sir Thos. Wynn and his lady.*

*7-Feb.: Dr. Hunter came with Sir John Pringle, Dr. Heberden, Dr. Watson and about twelve more fellows of The Royal Society.*

*11-Feb.: Dr. Hunter came with Dr. Solander, Dr.——, Mr. Banks and another gentleman. I unlocked the glasses to clean the face and legs with spirits of wine and oil of lavender.*

*12-Feb.: Dr. Hunter came to look at the neck and shoulders.*

*13-Feb.: I put four ounces of camphored spirits into the box and on both sides of neck and six pounds of plaster.*

*16-Feb.: I put four ounces oil of lavender, an ounce of rosemary and ½ ounce of oil of camomile flowers (the last cost four Sh.) on sides of the face and three ounces of very dry camomile flowers on the breast, neck, and shoulders.*

The body was said to resemble a Guanche or Peruvian mummy and was very dry and shrunken.

### John Hunter, M.D.

John Hunter (1728–1793) was born in Scotland, the younger brother of William Hunter, in whose anatomy classes he first proved so adept. After studying under the great surgeons of his time, he was appointed to hospital staffs and lectured on anatomy. A region of the body he described was named in his honor: "Hunter's canal." He served as a surgeon in the British army during the campaign in Portugal (1761–1763) and, on his discharge from the service, settled in general practice in London. There he continued the collection and study of anatomical and natural subjects. He was a most brilliant and prolific writer on all phases of medicine and surgery and later founded his own private anatomy classes, which were unexcelled for the number of students who later distinguished themselves in medicine. Among these students were Jenner, Abernathy, Carlisle, Chevalier, Cline, Coleman, Astley Cooper, Home, Lynn, and Macartney.

In 1776, Hunter was honored by appointment as Surgeon-Extraordinary to the King of England. In 1782, he constructed a museum between his two homes in London to house his anatomical and natural history collections. These eventually contained nearly 14,000 items, and at his death, they were purchased by the British government for the Royal College of Surgeons. The main exhibit hall, measuring 52 by 28 feet, was lighted from above and had a gallery for visitors.

Many stories are told of body stealing for dissection and for securing specimens for collections. None would better illustrate this than John Hunter's acquisition of the body of the

Irish giant O'Brien in 1783, at a cost to him of about $2500.00. O'Brien, about 7 feet 7 inches in height and dreading dissection by Hunter had, shortly before his death, arranged with several of his friends that his corpse be transported to the sea and sunk in deep water. The undertaker, who it was said had entered into a pecuniary agreement with Hunter, managed that while the escort was drinking at a certain stage of the journey to the sea the coffin should be locked in a barn. Confederates, who the undertaker had concealed in the barn, speedily substituted an equivalent weight of stones for the body. At night, O'Brien's body was forwarded to Hunter who took it immediately to his museum, where it was dissected and boiled to procure the bones. The skeleton was on exhibit until May 1941, when three-fourths of the museum of the Royal College of Surgeons, London, was destroyed by German bombers. Joshua Reynold's portrait of John Hunter displays the huge skeletal feet of O'Brien in the background.

## Matthew Baillie

Baillie (1761–1823) was a nephew of William and John Hunter. He was educated by his uncles and became famous as a physician and writer on medical subjects. He modified the Hunterian method of embalming so as to provide as good preservation as ever in a shorter period. Using a solution of oil of turpentine, Venice turpentine, oil of chamomile, and oil of lavender (to which was added vermillion dye) he injected the femoral artery. He allowed several hours of elapse before he opened the body as in a postmortem examination and made a small incision in the bowel below the stomach, into which he inserted a small piece of pipe through which he introduced water to wash out the contents of the bowels. Then, ligating the rectum above the anus and the small bowel below the stomach, he filled the intestinal tract with camphorated spirits of wine. The lungs were filled with camphorated spirits of wine via the trachea. The bladder was opened and emptied of its contents and a powder of camphor, resin, and niter was dusted over the viscera and the incision was closed. The eyeballs were pierced and emptied of their contents and repacked to normal with the powder mixture, as were the mouth and ears. The body was rubbed with oil of rosemary or lavender and placed on a bed of deep plaster.

## Europe's Access to Cadavers

Continental European countries such as France, Germany, and Italy did not encounter the problems in supplying medical schools with cadavers as existed in Great Britain. Medical schools had access to bodies unclaimed for burial, a situation not present in the British Isles until after passage of the **Warburton Act** in 1832. The problem in continental Europe was different, consisting of securing a means to preserve cadavers for dissection with nonpoisonous chemicals. In France, for example, medical schools in the north had scheduled anatomical dissection classes during the cold months of the year as the cadavers were unembalmed.

By the late eighteenth and early nineteenth centuries, France and Italy had a number of different techniques and chemicals for embalming proposed by members of the medical or scientific communities.

**Giuseppe Tranchina** (1797–1837) of Palermo, Italy, openly advocated and successfully used arsenical solutions, arterially injected, to preserve bodies for both funeral and anatomical purposes. An anatomist at the Royal University, he used a method involving an injection into the carotid artery. It is known he used this method as early as 1833 on the body of Prince Corrado Valguarnera of Niscemi and, later, on that of Cardinal Giacinto Placido Zurla (1834). The ingredients he used were revealed during a demonstration in the Naples Military Hospital in 1835 and consisted of a solution of white arsenic diluted in water or alcohol and then colored with either cinnabar or red lead oxide. No evisceration, drainage, or cavity treatment was performed. Tranchina's technique, which would lead to a perfect body exposure for 3 or 4 months, represents the very first documented method that did not involve evisceration but was uniquely relying upon arterial injection.

**J. P. Sucquet of France** (mid-nineteenth century) was one of the earliest proponents of the use of zinc chloride as a preservative agent. He injected about 5 quarts of a 20% solution of zinc chloride in water through the popliteal artery and also introduced some of this solution into the abdomen. One body prepared in this way was buried for 2 years, then disinterred and found to be in an excellent state of preservation. About 1845, an agent representing Sucquet sold the U.S. rights to his method and chemical to Chas. D. Brown and Joseph Alexander of New York City.

**Jean Nicolas Gannal** (1791–1852), a chemist in France (**Fig. 5**), began his life's work as an apothecary's assistant. From 1808 to 1812, he served in the medical department of

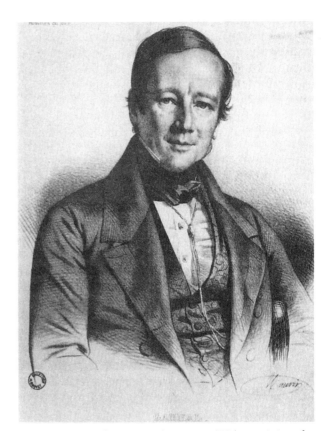

**Figure 5.** Portrait of J. N. Gannal at age 40. (*With permission of Ordre National des Pharmaciens. © Fonds de dotation pour la gestion et la valorisation du patrimoine pharmaceutique.*)

the French Army, including the Russian campaign under Napoleon. After his discharge from the army, he reentered the field of chemistry and was appointed assistant to the great French chemistry teacher Thenard. He later became interested in industrial chemistry and did research on methods of refining borax and improving the quality of glues and gelatins. In 1827, he was awarded the Montyon science prize for developing a method of treating catarrh and tuberculosis with chlorine gas. In 1831, he was asked to devote his time to devising an improved method of preserving cadavers for anatomical purposes. Close application to the problem resulted in success, which was recognized in 1836 by the award to Gannal of a second Montyon science prize.

His experiments included the use of solutions of acids (acetic–arsenous–nitric–hydrochloric), alkali salts (copper–mercury–alum), tannin–creosote–alcohol, and various combinations such as alum, sodium chloride, and nitrate of potash, and acetate of alumina and the chloride of alumina, the latter of which obliterated the lumen of blood vessels. His perfected method of embalming cadavers for anatomical purposes comprised the injection of about 6 quarts of a solution of acetate of alumina through the carotid artery without drainage of any blood. No evisceration or other treatment was used, although occasionally the bodies were immersed in the injecting solution until ready for dissection. Gannal used practically the same solution for embalming bodies for funeral purposes, although he did add a small quantity of arsenic and carmine to the solution. He injected about 2 gallons of this mixture, first upward and then downward in the carotid artery in less than one-half hour. No special treatment was given to the trunk viscera. In his book *History of Embalming*, he cited case histories of bodies he had embalmed and subsequently disinterred from 3 to 13 months after burial. Gannal states that in every such case, the body was found in exactly the same state of preservation and appearance as when buried.

Gannal was involved in several precedent-making events. In mid-April 1840, a Paris newspaper published the following article:

> *The young boy found murdered in a field near Villete not having been recognized and the process of decomposition having commenced, the Magistrates ordered it to be embalmed by M. Gannal's simple method of injection through the carotid arteries, so that this evidence of the crime may remain producible. This is the first operation of the kind performed by order of the Justices, and it was completed in a quarter of an hour.*

In his translation of Gannal's *History of Embalming* (1840) (**Fig. 6**), Harlan mentions that the Paris police have access to Gannal's embalming process to preserve bodies in the Paris morgue where murder has been suspected.

Gannal was indirectly responsible for the passage of the first law prohibiting the use of arsenic in embalming solutions in 1846 (to which the use of dichloride of mercury was also prohibited in 1848).

There are several versions of the story. In one, Gannal had omitted stating that a portion of arsenic was added to his alumina salts embalming chemical, and when this solution was analyzed and arsenic was found, the medical community was enraged and compelled the law to be decreed. The other tale, never documented, relates that Gannal was retained to embalm the corpse of a member of the nobility who died suddenly. The members of the nobleman's family accused the decedent's mistress of poisoning him with arsenic. Under French law, she was arrested and tried, the burden of her defense on her shoulders. Gannal followed the progress of the trial in the Paris newspapers and noted that the accused mistress was unable to prove her innocence. Finally, at the last possible moment, Gannal appeared at the trial and requested permission to testify on her behalf. He states that in his opinion the arsenic found in the body tissues of the deceased came there during the embalming with his embalming solution, as it contained arsenic. She was freed and the legal community petitioned for the abolition of arsenic in embalming solutions.

HISTORY

OF

EMBALMING,

AND OF

PREPARATIONS IN ANATOMY, PATHOLOGY

AND NATURAL HISTORY;

INCLUDING

An Account Of A New Process

For Embalming.

BY J. N. GANNAL.

Paris, 1838.

Translated From The French, With

Notes And Additions.

By R. Harlan, M.D.

PHILADELPHIA;

PUBLISHED BY JUDAH DOBSON,

NO. 106 CHESNUT STREET.

...........

1840

**Figure 6.** Title page of Harlan's translation of the History of Embalming.

Gannal had two sons, Adolphe Antoine and Felix, who became physicians and continued the embalming practice after his death. They embalmed many famous people including De Lessups, who constructed the Suez Canal. The sons died in the early 1900s.

**Richard Harlan** (1796–1843) of Philadelphia, Pennsylvania, graduated from the Pennsylvania Medical College in 1818 and was placed in charge of Joseph Parrish's private anatomical dissection rooms in Philadelphia. After engaging in various projects in company with other Philadelphia physicians, he became a member of the city health council. In 1838, he traveled to Europe and spent a portion of his time in Paris visiting various medical facilities and meeting local savants, among whom was J. N. Gannal. After being presented with a copy of Gannal's *History of Embalming*, he became so fascinated with it that he requested and received permission to publish an American edition translated into English. **The book, devoted entirely to embalming procedures, which was published in the United States in English** (Fig. 6).

## Other Physicians and Anatomists
### Girolamo Segato (1792–1836)
A naturalist, explorer, and cartographer residing in Florence, Italy, Segato is known to have converted the human body to stone ("petrification"), allegedly by infiltrating the bodily tissues with a solution of silicate of potash and succeeded this treatment by immersion of the body in a weak acid solution. The exact modus operandi is unknown. His technique was emulated by other notable Italian scientists, including Bartolommeo Zanon, Giovan Battista Rini, Giambattista Messedaglia, Paolo Gorini, and Efisio Marini.

### Thomas Joseph Pettigrew.
A London physician and surgeon, graduate of Guys Hospital, and fellow of the Royal College of Surgeons, Pettigrew (1791–1865), was one of the great historians of the science of embalming. His treatise *History of Egyptian Mummies*, published in London in 1834, is a masterpiece revealing Pettigrew's ability to accurately observe and minutely describe objects and processes of interest to students and practitioners of the art of embalming. This volume is to this day considered one of the finest works on Egyptian embalming methods and customs. In 1854, he withdrew from the practice of medicine and devoted his entire energy to the study of archaeology.

### Dr. Falconi
A French physician of the mid-nineteenth century, Falconi employed a means of preservation of cadavers for anatomical purposes, which is of interest because of its simplicity. The corpse was placed on a bed of dry saw dust to which about a gallon of powdered zinc sulfate had been added. No injections, incisions, baths, or any additional treatment were used. The bodies so treated were said to have remained flexible for about 40 days, after which time they dried and assumed the appearance of mummies.

### Dr. John Morgan (Circa 1863)
A professor of anatomy at the University of Dublin, Morgan made use of two principles that are widely recognized as necessary to achieve the best embalming results: (1) the use of the largest possible artery for injection and (2) the use of force or pressure to push the preserving fluid through the blood vessels. Also noted are his use of a pre-injection solution (the earliest mention found) and his controlled technique of drainage. Morgan cut the sternum down its center, opened the pericardium to expose the heart, made an incision into the left ventricle or into the aorta, and inserted a piece of pipe about 8 inches long. This injecting pipe was connected by 15 feet of tubing to a fluid container that was maintained 12 feet above the corpse, thereby producing about 5 pounds of pressure (**Fig. 7**).

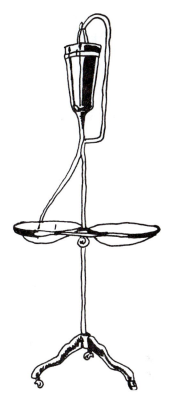

**Figure 7.** Gravity fluid injector. The jar filled with arterial chemical could be elevated several feet above the corpse, thus creating pressure for injection. (*Used with permission of Paula Johnson De Smet.*)

The tip of the right auricular appendage was clipped off to allow blood drainage. The first injection was composed of $1/2$ gallon of a saturated salt solution to which was added 4 ounces of niter. After this solution was allowed to "rush" through the circulatory system, a clamp was fastened over the auricular appendage when the drainage stopped. Several more gallons of a solution of common salt, niter, alum, and arsenate of potash were injected until the body was thoroughly saturated with the fluid. No special treatment of the internal organs or viscera was mentioned.

At this time, there was virtually no embalming of the dead for funeral purposes available for the largest percentage of deaths. Many books were written regarding the dangers to the living of exposure to the dead buried or entombed (unembalmed) in churches or in city cemeteries. There was also concern for those who handled the dead.

### Alfredo Salafia
One of the world's oldest and best-known examples of modern day embalming is a 2-year-old child by the name of Rosalia Lombardo. Little Rosalia died in December of 1920 in Palermo, Italy. Her father, full of grief over the loss of his child, called upon a local embalmer with more than 20 years of embalming experience to prepare his daughter. Today, Rosalia is known as "Sleeping Beauty" as she appears to just be sleeping.

It is not known how Salafia became interested in embalming. He worked with Francesco Randacio, a professor of anatomy at Palermo University, where he achieved excellent results after he was granted permission to apply his embalming procedure to unclaimed human bodies. His embalming skills were extraordinary. He was able to restore the remains of

Francesco Crispi, the Italian Premier, in 1902, after the original embalming had failed to preserve his body. He worked for months using hypodermic injections, performing restorative art by replacing the eyeballs with glass eyes and reattaching the hair and beard that had fallen out. He injected paraffin into the facial features to "regain the form and lost volume." The local press wrote of his work that allowed the body to be viewed three times from 1902 to 1914 following exhumation.

Salafia manufactured embalming chemicals through his "Salafia Permanent Method Embalming Company." He came to New York City on multiple visits to give demonstrations and sell his fluid. The company provided embalming using Salafia Perfection Fluid. The method he used was a single-point injection through the carotid artery using 1.5 gallons of his non-poisonous chemical.

Along with his nephews Oreste Maggio and Achille Salamone (who went to the Renouard School of Embalming and opened a funeral home), Salafia would demonstrate his chemicals and method on unclaimed bodies on two occasions. The first was in April of 1910. The body was embalmed and then enclosed in a glass case for 6 months. It was examined by a group of leading embalmers including Professor William P. Hohenschuch along with Frank E. Campbell, Charles F. Moadinger, Jr., and Fred Hulberg, Jr. The autopsy revealed well-preserved tissue throughout with no decomposition. It was proclaimed a success. He demonstrated it again in September of 1910 for the New York Embalmers Association. Again, the body was embalmed and examined 6 months. It was also found to be in an excellent state of preservation. Although he sold chemicals throughout the United States from this point through 1911, there was no further evidence of his corporation after December, 1911.

Although he never revealed his chemical formulation before his death, he did keep a beautifully handwritten and illustrated memoir. This memoir contained accounts of his embalming and formula. Through the generosity of his family, the memoir was shared with researchers at EURAC in Bolzano, Italy. His formulation included formaldehyde, possibly the first use in Europe. Professor Salafia understood not only the chemistry of preservation but also the sentiment of what embalmers do. He wrote in the opening of his memoir "A Noble Tradition. The sentiment of the people is innate with human nature and it is not always the real determinant of civil progress. The proof can be found in the most ancient of peoples where we find nobler traditions, much more moving than we do in the people of today, too evolved and too calculating and thus too cold. To hand down to the posterity the intact appearance of dear ones just as they were when they left us at the moment eternal departure, it is among these compassionate customs that antiquity has handed down to us and that time has preserved."

### Bernardino Ramazzini
The founder of occupational medicine, Ramazzini (1633–1714) wrote the *Diseases of Workers* in 1700, and an enlarged edition of that text was published in 1713. The latter edition contained a chapter on the disease of corpse bearers.

Numerous publications varying in size from leaflets to bound books were printed inveighing against existing burial practices. A few relevant titles are *Considerations on the Indecent and Dangerous Custom of Burying in Churches and Churchyards etc.*, 1721, London, A. Batesworth; *Blame of Kirk Burial, Tending to Persuade Cemeterial Civility,* 1606 NP, Rev. William Birnie; *Gatherings from Graveyards, Particularly Those of London etc.*, 1830, G. A. Walker, surgeon, London; and *Sepulture, History, Methods and Sanitary Requisites,* 1884, Stephen Wickes, Philadelphia. The astonishing accounts contained in these or similar works should convince even the most skeptical opponent of embalming of the sanitary value of the embalming process.

### From Europe to the Colonies
The transfer of embalming knowledge from Europe to the colonies in what today is the United States was accomplished by several means.

Anatomical study in the colonies as early as 1676 in Boston and again in 1750 recorded that "Drs. John Bard and Peter Middleton injected and dissected the body of an executed criminal for the instruction of young men engaged in the study of medicine." In 1752, the *N.Y. Weekly Post-Boy* carried an advertisement offering anatomy instruction by Dr. Thomas Wood. From 1754 to 1756, William Hunter, physician and student of the famed anatomy teacher Alexander Monroe I of Edinburgh, Scotland (and a relative of the Hunter brothers), lectured on anatomy at Newport, Rhode Island. Doctors William Shippen and John Morgan of Philadelphia studied medicine in Europe and anatomy under British anatomists. On their return to the United States between 1762 and 1765, they became engaged in teaching medical subjects, especially anatomy, in Philadelphia.

In 1840, the translation of Gannal's book, *The History of Embalming*, into English was to provide the first text in English printed in the United States devoted to embalming. In the mid-1840s, the acquisition of Sucquet's embalming technique and chemicals as a franchise by Dr. Charles D. Brown and Dr. Joseph Alexander of New York City added to the increasing amount of embalming knowledge transferred to the United States.

## MODERN PERIOD

By the year 1861 and the onset of the Civil War, the transfer of embalming knowledge from Europe to the United States was virtually concluded. A small group of medically trained embalmers existed together with printed information such as Harlan's translation of Gannal's textbook and various European embalming formulas and techniques that had been acquired.

Until the Civil War, however, little or no embalming was performed for funeral purposes. Most preservation, such as it was, for brief periods was provided by ice refrigeration when available.

With the outbreak of the Civil War in April 1861, there began the raising of troops by the North and South to prosecute the war. Little, if any, embalming was available to the Southerners during the war. Virtually all embalming was done by Northerners. As Washington, D.C. was the capital city of the north, it became a center for troop concentration both to protect the city and to serve as a marshaling point for the armies moving against the south.

Northern troops composed of individual companies from small geographical areas and regiments from individual states as disparate as Vermont and Maine, Minnesota and

Wisconsin, and Ohio, Pennsylvania, and New York crowded into the Washington, D.C. area. Civilian embalmers Dr. Thomas Holmes, William J. Bunnell, Dr. Charles Da Costa Brown, Dr. Joseph B. Alexander, Dr. Richard Burr, Dr. Daniel H. Prunk, Frank A. Hutton, G. W. Scollay, C. B. Chamberlain, Henry P. Cattell, Dr. Benjamin Lyford, Samuel Rodgers, Dr. E. C. Lewis, W. P. Cornelius, and Prince Greer are known to have embalmed during the Civil War. There are others who, to this day, remain anonymous.

None of the embalming surgeons, as they were called, were ever employed in the military as embalmers. Some had been or would become military surgeons but did not perform embalming while in the military service.

## Civil War Times

At the beginning of the Civil War, as in all previous wars fought by the United States, there was no provision for return of the dead to their homes. In the Seminole Indian Wars (during the 1830s), the Mexican War (1846–1848), and the campaigns against the Indians up to the outbreak of the Civil War, the military dead were buried in the field near where they fell in battle. It was possible for the relatives to have the remains returned to their home for local burial under certain conditions:

1. The next of kin was to request the disinterment and return of the body in a written request to the Quartermaster General.
2. On military authority confirmation that the burial place was known and disinterment could be effected, the family was advised to send a coffin capable of being hermetically sealed to a designated Quartermaster Officer nearest the place of burial.
3. Such Quartermaster Officer would provide a force of men to take the coffin to the grave, disinter the remains, and place them in the coffin and seal it. The coffined remains would then be returned to the place of ultimate reinterment.

During the early days of the Civil War and less frequently as the war dragged on, some family members of the deceased personally went to hospitals and battlefields to search for their dead and bring them home for burial. Civil War embalming was carried out with various chemicals and techniques. Arterial embalming was applied when possible. An artery, usually the femoral or carotid, was raised and injected without any venous drainage in most cases. Usually, no cavity treatment was administered. When arterial embalming was believed impossible because of the nature of wounds or decomposition, other means of preparation of the body for transport were resorted to. In some cases, the trunk was eviscerated and the cavity filled with sawdust or powdered charcoal or lime. The body was then placed in a coffin completely imbedded in sawdust or similar material. In other cases, the body was coffined as mentioned without evisceration.

Chemicals employed during the Civil War were totally self-manufactured by the embalmer and included, as basic preservatives, arsenicals, zinc chloride, dichloride of mercury, salts of alumina, sugar of lead, and a host of salts, alkalies, and acids. An example of fluid manufacture of one of the most popular embalming chemicals, zinc chloride, was the immersion of sheets of zinc in hydrochloric acid until a saturated solution was obtained. The resulting zinc chloride solution was injected without further dilution. Many of the injection pumps employed were quite similar to what would be described as greatly enlarged hypodermic syringes. Many required filling of the syringe, attachment of a cannula, emptying of the syringe, unfastening of the syringe, and refilling. It was an extremely slow process! A few pumps were designed to provide continuous flow, aspirating the embalming chemical continuously from a large source into the pump during the injection process. Others, such as the Holmes invention, were designed to fit over a bucket that could hold a gallon or more of liquid.

On May 24, 1861, 24-year-old Colonel Elmer Ellsworth, commander of the 11th N.Y. Volunteer Infantry, was shot to death in Alexandria, Virginia, as he seized a confederate flag displayed atop the Marshall House Hotel. He became the first prominent military figure killed in the war. His body was embalmed by Dr. Thomas Holmes, who had set up an embalming establishment in Washington, D.C. Funeral services for Colonel Ellsworth were performed in the White House, in New York City, and in Albany, New York, and he was buried in his home town of Mechanicsburg, New York. His funeral set a pattern to be followed by prominent members of the military, culminating in President Lincoln's historic funeral services. Colonel Ellsworth's embalming and viewable appearance were widely and favorably commented on in the press and did much to familiarize the previously uninformed public with embalming.

The Army issued only two sets of orders relative to fatal casualties in the early stages of the war. On September 11, 1861, War Department General Order 75 directed the Quartermaster Department to supply all general and post hospitals with blank books and forms for the preservation of accurate death records and to provide material for headboards to be erected over soldiers' graves. On April 3, 1862, Section II of War Department General Order 33 stated:

> In order to secure as far as possible the decent interment of those who have fallen, or may fall in battle, it is made the duty of commanding generals to lay off lots of ground in some suitable spot near every battlefield, as soon as it may be in their power, and to cause the remains of those killed to be interred, with head boards to the graves bearing numbers, and when practicable the names of the persons buried in them. A register for each burial ground will be preserved, in which will be noted the marks corresponding with the headboards.

**This was the origin of what was to become the National Cemetery System.**

### Embalming Surgeons of the Civil War

*Dr. Thomas Holmes (1817–1900).*
Holmes was born in New York City in 1817 and educated in local public schools and New York University Medical College, though the records of the period are incomplete and document only his attendance, not his graduation. He did practice medicine and was a coroner's physician in New York during the 1850s as numerous newspaper stories attest. He apparently moved to Williamsburg (now Brooklyn) and experimented with various chemicals for embalming and techniques. When the Civil War broke out, he opened an embalming office in Washington, D.C. and Colonel Ellsworth became his first prominent client.

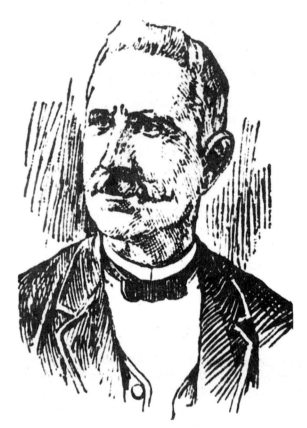

**DR. THOMAS H. HOLMES.**

**Figure 8.** Portrait of Thomas H. Holmes.

Holmes subsequently embalmed Colonel E. D. Baker, a prominent politician and soldier killed in battle. This case brought more publicity both for Holmes and for embalming (**Fig. 8**).

Holmes ultimately prepared about 4000 bodies (including eight generals) and patented many inventions relating to embalming during his lifetime. One, in particular, a rubber-coated canvas removal bag, was far ahead of its time (**Fig. 9**).

When the war ended, Dr. Holmes returned home to Brooklyn and only occasionally practiced embalming. He operated a drugstore and manufactured various products as diverse as embalming fluid and root beer! He invested heavily in a health resort and lost the investment. He wrote little about embalming, did not teach, and had no children. After a serious fall in his home, he became periodically psychotic and occasionally required confinement. When he died in 1900, it was said that he wanted no embalming.

### William J. Bunnell (1823–1891)

Bunnell was born in New Jersey, moved to New York City, and in the 1850s became acquainted with Dr. Holmes and married his sister. Dr. Holmes found him employment as an anatomy technician for some New York medical schools while teaching him embalming. When war broke out, Bunnell did not work directly with Dr. Holmes but formed his own Embalming Surgeon's organization with Dr. R. B. Heintzelman from Philadelphia as his active partner. Holmes and Bunnell did occasionally work together during the war at Gettysburg and at City Point, Virginia. After the war, it was reported that Bunnell was

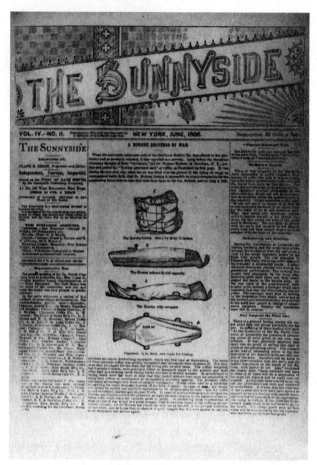

**Figure 9.** Front page of The Sunnyside, June 1886, featuring an article on Holmes's removal bag, citing its all-around utility as a sleeping bag and stretcher, its ability to be inflated as a raft, and, of course, its use as a corpse removal bag or coffin.

practicing medicine briefly in Omaha, Nebraska, and eventually opened an undertaking establishment in Jersey City, New Jersey. He became a marshall at the funeral of General Grant and became prominent in undertakers' associations. His son, George Holmes Bunnell (1855–1932), followed his father in the business and was given assistance by his uncle, Dr. Holmes. George H. Bunnell had twin sons: Milton became a funeral director, and Chester became a physician.

### Charles Da Costa Brown, Joseph B. Alexander, and Henry P. Cattell

Brown, Alexander, and Cattell were all active in the firm of Brown and Alexander, Embalming Surgeons. It is not known whether Brown and Alexander met in New York City in the late 1850s or in Washington, D.C. in early wartime. Cattell (**Fig. 10**) is believed to have been the stepson of Dr. Charles Brown's brother, as his mother married a brown in 1860. In any event, he entered the employment of the firm that embalmed Willie Lincoln, son of President Abraham Lincoln, and later embalmed the President Lincoln himself in 1865. After the war, Dr. Brown abandoned embalming, returned to New York City, practiced dentistry, and became very active in the Masonic Lodge. He died in 1896 and is buried in Greenwood Cemetery in Brooklyn.

Alexander died in 1871 in Washington, D.C. H. P. Cattell halted his embalming practice after the war, became

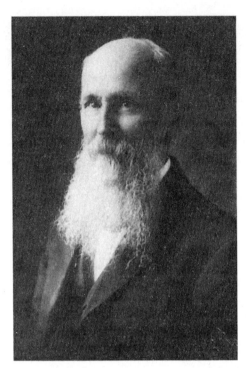

**Figure 10.** Portrait of Henry P. Cattell, an associate of Brown and Alexander, the embalming surgeons who embalmed Willie Lincoln in 1862 and President Lincoln in 1865.

a lithographer, and then entered the Washington, D.C. police force. None of his family was ever aware that he had embalmed President Lincoln. He died in 1915 and is buried in Washington, D.C.

In 2010 a new book regarding Abraham Lincoln was published that gave further insight into the embalming of the president. In James Swanson's book, *Blood Crimes: The Chase for Jefferson Davis and the Death Pageant for Lincoln's Corpse*, he details previously unknown information regarding the care of President Lincoln's body following his assassination. In this account, Henry P. Cattell of the Brown and Alexander Embalming Surgeons firm, is given credit for the embalming of Mr. Lincoln. Described by journalist George Alfred Townsend who viewed Mr. Lincoln's body at the White House, "No corpse in the world is better prepared according to its appearances." This was such an important event as well as long train ride until he reached his final resting place, that the "body men" were included among the dignitaries accompanying the President's body. "With so many dignitaries present at the station, the crowd failed to recognize two of the most important men on the passenger manifest. In the days to come, the success or failure of this vital mission would turn in large part upon their work. To accomplish it, they alone would have unfettered access to the president's corpse at any time of the day of night. These the body men, embalmer Dr. Charles Brown and undertaker Frank Sands. For the next 13 days, it was their job to keep at bay death's relentless companion, the decomposing flesh of Abraham Lincoln."

The account goes through the work these two men did to keep the remains in a presentable condition for all the public viewings that would take place over 13 days. One account of the viewing in New York City, "with practiced fingers," wrote on eyewitness, "the undertaker, Mr. F. G. Sands, and his assistance, Mr. G.W. Hawes, removed the dust from the face and habiliment's of the dead… and the lids was silently screwed down without form or ceremony, and with none but a few officers and orderlies and couple of reports as witnesses." On the day of his funeral in Springfield, Illinois Lincoln's coffin was opened for the last time. Dead for 18 days and not refrigerated, "only preservative chemicals and makeup had kept him presentable during the journey." The description goes on to make a note of his facial color changing over the time period and how each day the embalmers had to remove dust and dirt from his face and clothing. In addition to these descriptions of the president's physical body, there was also an account of the bill they presented to the government. "Drs. Brown and Alexander charged $100.00 for 'embalming remains of Abraham Lincoln late President of U.S.,' and $160.00 to ride the train: '16 days Services for self & Asst. @$10.00 per day." The cost for the President's funeral was totaled at $28,985.31, described as one of the most expensive funerals in American History at the time.

### Frank A. Hutton

Little is known of Hutton's personal biography. Born in or near Harrisburg, Pennsylvania, about 1835, he was a pharmacist by occupation. He had military service in the 110th Pennsylvania Volunteer Infantry ending in June 1862, was discharged in Washington, D.C., and became a partner in the firm of Chamberlain and Hutton, Surgeons. This partnership did not last long and Hutton withdrew in February 1863. He formed the firm of Hutton and Company with E. A. Williams, son of a Washington, D.C. undertaker as his partner. Hutton advertised in the Washington City Directory, taking a full-page space to extol his embalming expertise. He was also issued Patent 38,747 for an embalming fluid on June 1, 1863. The formula included alcohol, arsenic, dichloride of mercury, and zinc chloride.

During mid-April 1863, Hutton became embroiled in an argument with a client over charges for shipping his son's body to him. The client complained to Colonel L. C. Baker, provost marshall of the capitol, who, on April 20, 1863, arrested Hutton and seized the contents of his office as evidence. Hutton was confined in the Old Capitol Prison for about 10 days and then released. No details of his release or trial have been found. He subsequently relocated his quarters and continued in business with a much diminished clientele. Hutton is said to have returned to Harrisburg after the war ended and died there within a year.

### Daniel H. Prunk (1829–1923)

Born in Virginia in 1829, Prunk and his family migrated to Illinois where he attended college. After attending medical school in Cincinnati, he began medical practice in Illinois and in April 1861 moved to Indianapolis where he joined the 19th Indiana Volunteer Infantry as an assistant surgeon in September 1861. He was transferred to the 20th Indiana Volunteer Infantry in June 1862 and was arrested in November of that year and incarcerated in the Old Capitol Prison in Washington, D.C. for about 3 months for conduct unbecoming an officer. He was then dismissed from the service. From July to October 1863, he was acting assistant surgeon at the 2nd Division Army Hospital at Nashville, Tennessee, and subsequently requested permission to provide embalming services in Nashville. The request was

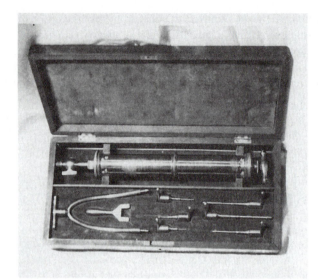

**Figure 11.** Injection syringe and cannulas of Daniel H. Prunk, Civil War embalming surgeon. (*Used with permission of the Illinois Funeral Directors' Foundation.*)

initially refused but finally granted late in 1863. He eventually had embalming establishments located not only in Nashville but also in Chattanooga and Knoxville in Tennessee; at East Point, Atlanta, Dalton, and Marietta in Georgia; and at Huntsville in Alabama (**Fig. 11**).

In 1865, Dr. Prunk was licensed by the Army to practice embalming and undertaking. (He was also engaged in a wholesale grocery business, cotton trading, and money lending.) He made his own embalming fluid by dissolving sheets of zinc in muriatic acid (hydrochloric acid) until a saturated solution of zinc chloride was obtained, to which a quantity of arsenious acid was added. The fluid obtained was injected quite warm without dilution or blood drainage.

Prunk sold all his embalming establishments in 1866 and returned to Indianapolis to practice medicine. It seems that he never engaged in embalming after his return to Indianapolis. He made one of the earliest written statements regarding the necessity of cavity treatment in a letter written in 1872, to Dr. J. P. Buckes to of San Jose, California.

> If I were going to ship a corpse from San Jose to New York City, we have advised for sometime the puncturing of the stomach to give vent to gases which accumulate at this time. In a subject with a large abdomen, where the bowels are discolored, the introduction of a couple of quarts into the peritoneal cavity by making a puncture near the umbilicus and throwing a thread of strong silk around it like a drawstring on a button cushion which can be readily closed after you are thru injecting.

### Dr. Richard Burr

Although little biographical information other than his rumored origin in Philadelphia is available concerning Burr (who apparently practiced during the period 1862–1865), he has achieved immortality as the embalmer photographed by the Civil War photographer Matthew Brady in front of his embalming tent while injecting a subject (**Fig. 12**). W. J. Bunnell complained about Burr's unprofessional conduct, alleging that, among other things, he set Bunnell's embalming tent on fire!

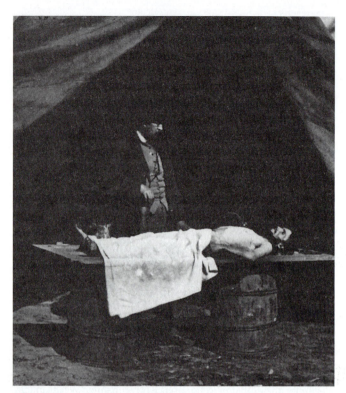

**Figure 12.** Richard Burr embalming near a battlefield during the Civil War. (*Source: Library of Congress.*)

He was also one of the men against whom complaints had been issued regarding inflated prices and poor services, which resulted in all embalmers being excluded from military areas by order of General U. S. Grant in January 1865. **This resulted in establishment of the first set of rules and regulations for the licensing of embalmers and undertakers in the United States.**

The final Army order for embalmers contained some of the suggestions made by Dr. Barnes, chief of the Army Medical Service in December 1863, to the effect that a performance bond should be posted by any embalmer desiring to practice. In addition, the requirement stipulated by the Provost Marshall General ordered the embalmer to furnish a list of his prices as charged for work or merchandise to the Provost Marshall General, the medical director of the department, and the Post Provost Marshall.

U.S. Army General Order 39 concerning embalmers (March 15, 1865) read as follows:

1. Here after no persons will be permitted to embalm or remove the bodies of deceased officers or soldiers unless acting under the special license of the Provost Marshall of the Army, department, or district in which the bodies may be.
2. Provost marshalls will restrict disinterments to seasons when they can be made without endangering the health of the troops. They will grant licenses only to such persons as furnish proof of skill and ability as embalmers, and will require bonds for the faithful performance of the orders given them. They will also establish a scale of prices by which embalmers are to be governed, with such other regulations as will protect the interest of the friends and relatives of deceased soldiers.

3. Applicants for license will apply directly to the Provost Marshall of the Army or department in which they may desire to pursue their business, submitting in distinct terms the process adopted by them, materials, length of time its preservative effect can be relied on and such other information as may be necessary to establish their proficiency and success. Medical directors will give such assistance in the examination of these applications as may be required by the Provost Marshall.

In the Army of the Cumberland, the following additional requirements were stipulated:
1. No disinterments will be permitted within the department between the 15th day of May and the 15th day of October.
2. The following scale of prices will be observed from and after this date: At Nashville and Memphis: for embalming bodies each at $15.00 to disinter, furnish metallic burial cases, well boxed, marked and delivered to the express office each at $75.00, zinc coffins and the above-listed services each at $40.00. An additional charge of $5.00 may be made for embalming and also for either of the above styles of coffins at Murfreesboro, Chattanooga, Knoxville, and Huntsville, Alabama, or in the field.
3. No person will be permitted to operate as an embalmer under any license issued to him until he shall have filed a bond in this office in the penal sum of $1000 conditioned for the faithful observance of this order, and for the skillful performance of such works he shall undertake by virtue of his license. [Such licenses were not transferable from one individual to another.]

By 1864, the Armory Square Military Hospital in Washington, D.C. had all its deceased patients routinely embalmed and the grave recorded so that the body could be disinterred and sent to family or friends when requested.

### C. B. Chamberlain

Chamberlain is said to have been born in Philadelphia. Although very little is known of the man, he definitely was an early partner of F. A. Hutton. He and Hutton apparently were not compatible, and he formed a new partnership with Ben Lyford. They both can be documented as practicing embalming surgeons on the scene at Gettysburg after the battle. Chamberlain is listed in Washington, D.C. City Directory as late as 1865 as a partner in Chamberlain and Waters Embalmers at 431 Pennsylvania Avenue. He is mentioned by F. C. Beinhauer, Pittsburgh undertaker, as being in the Pittsburgh area prior to and during the Civil War. Joseph H. Clarke also mentioned Chamberlain as a teacher of embalming in the post–Civil War period.

### Benjamin F. Lyford

Lyford was born in Vermont in 1841 and received public school education there. Lyford attended and graduated from Philadelphia University's 6-month course of medical studies. He first appeared on the Civil War scene as a partner of C. B. Chamberlain, who provided embalming after the Battle of Gettysburg. Later, he had altercations with Provost Marshall General Rudolf Patrick of the Army of the Potomac. This series of disagreements stimulated him to accept appointment on July 13, 1864, as assistant surgeon of the 68th Regiment of Infantry—U.S. Colored Troops. He reported to the unit in Missouri and subsequently served in Memphis. For a time, he served as commanding officer of a small cavalry and artillery contingent in southern Alabama.

He returned to his regiment stationed near New Orleans, Louisiana, and went on leave in New Orleans. He was arrested inside a bordello in full uniform and faced court-martial charges. Apparently found innocent of the charges, he was discharged from the Army on February 5, 1866, traveled to San Francisco, and opened an office for medical practice. One of his early patients was a wealthy widowed landowner who had an attractive daughter whom he fell in love with and married. The mother owned large tracts of land in Marin County across the bay north of San Francisco. Lyford built a health resort and dairy as well as his own home on this property and prospered.

In 1871, Lyford patented "An Improvement in Embalming," which was a very complicated system consisting of the introduction through the blood vessels of specially distilled chemicals (including creosote, zinc chloride, potassium nitrate, and alcohol) while the body was enclosed in a sealed container. The container that had the air within it alternatively evacuated to create a vacuum and reversed to create pressure. Finally, the body was eviscerated and the trunk cavity filled with an arsenical powder. His final recommendation was the use of cosmetics to color the features; he was one of the first to make this recommendation. In 1870, a local newspaper carried a story describing a body he had successfully embalmed. Lyford died in 1906 without issue and had a large, well-attended funeral.

### Dr. E. C. Lewis, W. P. Cornelius, and Prince Greer

This most interesting account of the Civil War embalming surgeons relates the method of the transmission of embalming technique from a medically trained practitioner to an undertaker, who, in turn, trained a layman in the skill. Dr. E. C. Lewis was a former U.S. Army surgeon, W. P. Cornelius (1824–1910) was a successful undertaker in Nashville, Tennessee, and Prince Greer was a former orderly, body servant, slave of a Colonel Greer of a Texas cavalry regiment who died in the fighting in Tennessee.

Thomas Holmes wrote:

*In the forepart of the war a young ex-Army doctor named E. C. Lewis called at my headquarters in Washington and wished me to instruct him in the embalming profession and sell him an outfit to go to the western Army and locate at Nashville. He offered as security a property holding in Georgetown, DC for any amount of fluid I would trust him for. I made a bargain with him and he used many barrels of fluid. I was often surprised at his large orders. [Note: Dr. Lewis's headquarters were at Mr. Cornelius's undertaking establishment in Nashville.]*

Cornelius stated:

*It was during the year 1862 that one Dr. E. C. Lewis came to me from the employ of Dr. Holmes and proposed to embalm bodies. It was new to me but I at once put him to work with the Holmes fluid and Holmes injector. He was quite an expert, but like many men could not stand prosperity and soon wanted to get into some other kind of business, which he did. When Lewis the embalmer quit, I then undertook the embalming myself with a colored assistant named Prince Greer.*

Cornelius explained that Prince Greer had earlier brought the body of Colonel Greer of a Texas cavalry regiment to Cornelius for shipment back to Texas. After shipping back the body, Prince Greer remained at Cornelius's premises and was asked what he wanted to do to earn his room and board. Prince Greer indicated he would do anything.

Cornelius continued:

*Prince Greer appeared to enjoy embalming so much that he himself became an expert, kept on at work embalming during the balance of the war, and was very successful at it. It was but a short time before he could raise an artery as quickly as anyone and was always careful, always of course coming to me in a difficult case. He remained with me until I quit the business in 1871.*

**Prince Greer is the first documented black embalmer in U.S. history.**

## Establishment of Embalming Schools

The incentive for embalming in the period AD 650 to 1861 was the preservation of anatomical material to further the study of and research in anatomy. Those who made the early strides in embalming were the anatomists, but about the time of J. N. Gannal (early nineteenth-century France) and Thomas H. Holmes (late nineteenth-century United States), general public interest was aroused in the preservation of the dead. This interest and the later demand for preservation for funeral purposes of all human dead grew far beyond the means and desires of the few, trained embalmers in the medical profession. During the late nineteenth century in the United States, schools of embalming instruction were established by experienced embalmers. Many funeral directors and doctors attended the schools to study embalming and to seek employment. By the beginning of the twentieth century in the United States, separation of the fields of embalming and medicine was complete. This brought about the advancement of both professions, particularly that of embalming, because it placed a complex art in the hands of specialists who are still striving to acquire more knowledge and skill in preserving the human dead.

## Public and Professional Acceptance

With the ending of the war and the assassination of President Lincoln, the Civil War's last major casualty, the public had been familiarized with the term *embalming* and obtained personal knowledge of the appearance of an embalmed body. This knowledge was acquired by the hundreds of thousands who viewed not only President Lincoln but also other prominent military and civilian figures as well as the ordinary soldiers embalmed and shipped to their homes.

Despite the end of the war and the establishment of peace, there was no wide adoption of embalming by civilian undertakers of the United States. There were many reasons for this apparent reluctance to adopt a worthwhile new practice. Undertakers in the United States at the end of the Civil War were an unorganized, largely rural group of individuals lacking a professional body of knowledge and skills. Specifically, they lacked textbooks of instruction on embalming, instructors and schools of embalming, professional journals, and professional associations. Until these necessities became available, embalming would not flourish.

The first step taken was to attempt the sale of embalming fluid to undertakers. Some Civil War embalming surgeons, such as Dr. Thomas Holmes, engaged in this endeavor on returning home. Holmes had a large local market (metropolitan New York City) for his preservative chemical, which he had named *Innominata*, and he promoted it well. Holmes, like other embalming chemical salesmen, realized quickly that the undertakers were interested in the preservative qualities of such chemicals but the clients were without knowledge of embalming techniques. Holmes, therefore, promoted the use of his Innominata as an external application, to wash the body and to saturate cloths to place over the face. His fluid was also poured into the mouth and nose to reach the lungs and stomach. Holmes' early practices were duplicated by other purveyors of embalming chemicals.

Examples of chemical embalming fluid patents include one issued to C. H. Crane of Burr Oak, Michigan, in September 1868. It was a powdered mixture of alum salt, ammonium chloride, arsenic, dichloride of mercury, camphor, and zinc chloride. It could be used as a dry powder or dissolved in water or alcohol to form an arterial solution and was named Crane's Electrodynamic Mummifier. In 1876, he sold the patent rights to this or a similar formulation to a Professor George M. Rhodes of Michigan. Another early embalming chemical manufacturer in 1877 was the Mills and Lacey Manufacturing Company of Grand Rapids, Michigan, whose embalming fluid featured arsenic as its preservative.

Instruments and chemicals available in the post–Civil War period included rubber gloves at $2 per pair (1877); anatomical syringes and three cannulas in a case for $20 to $22; surgical instruments in cases for $4 to $5; Rulon's wax eyecaps and mouth closers at $1 each; and Segestor embalming fluid for $4.50 per dozen pint bottles (1873). Professor George M. Rhodes was said to have sold 10,000 bottles of his dynamic Electro Balm in 1876 with more than 3000 undertakers using the product. Egyptian Embalmer Fluid (1877) sold for $6.50 per dozen pint bottles and was also available in 5 and 10 gallon kegs as well as $1/2$ and 1-gallon carboys at $3.00 per gallon.

Until the first quarter of the twentieth century, embalming was most frequently carried out in the home of the deceased or, in some communities, in the hospital where death occurred. There were early attempts in some funeral homes in the 1870s to provide both a preparation room and chapel space for the wake and services. In issues as early as 1876 of both *The Casket* and *The Sunnyside*,* there were accounts of the installation of preparation rooms. For example:

---

*The most significant impetus to spreading embalming knowledge was the founding of the professional journals The Sunnyside in 1871 and The Casket in 1876. Both, from their inception, carried advertisements for various embalming chemicals.

Hubbard and Searles Undertaking establishment at Auburn, New York, could provide seating for 100 persons at a service and had a cooling room with cement floor and marble slabs (2 × 8 feet) and running water connection.

Knowles Undertaking establishment at Providence, Rhode Island, had a preserver room and a corpse room where surgical procedures and postmortems were made.

### Dr. Auguste Renouard

In 1876, Dr. Renouard (1839–1912) became a regular contributor to *The Casket* of articles on all phases of embalming knowledge, which greatly implemented interest in embalming. He was born on a plantation in Point Coupee Parish, Louisiana, and received his early schooling locally. He is said to have attended the McDowell Medical School in St. Louis, Missouri, and, at the outbreak of the Civil War, to have returned to Louisiana to enlist in the Confederate Army. Despite his claim to military service in the confederate forces, no documented evidence has been found in some 50 years of searching. In the post-war period, he secured employment as a pharmacist in various cities such as New York, Memphis, and Chicago, where he was married. His son, Charles A. Renouard, was born shortly before the Chicago fire of 1871. Losing everything in the fire, Renouard traveled to Denver, Colorado, and secured employment as a bookkeeper for a combination furniture store and undertaking establishment. Because of its altitude, Denver at this time was regarded as a health resort for treatment of lung diseases.

The undertaking section of the firm returned many bodies to the east and south for hometown burial, and Renouard became interested in the procedures employed at his firm for shipment of the bodies. After studying the existing rudimentary system, he suggested to his employer that he be permitted to prepare the bodies for shipment by arterial embalming. This consent was given and it almost immediately produced a volume of letters from the receiving undertakers inquiring about the procedure used to create such beautiful corpses, which resembled a person asleep. Renouard graciously replied, explaining his chemicals and technique to the extent that it assumed the proportions of a correspondence course. Additionally, there were a number of individual undertakers who traveled to Denver to receive personal instruction in embalming from Renouard.

The publisher of *The Casket* urged Dr. Renouard to write a textbook on embalming and undertaking for use by undertakers. In 1878, he published *The Undertaker's Manual*, which contained 230 pages of detailed instruction on anatomy, chemistry, embalming procedures, instruments, and details of undertaking practice (**Fig. 13**). **This was the first book published specifically as an embalming textbook in the United States and followed by a horde of others.** In 1879, notices appeared in *The Casket* that undertakers in states such as Connecticut and Pennsylvania were agents for the sale of Auguste Renouard's chemical formulas and techniques (**Fig. 14**).

In 1881, Dr. Renouard was requested to open a school of embalming in Rochester, New York, but, for various reasons, this did not become a reality until early 1883. In 1880, the state of Michigan was the first to form an undertakers' association, which, in 1881, changed its name to Funeral Directors

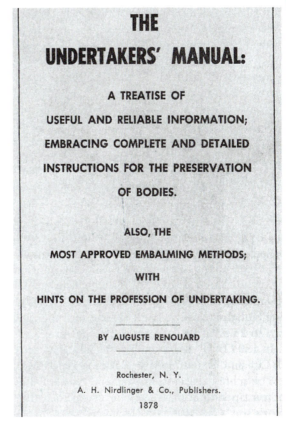

**Figure 13.** Title page of Auguste Renouard's first edition of The Undertaker's Manual.

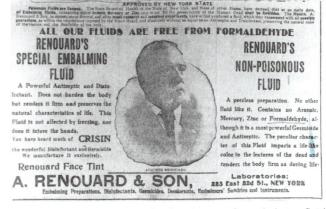

**Figure 14.** Auguste Renouard's advertisement for embalming fluid.

Association. Other states quickly followed the Michigan lead and organized state associations. **The various state associations met in 1882 in Rochester and organized the National Funeral Directors Association (NFDA), another important step toward professionalism.** Renouard provided demonstrations of embalming in Rochester at the first national convention of the Association. This set a pattern for many years of an obligatory embalming demonstration at state and national conventions. During the 1882 gathering, agents of an English firm (Dotridge Brothers, Funeral Supply Firm) offered Renouard a 5-year contract to teach embalming in London at $5000 per year, which he rejected.

The Rochester School of Embalming headed by Dr. Renouard under the auspices of the Egyptian Chemical Company opened in 1883 and he continued his affiliation with this school until December 1884. He then entered into an agreement with Hallett and Company Undertakers in Kansas City, Missouri, to locate his school, the School of Embalming and Organic Chemistry, on the company's premises. By mid-1886, he terminated his school in Kansas City and returned to Denver. He then began to travel to distant points such as Ft. Worth, Texas, and Toronto and Montreal, Canada, providing embalming instruction for periods ranging from 3 days to 2 weeks.

In 1894, Dr. Renouard made his final move to New York City and established the U.S. College of Embalming. The school had no fixed-term classes and the student remained until he was able to embalm. In 1889, the doctor's son, Charles A. Renouard, was reported to be a shipping clerk with the firm of Dolge and Huncke—Embalming Chemical Manufacturers. Early in 1899, Charles Renouard opened the Renouard Training School for Embalmers in New York City, and in February, 1900, Auguste Renouard closed the U.S. College of Embalming and joined Charles at his school. Charles provided several months of embalming instruction in London, England, on behalf of the O. K. Buckhout Chemical Company of Grand Rapids, Michigan. In 1906, Auguste traveled to England and continental Europe where he was most graciously received and entertained.

Auguste Renouard died in his home in 1912. A monument paid for by voluntary subscription of his former students was an example of the esteem in which he was held by those he instructed. **He can, without question, be regarded as the first major figure to provide embalming instruction for undertakers in the United States.** His son Charles continued the Renouard Training School for Embalmers until his death in 1950.

### Joseph Henry Clarke

Born in Connersville, Indiana, Joseph Henry Clarke (1840–1916) received his early education in pharmacy and enrolled as a student in a medical college in Keokuk, Iowa. His studies, however, were interrupted by the Civil War. He volunteered for service with the Union Army but was rejected because of physical defects. He was permitted to serve as a civilian and later held the position of assistant hospital steward in the Fifth Iowa Infantry. After the death of his father, he returned home before the end of the war to support his family. He married and secured employment as a casket salesman. During the course of his travel, he became acquainted with a fluid manufacturer and became sufficiently interested in embalming to sell embalming fluids as a sideline. His interest in embalming grew as he realized the need to demonstrate the method of use of the fluid he hoped to sell to his patrons. This, in turn, led to his study of and experimentation with embalming chemicals to solve problems relating to the preservation of the dead. He enrolled in an anatomy course conducted by Dr. C. M. Lukens of the Pulte Medical College in Cincinnati, Ohio, which broadened into a lifetime friendship and professional partnership in the founding of the Clarke School of Embalming at Cincinnati in 1882 (**Fig. 15**).

The school lacked permanence because Mr. Clarke traveled most of the year giving courses of instruction, each course

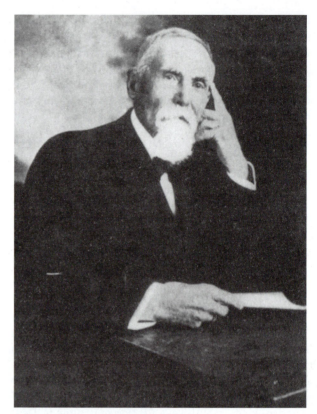

**Figure 15.** Portrait of Joseph Henry Clarke, founder of the Cincinnati College of Embalming.

varying in length from 2 to 7 days. His second course of instruction away from Cincinnati was presented in New York City. One class member was Felix A. Sullivan, who later became a well-known teacher and writer in the embalming field. Sullivan and Clarke became rivals and bitter enemies. One major clash occurred when General and ex-President Ulysses S. Grant died on July 23, 1885, at Mt. McGregor, New York. Clarke had been advised by the Holmes Undertaking Company (no relation to Thomas Holmes) of Saratoga, New York, that the company would be retained to handle the funeral of General Grant and that they wanted Clarke to do the embalming. Clarke was in Baltimore on the day of Grant's death, but he became ill and went to his Springfield, Ohio, home where he was bedridden for 3 to 4 weeks. The embalming was accordingly performed by one member of the Holmes Undertaking Company family and Dr. McEwen using Clarke's proprietary embalming chemical (**Fig. 16**).

After the body had been embalmed, Rev. Stephen Merritt, clergyman and undertaker of New York City and also General Grant's religious adviser, arrived together with Felix A. Sullivan and announced that they were to take charge. The Holmes personnel withdrew from the premises and Sullivan proceeded to reembalm the body. He claimed he withdrew all previously injected arterial fluid and replaced it with the chemical made by the company he represented. Clarke rebuffed these claims in professional journals. A reporter from *The New York Times* wrote that Mr. Holmes (of Saratoga, New York) was too drunk to carry out the necessary preparation of the body. *The New York Times* was subsequently sued for libel and lost the case, and Mr. Holmes was awarded several thousand dollars in damages.

**Figure 16.** Title page of an article by Joseph Henry Clarke for The Sunnyside.

The name of the embalming school was changed to the Cincinnati College of Embalming in 1899 and was established on a permanent basis. Mr. Clarke conducted only occasional lecture tours at that time. He was ably assisted in the management of the school by his son, C. Horace Clarke. In 1907, Charles O. Dhonau became associated with him and later took over operation of the school. Mr. Clarke was a capable teacher, lecturer, and author of several texts on embalming, and he held several patents in the embalming field. He retired in 1909 to San Diego, California, where he died in 1916.

### Felix Aloysius Sullivan (1843–1931)

Sullivan was born in Toronto, Ontario, Canada, in 1843, the son of a Scottish immigrant undertaker and an Irish mother. He unquestionably had the most interesting, controversial, riotous, and successful career as a practitioner, writer, teacher, and lecturer of embalming and related subjects. His career was so full of incidents that it would be impossible to recount all but a few highlights.

After the Civil War, he followed various occupations and traveled. He eventually drifted to New York City where he secured employment with various casket companies and finally became a funeral director for hire. He studied anatomy and other medical sciences and, by 1881, became an embalmer of some local repute. He was hired to go to Cleveland, Ohio, to reembalm President Garfield, who died from an assassin's bullet, and seems to have been successful in this venture. Sullivan attended Clarke's embalming class in New York City in 1882 to learn how such a class of instruction was conducted. Sullivan, together with W. G. Robinson, opened the New York School of Embalming in 1884 and a year later was again involved in the embalming of a president, this time President Ulysses Grant (see previous information on Clarke's career). He then entered and left a long list of employers. In 1887, he was in Chicago when the anarchists who bombed the police in 1886, killing and wounding police and civilians, were condemned to die. One exploded a dynamite cap in his mouth in jail and the others were hung. He prepared all bodies and was praised for his plastic surgery on the "mad bomber."

Sullivan continued his erratic employment or work habits, working for one firm, quitting, and then working for another. By 1891, he was again a lecturer/demonstrator, this time for the Egyptian Chemical Company. By 1892, he reached the height of his career as a lecturer, speaking and teaching in more cities to larger classes than anyone previously had. He was expelled from the State Funeral Directors convention in 1893 in St. Louis, Missouri, and a resolution was passed to forbid ever inviting his return. Sullivan settled in Chicago and opened a school of embalming. Local papers relate his arrest there together with a female companion (not his wife) on charges of adultery and wife and child desertion. When he finally settled the charges, he underwent a cure for alcoholism and resumed teaching in a succession of short-lived appointments at various schools.

In 1900, the O. K. Buckhout Company of Michigan, a manufacturer of embalming chemicals, had Charles A. Renouard under contract to lecture and sent him to London, England, to present a 3-week course of instruction that was very well received. Renouard returned home to attend similar engagements in the United States. The Buckhout Company had to find someone to continue the successful course of instruction in England, and the position was offered to Sullivan, who immediately accepted. Sullivan began teaching in London on October 8, 1900, a career that would extend to 1903. He lectured throughout the British Isles and helped to organize the British Embalmers Society as well as a journal entitled the *British Embalmer*.

He related that when Queen Victoria died in 1901, he was consulted about the possibility of embalming her. He recommended against it because it was impossible to guarantee perfect results. When he returned to the United States, he purchased an embalming school in St. Louis, Missouri, but the venture proved unprofitable. He then moved to Denver and Salt Lake City and eventually back to St. Louis, where he died. Sullivan wrote hundreds of articles plus eight books, taught thousands to embalm, and probably received more gifts from his classes than any other teacher before or since his time.

### A. Johnson Dodge (1848–1926)

Little did A. Johnson Dodge know in 1889 that he and his family were about to embark on a remarkable history of service to the funeral profession. At that time, he was a Maine legislator and general store owner, while his brother George B. Dodge ran a printing company in Boston. When the owner of the

Egyptian Chemical Company was not able to pay a bill to the printing company, George was given the company to pay the indebtedness. A. J. was an avid student of anatomy and chemistry and George knew that he had always dreamed of being physician. By 1890, George had convinced A. J. to close the store and come to Boston to learn embalming. His love of knowledge and learning went hand in hand with his ability to teach. He authored three textbooks of the day: *The Embalmer's Guide*, *The Essentials of Anatomy*, and *Sanitary Science and Embalming and the Practical Embalmer*.

Embalming instruction in those days was provided by embalming chemical companies through teachers who traveled around the country giving 2-day courses. In 1893, George and A. J. Dodge bought the Oriental School of Embalming, a traveling school based in Boston. By the end of that year, A. J. Dodge had resigned from the Egyptian Chemical Company but continued with the Oriental School. The school was renamed the Massachusetts College of Embalming in 1895 and incorporated under the Massachusetts nonprofit educational act. A. J. Dodge founded a new school in 1907, the New England Institute of Anatomy, Sanitary Science and Embalming, after selling his interest in the Massachusetts College. The New England Institute was chartered by the Commonwealth of Massachusetts as a nonprofit educational institution in 1910 and is still in operation today. In addition to these activities, A. J. Dodge served as a principal lecturer at the Barnes School of Anatomy and had founded his own manufacturing company after leaving the Egyptian Company.

A. J. Dodge's son, Walter Dodge, continued the family business by learning embalming and taking his skills to Detroit where he opened the Dodge Chemical Company. At the same time, his father was also opening the Dodge Chemical Company in Boston. They decided to join forces and the first plant was run out of A. J.'s home. A. J.'s knowledge of chemistry [leads] led him to develop a research arm of the company while still conducting all the lectures on the road. He traveled by train to various cities where he would arrange for demonstrations when bodies were available. By 1913 A. J.'s younger son George B. Dodge II joined the firm as a very successful salesman for the company.

The facilities for manufacturing at the home were becoming inadequate to keep up with the demand for their products. The next four decades saw tremendous growth of the company, leading to the move to its present location in Cambridge, Massachusetts. During this time, not only was the company expanding locally in the Boston area but it was also opening branch offices in other U.S. cities and Canada as well. Branch offices and warehouses were opened in Los Angeles, Fort Worth, Texas, and Chicago to provide its customers all over the country with prompt service. The Dodge Chemical Company (Canada) was formed in Toronto and had complete manufacturing facilities. By 1982, the company had expanded to Europe and now also has distributors in Australia, New Zealand, Mexico, and Japan.

One thing that A. J. Dodge clearly understood from very early on was the importance of research. He was always striving to create better products and techniques for the embalmer. To this end, he hired a full-time graduate chemist from Yale University, William B. O'Brien. O'Brien remained with Dodge until the time of his death. Research was to continue as an important part of the manufacturing process throughout the company's history. Important studies and discoveries were made by the likes of Louis McDonald, Dr. Jerome Frederick, and Margaret Boothe.

Even after A. J. Dodge's death, the family continued to devote significant time and resources to continuing education for embalmers and funeral directors. Today, the Dodge Company is still owned and operated by the Dodge family. They have remained true to A. J.'s vision of service to the funeral profession in everything they do.

## Increase in Embalming Schools

Some early "graduates" of embalming courses of instruction gave up regular employment at an undertaking establishment to provide embalming service to a number of undertakers who had no staff member trained to embalm. **This is how the terms *embalmer to the trade* or *trade embalmer* originated.**

Many undertakers and/or their assistants were eager to learn to embalm but were unable to absent themselves from their business or employment to take advantage of such training. Some, however, managed to attend the 3- to 5-day schools, sponsored by the embalming chemical companies, in their city where they were taught the basic skills by the itinerant instructors. Others augmented their meager knowledge by enrolling in home study courses offered by many of the established schools of embalming.

Schools of instruction in embalming increased in number and activity by the beginning of the twentieth century. Many manufacturers of embalming chemicals entered into the business of teaching embalming to maintain and increase the market for their products. Although the repair of injuries to the dead caused by disease or trauma had been dealt with since Egyptian times, it was not until 1912 that a systematic treatment for such cases was developed by a New York City embalmer, Joel E. Crandall (1878–1942). From this time on, the schools of embalming slowly began to adopt instruction in this special phase of embalming treatment. Today, the subject area is commonly referred to as **restorative art.** It would be impossible to list in this text every personality who became an embalming professor or every school that was established, but a few should be mentioned.

### *Carl Lewis Barnes*

Born into a family that operated an undertaking establishment in Connellsville, Pennsylvania, Barnes (1872–1927) studied medicine in Indiana, opened an embalming school there (**Fig. 17**), and moved it to Chicago. He manufactured embalming chemicals, wrote many books and articles on the subject, and had the largest chain of fixed-location schools in history in New York, Chicago, Boston, Minneapolis, and Dallas. While serving overseas as a medical colonel in the U.S. Army in World War I, his business failed. He never reopened the schools, continuing the practice of medicine until his death (**Fig. 18**).

### *Albert H. Worsham*

Worsham (1868–1939) attended Barnes's school and was on the faculty from 1903 to 1911 when he opened his own school

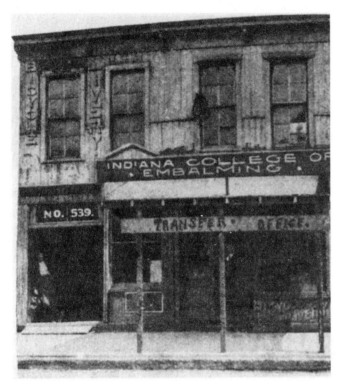

**Figure 17.** Old Indianapolis College of Embalming, Indianapolis, Indiana.

in Chicago, with his wife Laura and brother Robert as faculty members. He lectured widely and was noted principally for contributing to the early foundation of postmortem plastic surgery.

### Howard S. Eckels

Eckels (1865–1937) was a manufacturer of embalming chemicals and the founder of Eckels College of Embalming in Philadelphia, Pennsylvania. *(The school and chemical plant were in the same building, which was not an uncommon arrangement.)* Eckels wrote many articles and books, was successfully sued for plagiarism, and was not adverse to engaging in prolonged debates in the press. After his death, his son John managed the school well into the post–World War II period when it closed after a period of affiliation with Temple University.

### William Peter Hohenschuh

Born in Iowa City, Iowa, the son of an undertaker, Hohenschuh (1858–1920) took over the family business on the death of his father and began to teach embalming, which he had learned by correspondence from Auguste Renouard in the mid-1870s. Hohenschuh was active in the Iowa State Association and was elected president to the NFDA. He operated an embalming school in Chicago and, in 1900, in partnership with Dr. William S. Carpenter (1871–1944), opened the Hohenschuh-Carpenter School of Embalming in Des Moines, Iowa. He also operated funeral home. In 1930, Dr. Carpenter moved the school to St. Louis and merged it with the Moribund American College of Embalming owned by F. A. Sullivan. After Dr. Carpenter's death, his daughter Helene Craig and her son Golden Craig operated the school as well as the American Academy in New York City. This continued well into the post–World War II period.

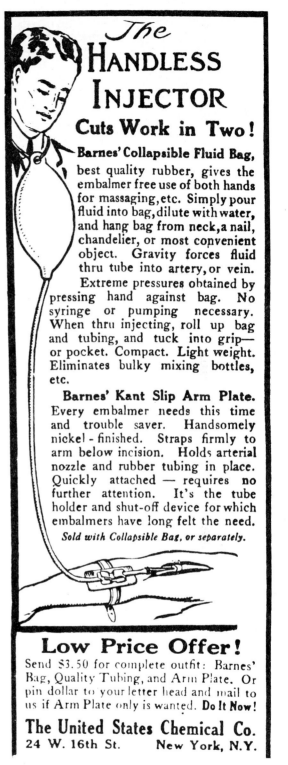

**Figure 18.** Advertisement for Barnes's handless injector.

### Clarence G. Strub

Born in Iowa on March 1, 1906, Strub attended the University of Iowa in Iowa City, Washington University in St. Louis, Missouri, and the Hohenschuh-Carpenter College of Embalming in Des Moines, Iowa. He became an instructor at the Hohenschuh-Carpenter College in 1929. In 1930, the school was moved to St. Louis where it merged with the American College of Embalming and operated under the name of the St. Louis College

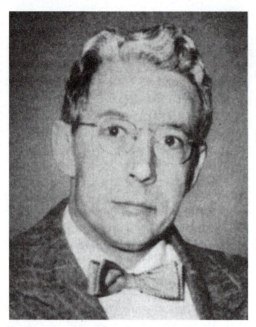

**Figure 19.** Photograph of Clarence G. Strub.

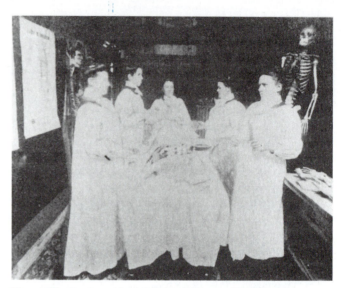

**Figure 20.** Anatomy class at Odou Institute of Embalming, New York, circa 1900 (*Professor Odou at center of group*).

of Mortuary Science. In 1934, he became a member of the staff of the Undertaker's Supply Company of Chicago and conducted clinics and demonstrations throughout the United States and Canada. He taught embalming and funeral management at the University of Minnesota and the Wisconsin Institute of Mortuary Science and was the director of research for the Royal Bond Chemical Company for many years (**Fig. 19**).

His greatest contributions to embalming lie in his ability to write clearly and simply, explaining embalming theory and practices. During his career, he published well over 1000 articles as well as many teaching outlines and quiz compendia. His little text, *The Principles of Restorative Art*, was the true prototype of all present-day texts on the subject. He also authored the monumental textbook *Principles and Practice of Embalming*, published by L. G. "Darko" Fredericks, which became the standard embalming text used by most colleges of mortuary science. Strub also wrote several technical movies such as the *Conquest of Jaundice* and *The Eye Bank Story* as well as many children's stories and movies. He was the architect of the Eye Bank System in Iowa, which set the national pattern, as well as the curator of the state of Iowa's anatomical donation program. He died in Iowa City, Iowa, on August 6, 1974.

### Women Embalmers

Women as well as men were trained as embalmers and not only practiced embalming but founded schools of instruction. Among these women were **Mrs. E. G. Bernard** of Newark, New Jersey, who founded the Bernard School of Embalming; **Mme. Lina D. Odou**, who founded the Odou Embalming Institute in New York City (**Fig. 20**); and **Lena R. Simmons**, who founded and operated the Simmons School of Embalming in Syracuse, New York, until her son Baxter took over the management.

## MORTUARY EDUCATION

The American Board of Funeral Service Education oversees the basic course content in embalming as a foundation for uniform performance standards in the preparation of all bodies embalmed in the United States. This basic course content also allows the Conference of Funeral Service Examining Boards to administer a uniform objective examination to those who are candidates for a license. As an introduction to this chapter, we are going to take an overview of the development of the basic course content in embalming, as it lays the foundation for professional performance standards.

Mortuary colleges and funeral service schools are relatively recent in origin. The development of mortuary education has followed the general pattern common to all professional fields. It emerged slowly from a period in which knowledge was transmitted from preceptor to student by means of observation and informal discussion, to its present academic status.

Following the American Civil War, when funeral homes first came into existence, the pioneers in funeral service experimented with materials, equipment, and methods for their use. There were no channels for wide distribution of the knowledge they gained through trial and error. Training was conducted solely by means of apprenticeship.

As the scope of funeral service expanded and as embalming came into wider use, commercial companies were organized to supply the needs of the embalmer and funeral director. Research was directed to developing better products, and this resulted in a rapid increase in knowledge of what today is termed *mortuary science*. During the latter decades of the nineteenth century, the establishment of trade journals made possible a wider distribution of this knowledge. These same companies employed skilled lecturers and demonstrators to instruct funeral directors in the use of these products and in improved methods of embalming. These early "classes," lasting from a few hours to a few days, provided the first formal vocational instruction.

As the public health and welfare aspects of funeral service became more widely recognized, state licensing laws were established. For the first time, educational requirements were formulated and a definite course of training was legally prescribed. At about this same time, educators established the first schools of embalming to train students in a relatively new art. Over the years, these pioneers in mortuary education expanded and improved the scope of training, often keeping far ahead of requirements prescribed by law and by licensing authorities.

A system for national accreditation of mortuary schools was first introduced in 1927 by the Conference of Funeral Service Examining Boards, a national association of state licensing boards. Higher standards governing qualifications of faculty, the curriculum, and teaching facilities were established and enforced. Details of the development of mortuary schools can be found in Part II of this textbook.

The National Council on Mortuary Education was established in 1942 by the NFDA and the National Association of Embalming Schools and Colleges. After World War II, with the termination of restrictions on assembly, a formal meeting was held in December of 1945 in Cleveland, Ohio. Officers for the Council were Chairman, Ralph Millard; Vice-Chairman, Jacob Van't Hof; and Secretary Treasurer, R. P. Mac Fate. The Council was attended by 62 school administrators, faculty members, state board authorities, and various funeral service association officers. The program committee comprised John Eckles, Jacob Van't Hof, and Otto Margolis. This meeting gave a fresh impetus to progress toward educational competence and professional status in funeral service. In March of 1947, the First National Teacher's Institute was held in Cincinnati, Ohio. Forty-four representatives from 14 schools met to lay the foundation for the course content in Chemistry and Mortuary Administration. Charles O. Dhonau of the Cincinnati College of Embalming presided over the meeting. In November of 1947, the Second Teacher's Institute was held in Pittsburgh, Pennsylvania (**Fig. 21**). More than 75 individuals from 23 schools and associations were present. Adopted at this meeting was the first basic course content syllabus for anatomy and embalming and the Mortician's Oath (drafted by R. P. Mac Fate). The Oath has been administered to all graduates of a mortuary college since 1948. Dr. Emory S. James of Pittsburgh was chair of the anatomy course content committee. The committee on the basic course content in embalming consisted of R. H. Hannum (Cleveland), L. G. Frederick (Dallas), R. Victor Landig (Houston), J. E. Shea (Boston), and E. L. Heidenreich (Wisconsin). The formulation and analysis of the embalming basic course content were brought about through the efforts of mortuary colleges, state boards, state associations, and the profession in general. The task was difficult because it meant resolving many individualistic teaching procedures into one common, sound educational basis. Once the basic course content was established, it was immediately recognized there would be an imperative need to review and update the curriculum every few years. Revision of the course content has continued over the years and is currently overseen by the American Board of Funeral Service Education. In their July 1994 meeting in Denver, Colorado, a glossary of terminology was appended to the basic course content in embalming. In a meeting in Denver as late as July of 2000, the basic course content in embalming was again reviewed, amended, and prepared for editing and input by the member schools of the American Board of Funeral Service Education. This basic course content is an example of a professional performance standard in the field of embalming in America.

## CONCERN FOR TREATMENT

Early embalming reports concerning arterial injection indicated some concern for special treatment of the trunk viscera. Most such treatments consisted of removal, treatment, and replacement of viscera in the trunk cavity together with some preservative material, either powdered or liquid. Other reports, such as those of the Gannal-Sucquet era, indicate dependence

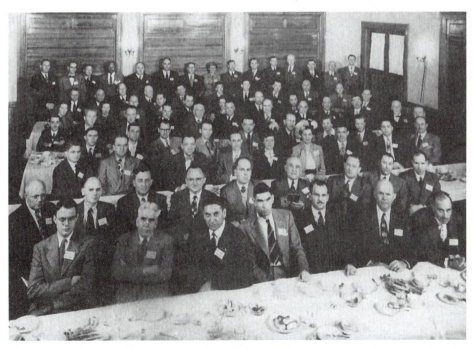

**Figure 21.** Educators from across the United States gathered for the Second Teachers Institute held in Pittsburgh, Pennsylvania, November 8 and 9, 1947. At this meeting, the first curriculum in anatomy and embalming was established and the Mortician's Oath was adopted. (*Used with permission of the Pittsburgh Institute of Mortuary Science, Pittsburgh, Pennsylvania.*)

for total preservation solely on the arterial injection unaccompanied by any special treatment for the trunk cavities. Gabriel Clauderus had advocated preservation based on introduction of his preservative chemical into the trunk cavity followed by immersion of the entire body in the preservative.

It was not until the mid-1870s that a "modern" system of treatment for the cavities was designed. The inventor of the trocar, Samuel Rodgers (listing Los Angeles, New York City, and San Francisco as his residences), secured two patents for the trocar, one in 1878 and the second in 1880. The 1878 patent described the trocar much as it exists today. The 1880 patent was issued for a system of embalming that consisted of introduction of his trocar, thrust through a single point in the navel into all the organs of the trunk to distribute a preservative fluid throughout the trunk viscera. The simplicity of this treatment and its modest success made it appealing to those who, for whatever reason, did not adopt arterial embalming, which required greater knowledge of anatomy and surgical skill. The inevitable result was a confrontation between "belly punchers" (cavity treatment advocates) and "throat cutters" (arterial embalmers) concerning the merits of their respective means of preservation.

It slowly became evident that neither system was always completely successful and that combination of the two systems, arterial injection followed by cavity treatment, offered the greatest promise of embalming success. Although Rodgers did not mention aspiration prior to injection of preservative chemicals in his process, Auguste Renouard did specifically recommend this in his *Undertaker's Manual*. Rodgers's method of a single-entrance opening into the trunk cavity was a brilliant concept not followed by all his contemporary "authorities." Espy's and Taylor's books of embalming instruction, for example, advocated multiple (three to four) points of insertion through the trunk wall for the trocar. Rodgers formulated an embalming preservative chemical named *Alekton*, which was believed to have phenol as its principal preservative. He also recommended cavity treatment followed by hypodermic injections using his trocar, inserted into the limbs of the corpse.

Since the introduction of arterial injection of the blood vessels in the late seventeenth century, no other system of corpse preservation explored had ever been seriously used. In 1884, a British physician, Dr. B. W. Richardson, devised what he termed **needle embalming**. The process consisted of inserting a trocar (the needle), such as Rodgers's invention, at the medial corner of the eye socket and forcing it into the brain area, where the injection process was repeated. After removal of the trocar from the brain area, cavity treatment, aspiration, and injection were carried out. This process was most often referred to as the **eye process**. Rodgers in his early patent had proposed insertion of his trocar through the nose to inject preservative chemicals into the brain area, but did not suggest that this process would preserve the entire body as Richardson contended. It eventually was to be called the **nasal process**. Professor Sullivan, ever alert for any new procedure to interest his students, adopted Richardson's eye process and exploited its simplicity to the maximum.

Carl Barnes offered a variation of the procedure by inserting the trocar through the neck and into the brain via the foramen magnum. T. B. Barnes, his brother and school instructor associate, inserted the trocar between dorsal vertebrae into the spinal canal. In this method, Dr. Eliab Meyers drilled a hole through the center of the vertex of the skull, permitting direct access for a small trocar into the superior sagittal sinus. The process, regardless of point of access, is said to have delivered the preservative chemical eventually into blood vessels within the cranium and then to the rest of the body.

A dramatic test demonstration of the process is both described and illustrated in Barnes' textbook, *The Art and Science of Embalming*. A severed head of a dissection room subject had trocars inserted into the brain area through the eye socket route. Rubber tubes connected the carotid arteries and jugular veins with collecting bottles. As fluid was injected through the trocars into the brain area, fluid flowed into the collecting bottles via the carotid arteries and jugular veins. The process achieved moderate popularity until about 1905, when it became extinct. Not all teachers of embalming were advocates of it, and J. H. Clarke was a vigorous critic.

A variation of the process was the short-lived attempt to insert the trocar into the left ventricle of the heart and inject the arterial system. The great difficulty encountered in positively locating the left ventricle quickly discouraged this procedure. The intentional application of an electric current directly to a corpse for the intended purpose of simulating the effect of lightning or accidental electrocution on the blood—destruction of blood coagulation—has been attempted many times without any appreciable success.

One early experimenter was Charles T. Schade of McAlester, Oklahoma, who as early as 1909 conceived the idea of applying an electric current, powered by dry cell batteries, to the body surface, in the belief that this would cause small muscles to contract and hence force blood out of the areas of discoloration. No effect was noted concerning the ability of an electric current applied externally to a corpse to prevent normal postmortem blood coagulation or promote dissolution of any existing intravascular clots. Similar attempts to accomplish this desirable effect have been attempted through the years down to the present, both in the United States and in England without success. Those who have experimented have concluded that the dead human body does not conduct an electrical current well enough to accomplish the intended purpose.

Toward the end of the nineteenth century and on into the twentieth century, a number of events were to occur that would accelerate embalming toward the level of professionalism. A convergence of two movements became apparent around 1897, with the appearance of advertisements by embalming fluid companies stating that their fluid contained formalin. For some years, there had been arguments to eliminate arsenic and other poisons from inclusion in embalming fluid formulas for the same medicolegal reason that the French prohibited arsenic in 1846 and bichloride of mercury in 1848. Now that a powerful disinfectant, **formalin**, was available and reasonably priced, the opportunity to eliminate poisonous chemicals was at hand. The state of Michigan led the way in 1901 and was followed by other states.

The second movement was to require regulations for both licensing and governing those who practiced embalming, and in 1893–1894, the state of Virginia became the first state to do so. Formalin content fluids were not a total blessing and were not as favorably received as might have been expected. Embalmers of the period were unaccustomed to the very different characteristics of the new preservative. For example, bodies embalmed with arsenic were said to have been relatively supple, making dressing and positioning relatively easy. Many of the poisonous chemicals had bleaching qualities and left the body quite white. Only a few left any undesirable coloration, such as those reported to contain copper, which tended to produce a bluish color in the skin. Then too, little or no problem was reportedly encountered to the penetration of all the body tissues, with or without blood drainage. There was also the proven ability of such poisonous chemicals to preserve the body tissues. There were, of course, some negatives such as the possible absorption of poisonous chemicals through the embalmer's unprotected skin, various skin irritations, and thickened and cracked fingernails.

Embalmers beginning to experiment with the formalin-based embalming fluids had to learn that they must remove the blood in all cases and began to use low-formalin-content or nonformalin fluids to wash the blood out before injection of the preservative formalin-based solutions. They also learned that they had to position the body properly before injection and the hardening effected by formalin or they would encounter serious problems later in trying to properly position hands together. To their astonishment, embalmers also discovered that formalin reacted with the bile pigments present in the skin of jaundiced bodies to produce an unsightly green-colored skin.

The opponents of formalin fluids were highly critical of the formaldehyde fumes, which irritated mucous membranes, claiming these effects were more dangerous to health than the poisonous chemicals. Reason and science prevailed, and the embalming fluid formulas were improved to overcome most of the early problems. With the eventual transfer of the site of embalming from the family home bedroom to the funeral home preparation room, proper ventilation tended to eliminate most of the irritation problem. Chemicals became more diverse. For example, different formulas were developed for specific uses, such as arterial and cavity, pre-injection, coinjection, and for special purposes as in decomposing cases. The delivery of embalming fluids in concentrated form, to be added to water to create the desired dilution strength, was a distinct contrast to the former embalming chemical packaging, which was delivered in containers already combined with water ready to inject. Thus, embalmers had to become more experienced and intelligent in the mixing of the formalin embalming solution than they had formerly been.

## UTILIZATION OF NEW DEVICES

Over the years of embalming in bedrooms of the home of the deceased, little in the way of improvements was instituted in injection pumps or aspirating devices. With the transfer of the majority of embalming preparations to the funeral home, however, new devices could be used. In the last quarter of the nineteenth century, most embalming pumps or injectors were based on the gravity bowl, the hand pump, or the rubber bulb syringe. The gravity bowl was simply a container suspended above the body and connected to the arterial tube by a length of rubber tubing. The height of the bowl above the body determined the pressure. Its main advantage was that it did not require the constant pumping by the embalmer and, therefore, left hands free to perform other tasks. The hand pump could produce either pressure or vacuum for injection or aspiration into or from a glass container.

When the preparation of the body was moved to the funeral home, water pressure was used to create suction to aspirate. Special aspirators, such as the Penberthy, Worsham, and Slaughter models, generated suction by water pressure and were made to attach to preparation room sink faucets, connected by rubber tubing to the trocar. Later in the 1950s, special electric motor-driven aspirators were devised and were found to overcome the aggravation encountered by low water pressure during high-water-use periods. *Most communities today have requirements relating to the need for preventing suction of aspirated material into the water system.*

At a New York state convention in 1914, a battery-powered electric pump, the Falcon Electric Embalmer for injecting embalming chemicals, was demonstrated but was not widely adopted. Some new instruments devised to simplify or improve certain embalming procedures were developed in the 1920s and 1930s. A new method of jaw closure was devised involving "barbed tacks" driven into the mandible and maxillae by a spring-propelled hammer. Wires attached to the "tacks" were then twisted together to secure the desired degree of jaw closure. A plastic, threaded, screw-like device called the **trocar button** became the most useful waterproof seal for trocar punctures, bullet wounds, and even for intravenous needle punctures (when surgically enlarged). A metal dispensing device that was attached directly to any standard 16-ounce bottle of cavity fluid (by screwing it into the bottle opening in place of the cap) simplified cavity fluid injection. The dispenser was connected to the trocar by a length of rubber hose and injection was accomplished by gravity after the cavity fluid bottle was elevated and inverted.

It was not until the mid-1930s that electric-powered injection machines were available and in use. Some were simply electric motors with fittings to produce pressure or vacuum-connected to suitable containers by rubber tubing. One of the first "self-contained" embalming fluid injection machines put on the market in the 1930s was the Snyder–Westberg device. It was originally designed to hold one-half gallon of embalming fluid. The machine was compact, durable, and trouble-free, and was originally designed with motor and the fluid container side by side. Model II of the Snyder–Westberg device was designed so that the fluid container was placed above the injection motor; thus, the fluid was "gravity fed" to the pump. This arrangement has become standard on all self-contained units. In 1937, the Slaughter Company developed an all-metal fluid injection tank equipped with a pressure gauge; in 1938, the Flow master electric-powered injection machine was announced; in 1939, the Frigid Fluid Company developed a pressure injector consisting of a metal container for holding embalming fluid complete with exit connection with shut-off and a carbon dioxide gas cylinder to create the necessary pressure to inject the fluid. **In mid-1939, the Turner Company announced the availability** of the Porti-Boy, which was to become the all-time most popular injection machine. Several improvements over the years included a pulsator device, a larger fluid tank, and the ability to produce extreme high-pressure injections. By the 1960s, extreme high-pressure injection machines such as the Sawyer were available and in use.

## AVAILABILITY OF MODERN MATERIALS

With the end of World War II, metal and other materials became available to produce various new embalming devices. The concept of using externally generated agitation to assist in blood removal became popular. Some embalming tables had such pulsating devices built-in as an integral part of the structure. Other pulsating devices were devised to be attached to existing operating tables or were handheld devices to be applied to the body over the course of the major blood vessels. Disillusionment with this development came after a short period of use. The vibrations produced by such devices made it impossible to keep instruments, and even the body itself, from sliding downward toward the foot of the table.

Another innovation was the development of a conventional embalming fluid by the Switzer Corporation of Cleveland that contained a large quantity of fluorescent dye. The dye was to act as a tracer or indicator of the degree of circulation or penetration of the embalming fluid when viewed under an ultraviolet light illuminator furnished with the embalming fluid. Although the system did indeed disclose the extent of the distribution of the embalming chemical and its fluorescent dye, it never was proof positive that areas of the body beneath the skin were thoroughly embalmed.

In the wake of Hiroshima and Nagasaki and other major disasters such as airline crashes, earthquakes, mudslides, and building collapses, a search was instituted for some new means of quickly processing (preserving) huge numbers of dead. Over the years, different means of processing (preserving) the victims of such tragedies were devised, tested, and found unsuitable for various reasons. Experiments were conducted with processes using ultrasound, radiation, atomic bombardment, and ultracold. No process tried seemed to be capable of preserving a tremendous number of bodies in a brief period. The search continues!

Indisputably, the greatest change in embalming procedures began in the 1980s by the intervention of federal government agencies. The Federal Trade Commission (FTC) adopted rules concerning the necessity for embalming and the securing of consent for same. The Occupational Safety and Health Administration (OSHA) adopted rules relating to embalming procedures, funeral home personnel protection, and similar public health and hygienic measures. The Environmental Protection Agency (EPA) issued rules concerning the use and control of formaldehyde and chemicals used by embalmers.

Although it has been generally conceded that formaldehyde-based fluids performed well as preserving and fixing agents for the embalming process, chemical research for an improvement in embalming chemicals has always been active.

During the 1930s, Hilton Ira Jones of the Hizone Company performed extensive research on glyoxal, a chemical that seemed to display much promise for use in an embalming formula. World War II, however, reduced the available supply and thus the research in this direction.

Another chemical, glutaraldehyde, was thoroughly researched and developed into an embalming formula by the Champion Company. Several embalming fluid companies now have formulations that replace formaldehyde in embalming solutions. The concept for a computerized embalming machine, the Embalmatron, was initiated by Trinity Fluids, LLC to create a closed system of delivery for the chemical solution using a computer-based system. The closed delivery system would eliminate chemical fumes. The search has intensified to substitute formaldehyde with less hazardous options.

## PROFESSIONALISM IN EMBALMING

In many states, a single license to practice as a funeral director and embalmer is issued. The remaining states issue a separate license for embalming and a separate license for funeral directing. As a result, members of large funeral directors' state associations and trade associations such as the NFDA, International Order of the Golden Rule (OGR), International Cemetery, Cremation and Funeral Association (ICCFA), or Selected Funeral Directors Association include individuals who are both embalmers and funeral directors. Their educational and convention programs attempt to include both groups. However, in more recent years, programming emphasis has been placed on the subjects related to funeral directing.

Trade associations devoted solely to embalmers are very few in number. The oldest international association (and by far the largest with over 1300 members in Britain alone) is the British Institute of Embalmers (BIE) founded in 1927. It has 14 divisions; 9 divisions within England and Scotland, while other divisions include Ireland, Belgium, Australia, Overseas, and the latest the North American division established in 1994. In the United States, the Ohio Embalmers Association founded in 1931 is the oldest and one of the largest. The second oldest is the Academy of Graduate Embalmers in Georgia founded in 1955. The Michigan Embalmers Society was founded in 1991. In 2004, The American Society of Embalmers was established. These organizations provide educational programs for their members along with publications and Web sites with resources for the embalmer.

With many states beginning to require continuing education for licensees and with the increasing difficulty of the types of embalming cases being seen in preparation rooms around the country, there became the need for embalming seminars for mortuary school graduates.

The Dodge Seminars have been providing funeral directors and embalmers with educational seminars since the 1950s. With lectures and demonstrations by men like Ray Slocum, Louis Fitzpatrick, and other Dodge staff members, they have kept education as an important part of their mission. In 1921, the company began producing a house journal that published articles on various subjects on both embalming and funeral directing and continues today as *The Dodge Magazine*.

Vernie Fountain's Fountain National Academy in Springfield, Missouri, focuses on difficult case embalming. He brings in attendees from around the world for extended day preparation room sessions. In 2010, he organized the first international embalmers conference. *See History of Modern Restorative Art for further information.*

Since the Civil War period, the transportation of the deceased from the place of death back to their home has been on the increase. From the days when train transportation was the most common method of transportation within the United States to today when we transport remains around the world, embalming is the best way to preserve the deceased for this purpose. Traveling to foreign countries can take more than 14 days to accomplish due to individual foreign country laws. Many of these laws are outdated but still must be followed or risk having the deceased returned to the funeral director of shipping origin. One of the concerns that were observed here in the United States during the late 1940s and early 1950s was that a family that had a death away from home would be paying for services and merchandise they did not need or necessarily want. To transfer the deceased to their home, they would be purchasing caskets as a means to enclose the deceased during the transport period. The invention of the combination shipping air tray benefited both funeral service and families. This allowed protection of the deceased and the ability of the family to purchase the casket of their choice with the local funeral home. During this time frame, we begin to see the "shipping specialist" emerge. Either local funeral homes that would help to minimize the cost for the family and local funeral home or a company that would have a network of funeral homes that they worked with to affect the speedy and competent preparation of the deceased. The first of these was Inman Nationwide Shipping founded by Robert J. Inman of Cleveland, Ohio. Other companies had been formed but not to the extent that Mr. Inman had successfully created. He eventually expanded services into the international shipping arena as this need arose. Today, the shipping of human remains is done approximately 25 to 30,000 times per year. There are no firm statistics, but this is based on information from the major airlines that handle the majority of human remains shipments.

## DISTANCE OR WEB-BASED MORTUARY SCIENCE EDUCATION

In the mid-2000s, funeral service education became widely accessible through distance and web-based education. In 2007, the American Board of Funeral Service Education (ABFSE) received approval from the U.S. Department of Education to offer distance-learning education. The American Academy McAllister Institute (AAMI) was the first to initiate an online education program. Distance education is now a mainstay in the curriculum of funeral service education.

Of historical interest is a glance back to the early 1900s when both Dr. Auguste Renouard and Madame Lina Odou both offered correspondence courses. Madame Odou's advertised her correspondence course from 1903 to 1905 in the professional journals of the day for $35.00.

## EMBALMING PERSPECTIVES AROUND THE GLOBE

Embalming has been practiced in numerous countries around the world for years using different methods of preparation. Many embalming chemical companies in the United States are sponsoring seminars and providing training in those countries. In the past 10 years, a large number of embalmers from around the world have traveled to the United States for continued education and training. In turn, some of these embalmers have set out to introduce embalming education courses in their home countries. Below are updates of how some countries are addressing embalming education.

### Australia (and South East Asia)—Jan Field

For more than 20 years the Australian Institute of Embalmers has been an educational resource in the South Pacific and South Asia. Their website states, "The AIE, through its Council, negotiates with various agencies and authorities to ensure that only the finest practices are accepted and that professional status is recognized. The presence of the AIE has produced a culture in Australia where embalming is an accepted part of the funeral process." The British Institute of Embalmers has had a presence in this part of the world through their Australasian Division for more than a decade. Education is provided to members in Australia, New Zealand and Tasmania.

Both of AIE and BIE Australasian Division in collaboration with embalming chemical companies provide embalming and restorative art education multiple times throughout each year. These seminars draw attendees from many countries throughout the South Seas and South Asia.

In recent years, specialized hands-on restorative art seminars have provided additional tools to those who want to expand their knowledge and skills for those difficult trauma cases.

### Belgium and Europe—Alain Koninckx

In Europe, and more particularly in Belgium, embalming is a practice in full operation. It has long been marginal, and mainly used for repatriations or to solve sanitary problems, the presentation aspect has been unappreciated. Since the mid-2000s, I continue to emphasize the practice to funeral directors by highlighting the presentation aspect and the added value of an open casket viewing for the family. With this in mind, I am a teacher of embalming at state training centers for funeral directors. Where I try to change the mentality by advocating the open casket viewing, and for that the utility of embalming. This training attracts many young people wanting to optimize the presentation of the deceased.

In my early days, I was often confronted with heavy trauma cases, and I was helpless because of my lack of knowledge. I went to train with Vernie Fountain at the Fountain National Academy in Springfield, Missouri. And since then, I have been promoting facial reconstruction in Belgium and all over the world. For this I publish many works done in medical school (e.g., the use of fluorescein to inject bodies and better understand the RCI), and participate in many professional conferences around the world. I speak about it for other embalmers or emphasize the facial reconstruction with funeral directors who are not always informed that it is possible to present the deceased who have suffered major trauma.

It was quite natural in this context to create in 2013 a school of facial reconstruction and extreme cases: the European School of Embalming Skills, where we train embalmers from around the world in these techniques. The great satisfaction with this school is the return of our students who tell us they could present a severely traumatized deceased, something impossible before their training. With others, we try to have embalming recognized by our department to protect our art. I remain optimistic in the future because the new practitioner seems to have noble motives for serving families.

## Canada

Initial licensing requirements differ from province to province in Canada. Many of the provinces have mortuary science programs offered through local colleges. Many of these established embalming programs also offer continuing education once a student has completed a formal course. Additionally, the established funeral service association also offer continuing education programs that emphasize embalming. There are also a number of established programs that emphasize embalming education for difficult or trauma cases as well as advanced practice for restorative art. The goal of these programs is to bring state-of-the-art techniques to Canadian embalmers through classroom and hands-on education experiences.

## Ireland—Glyn Tallon

I feel it is all of our duty to give back to our communities and to provide support to those who need it, in whatever way we can, be that contribution big or small. Nurses, teachers, the shopkeeper at the corner shop; we all have our roles, our strengths, and weaknesses. For me, I saw and witnessed how death affected our families and our communities. I knew I had the ability to deal with death both physically and emotionally and saw the immense importance it played in the role of the Irish funeral and in our unique approach to death. To be able to give some sort of ease, some sort of comfort to those loved ones who are in grief or anguish, will remain the anchor for my entire work goals.

The value of the embalming process, to those who are bereaved is unquestionable for me; but I accredit working as an embalmer within the strict traditions of the Irish funeral and home wakes, as being an incredible motivator, in highlighting the immeasurable importance of the deceased.

Comments made, sometimes in jest, are frequently volunteered throughout the industry, how "the Irish sure know how to do a funeral" but for me, I believe there is huge testament to that statement. I personally believe that the greatest value of our Irish traditions; our need to see our loved one, bring our loved one's home; allows the grieving to act on our most fundamental psychological wants and needs. As humans, hurt and shocked and in pain, we need to see, to confront and to experience our loss. The Irish funeral may seem quite quick to other approaches, but it can be a very raw and intense experience for the bereaved.

Our loved ones can be removed from their homes or hospital beds mere hours from dying. It is not uncommon to be assisted by family members at any stage of this process. Families may often choose to accompany the funeral director back to premises where they understand their loved one will be prepared. On accounts some families have even waited outside during this time. The Irish accompany their dead, doing what they can, where they can at presentable stages; your importance will vary from the one to drop clothes to the funeral director, to those asked to make the sandwiches, but fundamentally, from the embalmer's perspective, the deceased is expected to be returned in timely fashions. At key services throughout the funeral process the deceased will be surrounded by friends and family, they may remain in their own homes or in repose at a local funeral home until the moment of final burial or cremation, with a daily stream of visitors in some cases 24 hours. This process may take place within 2–3 days.

The Irish embalmer works within tight schedules, with little room for error. Our deceased do not remain under our watchful eye for any more than a few hours before they are sent out to funeral directors or home to their own personal beds. Our work is vulnerable and exposed and it requires confidence in your skill to guarantee the work that you do, for sanitation and preservation as well as presentation, be thorough and sound. Having a loved one lie in repose in their home without the veil of the casket or a coffin, demands that the work you do, be to the best achievable standard.

Reconstruction work has not been an easy concept to introduce to Ireland. Requesting more time to work on the deceased initially concerned people, posing possible disruption to the typical time frame of our funerals and negotiations certainly had to be made to allow for the real value of reconstruction work to present itself. Over time the value of the work that you give to the community, becomes valuable to them and very slowly sought after. Small communities around Ireland remain intertwined and deeply rooted in our traditions. Though times modernize around us, the value of time spent mourning our loved ones remain an unchanging need with the people; it is a time to show support, to open your doors, to extend unquestionable aid, because we all experience death and in small towns and villages, a single loss can affect a multitude.

In the past "it's a closed coffin" spread on the lips about the industry and community, as a strong indication of how severe injuries may have been, an indication of the longitude of an illness and a general indication to all that the situation was most likely worse than what they could have imagined. It clouded the services and added more to the loss of the deceased. Personal requests to close a coffin and specify no viewing are 100% respected and honored, however as in life, death is not black and white and circumstances for the family to wish for a mere chance to say goodbye is often snatched from them.

The reconstruction services that I am able to offer our community has made possible what was previously deemed impossible. Cases of remains being out of doors, showing signs of animal interference, extreme cases of 42 days submerged in water, severe trauma from road traffic accidents, farming accidents, in many cases missing significant anatomical features altogether, the list is endless and though they require significant work, viewable remains are in fact achievable. Working within this, fast-paced, very tactile, very personal traditions of this country, sets huge responsibility on Irish embalmers. Irish embalmers work under immense pressure and in honesty, their work must leave the embalming room with the embalmer being confident that they have done all they can do to guarantee successful, sanitation, preservation, and presentation in mere hours. We do not have the luxury of other countries where we can check-in, in the morning to assess how the remains have changed or altered or take additional time to do small touch-ups. Our work must be presentable and with all precautions taken in a very small timeframe. Though the reconstruction work on many of the cases that come through my business are extreme in nature and will require significantly more work than the standard few hours, the pace is most certainly set by the waiting family. The grieving family are our business, our clients, the people we serve, and the ones to be considered as we do the work we do and here in Ireland they are the ultimate consideration when it comes to time. The family are, in so many cases, literally waiting to have their loved one returned. In many of my cases, this requires working throughout the night, to ensure the family may have their loved one returned in the early morning or afternoon. I am a firm believer that successful reconstruction work starts with thorough and precise embalming. Though cosmetic work will cover a multitude in the embalmers favor toward the end, in so many of my cases if the base canvas we are working on, is not a sound, well embalmed deceased, it will inevitably cause a domino effect that will be continuously problematic as the restoration continues. My emphasis in our college here in Navan is to establish very early on with my students that preservation is a fundamental that cannot be rushed or ignored. If my students can become confident that the deceased is well embalmed, then all the rest are skill sets that can be learned and perfected over their working careers.

To many in the profession, the concept of working long hours to slowly and tediously piece together what presents itself on my embalming table is dismissed and undervalued. They hold considerations of paying staff and delaying services above the value of 'the final goodbye'. The families I serve are the ultimate critics in my mind and over many years of service, it has become blatantly obvious by their comments, that the work that I do to restore their loved one, is not only well respected but now sought after. It is of value to them. They actively choose to allow for this time, in the hope of getting their goodbye. It is a complicated thing to put value on and in the end the only one who truly can, is the grieving family.

Death as a subject is examined and researched psychologically as much as it has been dissected anatomically and there are strong arguments that a chance to view your loved one and be granted a chance to say goodbye will not cure the loss but equip the bereaved with an understanding of the situation that aids them in continuing their grieving process in a healthier manner than those denied the chance. To be in a position to offer that chance to a family, even if the comfort were for one solitary individual, is an honor for me and a reason to constantly motivate myself to work hard and continually, at the work that I do.

From the perspective of the embalmer the longevity of your work, the sturdiness of your work, will always remain a priority and a concern during the time of repose, but the value of trying and attempting to restore a loved one so they can return to their family, resulting in a healthier way for the family to cope with their loss, should never be measured. Reconstruction work requires time. Repeat experience will allow you to become confident at your skills and to eventually become more confident and calculated in your decisions. Achieving ultimate perfection in reconstruction work is near impossible but it does not decrease the value of its impact. Identifiability offers a comfort to those who seek solace in a goodbye and any embalmer should work within the constraints of their capabilities to aim for their personal best, to achieve this. The families I work with work closely with me so a clear and transparent communication is established and we work together so they have an understanding on what I can work towards. When working through third parties this lack of unquestionable perfection as the end result, easily becomes a reason for some to deny a family the choice to decide if reconstruction would offer some comfort to them. Families are often denied their viewing because the deceased was deemed unviewable, by selective individuals and the very option was taken from them. Continued education on what is achievable and the importance of this work will hopefully result in families having more of a voice on their wishes and give them a chance to make decisions on the options available to them at this time.

While I continually aim to better my own education, I equally see that the real value for the education is to share it and spread it. When we aim to better each other's personal skills, we set a standard and it results in good work being done across our profession.

### South America—Camilio Andres Jaramillo

The origin of funeral service in Colombia and South America are very similar to those in the United States of America. Local carpenters and cabinet makers were appointed to make coffins upon request when someone in the comunity would pass away. Later on, they began to make extra coffins so they did not have make them in a rush. This began back in the mid 1800s when funeral homes in South America began to appear. During this time, embalming was not a common practice in South America.

There are a few instancies of medical embalmings performed for special cases but they were very rare in funeral practice in South America. Mexico, the Caribbean and Puerto Rico whose proximity with the United States, allowed them to have a closer relationship with embalming than the rest of South America that did not practice embalming at all.

Families would take care of their own dead. Women usually dressed the deceased and used flowers and essenses to mask any decomposition odors. It was believed that the smell of decomposition was a reliable indication that burial could be done with no risk of burying someone alive.

Funeral homes were more focused on selling and providing elaborate caskets, renting stands, furniture, and all the ítems necessary for a home wake. Providing quality monuments and marble headstones, even the use of horse drawn hearses was not as common until the beginning of the twentieth century. In many places people still prefer to carry caskets and coffins on their own shoulders.

The origins of embalming in South America begin with Jose Adán Rendon from Medellin, Colombia. Mr. Rendon attended Renouard's academy in New York in the late 1920s, it is believed he a close friend to the late Frank E. Campbell.

Funeraria Rendon in Medellin, mentions Campbell numerous times. Even famous Argentinian tango Singer Carlos Gardel's funeral was done by Mr. Rendon. The body was prepared and shipped by Frank E. Campbell to Argentina back in 1935.

Rendon Funeral Home was the first to open in Colombia back in 1870 and went closed back in 1974. Although Mr. Rendon was a qualified embalmer, he did any teaching. Some historians even say he seldom practiced embalming in Colombia, except for very special ship-out cases. Funeral practitioners when required to do any kind of "embalming" would simply hypodermically inject formalin and pack orifices with cotton. It is believed that there may have been attempted evisceration in some cases.

It was not only until 1967 that a funeral home was opened in Barranquilla, Colombia (Jardines del Recuerdo). This funeral home was operated by Americans. They brought American-trained embalmers and helped to train a few local morticians. The Americans went back to the home and a group of four local embalmers stayed on at the funeral home.

As time passed, those four embalmers moved to different firms and began showing their embalming techniques to local practitioners. Funeral homes did not have prep rooms, nor embalming equipment. These practitioners wanted to try embalming and had to adapt those techniques and instruments to whatever they had available. Preparations were made at home along with visitations for a long period of time. Today, very few places still do home preparations and wakes.

It was only until the late 1970s and 80s that a Colombian Funeral Home (San Vicente Funeral home) from Medellin regained interest in embalming and invited American and Puerto Rican embalmers to do in-house seminars for local practitioners. San Vicente also imported instruments, injecting machines and all the required equipment for home embalmings as well as prep room supplies. Soon after ALPAR (Latín American Association of Cemeteries and Funeral Homes) began doing embalming seminars for their associates.

Some of the embalmers that helped with the training were: Al Green and Mr. Albo (United States), Julio Lopez and Guadalupe Rivera (Puerto Rico), Mario Lacape (Guatemala) and Camilo A. Jaramillo (Colombia).

From these education events, embalming began to be a common practice in many Colombian funeral homes. The mentorship of American, Puerto Rican and Guatemalan licensed embalmers made it possible to have seminars and presentations, most of them held at San Vicente Funeral Home.

Back in 2001, the first program on embalming was officially opened at the Tecnologico de Antioquia, a four semester program focused on embalming and basic directing skills for practitioners. Before that, the Head of the Medical Examiner's office of Colombia had (and still has) a diploma program for embalmers that offers two 120-hour seminars a year.

Colombia does not require a license for practitioners but it is coming since a new law will be effective in the year 2020. It will govern all funeral homes, cemeteries, embalming, and crematory practitioners. The local government has also opened an embalming program for informal practitioners that want to be licensed in the near future. This program is exclusive for practitioners that are already working and find it difficult to attend college.

Now there is a large number of practitioners that are providing training for new embalmers all over South America but mainly in Colombia. Most of them have attended local schools or have attended numerous seminars that make embalming more wide spread in Colombia.

The advancements made in Colombia have echoed throughout South America, Brazil, Argentina, Ecuador, Bolivia, and Venezuela began implementing embalming after visiting and replicating the Colombian experience. Even Peru and Chile are now beginning to gain interest regarding embalming. There is still a long way to go for embalming in South America due to cultural issues, prices, and funeral customs. Embalming is not viewed as an important part of funeral practices. Yet some companies are beginning to slowly implement it. South America has a very strong European influence in funeral service traditions found mainly in Spain, Italy, and Portugal. Embalming is still not practiced very frequently in these countries.

It is astonishing what has been achieved in the embalming field in nearly 5000 years of growth of knowledge, skill, and experience. Naturally, what the future holds is unknown, but those working in the field feel it will be as exciting and rewarding as the past millennia.

## BIBLIOGRAPHY

Beverly R. *History of Virginia.* 1922:185.

McClelland EH. *Bibliography on Embalming.* New York: National Association of Mortuary Science, 1949. [Mimeographed copy, limited to 100 copies]

McCurdy CW. *Embalming and Embalming Fluids—With Bibliography of Embalming.* Wooster, OH: Herald Printing, 1896.

Oatfield H. *Literature of the Chemical Periphery—Embalming.* Advances in Chemistry Series, No. 16. Washington, DC: American Chemical Society. [A key to pharmaceutical and medicinal chemistry literature]

Pinkerton J. *Collection of Voyages,* Vol. 13, 1812.

*Surgeon General's Catalogue.* Washington, DC: U.S. Army, 1883–1884.

Townshend J. *Grave Literature.* New York (private collection), 1887. [A catalogue of some books relating to the disposal of bodies and perpetuating the memories of the dead]

### Egypt

Aliki. *Mummies Made in Egypt.* New York: Thomas J. Crowell, 1979.

Arcieri GP. *Note E Ricordi—Sulla Preservatione Del Corppo Umano,* No. 1. Florence, Italy: Rivista Di Storia Delle Scienze Medicine E Naturoli, 1956.

Bardeen CR. Anatomy in America. *Bulletin of University of Wisconsin* September 1905, No. 115.

Brier B, Wade RS. The use of natron in human mummification: A modern experiment. *ZAS,* No. 124, 1997.

Brier B, Wade RS, Zimmerman MR. Brief communication: Twentieth-century replication of an Egyptian mummy: Implications of paleopathology. *American Journal of Physical Anthropology* 1998;107.

Budge EAW. *The Mummy.* Cambridge, UK: Cambridge University Press, 1893.

Choulant L. *History and Bibliography of Anatomical Illustration.* New York, 1962. [Reprint]

David AR, ed. *Manchester Museum Mummy Project.* Manchester, UK: Maney and Sons, 1979.

Harris JE, Weeks KR. *X-Raying the Pharaohs.* New York: Charles Scribner's Sons, 1973.

Hemneter E. *Embalming in Ancient Egypt. Ciba Symposia;* Vol. 1, No. 10. Summit, NJ: Ciba Pharmaceuticals, January 1940.

Herodotus. *History.* Rawlinson G, trans. New York: Dial and Tudor Presses, 1928.

Liebling R, et al. *Time Line of Culture in the Nile Valley and Its Relationship to Other Countries.* New York: Metropolitan Museum of Art, 1978.

Martin RA. *Mummies.* Anthropology Leaflet No. 36. Chicago: Chicago Natural History Museum Press, 1945.

Mendelsohn S. *Embalming.* Ciba Symposia, Vol. 6, No. 2. Summit, NJ: Ciba Pharmaceuticals, May 1944.

Moodie RL. *Anthropology Memoir, Vol. III: Roentgenologic Studies of Egyptian and Peruvian Mummies.* Chicago: Field Museum Press, 1931.

Pettigrew TJ. *History of Egyptian Mummies.* London: Long-man, Rees, 1834.

Piombino-Mascali D. *Il Maestro del Sonno Eterno.* La Zisa, Palermo, 2009.

Piombino-Mascali D, Williams, MJ. Rosalia Lombardo and her Master Embalmer. *The Director* July 2009.

Pons A. *Les Origines de L'Embaumement et L'Egypte Predynastique.* Montpelier, France: Imprimerie Grollier, 1910.

Smith GE, Dawson WR. *Egyptian Mummies.* New York: Dial Press, 1924.

Steuer RO, Saunders JB de CM. *Ancient Egyptian and Indian Medicine.* Berkeley–Los Angeles: University of California Press, 1959.

Touchette N. MUMAB, The Making of a Modern Mummy. *ChemMatters* February 1996.

Wade RS. Medical mummies: The history of the Burns Collection. *The Anatomical Record,* 1998.

## Peru*

Garcillaso de la Vega. *Royal Commentaries of Peru.* Rycant P, trans. London, 1688.

Prescott WH. *History of the Conquest of Peru,* 2 vols. Philadelphia: J.B. Lippincott, 1882.

Rivero ME, Von Tschudi JJ. *Peruvian Antiquities.* Hawks FL, trans. New York: George Putnam, 1853.

Von Hagen VW. *Realm of the Incas.* New York: New American Library of World Literature, 1957.

## Alaska and Aleutian Islands

Quimby GI. *Aleutian Islanders.* Anthropology Leaflet, No. 35. Chicago: Natural History Museum, 1944.

## North American Indians

Yarrow HC. *Study of Mortuary Customs among the North American Indians.* Washington, DC: U.S. Government Printing Office, 1880.

## Ecuador—Jivaro Indians

Cottlow LN. *Amazon Head Hunters.* New York: Signet. Book/Henry Holt, 1953.

Flornoy B. *Jivaro.* New York: Library Publishers, 1954.

## Canary Islands

De Espinosa A. *The Guanches of Tenerife.* London: Hakluyt Society, 1907.

Hooton EA. *The Ancient Inhabitants of the Canary Islands.* Harvard African Studies, Vol. II. Cambridge, MA: Harvard University Press, 1925.

## Europe (Early Period)

Bradford CA. *Heart Burial.* London: Allen & Unwin, 1933.

Castiglioni A, Robinson V. *The Anatomical Theater.* Ciba Symposia, Vol. 3, No. 4. Summit, NJ: Ciba Pharmaceuticals, May 1941.

Clauderus G. *Methodus Balsamundi Corpora Humane Aliaque Majora sine Evisceratione et Sectione Hucusque Solita.* Altenberg, Germany: G. Richterum, 1679.

De Villihardouin G, DeJoinville J. *Memoirs of the Crusades.* New York: E. P. Dutton, 1938.

Dionis M. *Cours D'Operations de Chirurqie.* Paris: d'Houry, 1746.

Dobson J. Some eighteenth century experiments in embalming. *Journal of the History of Medicine* 1953.

Garrison FH. *Introduction to the History of Medicine.* Philadelphia, 1929.

Greenhill T. *Nekrokadeia—Or the Art of Embalming.* London: printed for the author; 1705.

Guichard C. *Des Funerailles et diverses Manieres.* Lyon, France: D'ensevelir, 1582.

Guichard C. *Funerailles.* Lyon, France: Jean de Tovrnes, 1581.

Guybert P. The charitable physitian showing the manner to embalm a dead corpse. In *The Charitable Physitian.* London: Thomas Harper Printer, 1639.

Paré A. *How to Make Reports and to Embalm the Dead* (translated). London: Cotes & Young, 1634.

Pilcher LS. The Mondino myth (reprint). *Medical Library and History Journal* 1906;4(4, December).

The art and science of embalming dead bodies. In Offen-bach P, M.D. *A New Medical Treatise.* Frankfort: Zacharian Palthenium, 1605. [Taken from the 29th book of Peter Forestus and translated from the Latin into German]

Treece H. *The Crusades.* New York: Random House, 1962.

Walsh JJ. *The Popes and Science.* New York: Fordham University Press, 1908.

Walsh JJ. *The 13th—Greatest of Centuries.* New York: Catholic Summer School Press, 1907.

Wellcome HS. *The Evolution of Antiseptic Surgery.* London: Burroughs Wellcome, 1910.

Young S. *The Annals of the Barber Surgeons of London.* London: Blades East & Blades, 1890.

## Europe (Late Period)

Bailey JB. *The Diary of a Resurrectionist 1811–1812.* London: Swan-Sonnenschein, 1896.

Ball JM. *The Sack em Up Men.* London: Oliver & Boyd, 1928.

Bayle DC. *L'Embaumement.* Paris: Adrien Delahaye, 1873.

Blanchard S. *Anatomia Reformata—Balsamatione, Novus Methodus.* Leiden: Boutesteyn & Lughtmans, 1687.

Cole FJ. *A History of Comparative Anatomy.* London: MacMillan, 1944.

Coliez A. *Conservation Artificielle des Corps.* Paris: Amedee Legrand, 1927.

Cope Z. *The History of the Royal College of Surgeons.* Spring-field, IL: Charles C. Thomas, 1959.

Dawson WR. Life and times of Thomas J. Pettigrew. *Med Life* (3 issues) 1931;38(1–3, January–February–March).

DeLint JG. *Atlas of the History of Medicine,* Vol. I. London: H. K. Lewis, 1926.

Eriksson R, ed., trans. *Andreas Vesalius 1st Public Anatomy at Bologna—1540.* Uppsala, Sweden: Almquist & Wikselle, 1959.

Gannal JN. *Histoire des Embaumements.* Paris: Ferra Librairie, 1838.

Gannal JN. Harlan R, trans. *History of Embalming.* Philadelphia: Judah Dobson, 1840.

Gerlt-Wernich-Hirsch. *Biographisches Lexikon Der Herrvor-ragenden Arzte Aller Zeiten und Volker.* Berlin: Urban & Schwarzenberg, 1932.

Laskowski S. *L'Embaumement, la conservatione des Sujets et les Preparations Anatomiques.* Geneva: H. Georg, 1886.

Mann G. The anatomical collections of Fredrick Ruysch at Leningrad. *Bull Cleve Med Library* 1964;11 (1, January).

---

*Also see Moodie in list under Egypt.

Nordenskiold E. *The History of Biology.* New York: Tudor, 1928.

Paget S. *John Hunter.* London: T. Fisher University, 1898.

Peachy GC. *The Homes of Hunter in London.* London: Bailliere, Tindall & Cox, 1928.

Pettigrew JT. Fredrick Ruysch. In *Pettigrew's Medical Portrait Gallery.* London: Whitaker, 1840.

Ramazzini B. *De Morbio Artificum* (2nd ed., 1713). *Diseases of Workers.* Wright WC, trans. New York: Hafner, 1964.

Richardson BW. The art of embalming. In *Wood's Medical and Surgical Monographs*, Vol. III. New York: 1889.

Sigerist HE. *The Great Doctors.* Garden City, NY: Doubleday; 1958.

Singer C. *Studies in the History and Method of Science,* Vol I.—1917, Vol II.—1921. Oxford, England: Clarendon Press.

Sucquet JP. *De L'embaumement et des conservation pour l'etude de l'anatomie.* Paris: Adrien Delahaye, 1872.

Sucquet JP. *Traits du visage dans l'embaumement.* Paris: Adrien Delahaye, 1862.

## United States

Barnes CL. *The Art and Science of Embalming.* Chicago: Trade Periodical, 1905.

Clarke CH. *Practical Embalming.* Cincinnati, OH: C. H. Clarke, 1917.

Clarke JH. Reminiscences of Early Embalming. *The Sunnyside,* 1917.

Crane EH. *Manual of Instructions to Undertakers,* 8th ed. Kalamazoo, MI: Kalamazoo, 1888.

Dodge AJ. *The Practical Embalmer.* Boston: A. Johnson Dodge, 1908.

Eckels HS. *Practical Embalmer.* Philadelphia: H. S. Eckels Co., 1903.

Espy JB. *Espy's Embalmer.* Springfield, OH: Espy Fluid Co., 1895.

The Faculty of the Cincinnati School for Embalming. In Lukens CM, Clarke JH. *Textbook on Embalming.* Springfield, OH: Limbocker, 1883.

Gallagher T. The body snatchers. *American Heritage* June 1967.

Johnson EC. Civil war embalming. *Funeral Directors Rev* June–July–August 1965.

Johnson EC, Johnson GR. A Civil War Embalming Surgeon—the story of Dr. Daniel H. Prunk. *The Director* (NFDA publication) January 1970.

Johnson EC, Johnson GR. *Alone in His Glory.* Unpublished manuscript, Civil War Mortuary Practices.

Johnson EC, Johnson GR. *Prince Greer—America's First Negro Embalmer.* Liaison Bulletin, International Federation of Thanatopractic Association, Paris, April 1973.

Johnson EC, Johnson GR. The undertakers manual. *Canadian Funeral News* July 1980.

Johnson EC, Johnson GR, Johnson M. Dr. Thomas Holmes—pioneer embalmer. *American Funeral Director* July–August 1984.

Johnson EC, Johnson GR, Johnson WM. Dr. Renouard's role in embalming history. *American Funeral Director* August 1987.

Johnson EC, Johnson GR, Johnson WM. History of modern restorative art. *American Funeral Director* January–April 1988.

Johnson EC, Johnson GR, Johnson WM. The trial, execution and embalming of two Civil War soldiers. *American Funeral Director* December 1986.

Johnson EC, Johnson M. H. Rhodes—conscientious caretaker of Arlington National Cemetery. *American Funeral Director* January 1984.

Johnson M. A historic precedent to the FTC rules of 1977 (Civil War licensing for embalmer requirements). *NFDA Bulletin* 1979.

Johnson M, Lena R. Simmons—The grand dame of early embalmers. *American Funeral Director* January 1977.

Johnson M, Lina D. Odou—Embalmer. July 1977.

Keen WW. *Addresses and Other Papers.* Philadelphia: Saunders, 1905.

Mendelsohn S. *Embalming Fluids.* New York: Chemical Publishing, 1940.

Mills and Lacey Mfg. Co. *Practical Directions for Embalming the Dead.* Grand Rapids, MI: Stevens, Cornell and Dean, 1881. [No author stated]

Myers E. *Champion Textbook on Embalming.* Springfield, OH: Champion Chemical Co., 1908.

Renouard A. *Undertakers Manual.* Rochester, NY: A. Nirdlinger, 1878.

Renouard CA, ed. *Taylor's Art of Embalming.* New York: H. E. Taylor, 1903.

Samson H, Crane ON, Perrigo AB, et al. *Pharmaceutical, Anatomical and Chemical Lexicon.* Chicago: Donohue & Henneberry, 1886. (The NFDA official textbook.)

Strub CA, Frederick LG. *The Principles and Practice of Embalming,* 4th ed. Dallas, TX: L. G. Frederick, 1986.

Sullivan FA. *Practical Embalming.* Boston: Egyptian Chemical Co., 1887.

Swason, James. *Bloody Crimes: The Chase for Jefferson Davis and the Death Pageant for Lincoln's Corpse.* Harper Collins, 2010.

https://www.nationalgeographic.com/magazine/2019/05/leonardo-da-vinci-artistic-brilliance-endures-500-years-after-death/.

War Department. General Order 75, September 11, 1861.

War Department. General Order 33, April 3, 1862.

War Department. General Order 39, March 15, 1865.

Wightman SK. In search of my son (Civil War). *American Heritage* February 1963.

## International Embalming Associations

| | |
|---|---|
| Australian Institute of Embalmers | www.aieptyltd.org/ |
| British Institute of Embalmers | www.bioe.co.uk |
| European Association of Embalmers | http://europeanembalmers.eu/ |
| European School of Embalming Skills | http://eses.be/english.html |

# PART III

## History of Modern Restorative Art

Edward C. Johnson, Gail R. Johnson, and Melissa J. Williams

The reader is encouraged to revisit the section on Egyptian embalming procedures, entitled Ancient Restorative Art, found in the preceding section of this text. Virtually all documented reports of embalming in the anatomical or middle period in Europe included the practice of enclosing the preserved body within a metal-lined, hermetically sealed coffin, which precluded viewing. To satisfy some medieval customs relating to funeral practices and chivalry, an imago or effigy of the decedent was created by preparing a death mask as the basis for the head. The features were painted to closely resemble the normal lifelike appearance, and effigies were often adorned with a wig. The completed head was attached to a torso, complete with arms and legs, proportional to the life size of the decedent. The effigy was dressed in the clothing or armor of the decedent and placed on the coffin containing the corpse, where it remained during the entire period preceding actual interment (**Fig. 1**).

A recent discovery suggests that in the early 1900s, there was a concern for the appearance of the deceased in Europe. Alfredo Salafia, a prolific embalmer from Palermo, Italy, describes his attention to former Italian Premier, Francesco Crispi, who died in Naples. Crispi was to be returned to Palermo and was unsuccessfully embalmed by another practitioner. Salafia reembalmed the body (possibly the first indication that this is a successful procedure) and replaced the eyes with glass eyeballs, reattached the hair and beard that had fallen out, and filled out the facial features with injections of paraffin to "regain the form and the lost volume."

During the U.S. Civil War, a few documents indicated that some effort was made to repair traumatic injuries. One such document in the Frank Hutton collection was a letter from the family of a Union Army soldier who was embalmed and sent home for burial. The family wrote in their letter to Hutton that the corpse "looked pretty good for being dragged by mules."

By and large, however, it can be stated without fear of contradiction that very little of what is referred to today as restorative art was practiced until the second decade of the twentieth century. There were exceptions occasionally, such as the treatment of the anarchist bomber's suicide in Chicago briefly described in the section on Felix Aloysius Sullivan (see the preceding section). Joseph H. Clarke briefly mentions the treatment of a tumor case in his book *Reminiscences of Early Embalming*.

What is termed restorative art today represents the greatest remaining challenge to the skill, the ability to improvise, and the courage of the practicing embalmer. It is the last frontier and poses problems to test those who choose to grapple with its manifest difficulties. Formerly known most commonly by several popular terms such as plastic surgery, demisurgery, and dermasurgery, it is today most commonly referred to as restorative art.

The term *restorative art*, not adopted until the early 1930s, is in reality a poorly contrived label for specialized postmortem treatment accorded those dying of trauma or debilitating disease, the practice of which is most often believed to have originated entirely in the United States in recent years. Such a premise is false inasmuch as the practice of restorative art is dependent on and inseparable from the embalming procedure. Thus, one realizes that restorative art has been practiced from the origin of embalming in Egypt and so it was (**Fig. 2**).

The year 1912 marks the establishment of the modern era of what is today known as restorative art. The first articles appeared in the April 19, 1912, issue of *The Sunnyside*. *Demisurgery*, termed by its founder, was "the art of building or creating parts of the body which have been destroyed by accident, disease, decomposition or discoloration, and making the body perfectly natural and life-like."

The science of restorative art as known today was founded by one man, Joel E. Crandall, then an embalmer in New York City. Although many others made important contributions to this science through the years, no other one person can claim the honor of stimulating the interest of fellow embalmers in this most difficult technical subject area.

An editorial in the April 19, 1912, issue of *The Sunnyside* stated that "the photographs of before and after appearance of a mutilated body show what can and should be done. The originator of the new art of demisurgery is Joel E. Crandall of New York City and his first article on the new technique appears in the pages of this issue of *The Sunnyside* " (**Fig. 3**).

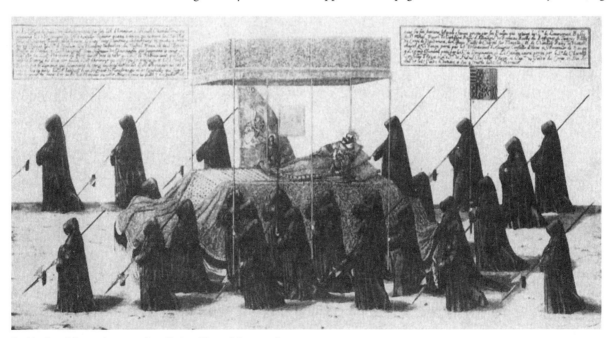

**Figure 1.** Medieval funeral procession. Note effigy of deceased.

**388** Embalming: History, Theory, and Practice

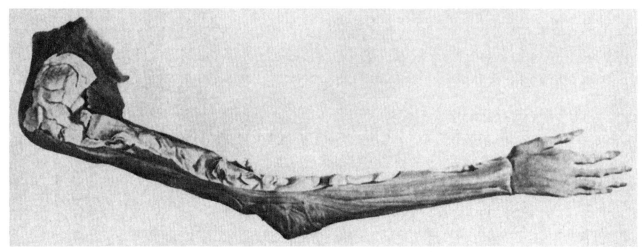

**Figure 2.** Arm of a mummy of the Egypt's twenty-first dynasty, showing the packing material.

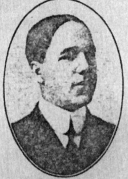

**Figure 3.** Crandall's advertisement for his services.

Howard S. Eckels in a letter published in the May 14, 1914, issue of *The Sunnyside*, stating that the science of demisurgery was indeed founded by Joel E. Crandall, made an early acknowledgment of Crandall's primacy in the field.

A. Johnson Dodge, quoted in the June 1, 1917, issue of *The Casket*, states:

> How to care for mutilated or postmortem cases, or bodies which from any cause have become unsightly and make them presentable, should constitute a part of the education of the embalmer. Thorough instruction in this difficult part of the art should be given by the instructors in our schools. But this part of the work requires special experience and some study either to practice or teach it successfully. It was first taught as a specialty by Mr. Joel E. Crandall of New York City, and to him belongs the credit of introducing it. We think Mr. Crandall is the only person who has attained any great degree of success in the practice of this art, and would recommend the student who wishes to attain a high degree of proficiency in this part of his profession to apply to Mr. Crandall for instruction, as he appears to be the only known person really competent to teach it.

Joel E. Crandall (1878–1942) was born on September 16, 1878, in Whitesville, New York. Approximately at 20 years of age, he began working for a New York City undertaker. Deeply interested in embalming and becoming increasingly skillful, his services were much in demand and he was employed by both Frank E. Campbell and Stephen Merritt undertaking establishments as well as the National Casket Company.

Writing in 1912 about his efforts to repair mutilated cases, he stated that he had studied the problems over a period of 10 years. His early efforts to use conventional materials such as plaster of paris were abandoned for any use except as an interior deep filler in contact with bone. He formulated covering cosmetics and a waxlike putty to fill in missing or damaged areas.

His earliest experiments were on severely mutilated bodies that neither the family nor the undertaker believed could be restored to viewability. Little by little, over the years, by trial and error, he developed a successful system for treatment of mutilated cases that eventually embodied most present-day principles or techniques.

Among the requirements Crandall advocated were a recent photograph of the decedent as a reference for the restoration, hardening of the soft tissues of the face as a prerequisite to demisurgery, and enough working time to carry out the entire treatment. Crandall also made the earliest mention of the use of "concealed stitches" to close lacerations and "corrective surgery" to remove remnants of features or tissue impossible to incorporate into the restoration. For his early research, he made use of plaster life-size heads that he mutilated and repaired: a procedure that was eventually adopted in one form or another by most embalming schools for laboratory practice and is generally used to this day.

Crandall began his career in demisurgery by offering his services anywhere within a 400-mile radius of New York City. Gradually, by demand, he was compelled to offer instruction in demisurgery. Each class was limited to 25 students for a 1-month period of instruction.

About the same time, he manufactured and sold the first demisurgical grip containing all required instruments, cosmetics, brushes, prefabricated mustaches and eyelashes, and preformed facial features of wax.

The use of prefabricated features as a base for individual modification of the decedent's facial topography enabled the unskilled or untrained embalmer to perform a reasonable restoration that is otherwise impossible. Crandall's brilliant concept was to be duplicated by others a number of times over the ensuing years.

A report of a restoration in 1924 mentions the use of prefabricated eyes and nose. The manufacturer of the parts, William Collier of New York City, advertised a kit containing prefabricated features in 1929 and patented the same in 1931. The Eckels Company of Philadelphia offered a similar kit in October of 1930 (**Fig. 4**), as did the Paasche Airbrush Company of Chicago in 1936. An interesting improvement on prefabricated features was developed by a dental plastic surgeon named C. J. Speas, who taught restorative art at Gupton-Jones College of Mortuary Science in Nashville, Tennessee, in the late 1940s. The basic concept was the "family resemblance theory," that is, members of the same family frequently resemble one another very closely. Thus, for example, when a nose is destroyed, a mold is made of the nose of a family member most closely resembling the decedent, cast in wax, and fitted into the decedent's face. Thus, a custom-made prefabrication is created.

Crandall purchased the Clerihew Undertaking Company located at 133 Broadway, Paterson, New Jersey, in 1913, and continued to maintain premises in New York City for his demisurgical supply company and school. Crandall must have written at some length on the subject of demisurgery, because *The Funeral Director's Encyclopedia*, a proposed three-volume work, each volume supposed to contain about 600 pages, was described in *The Sunnyside* in 1916 as having 100 pages on the art of demisurgery by Joel E. Crandall. No copies of this three-volume encyclopedia are known to exist, and it is suspected that it was never published. The 100 pages on demisurgery referred to were most likely the basic lectures by Crandall in the resident course of instruction at the Demisurgical Institute of New York and the teaching text in his correspondence course in 1918 (**Fig. 5**).

The greatest impact of Crandall's influence on the embalmers of America resulted from his published photographs of mutilated cases taken before and after treatment, most of which were extremely difficult to restore even by today's standards. His work was exceptionally well done and was an inspiration to embalmers who desired to improve their skills, for he showed and proved that difficult cases could be restored to a viewable condition.

The effect of Crandall's announcement of the founding of the art of demisurgery on the embalming schools of the country varied. Some heads of schools such as Robbins of Boston, Charles O. Dhonau of Cincinnati, and Thorton Barnes of New York were rather vocal in their protest concerning Crandall's claim that he was the founder of the science (**Fig. 6**). All three claimed that their schools had taught the subject for years, although in truth, no mention of the matter in advertising nor listing of the subject matter in the school curricula is noted prior

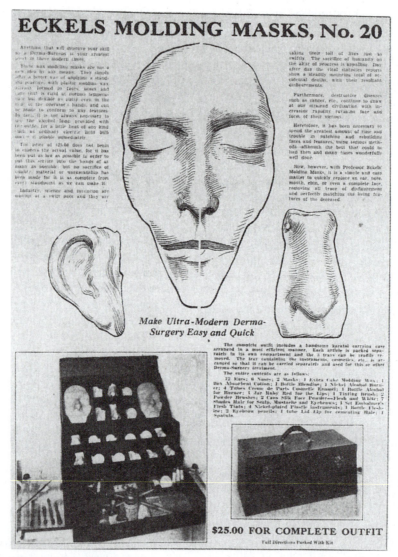

**Figure 4.** Advertisement for Eckels molding masks.

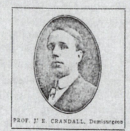

**Figure 5.** Copy of the first ad for demisurgery in 1918.

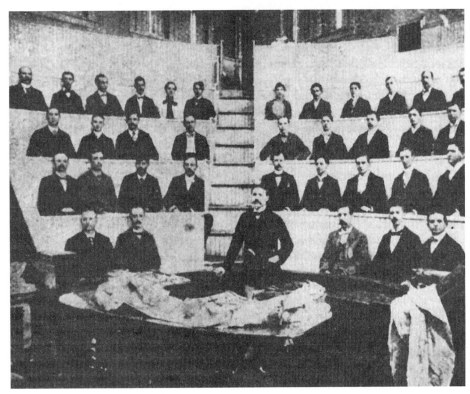

**Figure 6.** Carl L. Barnes (center) giving a demonstration in the Cook County Morgue, contiguous to the Barnes College building.

to April 1912. Barnes Schools began to advertise the teaching of DeMort-Ology, and the Cincinnati School added a course in demisurgery, whereas Robbins stated that his school taught artistic embalming, decoloration, and postmortem surgery. C. A. Renouard stated that he neither taught nor recommended the use of cosmetics and, further, that much of demisurgery was unnecessary and unwelcome. Before his death, in 1953, Renouard was to reverse his opinion to the extent of even providing special short-term courses in restorative art.

Dhonau additionally accused Crandall of publishing retouched photographs of his restored cases. This so incensed Crandall that he secured affidavits from everyone concerned—the undertaker, the photographer, lawyers, and family representatives, who attested to the authenticity of his work as represented by the case photographs.

The interest in the new art of demisurgery was immediate and has continued to the present day. The professional journals increasingly carried both photographs and case reports of successful treatment of mutilated cases, while advertisements multiplied for cosmetics, instruments, and demisurgical materials.

Among the cases Crandall treated was the famous Colonel Jacob Astor, who died at sea in 1912 as a passenger on the *Titanic*. His body, like hundreds of others, was taken from the sea near the site of the sinking and transported to Halifax, Nova Scotia, and from there returned to New York City for burial. Crandall was called by the New York undertaker in charge to treat Astor's badly discolored face. By means of Crandall's cosmetic skill, the casket was open for viewing of the body as it lay in state at the Astor estate near Rhinebeck, New York.

The February 1917 issue of *The Sunnyside* carried a notice that Crandall had taken motion pictures of a number of his demisurgical cases and that the films would be available for teaching purposes and presentations at conventions. Historically, this is the first known recording of any restorative procedures in motion pictures.

By 1918, the effect of World War I on the funeral profession was becoming evident and Crandall was interviewed by *The Sunnyside* for his views on the application of demisurgery to U.S. war casualties. He was most forthright in his conviction that all our war dead should be embalmed shortly after death and restored later at a convenient time and place.

From 1923 onward, however, Crandall faded in national mention, although he continued to operate his Paterson, New Jersey, funeral home until his death on July 19, 1942.

Joel E. Crandall demonstrated that any case, no matter how badly mutilated, could be restored to viewability. Furthermore, he devised not only the materials for his newly created science of demisurgery but also the technical instructions to accomplish this new skill.

All practicing embalmers owe a debt of gratitude to Joel E. Crandall, demisurgeon and founder of demisurgery, known today as restorative art.

The sudden and unforeseen arrival of Joel E. Crandall on the educational scene as the founder of the new art of demisurgery created the problem of partial loss of educational leadership for the American embalming schools. Recovering quickly from this threat, most schools began to teach the subject, although some, out of pride or vanity, refused to give the new art Crandall's title of demisurgery.

The immediate exception was Cincinnati College, which called the subject demisurgery but insisted that the subject had been taught there for years. Eckels College used the term "demisurgery" and acknowledged Crandall as the founder. Boston College called the course "postmortem surgery and the art of decoloration," and the Barnes School dubbed it DerMort-Ology *and* dermasurgery. An article describing Albert Worsham's demonstration of demisurgery calls it *plastic work*. The terms "dermasurgery" and "plastic surgery" also were noted as descriptive titles for the art, although one of the most original titles was used in 1917 by the New York School of Embalming (formerly Barnes School), which advertised derma sculpture taught by a sculptor and demisurgery taught by an embalmer. An advertisement for Dermatol Cosmetics in 1913 stated that it was not necessary to go to school to learn demisurgery or cosmetic application as everything one needed to know was in the pamphlet wrapped around each jar of cosmetics.

From 1912 onward, the pages of our professional journals disclose early contributions to the science of what today is termed restorative art. More and more advertisements are seen for cosmetics, demisurgery kits, and equipment (**Fig. 7**). Before-and-after case photos, pioneered by Crandall, appeared with some frequency in product advertisements as well as in articles. Demonstration of demisurgery at meetings and conventions became every bit as popular and as well attended as embalming demonstrations had been 30 years earlier.

Many prominent teachers and heads of embalming colleges wrote about the "new art." Some made first mention of standard basic procedures or techniques still employed today. Others advanced practices that were proven later to have little real value; for example, Robbins, in 1912, advocated the grafting of skin from another area of the body to replace damaged skin on the head. Such procedures were seldom very successful.

In 1912, Robbins, together with Lena Simmons, mentioned invisible or blind stitching (subcutaneous sutures), and C. O. Dhonau in the same year recommended baseball stitching with wax covering and concealing the sutured area, a rather unsatisfactory technique. Razorless shaving cream (a depilatory) made a brief but unsuccessful appearance in 1914, as it had a number of times since then.

Basic principles of demisurgery practice, such as using very concentrated fluid to produce firm tissue as ideal for final restoration and performing basic restoration to a near-normal anatomical relationship prior to arterial injection, were reiterated by C. O. Dhonau, Robbins, Worsham, Lena Simmons, and others. Some recommended removal of tumors and other surgical procedures prior to embalming, but Worsham and most modern authorities recommended that this be done after arterial injection. Most early authorities agreed that it was necessary to wait between completion of the arterial treatment and the final application of wax and cosmetics. Most recommended a minimum of 6 to 10 hours' time-lapse to ensure drying and halting of leakage from torn tissues.

In 1915, Worsham mentioned using cotton and collodion as a cavity filler to within one-sixteenth of an inch of the normal surface and then covering this surface with wax. He also used the cotton and collodion to form such basic features as lips, ears, nose, and eyelids.

Dhonau, writing at some length on demisurgery in 1915, called attention to the individuality of the human face, the differences in the lateral halves, as well as cosmetic skin variations. His suggestion, noted for the first time, to do the "work in the same light as that in which the body will rest until its final disposition," is still heeded today. In 1915, he demonstrated modeling of the facial features on a plaster skull, a technique that is today fairly standard throughout the schools for the teaching of restorative art.

One of the more dramatic demisurgical cases of the era was that treated by Worsham in Chicago in mid-1917. A lion tamer was attacked, mangled, and killed while performing in the lions' cage. A Chicago undertaker, Lafayette C. Ball, who was present at the place of attack, ran to his nearby funeral home, secured several bottles of formalin-based cavity fluid, returned to the circus cage, and poured the contents of the bottles over the dead lion tamer's torn body. This ingenious technique stopped the lions from further mangling the body and permitted the circus personnel to retrieve it. Worsham, called on to prepare the body, was confronted with the need to replace both ears, much of the face, and both arms and to close the torn open abdomen from which some viscera had been devoured. Before-and-after photos disclose a reasonable restoration.

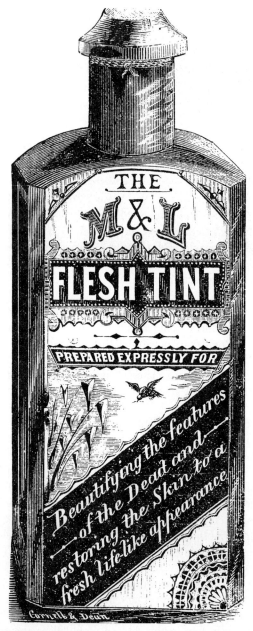

**Figure 7.** This preparation, although not a preservative, is a valuable aid to the embalmer's art.

Practicing embalmers were stimulated to try to repair difficult cases too. *The Sunnyside* issue of September 15, 1914, published a story and before-and-after photos of two cases, a murder and suicide by shotgun. In both cases, the skulls had been shattered by a 16-gauge shotgun. Mr. and Mrs. G. A. Rousevell of Lead, South Dakota, restored the bodies to a virtually normal appearance.

In 1917, C. O. Dhonau announced a new technique for treating swollen, blackened eyes. He incised the underside of the affected lid or lids, pressed out the accumulated blood and serum, and then applied 50% phenol solution to shrink and bleach the area.

At this time, the schools, which conducted courses of instruction of quite varying lengths averaging 3 months' duration at most, allotted some instruction time to demisurgery. Some schools scheduled regular periods in the laboratory for learning to form facial features in wax or clay on a plaster skull. Unique among these courses was that taught by Worsham, whose class in demisurgery was most often given at the end of the entire course of instruction. By the 1930s, it amounted to 25–40 total hours of laboratory work. The actual practice was carried out on mutilated human heads leftover from the anatomy dissection classes. The heads were stored in preservative fluid between class sessions and were, of course, rather wet, distorted, and chemically malodorous. The actual practice, however, was realistic, as all suturing, cavity filling, feature forming, and cosmetizing were practiced just as on an actual case.

In 1948, at the Postgraduate Institute of Restorative Art of Chicago, the laboratory teaching system was modified by the recreation of dozens of mutilated heads in plastic and rubber, which permitted suturing, waxing, and cosmetizing. The school was headed by Dean Edward C. Johnson.

Before-and-after photos of a case handled by the faculty and students of the Simmons School in 1921 indicate good results. In 1924, Cincinnati College featured its postmortem plastic surgery laboratory in an advertisement for the first time. In 1926, Dhonau criticized fluid manufacturers for issuing diplomas in demisurgery to those in attendance at their free clinics. This was a throwback to 35 years earlier when fluid manufacturers were criticized for issuing diplomas to those attending their embalming clinics.

Virtually every issue of *Casket and Sunnyside* during the 1920s carried at least one feature article about demisurgery, whether a case history, before-and-after photos, new products for the demisurgeon, or editorial praise and commendation for the procedure. In 1925, an advertisement appeared announcing that Clyde E. Richardson of Paterson, New Jersey, was available for dermasurgical cases. It is believed that he was trained by Joel E. Crandall. The April 1, 1925, issue of *Casket and Sunnyside* had a four-page insert by the Eckels Chemical Company of Philadelphia on dermasurgery. The copy was a combination of a sales pitch for the Eckels Company's cosmetics, instruments, and other materials and technical advice on case treatment.

Three notorious criminals—John Dillinger, Bonnie Parker, and Clyde Barrow—died at the hands of law enforcement agents in July 1934. Dillinger, dead from bullet wounds in a Chicago alley, was taken to the Cook County morgue, where a Worsham College of Mortuary Science instructor, Don Asheworth, was requested to make a death mask of Dillinger for the FBI. As he worth related to the writers that he was visited by the FBI at 2 AM and that he was persuaded to hand over the extra mask.

Bonnie and Clyde were slain near Arcadia, Louisiana, and taken to a mortuary there. Both were embalmed in Louisiana, but Clyde was taken to the Sparkman–Holly–Brand Mortuary in Dallas, whereas Bonnie was taken to McKamy–Campbell Funeral Home, also in Dallas. Clyde, his head shattered, received more than 100 bullet or shotgun pellet wounds; Bonnie received more than 50 bullet wounds. Both bodies were restored and viewed in their respective caskets by approximately 50,000 people.

In 1936, Bruno Hauptmann, the convicted kidnapper and murderer of Charles A. Lindbergh's baby, was executed by electrocution. Reports of his preparation state that restorative art procedures were required to repair burns on his face and head. Services were private, however, and followed by cremation.

In the December 1926 issue of *Casket and Sunnyside* appeared the first advertisement for the electricheated spatula, manufactured by the Montez Manufacturing Company, Addison, Michigan (**Fig. 8**). This device, highly touted when first developed as an excellent spatula to smooth and model wax as well as to reduce swollen areas, was less effective than anticipated. The heat of the iron had a tendency to melt wax and leave an unnaturally shiny surface. When used to reduce swelling, the device produced only a very minor evident reduction after much effort. Perhaps its best use was to "iron" tissue.

In August 1927, during the Minnesota 37th State Convention at St. Paul, the term "restorative art" was first used. The Worsham College advertisement of December 1927 used the term "restorative art" but later reverted to the term "dermasurgery." In 1929, the McAllister School listed Robert C. Harper as professor of restorative art. In November 1928, William G. Collier, Collier School, New York City, stated in an address, "Any man can be taught the principles of this restorative art." It was to take some years, however, before the term *restorative art* was adopted and uniformly applied to the subject area first termed demisurgery by Joel E. Crandall in 1912.

By the mid-1920s, articles by teachers and practitioners of embalming on restorative art appeared with frequency in most professional journals and house organs of chemical manufacturers and supply companies. One such writer and practitioner was William G. Collier, a trade embalmer of New York City, who became a prolific author of articles on restorative art. Collier, scion of a well-established funeral service family, first appeared in print in *Casket and Sunnyside* in 1925 with an article on jaundice treatment. From that moment, he was a more or less regular contributor of articles dealing with treatment of facial cancer, decapitation, general demisurgical procedures, and cosmetics.

Collier founded both a school of embalming instruction and a shipping service in New York City and was the holder of several patents for restorative wound fillers and preformed facial features. Collier is remembered as a patient teacher, excellent speaker, and excruciating writer.

The Champion Company in March 1929 introduced the subject area to the readers of its house organ, *Champion Expanding Encyclopedia of Mortuary Practice*, with an article entitled "The Art of Plastic Surgery." Such articles by the supervising

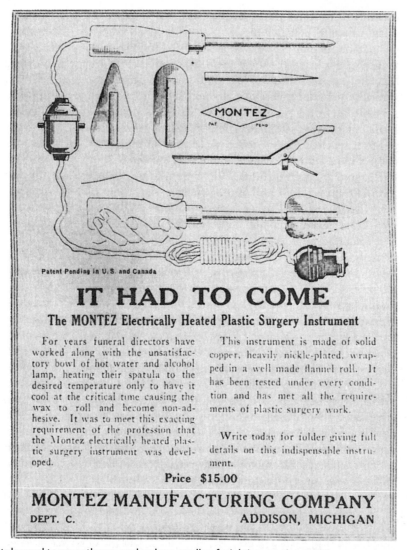

**Figure 8.** Early heated spatula used to smooth wax and reduce swollen facial tissues, circa 1926.

chemist, A. O. Spriggs, on a variety of subjects (e.g., treatment of gunshot cases, subcutaneous suture, and hypodermic injection of tissue filler cream), were assembled into a textbook in 1934, which is still available today under the title *Champion Restorative Art*.

As early as 1927, C. F. Callaway was lecturing, demonstrating, and writing on the subject of restorative art. Callaway became a special representative of the Undertaker's Supply Company of Chicago and wrote many articles on plastic surgery for its house organ as well as trade publications. Ten years later, he was joined in these activities by Ralph Hensen, who later taught mortuary science subjects at the College of Mortuary Science at St. Louis, and by Clarence G. Strub (**Fig. 9**), whose last years in a long and distinguished professional career in funeral service were spent with the University of Iowa as curator of the Anatomy Department of the Iowa Medical College eye enucleation training program. Strub's early contribution to restorative art was his publication of a small textbook of 32 pages entitled *The Principles of Restorative Art As the Embalmer Should Know Them* in 1932 (**Fig. 10**). The little text was extremely well written in a simple and direct style with emphasis on the practical application of technique, although

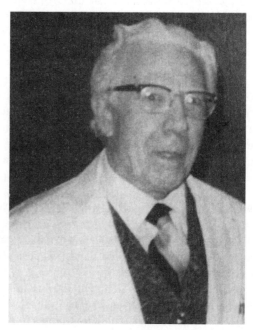

**Figure 9.** Photograph of Clarence G. Strub.

The Principles of Restorative Art
As the Embalmer Should Know Them

By

CLARENCE G. STRUB

Professor of Embalming and Plastic Surgery,
Hohenschuh-Carpenter College of Embalming, St. Louis, Mo.

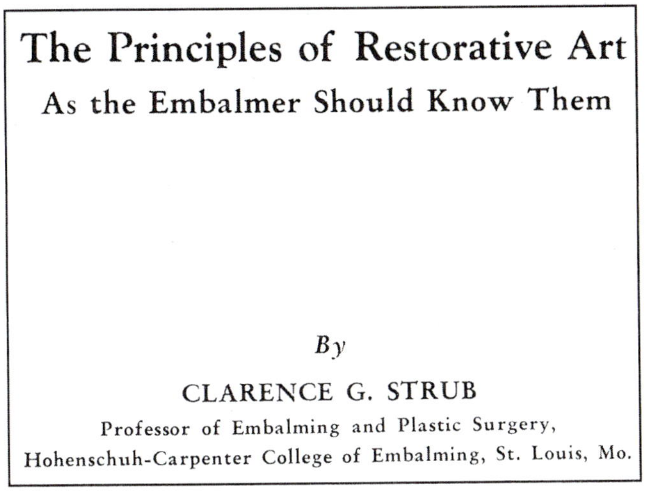

**Figure 10.** Title page of Clarence G. Strub's book.

it did embody some elements of theory. Taken as a whole, the book can be recognized as the true prototype of the best contemporary restorative art textbook.

The Dodge Chemical Company, during this period, also had a team of talented writers, lecturers, and demonstrators in the persons of Frank Stallard, a voluminous writer whose articles appeared for years in trade publications and the Dodge Chemical Company house organ, and Ray Slocum, a most popular embalming and restorative art demonstrator on the Dodge "faculty." Both Stallard and Slocum produced pamphlets of instruction on the subject of embalming and restorative art, which were much sought after and highly prized by practicing embalmers.

In 1945, *Casket and Sunnyside* inaugurated a monthly feature, "Restoration Clinic," by E. C. Johnson. Each monthly article described treatment for a particular type of case and was illustrated by before-and-after photographs of each case. The series continued monthly for more than 14 years.

The spring of 1931 was marked by the untimely death of one of the early full-time embalming college teachers of restorative art, Ivan P. Bowsher. Bowsher, dying at age 33, was a World War I veteran who had graduated from Cincinnati College in the class of 1921. While a student at the college, he was recognized as a gifted artist and was invited to join the faculty, on graduation, as a teacher of restorative art. For 10 brief years, he gave the students of Cincinnati College one of the best courses of instruction in restorative art available. On his death, the college instituted the Ivan P. Bowsher Medal for outstanding achievement in restorative art to be awarded to one member of each graduating class. Cincinnati College had another outstanding teacher of restorative art, G. Joseph Prager, who with Dean C. O. Dhonau wrote an excellent textbook entitled *Manual of Restorative Art*, published in 1934. Prager continued and expanded the restorative art curriculum inaugurated by Bowsher and in 1955 published another textbook entitled *Post Mortem Restorative Art.*

An excellent book that deals with a very limited area of the field of restorative art, written by Gladys P. Curry of Boston in 1947, is titled *A Textbook of Facial Reconstruction.* Gladys Curry was an internationally recognized authority on the identification of the dead, and her expertise was often requested

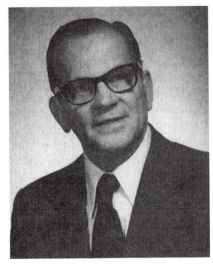

**Figure 11.** Photograph of J. Sheridan Mayer.

in disasters such as the infamous Coconut Grove nightclub fire, which claimed more than 500 victims, and the recovery of decomposing bodies of the crew members of the submarine *Squalus* lost in U.S. waters in 1939.

The Curry text is devoted solely to instruction in reconstruction of the soft tissues of the head and neck with clay or wax and is devoid of any instruction on or concern with the ordinary restorative problems or embalming of such cases. This text is highly recommended as an invaluable addition to an embalmer's library for reference on modeling and identification techniques.

The contemporary standard textbook on restorative art was written by the late Sheridan Mayer (**Fig. 11**), published as a lengthy treatise in 1940 and as a fully hardbound textbook in 1943 entitled simply *Restorative Art.* This work has gone through many revisions and is now used in most mortuary science college programs. Mayer also wrote the treatises *Workbook on Color* published in 1947 and *Mortuary Cosmetology* published in 1948. In 1973, he published the textbook *Color and Cosmetics*, which is in use in mortuary science college programs.

It is noteworthy and to his great credit that Mayer overcame the handicap of not being a practicing embalmer and yet was able to impart instruction intelligently. Mayer is one of the very few, if not the only, truly successful teachers who had never been a practicing embalmer.

His introduction to the teaching of restorative art was at a clinic at the Eckels College of Mortuary Science in Philadelphia, September 6–8, 1939, where he appeared on the program with the famed Covermark cosmetic formulator Lydia O'Leary. His dynamic and informative presentation was so well received by all in attendance that he was offered a position on the faculty, which he accepted and retained until 1947.

In 1947, he joined the faculty of the Pittsburgh Institute of Mortuary Science, where he met Otto S. Margolis and formed an admiration for him. In 1951, when Margolis assumed control of the American Academy of Mortuary Science in New York City, Mayer accompanied him there to strengthen the faculty. The American Academy merged with the McAllister Institute in 1964.

Mayer has written extensively on the subject of cosmetics and restorative art and has written articles for many professional journals. His greatest contribution to the subject of restorative art, however, has been his influence and steady guidance of mortuary colleges toward the development and acceptance of a uniform course of instruction, as well as the adoption of uniform standards of facilities for such instruction and relevant examination questions. He has been the chairman of the restorative art course content committee of mortuary science schools and colleges for many years, where he accomplished monumental tasks in curriculum studies and syllabus preparation and screening of a bank of examination questions on the subject of restorative art. Mayer taught until 1975. In December of 1993, he died in Cincinnati, Ohio, where he had retired.

The words of A. Johnson Dodge, as so well stated in 1917, are still valid today: "How to care for mutilated bodies and make them presentable should constitute a part of the education of the embalmer. Thorough instruction in this difficult art should be given by instructors in our schools. But this part of the work required *special experience* and some study either to practice or teach it successfully."

One area of instruction in restorative art that has been recognized increasingly as a valuable practical working asset is the study of physical anthropology. Physical anthropology has been defined as a science that deals with the physical likenesses and differences of the races and sexes as well as the changes wrought by age and disease of humans. Such study has been most helpful in the practice of restorative art. It has been particularly invaluable in identification and reconstruction of skeletal remains. Study of skeletal remains can reveal sex, race, age, general height range, and individual characteristics such as right- or left-handedness, old trauma, (e.g., healed fractures), and diseases. Perhaps, the most interesting use of such knowledge is the reconstruction of the face on a fleshless skull.

The technique used today by experts such as Betty Catliff, assistant to Clyde Snow, physical anthropologist, retired Chief of the Federal Aviation Authority, Physical Anthropology Unit, at Norman, Oklahoma, is virtually identical to the original system devised by Wilhelm His of Leipzig University in Germany.

In brief, in 1895, His was compelled to devise a method of identifying a skull as to whether or not it and its associated bones were the remains of the renowned composer Johann Sebastian Bach. The bones had been disinterred from the church cemetery during enlargement of the church of St. John and a new more elaborate grave and monument for the remains, if indeed they were his, were planned. Proof of the identity was imperative.

His began assembling measurements of the key points from the numerous undissected cadavers in his laboratory. He recorded each point thickness for each corpse and then averaged these measurements to secure a single working measurement for each such point. He had small metal markers constructed, which were labeled A, B, and so on, to correspond with the tissue thickness at that point.

He secured the services of a well-known sculptor who agreed to undertake the project of reconstruction of the skull using the His technique. The metal markers were put in position on the skull and embedded in clay. When they were all correctly placed, strips of clay were applied connecting the points, and these in turn were interconnected. Finally, the vacant spaces were filled in and the features formed. The reconstructed skull appearance obtained closely resembled contemporary portraits and sculptures of Bach, and the committee for construction of the new tomb and monument was satisfied.

This technique has been updated from time to time by creating new tables, as His did, of females and other races. The technique has produced good results even by those using the procedure for the first time.

Through the years, special schools were founded to teach cosmetic application and restorative art. An example of such a school, unaffiliated with an existing school of mortuary science, was the Embalmers Graduate College formed in Chicago in 1937 by L. Roy Davenport and Honora D. Mannix, which offered 30 hours of instruction and practice in both cosmetology and restorative art.

Edward C. Johnson (1914–2000) was recognized nationally and internationally as an educator, writer, and demonstrator in the field of embalming and restorative art. He was born in Chicago in 1914 and worked for 66 years in funeral service throughout the greater Chicago area. He graduated in 1936 from the Worsham College of Mortuary Science in Chicago. He worked at this time for Oscar G. Merager, a Chicago undertaker. He developed an interest in restorative art. This was during a time when bodies were still embalmed in the home without gloves, in front of the family of the deceased!

Johnson taught embalming, restorative art, and the history of embalming at the Worsham College and served at its associate dean. Years later, he taught in the mortuary program at Malcolm X Community College in Chicago. Over his teaching career, he taught more than 10,000 students. He authored more than 650 scholarly articles on the history of embalming and American funeral service. In 1950, he was a major contributor to the National Funeral Directors Association publications, *Funeral Customs the World Over* and *The History of American Funeral Directing*.

In 1948, Professor Johnson organized the Postgraduate Institute of Restorative in Chicago. The curriculum included a short 2-week course and the standard 7-month course that offered 25 hours per week of instruction. When the school was merged into Worsham College in 1955, the course had been taken by 16 mortuary college restorative art instructors or their assistants.

Following his death, more than 90 boxes of books and educational materials were given by his family to the Museum of Funeral Customs in Springfield, Illinois. Edward Johnson was truly an indefatigable educator and practitioner in the fields of embalming, embalming history, and restorative art.

***Restorative Art—Educational and In-Use Materials.***
Education of embalmers at all levels of skill in restorative art has been enhanced by the production of photographic records of actual restorative procedures. Some of these productions were in black and white, some in full color, some in motion, and others in still pictures. Most are silent and very few have either sound or voice accompaniment.

The truly classic motion picture on restorative procedures was produced in color in the early 1930s by the late Earle K. Angstadt (**Fig. 12**) of the Auman Funeral Home of Reading,

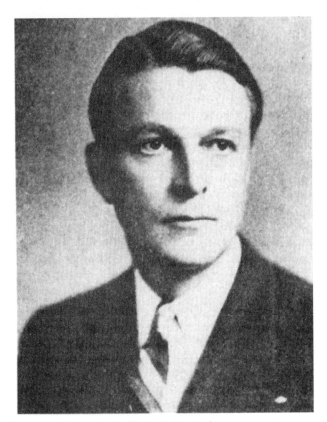

**Figure 12.** Photograph of Earle K. Angstadt.

Pennsylvania, who also performed all the actual restorative art techniques displayed in the film. The silent film has subtitles and is expertly photographed. It depicts classic technique, flawlessly performed, during the restoration of a surgically removed mandible, reduction of facial swelling, hypodermic tissue filling of face and hand, and replacement of eyelids and eyelashes damaged beyond salvage by an infection. This film, still available from the National Funeral Directors Association headquarters, will never be improved on.

Another much longer film, recording many more cases of severe trauma, was produced in the late 1930s by the late R. Victor Landig, founder of the Landig College of Mortuary Science at Houston. The photography of the 10 or 12 cases recorded on the film varies widely from poor to good, with respect to color fidelity, focus, and technique, whereas restorative skill is uniformly good except for the handling of hair restorations.

The Los Angeles College of Mortuary Science produced a fine color motion picture complete with sound and voice in the late 1940s. The film depicts no actual cases but does show how to produce plaster practice masks and provides excellent modeling instruction for producing the individual facial features. The Champion Company of Ohio has a motion picture in color made in the 1940s by A. O. Spriggs, featuring his technique in treating a small group of actual restorative cases. E. C. Johnson has slides recording the treatment of several hundred cases, including virtually every conceivable problem requiring restorative art treatment.

Our profession desperately needs more visual aids such as the foregoing to provide wider exposure of our practitioners to successful techniques at conventions, meetings, seminars, and workshops.

In 1933, the Hydrol Chemical Company made a most significant announcement in the trade journals concerning the patenting of liquid tissue builder that coagulated or jelled on being hypodermically introduced into the body tissue. This, of course, was a vast improvement over ordinary liquids such as glycerin, then in use for this purpose, as such liquids, remaining liquid, tended to settle away from the high point in response to the pull of gravity. This failure of the hypodermically deposited material to maintain its position obviously ultimately destroyed the effect of such treatment.

Another equally vexatious problem resulting from the use of such permanent liquid-state tissue builders was the most disturbing occurrence of seepage from the point of insertion of the hypodermic needle. Both of these problems were corrected by the new jelling tissue builder as it would neither seep nor shift its position due to the change in its structure from liquid to semisolid to solid.

An alternative material such as hand cream or petroleum jelly had been used, but the technique for successful use required that both the filled syringe and the large-diameter needle be kept warm to permit a free flow of the semisolid material. Special hypodermic syringes with screw-threaded plungers were devised to make the ejection of thick creams easier, but they never did become very popular, and after introduction of coagulable liquid filler, they virtually disappeared from the market (**Fig. 13**).

In 1935, the Dodge Chemical Company introduced De-Ce-Co needle injector and needles as an improved means of securing mouth closure and in 1937 offered a complete set of eight specially designed restorative art instruments. In addition, the company, like many others, offered a complete range of cosmetics, waxes, and restorative art chemicals.

Methods of cosmetic application, but primarily application of highlight or accent cosmetics over waxed areas, had always required improvement. The difficulty in applying accent cosmetics evenly and naturally on waxed surfaces is a problem familiar to all experienced embalmers. The best solution is to apply the cosmetics with an airbrush or power sprayer. By these means, the cosmetics are literally floated into position, and disturbance of either the underlying base cosmetics or the wax surface is completely avoided.

As far back as 1911, spray applicators, powered by carbon dioxide cylinders, were available to the embalmer for cosmetic application, but it was not until the 1930s that the need and desire for sprayer-applied cosmetics became popular.

In 1934, the Undertaker's Supply Company announced the availability of the E-Z Way manually operated spray cosmetic applicator and a compatible cosmetic. The device was well received because it was most efficient and was generally conceded to be the best of the nonpower-operated sprayers, many of which are still in use today.

In 1936, the Paasche Company of Chicago, a manufacturer of industrial and artistic airbrush equipment, offered a restorative art airbrush kit designed for embalmers' use (**Fig. 14**). The kit contained an electric-powered air compressor; an airbrush applicator of high quality; restorative art wax; cosmetic instruments, preformed features such as ears, nose, and lips; and an instruction pamphlet. The Nuance AireTynt cosmetic applicator was advertised in 1937 by J. Horace Griggs of Amarillo,

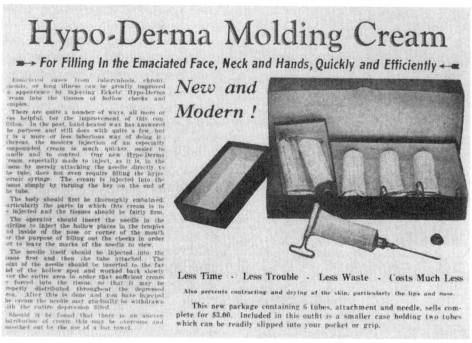

**Figure 13.** Tissue filler using cream, circa 1930.

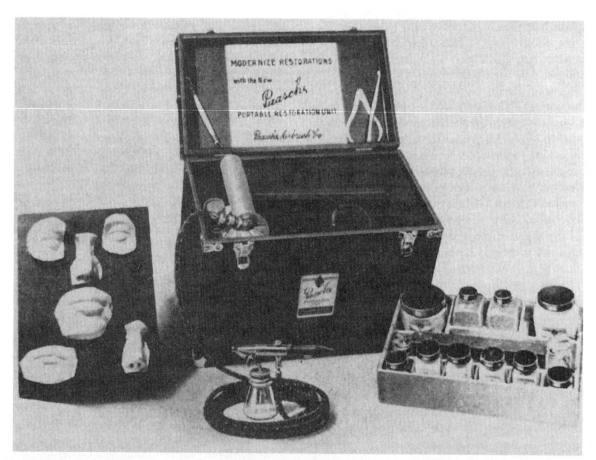

**Figure 14.** Paasche Company's restorative art airbrush kit designed for embalmers' use.

Texas (**Fig. 15**). The airbrush applicator could be adapted to apply cosmetics, whether powered by a manually operated pump, an electric-powered air compressor, or a carbonic gas cylinder.

Today, many embalmers have been using, when the need arises, inexpensive easily available handheld model paint sprayers that are powered by small replaceable containers of Freon gas. These units, readily available in hobby shops, hardware stores,

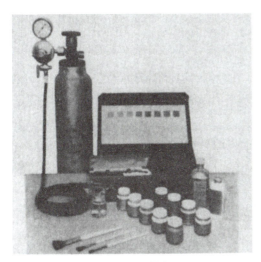

**Figure 15.** Master Nuance Aire-Tynt Unit.

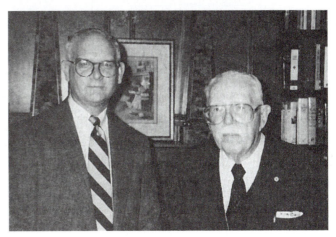

**Figure 17.** Robert G. Mayer (left) and Edward C. Johnson are instructors of embalming and restorative art. They are the primary authors of *Embalming: History, Theory, and Practice*.

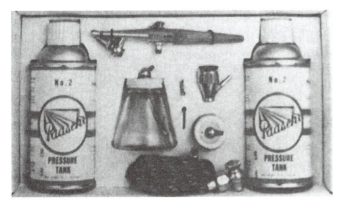

**Figure 16.** Handheld model paint sprayer powered by small replaceable containers of Freon gas.

or paint stores, serve the purpose equally as well as the more expensive air compressor-powered sprayers (**Fig. 16**).

Restorative art was considered of sufficient importance in 1945 to have Richard G. Reichle, registrar of Worsham College, address the National Funeral Directors Association convention in Chicago on the continuing value and need for these procedures.

Now, as in the origin of the art, it is necessary for the individual embalmer, in charge of the case, to initiate the restoration of that case and to bring it to a successful conclusion. No amount of material, equipment, or training can substitute for the individual will and determination to overcome a most distressing case. The individual, now as always, is the key to success. The will to succeed and the ability to improvise are more often of value than any other asset.

It is therefore necessary that we in funeral service rededicate ourselves to the fulfillment, to the very best of our ability, of the American way—the funeral with the body present and viewable (**Fig. 17**).

### Restorative Art and Emerging Technology

Within the last 40 years, three-dimensional printing (3-D) has revolutionized technology and manufacturing sectors. Endless applications exist for the use of this technology in the field of restorative art. Feature restoration using 3-D printed replicas promises suitable and accurate facial and other anatomical feature replacements. Historically, mass-produced latex ears and noses served as replacements and were difficult to scale for acceptable fit. Embalmers in Guangzhou, China developed a program to recreate facial features and hands in a laboratory; a facial mask created using 3-D technology is displayed in the funeral service center.

## BIBLIOGRAPHY

Benkard E. *Undying Faces*. London: Hogurth Press, 1929. [A collection of death masks from the fifteenth century to the present]

Clarke CH. *Practical Embalming*. Cincinnati, OH: C. H. Clarke, 1917.

Crane EH. *Manual of Instruction to Undertakers*, 8th ed. Kalamazoo, MI: Kalamazoo, 1888.

Curry GP. *Facial Reconstruction*. Boston, MA, 1947.

Dhonau CO, Prager GJ. *Manual of Restorative Art*. Cincinnati, OH: Embalming Book Co., 1932.

Dodge AJ. *The Practical Embalmer*. Boston, MA: A. Johnson Dodge, 1908.

Dutra FR. Identification of person and determination of cause of death. *Archives of Pathology* 1944;38:339.

Eckles HS. *Derma Surgery*. Philadelphia, PA: H. S. Eckles, 1925.

Espy JB. *Espy's Embalmer*. Springfield, OH: Espy's Fluid Co., 1895.

Gerasimov MM. *The Face Finder*. Philadelphia, PA/New York, NY: Lippincott, 1971.

Gradwohl RBH. *Legal Medicine*. St. Louis, MO: C.V. Mosby, 1954.

His W. *Anatomische Forschungen ü ber Johann Sebastian Bach's Gegeine und Antlitz Nebst Bermerkungen über dessin Bilder*. Leipzig: S. Hirzel, 1895.

Hooten EA. *Up from the Ape*. New York, NY: Macmillan, 1946.

Johnson EC. *Restorative Art*. Chicago, IL: Worsham College, 1948.

Krogman W. *A Guide to the Identification of Human Skeletal Material*. Washington, DC: FBI Law Enforcement Bulletin, 1939.

Krogman W. *The Human Skeleton in Forensic Medicine*. Springfield, IL: Charles C. Thomas, 1962.

Mayer JS. *Workbook on Color*. Philadelphia, PA: Westbrook Publishing Co., 1947.

Mayer JS. *Mortuary Cosmetology*. Philadelphia, PA: West-brook Publishing Co., 1948.

Mayer JS. *Color and Cosmetics*. Bergenfield, NJ: Paul Publishing, 1973.

Mayer JS. *Restorative Art*. Dallas, TX: Professional Training Schools, 1993.

Michel G. *Scientific Embalmer.* Cleveland, OH, 1922.

Piombino-Mascali D, Williams MJ. Rosalia Lombardo and her master embalmer. *The Director*, July, 2009.

Quiring DP. "Skeletal identification." Address to Ohio State Coroners Association, May 23, 1951.

Reichle RG. "Practical problems in restorative art." Lecture National Funeral Directors Association 63rd Convention, Chicago, 1945.

Smith E, Dawson WR. *Egyptian Mummies.* New York, NY: Dial Press, 1924.

Spriggs AO. *Plastic Surgery*, 4th ed. Springfield, OH: Champion Chemical Co., 1946.

Stewart TD. *Essentials of Forensic Anthropology.* Springfield, IL: Charles C. Thomas, 1979.

Strub CG. The principles of restorative art. *Embalmer's Monthly*, 1932.

Wentworth B, Wilder HH. *Personal Identification.* Chicago, IL: T. G. Cooke Fingerprint, 1932.

https://3dprint.com/240838/chinese-morticians-improving-facial-reconstruction-3d-printing/

# PART IV

## Selected Readings

The following articles have appeared in various professional publications and are reprinted for the purpose of supplemental reading. Suggested practices, products, and viewpoints are solely the expression of the authors.

1. Summary of Guidelines Submitted to OSHA from the National Funeral Directors Association Committee on Infectious Disease (Summer, 1989)
2. Mortuary Care of Armed Forces Service Members. Excerpted from: Standards for Department of Defense (DOD) Mortuary Facilities and for Drafting a Performance Work Statement (PWS) for DOD Contracted Mortuary Services, March 2019
3. Identification: An Essential Part of What We Do, by Michael Kubasak (2002)
4. *The Mathematics of Embalming Chemistry: Part I. A Critical Evaluation of "One Bottle" Embalming Claims,* by Jerome F. Frederick (1968)
5. The Measurement of Formaldehyde Retention in the Tissues of Embalmed Bodies, by John Kroshus, Joseph McConnell, Jay Bardole (1983)
6. The Two-Year Fix: Long-Term Preservation for Delayed Viewing, by Kerry Don Peterson (1992)
7. Occupational Exposure to Formaldehyde in Mortuaries, by L. Lamont Moore and Eugene C. Ogrodnik (1986)
8. The Strange Case of Dr. Jekyll and Formaldehyde (Is It Good or Evil), by Maureen Robinson (2009)
9. The Preparation Room: Ventilation, by Jack Adams, CFSP (2004)
10. Risk of Infection and tracking of work-related infectious diseases in the funeral industry, by Susan Salter Davidson and William H. Benjamin, Jr. (2006)
11. Creutzfeldt-Jakob Disease, by Ruth Carrico, Christian Davis Furman, Curtis Rostad and Dorothy Cannan Hyde (2005)
12. Hepatitis from A to G, by Kim Collison (1999)
13. The Increase in MRSA and VRE, by Mike Cloud, Jr. (1999)
14. The Antimicrobial Activity of Embalming Chemicals and Topical Disinfectants on the Microbial Flora of Human Remains, by Peter A. Burke and A. L. Sheffner (1976)
15. The Microbiologic Evaluation and Enumeration of Postmortem Specimens from Human Remains, by Gordon W. Rose and Robert N. Hockett (1970)
16. Professional Hair Care for Human Remains, by Darla A. Tripoli (2010)
17. Restricted Cervical Injection as a Primary Injection Method, by Ben Whitworth (2021)
18. Enhance Emaciated Features Arterially Using Split Injection and Restricted Drainage, by Sharon L. Gee (2005)
19. Embalming—United Kingdom and European, by Peter J. Ball (2005)
20. The Art of Embalming and Its Purpose, by Ron Hast (2006)
21. Embalming COVID-19: Infection Control and Storage, by Jzyk S. Ennis, PhD (2020)
22. Cosmetic Airbrushing of Un-embalmed Decedents, by Daryl M. Hammond (2019)

**Summary of Guidelines Submitted to OSHA from the National Funeral Directors Association Committee on Infectious Disease (Summer, 1989)**

# PUBLIC HEALTH PRECAUTIONARY REQUIREMENTS AND STANDARDS

## I. Background.

Prevention of the transmission of recognized classical and/or opportunistic pathogens from human remains to the embalmer, from the embalmer to his or her family, and to the families and friends of the deceased is a reasonable public health expectation.

Many of the infectious agents associated with medical and paramedical environments are classified as "opportunistic" pathogens or microbial agents considered to be of lower or reduced virulence. The increasing association of "opportunistic" pathogens with symptomatic infectious diseases has all but eliminated the reference to the category "nonpathogen."

The implementation of minimum professional practice standards in embalming is necessary to provide a standard of quality control and quality assurance in the preservation and disinfection of human remains. It is important that when embalming is performed, a significant measure of uniformity of professional skills will be employed by all funeral service practitioners.

Following somatic or functional death, normally structurally intact epithelial, facial, and other tissue barriers undergo a loss of structural integrity and permit the body-wide translocation and distribution of systemic microflora and create alternate body fluid and body tissue reservoir sites of host contamination.

During life, the body fluids or body secretions most frequently associated with the transmission of potentially infectious doses or densities are quite definable. After death, this is no longer true. All body fluids and body tissues may become reservoirs of infectious agents within a relatively short postmortem interval.

Cellular death may not be complete for up to 12 hours after somatic or functional death. During this postmortem interval, the viability and potential infectivity of blood-borne viruses, for example, HIV and hepatitis B, may persist, and the exiting of the agents from any body opening, natural or artificial, may occur.

Funeral service practitioners normally have more than casual contact with parenteral (including open wound) and mucous membrane exposure to blood and body tissues. Such individuals occupationally exposed to blood, body fluid, or tissues can be protected from the recognized risks of blood-borne agents such as HIV and HBV (hepatitis B virus) by imposing barriers in the form of engineering controls, work practices, in-service training, and protective equipment and attire.

## II. Recommendations.

It is recommended that every funeral service firm/facility in the United States adopt the following policies and guidelines for implementation: (1) public health guidelines, (2) personnel health precautions for the prevention of blood-borne microbial agent(s) and infections, and (3) minimum standards for the embalming and disinfection of human remains. The recommendations and guidelines within each of the three categories described above are as follows.

## 1. PUBLIC HEALTH GUIDELINES

***A. Care of the Human Remains.*** Thoroughly cleanse and disinfect the body surface and natural or artificial body orifices/body openings with a suitable EPA-registered, hospital, or health care facility acceptable agent, for example, tuberculocidal, germicidal detergent. The tuberculocidal germicidal detergent, for example, a phenylphenol or a third-generation quaternary ammonium compound complex, should be an EPA-registered product offering confirmatory evidence of all label claims, including the recommended use dilution. The disinfected body surfaces should be thoroughly rinsed following a minimum of a 10-minute exposure interval.

Injection and drainage procedures should include (1) multisite injection and drainage procedures, (2) intermittent or restricted drainage, (3) the use of a 3.0% v/v formaldehyde-based arterial injection solution or a 2.0% glutaraldehyde-based solution, and (4) the use of 1 pint of concentrated cavity chemical per major or primary body cavity, for example, abdominal, pelvic, and thoracic, or 1 pint of concentrated cavity chemical per 50 pounds of body weight.

***B. The Embalmer (Universal Precautions).*** This category of barrier attire utilization and precautions has replaced the health care facility category of Blood and Body Fluid Precautions. The category requires the *minimum* barrier attire utilization of a whole-body gown or apron and gloves. The wraparound, moisture-repellent, or moisture-proof gown or apron of rubber, plastic, or impregnated fabric is considered to be disposable or a single-use barrier attire item. The same is true for the gloves. Double rubber or plastic gloves are recommended for funeral service personnel.

This minimum standard of barrier attire protection is to be employed in the preparation of *all* human remains, no matter what the indicated cause of death reported. The risk of blood and body fluid exposure is significantly high for all funeral service personnel, and frequently, the infectious disease status of the deceased is unknown. Therefore, it is recommended that all persons performing postmortem procedures consider the use of additional barrier attire items such as protective eyewear, oral–nasal masks, and shoe and head covers.

Hands should be thoroughly scrubbed, using an EPA-registered* medicated liquid soap, before and after gloving. If a glove is penetrated by a sharp or the uneven edge of a bone, the glove is to be removed and replaced as soon as possible.

All instruments employed during the embalming should be sterilized or disinfected prior to reuse. A high-level disinfecting liquid immersant may be employed in lieu of a steam sterilizer if the latter is not available. Chemical germicidal detergents registered with EPA as "cold chemical sterilants" can be used either for sterilization or for high-level disinfection, depending on the interval or contact.

***C. Air Handling Within the Environment "at Risk."*** An efficient air supply and air exhaust system or an air purification system must be operative within the embalming environment. The air handling system should protect the embalmer from a hazardous airborne density of biologic particulates as well as from the accumulation of formaldehyde monomers exceeding 0.75 ppm, the permissible exposure limit or 8-hour time-weighted average (TWA) concentration. The TWA "action level" is 0.5 ppm of formaldehyde monomer concentration.

***D. Terminal Disinfection and Decontamination.*** All instruments; horizontal surfaces such as floor, operating table, sink, and countertop; waste receptacles; and any other surface in direct or indirect contact with the preparation site must be cleansed and disinfected upon removal of the human remains from the preparation environment.

All instruments, including trocars and venous drainage tubes, must either be steam-sterilized or immersed in a suitable cold chemical sterilant. *Note*: The use of a hypochlorite, 1000–5000 ppm, may be used for the "spot" disinfection of body fluid spills on hard, nonporous surfaces. However, immediate rinsing is necessary to prevent the formation of BCME (bischloromethyl ether), a confirmed carcinogen, in the presence of formaldehyde monomers.

***E. Solid Waste Management.*** Potentially infective, contaminated solid wastes associated with the preparation of human remains should be placed in "alert" colored plastic bags, for example, red, the bag twist-closed and securely tied prior to ultimate disposition. Local codes permitting bulk blood and suctioned/aspirated fluids may be carefully drained into the sanitary sewer system, and vacuum breakers must be installed on all involved water lines to prevent the back-siphoning of contaminated liquids into potable water supply lines.

***F. Hearse/First Call Vehicles.*** Cleanse and disinfect all mortuary cots or trays following exposure to the unembalmed human remains. Employ cleansed and disinfected cot or tray covers for each transfer of unembalmed human remains from the home or from the health care facility to the preparation room. Cleanse and sanitize the internal horizontal surfaces of the hearse/first call vehicle following the transfer of the remains to the preparation room.

***G. Funeral Service Personnel Health Recommendations.***
1. Annual physical examination
2. Annual TB skin testing
3. Immunizations—annual influenza, single-dose/single-series Pneumovax, hepatitis B, Rubella vaccine—are recommended for all women of pregnancy age if not protected and for all male employees because they can transmit to the female employee.

## 2. PERSONNEL HEALTH PRECAUTIONS FOR PREVENTION OF BLOOD-BORNE AGENT(S) AND INFECTIONS

***A. Removal/Transfer of Human Remains.***
1. Removal personnel (licensees, resident trainees, nonlicensees, and nonresident trainees)—disposable whole-body barrier attire and plastic or rubber gloves.
2. Avoid contact with covering of remains at sites of body fluid or exudative contamination. Place the remains in an impervious plastic whole-body pouch and effect zipper closure.
3. Sanitize the transfer vehicle following the transfer of remains to the preparation room.

---
*For example, *para*-Chloro-*meta*-xylenol (PCMX) or chlorhexidene gluconate (CHG) biocidal additive.

**B. Transfer of the Remains to the Preparation Room, Using a Team of Two Employees.** Transfer the pouched remains to the preparation room table, open pouch, and loosen body coverings. Allow the body coverings to fall into the pouch. Carefully position the remains from side to side for the careful removal of the pouch and contents. Dispose of the pouch and contents as contaminated solid wastes.

**C. Terminal Disinfection.**

1. Disinfect all horizontal inanimate surfaces in direct or indirect contact with preparation site.
2. Sterilize or disinfect all instruments by cold chemical sterilizer immersion or by steam sterilization.
3. Remove all barrier attire items, place in plastic bag, and treat as contaminated solid wastes in terms of final disposition.
4. Scrub ungloved hands and wrists with a medicated liquid soap preparation, preferably one that is recommended as a health care personnel hand wash.
5. Complete whole-body bathing or showering and shampooing prior to return to home or office.

**3. MINIMUM STANDARDS FOR THE EMBALMING AND DISINFECTION OF HUMAN REMAINS.** The following professional profile of standards for embalming practices and procedures is based on laboratory evaluations and post-embalming observations.

**A. Multiple-Site Injection and Drainage.** Multiple-site (two or more) injection and drainage procedures assure a more consistent distribution and ultimate diffusion of the disinfection and preservation chemicals to all receptive tissue sites, deep and superficial. This will more consistently provide public health protection as expected from the thorough preparation of human remains for ultimate disposition.

**B. Rate of Flow of Arterial Injection Chemicals.** A moderate rate of flow, 12–15 minutes per gallon of arterial injection solution, accompanied by a sufficient arterial injection pressure to maintain the desired rate of flow, 2–10 psi, are recommended for the assurance of distribution and diffusion of the arterial injection chemicals.

**C. Intermittent or Restricted Drainage.** This method of venous drainage should produce maximum preservation and disinfection. It is considered to be one of the most effective procedures for the assurance of adequate distribution of arterial injection solution(s). It is especially recommended following the removal of surface discolorations.

**D. Total Volume of Arterial Injection Solution Employed.** Consideration should be given to the use of a minimum of 3–4 gallons of arterial injection solution in adult remains weighing 125–175 pounds. Injection and drainage procedures may involve the removal of 4–6 quarts of body fluids. To properly restore the loss of body fluids and overcome the loss, through drainage, of arterial injection chemicals, it becomes necessary to employ the recommended volume of arterial injection solution, for example, 1 gallon per 50 pounds of body weight, exclusive of the primary injection solution(s) volume.

**E. Use of Supplemental Injection Chemicals.** The enhancement of the arterial distribution of the arterial injection solution may often require the use of supplemental additives, for example, modifying and surface tension-reducing additives and water softeners. The use of such additives may increase the efficacy of injection solution distribution as well as the efficacy of venous drainage.

**F. Concentration (%) of Preservative/Disinfecting Chemicals in the Arterial Injection Solution.** Laboratory investigative data indicate that the percent of formaldehyde v/v in the formaldehyde-based arterial injection solution should not be less than 2.0. Formaldehyde concentrations ranging from 2.3% to 3.0% v/v will inactivate resident bacterial densities 95% or more. Formaldehyde concentrations less than 2.0%, for example, 1.0% v/v, may produce expected tissue fixation, but may not produce the desired level of microbial inactivation. Significant reduction in the endogenous microbial populations should always exceed 70% if public health expectations are to be fulfilled on a consistent basis.

Formaldehyde is categorized as an "intermediate" to a "high-level" chemical disinfectant when employed in concentrations ranging from 3.0% to 8.0% v/v. The recommended use of a minimum 2.0% v/v concentration of formaldehyde is based on this categorization as well as investigative data.

**G. Cavity Chemical Utilization.** Following the thorough treatment of the thoracic, abdominal, and pelvic cavities, including the aspiration of liquids and semisolids from non-autopsied remains, the injection of 1 pint (16 oz) of undiluted cavity chemical into each of the three trocar-prepared cavities is recommended. In remains weighing in excess of 150 to 200 pounds, it is recommended that the embalmer use 1 pint of concentrated cavity chemical per 50 pounds of body weight. The weight of the body viscera may approximate 15% of the total body weight. The chemically targeted hollow and solid organ tissues require maximal chemical contact following the trocar penetration and separation to ensure the prevention of the microbial generation of putrefactive activity, including body opening purge.

**III. Administration.**

The funeral home owner/manager/employer should establish formal policies and procedures to ensure that all job-related tasks that involve an inherent potential for mucous membrane or skin contact with blood, body fluids, or tissues, or a potential for spills or splashes of blood or body fluids, will require appropriate preventive/protective measures. These preventive measures would be applicable to licensed, non-licensed, resident trainee, and nonresident trainee personnel. Engineering controls, work practices, and protective barrier attire are critical to minimize exposure to HBV, HIV, and other blood and body fluid-transmitted microbial agents and to prevent infection(s). It is essential that the funeral home employee be fully aware of the reasons for the required preventive measures. Therefore, employee education programs must be implemented to assure familiarity with applicable work practices.

The employer should establish the following formal policies:

1. Develop and provide in-service training programs for all employees whose responsibilities include the direct or indirect exposure(s) to blood, body fluids, or tissues.

2. Document the attendance of employees at all scheduled and announced in-service training programs. The in-service training course content should include the approved Standard Operating Procedures (SOPs) for embalming practices and the required items of protective equipment and personnel barrier attire items.
3. Assure the convenient availability of all items of protective equipment and barrier attire items.
4. Surveillance of the workplace to ensure that the required work practices are being observed and that the protective barrier attire items and equipment are conveniently available and properly used.
5. Investigation of known or suspected parenteral exposures to body fluids or tissues to establish the conditions associated with the exposure and to improve training, work practices, or preventive equipment to prevent a recurrence.

### IV. Training and Education.

As recommended under the heading "Administration," the employer must establish an initial and periodic training program for all employees who may sustain direct or indirect exposure to blood, body fluids, or tissues. The employee must understand the following as a result of adequate in-service training:

1. Modes of transmission of HBV, HIV, and other blood and body fluid-transmitted microbial agents.
2. The basis for the employment of the types of protective equipment and items of barrier attire.
3. The location of protective equipment and items of barrier attire, the procedures for the proper use of same and for the removal, decontamination, and disposition of contaminated barrier attire items or equipment.
4. The corrective actions necessary to disinfect blood and body fluid spills or splashes.
5. Concurrent and terminal disinfection and decontamination procedures. Disposable, puncture-resistant containers are to be employed for used needles, blades, and so on.

### V. Work Practices.

1. Work practices should be developed on the assumption that all body fluids and tissues are infectious.
2. Provision must be made for the safe removal, handling, decontamination, and disposition of protective clothing items, equipment, soiled linens, and so on.
3. Work practices and SOPs should provide guidance on procedures to follow in the event of spills or personal exposure to fluids or tissues.

### VI. Personal Protective Equipment.

A required minimum of choice of barrier attire items or protective equipment should be specified by the firm's SOPs. As more departments of public health require the reporting of infectious disease causes of death by category of precautions implemented by the health care facility, it becomes increasingly important for the funeral service firm to be aware of the infectious diseases included in a given category or patient isolation precautions. The following is a recommended listing of barrier attire items that should be employed for a reported category of health care patient isolation precautions:

| Category-Specific Health Care Facility | Recommended Funeral Service Personnel Barrier Precautions Attire |
|---|---|
| 1. Strict precautions | Masks (face covers), gowns, gloves (double plastic or rubber gloves are recommended), head covers, shoe covers, eye protectors |
| 2. Contact precautions | Gowns, gloves, shoe covers |
| 3. Respiratory precautions | Masks, gowns, gloves, head covers, shoe covers |
| 4. Enteric precautions | Gowns, gloves, shoe covers |
| 5. Blood and body fluid or **universal precautions** | Gowns, gloves, masks, head covers, shoe covers, eye protectors |

### VII. Medical.

The employer should make available, at no cost to the employee, the voluntary HBV immunization for all employees whose responsibilities involve the direct or indirect exposure to blood, body fluids, or tissues. The employer should also provide for the monitoring, at the request of the employee, for HBV or HIV antibodies following known or suspected parenteral exposure to blood, body fluids, or tissues.

### VIII. Record Keeping.

The employer should require the completion of a case report for the preparation of all remains. Each case report should include (1) health care facility reporting of category of patient isolation precautions implemented, if applicable; (2) sites of injection and drainage employed; (3) volumes and concentrations of arterial injection and cavity treatment chemicals; (4) protective equipment and barrier attire items employed; (5) pre-embalming appearance and condition of the remains; and (6) any other observations or procedure relating to the public health status of the remains.

---

**Mortuary Care of Armed Forces Service Members. From: Standards for Department of Defense (DOD) Mortuary Facilities and for Drafting a Performance Work Statement (PWS) for DOD Contracted Mortuary Services, March 2019.**

# 1. INTRODUCTION

This establishes the DoD standards for funeral homes under contract for DoD mortuary services, and shall apply to all Military Service components. The standards contained herein are not applicable to deaths where the person authorized to direct disposition (PADD), or where the person with authority to effect disposition (PAED) elects to make all arrangements for the disposition of remains.

# 2. GENERAL INFORMATION

This is a description of services for use by both DoD mortuary facilities and funeral homes contracted by DoD to provide mortuary services.

## 3. CLASSIFICATION OF REMAINS STANDARDS

### 3.1. General.

The embalmer will make a recommendation to the Military Service representative regarding the view ability of the deceased. Remains will be classified in one of three categories: viewable, viewable for identification, or nonviewable. Every attempt will be made to restore remains to a natural form and color that permits the person with the authority to direct or effect disposition to make the decision on whether the remains are to be viewed or not. The manner in which the remains are to be prepared will take into consideration cultural and religious customs and traditions of the deceased as well as the PADD's preferences.

#### 3.1.1. Viewable.

Remains are considered viewable when the face and hands have only minor or no trauma, edema, dehydration, or discoloration. Remains may be fully restored to a natural color or form. Condition of the remains allows for dressing in a uniform or other clothing selected by the PADD or PAED.

#### 3.1.2. Viewable for Identification.

Remains may or may not be fully intact with face and hands that may have trauma, edema, dehydration, or discoloration. Although remains may be missing limbs or have received other trauma, condition of remains allows for dressing in uniform or other clothing selected by the person with the authority to direct or effect disposition. Remains may be restored to an appearance suitable for visual recognition.

#### 3.1.3. Nonviewable.

Remains may or may not be fully intact; and may manifest extreme trauma, edema, dehydration, discoloration, or decomposition. Remains may not be able to be restored to an appearance suitable for visual recognition. Condition of remains may not allow for dressing in uniform or other clothing selected by the PADD or PAED.

**3.1.3.1. Head Wrap.** Remains are categorized as such when they are categorized as nonviewable with the face or head having severe trauma, edema, dehydration, or discoloration such that restoration to a condition of viewable recognition is not possible. However, the condition of remains allows for dressing in uniform or other clothing selected by the person with the authority to direct or effect disposition. The head wrap will be accomplished IAW paragraph 4.4.4.

**3.1.3.2. Full Body Wrap.** Remains categorized as nonviewable. The remains may not be intact or may have sustained severe trauma, edema, dehydration, or discoloration where restoration to a condition of viewable recognition is not possible and the remains cannot be dressed. In this situation, the remains will be prepared using a full body wrap. The full body wrap will be accomplished IAW paragraph 4.4.2 and 4.4.3.

## 4. EMBALMING STANDARDS

### 4.1. General:

DoD Mortuary Facilities and facilities under contract to provide DoD mortuary services will prepare and embalm the remains of all entitled personnel in accordance with the written instructions of the PADD/PAED and in accordance with law. The embalmer will verify PADD/PAED elections prior to beginning the preparation and embalming of the remains. No remains will be embalmed without written or oral instructions as outlined below. Oral instructions may be accepted if confirmed by the Military Service Casualty or Mortuary Affairs Office representative, however, follow-on written authorization must be obtained prior to the release of the remains, subsequent remains or retained organs. The Mortuary Officer will note in the case file who provided the oral instructions and when (date and time) they were provided. The written authorization will be obtained at the first reasonable opportunity and uploaded into the case file. Predeath directives authorizing embalming, duly executed by the deceased, shall be given full legal effect and shall constitute an effective authorization to embalm. Human remains prepared at a DoD Mortuary Facility or contracted facility may not receive final disposition for an extended period of time (10 or more days), and may have been subjected to extreme trauma, weather conditions, or have been transported over long distances. Therefore, all remains, whether viewable or nonviewable, require variations in preservation techniques and procedures to accomplish maximum disinfection, preservation, and restoration of all body tissues. The following procedures will be accomplished in the course of processing or reprocessing all viewable remains, and to the extent possible for nonviewable remains.

#### 4.1.1. Insect Treatment.

Disinfection and treatment as necessary with appropriate chemicals.

#### 4.1.2. Disinfecting.

All body orifices shall be treated with a nonastringent disinfectant chemical.

#### 4.1.3. Washing.

All body surfaces will be thoroughly washed with warm water and germicidal soap. Special attention will be given to the viewable surfaces, that is, the face and hands.

#### 4.1.4. Body Positioning.

The body will be positioned to appear comfortable and restful. The head will be positioned straight, without any turn, and hands will be positioned left over right. Deviation will be dependent upon the conditions of the remains at the discretion of the embalmer.

#### 4.1.5. Damaged Tissue.

The embalmer will determine when during the preparation process ulcerated, burned, and necrotic tissue, and/or bedsores, shall be excised and/or treated either by hypodermic injection or by cavity pack application of deodorizing/preserving chemicals. All excised tissues will be retained with the remains and not disposed of as medical waste. The excised tissue will be treated with the organs and placed in the body cavity.

**4.1.5.1. Prevent Leakage.** All lacerations, penetrating wounds, and autopsy incisions shall be sutured closed to prevent leakage. In cases where there has been significant loss of tissue due to dismemberment, blast damage or charring and the tissue is unable to be closed, the embalmer will ensure exposed tissue is thoroughly embalmed, dried, and packed with drying powders and secured with an absorbent material to prevent leakage and facilitate dressing in uniform or clothing provided by the PADD.

**4.1.5.2. General Full Body Wrap Guidance.** The use of full body wraps as prescribed in this document will be utilized as a last resort in cases where viewing would not be possible (e.g., severe charring of the upper torso, severe crushing of the head, and uncontrolled odor caused by decomposition). A full body wrap should not be used only to prevent leakage or to address missing limbs.

**4.1.5.3. Communication Required with Full Body Wrap.** The recommendation for the use of a full body wrap must be a collaborative effort between embalmer and Branch of Service liaison/case manager. Whenever possible, the Branch of Service liaison/case manager must view the remains and discuss preparation procedures with the DoD or contract embalmer so that they can effectively communicate condition of remains and reason for the recommendation of a Full Body Wrap with the PADD. All communication among the preparing embalmer, Branch of Service liaison/case manager and the PADD shall be documented in writing and entered in the appropriate mortuary case file.

### 4.1.6. Dressing Remains.
The PADD/PAED will be consulted and provided the opportunity to determine the clothing the deceased is to be dressed in, or which is to be displayed upon the top of wrapped remains, as the situation dictates. The contract funeral home or DoD facility providing mortuary services will be provided the clothing selected by the PADD/PAED, or will be provided a uniform by the Military Service. Prior to dressing, all remains will be placed in a white, opaque, or clear leak proof protective undergarment (one-piece plastic garment used to cover the entire body from the neck down to include the feet). Drying powder and/or preservative powders will be placed inside the protective undergarment to absorb any possible leakage or odors.

### 4.1.7. Grooming.
Military personnel who are dressed in their service uniform will be groomed in accordance with Military Service regulations and standards. Male facial and scalp hair shall be washed and groomed to conform to military standards; suitable hair preparation shall be accomplished for females to conform to military standards. If the PADD requests other accommodations, the preparing mortuary will consult with the appropriate Military Service to ensure compliance with Military Service standards. Fingernails shall be cleaned and trimmed. When the PADD has requested that the Service member not be dressed in the service uniform, the mortuary representative will check with the PADD to determine the correct attire. For nonmilitary personnel, the Military Service mortuary representative will check with the family to ascertain personal preferences.

### 4.1.8. Cosmetics.
Cosmetics shall be applied only in the amount necessary to produce natural color and texture. For female Service members, the cosmetics will conform to military standards unless expressly requested otherwise in writing by the PADD.

### 4.1.9. Setting Features.
The mouth will be securely closed by needle injector, muscular or mandibular suture, where the lips abut to form a natural expression. The eyes shall be securely closed by the use of eye caps or other appropriate means, with proper attention given to prevent wrinkling of the eyelids and a sunken appearance.

## 4.2. Preparation of Unembalmed Remains:
When the PADD/PAED has requested the deceased, be prepared for shipment to the receiving funeral home without embalming, the preparing mortuary will evaluate the condition of the remains and determine the feasibility of complying with the request based upon local and national regulations or laws at the place of origin and destination, and any restrictions imposed by available transportation methods, such as air, train, or hearse. Unless prohibited by law, regulation, or the availability of transportation options, the preparing mortuary will prepare unembalmed remains IAW paragraphs 4.1.1 through 4.1.9 above to the extent possible in IAW religious preparation practices or other preferences as directed by the PADD/PAED. This section applies to subsequent remains recovered and identified after mortuary processing or interment/inurnment has occurred.

## 4.3. Preparation of Viewable Remains:
### 4.3.1. General.
To obtain optimum results, a thorough pre-embalming case analysis will be completed by the embalmer utilizing the number of arterial injection sites necessary to ensure proper distribution of fluid. The only exception to this requirement is in the absence of a limb or the head. The arterial chemical solution injected into the remains shall contain a minimum 5% concentration, by volume, of formaldehyde or isomer of formaldehyde derivative preservative agent(s). The total volume of arterial solution injected shall not be less than 1 gallon per 50 pounds of body weight. Unless the decedent is edematous, a humectant must be added in equal volume to the arterial chemical, in the total fluid solution injected into the head and arms. It is permissible for a humectant based arterial chemical to be used in lieu of humectant additive being incorporated into the total fluid solution. For nonautopsied cases, the thoracic, abdominal, male genitals, and cranial cavities shall be thoroughly aspirated and injected with full-strength cavity chemicals having a 36-index (%) or greater. A minimum of 16 ounces of cavity chemical must be injected into the thoracic cavity, and a minimum of 16 ounces in the abdominal cavity and male genitals, and a minimum of 2 ounces of cavity chemical to ensure preservation of contents of the cranial cavity, having a 36-index (%) or greater. Hypodermic injections, packs, or other special treatments shall be accomplished, as required, to assure the disinfection and preservation of all body tissues. A suitable cream or lotion shall be applied on the face and hands to prevent dehydration.

### 4.3.2. Treatment of Scalp (Viewable Remains).
If the scalp was shaved because of medical treatment or surgery, processing or reprocessing shall be accomplished as specified for viewable remains, after which the cranium shall be wrapped with gauze or equivalent in a neat and professional

manner. The Military Service retains the ability to use an authorized uniform hat or beret, in lieu of gauze wrap. For remains requiring a partial head wrap the remains will be prepared IAW paragraph 4.4.4. The embalmer will ensure the tissue is firm, dry, and thoroughly preserved. The wrapping will be accomplished IAW paragraph 4.4.4., but will be limited to covering the affected area of trauma providing the possibility of viewing if desired by the person with authority to direct or effect disposition.

### 4.3.3. Disfigured Hands (Viewable Remains).
When the hands are disfigured, to the point that restoration is not possible, or discolorations are present that cannot be cleared, the hands shall be treated in a manner which shall render all tissue firm, dry, and thoroughly preserved. The hands, regardless of condition, will then be placed in opaque, leak proof gloves followed by white (military) cloth gloves.

### 4.3.4. Wounds, stains, and discolorations.
All lacerations, abrasions, incisions, excisions, and burn wounds shall be sealed and/or sutured to prevent leakage. Swollen or distorted features shall be reduced, if possible, to the normal contours. Applying packs and/or needle injection may be used to chemically bleach antemortem/postmortem stains. On viewable areas, masking cosmetics may be used to render stains/discolorations nondetectable.

## 4.4. Preparation of Nonviewable Remains.
### 4.4.1. General.
To obtain optimum results, a thorough pre-embalming case analysis will be completed. Each gallon of arterial fluid shall contain a minimum 10% concentration, by volume, of formaldehyde or isomer of formaldehyde derivative preservative agent(s).

### 4.4.1.1. Preservation treatment.
The total volume of arterial solution injected shall not be less than 1 gallon per 50 pounds of body weight. All body areas shall be further treated by means of hypodermic injection using undiluted cavity chemicals having a 36-index (%) or greater. In addition, packs, special gels, and/or dry sanitizers shall be used, as required, to ensure preservation, prevent leakage, and eliminate all offensive odors.

### 4.4.1.2. Cavity and genital treatment.
The thoracic, abdominal, male genitals, and cranial cavities shall be thoroughly aspirated and injected with full-strength cavity chemicals having a 36-index (%) or greater. A minimum of 16 ounces of cavity chemical must be injected into the thoracic cavity, and a minimum of 16 ounces in the abdominal cavity and male genitals, and a minimum of 2 ounces of cavity chemical to ensure preservation of contents of the cranial cavity, having a 36-index (%) or greater.

### 4.4.1.3. Procedure when arterial injection and/or cavity treatment is not possible.
When arterial injection and/or cavity treatment is not possible, all articulated and disarticulated anatomical portions shall be thoroughly disinfected and preserved via hypodermic injection and accessory chemical embalming techniques. Immersion and/or hypodermic injection with a trocar and/or syringe and needle, using full strength cavity chemicals 36-index (%) or greater is acceptable. Surface application of liquid, gel, or dry sanitizers and preservatives is also required to supplement primary needle and/or hypodermic injection techniques.

### 4.4.2. Nonviewable with Full Body Wrap.
Wrapped Remains. Remains that have been processed or reprocessed as outlined in paragraphs 4.3 or 4.4 and are traumatized to the extent that the remains cannot be dressed, shall be wrapped.

**4.4.2.1. Preparation for Full Body Wrap.** Wrapping shall be accomplished as follows: Polyethylene sheeting (5 mil or greater) and a wool blanket shall be furnished by the Military Service's mortuary representative. The military wool blanket shall be spread on the dressing table with opposing corners at the head and foot ends of the table. The blanket is then covered with white cotton sheet followed by a sheet of polyethylene. Cotton strips are laid down the center of the plastic sheet and liberally coated with a preservative/drying compound (hardening compound).

**4.4.2.1.1. Dorsal side preparation.** The dorsal side of the remains shall be liberally coated with a gel preservative followed by a liberal coating of drying compound (hardening compound), and then laid on top of the prepared wrapping material on the dressing table.

**4.4.2.1.2. Ventral side preparation.** The ventral side of the remains shall be liberally coated with a gel preservative followed by a liberal coating of drying compound (hardening compound).

**4.4.2.1.3. Strips, sheeting, and blanket preparation.** Additional cotton strips shall be placed over the remains, completely covering them. The polyethylene sheet is then folded in around the remains IAW paragraph 4.4.2.1. The folding of the polyethylene sheeting, white cotton sheet, and wool blanket shall be uniform, with the head and foot ends folded in first.

### 4.4.3. Full body Wrap Procedure.
The wrapping material on the left side of the remains shall be folded to the right. The right side then folded to the left side of the remains shall be secured with tape or pins, as applicable and described below. All seams in the polyethylene sheeting shall be sealed with nylon filament packing tape, to ensure no odor and/or fluid is emitted from the wrapping. When necessary, in extreme cases, duplicate layers of polyethylene sheets may be used. The white cotton sheet is then wrapped around the polyethylene-sheathed remains, secured with large safety pins (silver in color, 2–3 inches) placed no more than 4 inches apart. The wool blanket is then wrapped around the white cotton sheet, which shall have as few creases as possible, and secured with large safety pins (silver in color, 2–3 inches) placed no more than 4 inches apart. A tag identifying the deceased shall be attached to the foot end of the wrapped remains bearing the deceased name, rank, last four of the social security number or DoD identification number, and date of death. Remains that have been processed or reprocessed as outlined in paragraph 4.4.2 will be draped in the clothing provided by the Military Service mortuary representative.

### 4.4.4. Nonviewable Head Wrap.
Prior to beginning the wrapping process, all tissue and hair shall be rendered as dry as possible. During the embalming process, the tissue shall be prepared to present as natural a head shape as possible once the head wrap process is complete.

**4.4.4.1. Materials.** Required materials to accomplish the head wrap process include two (2) clear or semitransparent plastic

(.78 mil or greater) liner bags approximately 24″ by 23″, 2″ white surgical tape or 2″ clear strapping tape, 12 yards of 4.5″ (sterile or nonsterile) gauze bandage (approx. 3 rolls), cotton prep towels, (sterile or nonsterile) absorbent cotton or absorbent sheet product.

**4.4.4.2. Procedure.** Wrapping shall be accomplished as follows: the embalmer will place one clear or semitransparent bag over the head and tuck down into the full body, plastic garment, as required in paragraph 4.1.6. Ensure all air is removed from the bag before it is secured at the base of the neck with tape. Taping the bag around the forehead, over the nose and over the chin may provide a more aesthetically pleasing shape. The embalmer will place a second clear or semitransparent bag over the head and repeat the above steps, taking care not to lose shape of the facial features, if present. A minimum of three (3) strips of gauze bandage will be prepared side by side, overlapping .25 inch and centered over the crown of the head extending to the base of the skull and the base of the chin. The bandage will be tightly stretched and unobtrusively secured by tape. Beginning at the natural hairline on the left side of the head, the embalmer will secure the end of gauze bandage roll. Once secure, the gauze bandage will be wrapped around the head, overlapping the previous row of bandage by one half the width of the gauze bandage. This is done to ensure no visibility of the underlying plastic bag and to present a neat and professional appearance. The gauze bandage will continue to be wrapped around the head, down the neck until it reaches the base of the neck and will be secured with white surgical tape. The remains should then be dressed IAW paragraph 4.1.6, ensuring no tape is visible above the collar of the shirt or blouse. Trauma that is isolated to a specific area will be wrapped with gauze or equivalent in a neat and professional manner.

### 4.5. Preparation of Autopsied Remains:

If a partial or complete autopsy is performed, chemical injection and application with multisite drainage shall be accomplished, using the arterial chemical solutions requirements as specified in 4.3 or 4.4. Hypodermic injection of the thoracic and abdominal walls; back, buttocks, male genitals, shoulders, vertebral column with an undiluted cavity chemical having a 36-index (%) or greater is required. The scalp will be injected by syringe and needle with the chemical solution used for the arterial injection.

### 4.5.1. Internal Organs (Viscera).

All remains, including internal organs and partial remains, are not to be disposed of or destroyed. The viscera from remains that have had a cranial, thoracic and/or abdominal examination, shall be removed, cut into small portions and immersed in a undiluted cavity chemical having a 36-index (%) or greater, for an appropriate amount of time but typically a minimum of 2 hours. The inner surfaces of the body cavities shall be given a liberal application of gel formaldehyde or isomer of formaldehyde derivative preservative agent. The preserved organs are to be placed into the thoracic or abdominal cavities and liberally coated with a formaldehyde or isomer of formaldehyde derivative preservative agent and drying compound (hardening compound).

### 4.5.2. Cranial Cavity and scalp.

When a cranial autopsy is performed, the vertebral and internal carotid arteries must be sealed, the cranial cavity shall be packed with cotton and drying compound, both in the cranium and the calvarium secured by cranial clamps or wiring. The scalp shall be replaced over the calvarium, the incision will be coated with drying compound and tightly and neatly sutured to avoid leakage and unnatural appearance. The color of the suture cord should blend with the deceased's hair.

### 4.6. Embalmer Evaluation:

The DoD or contracted facility embalmer processing or reprocessing the remains shall critically evaluate the completed treatment to ensure all remains are effectively disinfected, uniformly preserved, and will arrive at its destination in excellent condition. The Military Service mortuary representative will authorize delivery or shipment of remains from a contracted facility when assured that the services and supplies furnished by the contractor including the signed DD Form 2062 (Record of Preparation and Disposition of Remains, DoD Mortuary Facility) or the signed DD Form 2063 (Record of Preparation and Disposition of Remains, Contracted Mortuary Facility) meets the PWS, DoD Standards within this document, and commercial item descriptions in their entirety.

### 4.7. Quality Assurance Evaluation:

Remains will be inspected after embalming, after dressing, and after placement of remains in a casket. If the remains do not pass inspection at any point in the process, corrective action will be taken to correct the deficiency and it will be documented in the case file. Additional actions that may be required to correct a deficiency may include any of the following: additional disinfectant or preservative treatment, redressing or rewrapping, or placement of remains in a new casket when the original casket is defective.

## 5. CREMATION.

Cremation of remains defined as whole body or a nonintact torso, may not be performed in a mortuary operated by a Military Service or through a funeral home or crematory under contract with a Military Service.

> **Identification: An Essential Part of What We Do***
>
> *Michael Kubasak*

Requests for both cremation and burial without formal ritual are becoming common in funeral homes throughout the country. As requests for these and other abbreviated services increase, so does the decision not to view the body. This poses several challenges for the funeral director:

- Regardless of what services are requested, we must perform certain legal functions. Everything we do in caring for a decedent and in serving a family has legal implications and carries liability.
- We cannot treat even minimal service requests casually.
- No matter how simple or complex the service, we must perform all duties in an ethical, professional manner.

---

*Reprinted from *Mortuary Management*, Vol. 89, No. 9, Monterey, CA: Abbott and Hast Publications, Inc.; 2002, with permission.

- Abbreviated services of any type carry a higher risk of misidentification than traditional (full) services.

Viewing is rarely an easy matter for newly bereaved families. As funeral directors, we can identify with a family's reluctance to view. At the same time, to fulfill our professional and legal responsibilities, we must involve the next of kin or their designated representative in verifying the identity of the body in our custody. We are like the physician who knows that in order to accomplish a beneficial outcome and give peace of mind to the patient or confirm a diagnosis, the patient may have to endure some discomfort.

Funeral directors offer a wide spectrum of services. *Identification is central to all of them.* Identification is imperative before performing a cremation or any type of abbreviated service without formal viewing, including burial, entombment, or shipping of the body. This makes sense from a risk-management point of view. We are responsible for preventing misidentification *even if the error was made before the body came into our custody.* If the wrong body is cremated, buried, or shipped, there is serious liability for the funeral home and for everyone who participated in the chain of custody.

The need for positive identification is not something new or unique in funeral service. The best funeral directors have always required it. Even in those states where it is not required by law, we have a clear responsibility to ensure the positive identification of every deceased person we serve, just as a surgeon must be sure of the patient's identity and the procedure planned before beginning. It is a standard of care. The only exception to requiring verification of the deceased *might* occur when the deceased dies at home in the presence of family or legal representative, and the funeral home transfers the deceased from the residence *directly* to the funeral home.

Identification makes sense professionally, practically and legally for several reasons:
1. Identification certifies that this is the right person beyond any doubt.
2. Identification underscores the professional responsibilities we assume in providing disposition.
3. Identification stresses the irreversibility of the cremation process.
4. Identification facilitates the process of grieving. The majority of memories are visual. Seeing the person dead is a powerful confrontation that undercuts the normal tendency to deny that a death has occurred. If at least one person in the family certifies personally to the death, it becomes easier for others to accept the finality of death and to proceed with their mourning. The "Missing person" phenomenon teaches us that the absence of positive identification can complicate bereavement.
5. Identification serves as a preventive mental health measure for the bereaved by establishing a basis for certifying the death has occurred and for setting in motion the supportive and therapeutic benefits of whatever ethnic, social, and spiritual services follow the death.

Some funeral directors take exception to having a firm policy on identification before disposition or treat it with indifference. However, today's litigious climate and the tendency of courts and juries to award enormous settlements make a profound statement. *Verifying the identity of the deceased prior to any disposition, especially when cremation is selected, is the foundation of all risk reduction methods.*

A recent legal case provides an example. A hospital released the wrong decedent to a funeral home. The funeral home cremated the body that was transferred into their custody. When it became known that the wrong body was cremated, the funeral home was sued. During a trial that received front-page newspaper coverage, the funeral home claimed it did not start the problem. The court agreed but determined that the funeral home "acted below the Standard of Care by not verifying the identity of the deceased," before performing cremation. The court further stated that they were the last ones that could have remedied the error, but failed to do so. In the *chain of custody*, the funeral director occupies a vital position that carries liabilities even for misidentification that may have occurred previously.

Practicing risk management, including identification, is not done merely for the funeral director but also for the survivors. Today, funeral service deals with a skeptical consumer. Any attempt to distance the family or their designated representative from the reality of our services, no matter how well intentioned, especially when cremation is chosen, or to save them from the need to verify the identity can come back to haunt us. For the family, a lack of understanding can contribute to doubts and mistaken assumptions.

For the funeral director, making funeral arrangements today is substantially different from what it was 30 years ago. Then we were making adjustments to comply with FTC regulations. Today, funeral service is scrutinized by Wall Street, the media, consumer watchdogs, and the legal community. As society becomes less trusting, families question what they once took for granted. We can no longer assume that people understand what we say or do. Most people are inexperienced in planning a cremation, burial service, or shipment of the body. They are well aware of reports of alleged wrongdoing by some in funeral service. To be more consumer-focused means more disclosure, more explanation and information about what we do, where it is done, and how it is accomplished. By explaining, we build trust. **A policy requiring verification of the identity of the deceased builds trust. It is the foundation of all risk reduction methods and the best way to ensure that the wrong person will never be cremated, buried, or shipped.**

Every funeral director has heard people raise doubt about whether the person really died. In the absence of viewing, it is easy for people to question the identity of the person buried or cremated. Many of us have experienced misidentification of remains from a medical center, nursing home, coroner's office, or other institution. We cannot put our reputation and business in someone else's hands. Trusting the name that is imprinted on a toe tag or wristband without question is no longer safe practice. Positive identification means having the next of kin or their legal representative *verify* that the identity is correct. I can recall two legal cases as examples. At a medical center, two males died on the same day. One occupied a room on the second floor, the other on the fifth floor. Unrelated to one another, they shared the same common last name. Hospital personnel were unaware of this unique situation, but correct wristbands and toe tags were attached after the death. As you might guess, at the time of transfer from the hospital, the morgue attendant and the funeral home representative only looked for comparison using the last name. This serious error was discovered at the funeral home the next day when a grandson wanted to place a handwritten letter with his grandpa. In the other case, two people died at a nursing facility, one male, the other female, only a few rooms apart. While preparing both for transfer, the nurse was sidetracked by an emergency. In her haste, she gave another nurse the body tags. The second nurse attached the wrong identification tags to each decedent. One body was mistakenly cremated. Three days later, out-of-town relatives arrived at the other funeral home to claim the body for transport and burial in a native American cemetery and discovered the mistake. Knowing nightmares like these can occur, how can you prevent them in your practice?

You can develop a policy of identification at your funeral home. Here are some guidelines to consider for each decedent that comes into your custody:

1. Identification should be performed by the next of kin or their *designated-in-writing* representative (relative, clergy, best friend) and presented as policy, NOT an option.
2. If identification is done by photograph, the funeral home should take the photograph after obtaining written permission to do so. If the family brings their own photograph, it must be recent enough for valid comparison and must be retained in the decedent's file. The person making the identification should sign the back of the photograph, noting the date and time the identification occurred.
3. Identification should take place at the funeral home in an appropriate room, such as a small chapel or slumber room. Viewing should *never* be done in a garage, flower room, storage room, preparation room, or carport area.
4. During the arrangement conference, families should be informed that identification viewing is not the same as formal viewing but is a very time-limited act, usually taking from several seconds to several minutes. Frank discussion reduces the possibility of misunderstanding about its purpose.
5. Whenever possible, identification should take place with the deceased in the casket or container to be used for the cremation, burial, entombment, or shipment.
6. Prepare the person who will be making the identification before it occurs. Inform them where it will take place, what they will see, and how the deceased is covered. Disclose that the body may not be embalmed, dressed in normal attire, or clean-shaven. If there was a postmortem examination or there are manifestations of trauma or disfigurement, mention this as well as any other relevant details.
7. Prepare a form on your letterhead stating the name of the deceased, date of death, and the name and relationship of the person with the right of disposition. If the next of kin designates another person to make the identification, *it should be done in writing*, noting the relationship of the person designated by the next of kin. Once the identification is complete, have the person making the identification sign the form and indicate the date and time it occurred.
8. If at all possible, after the identification has been performed, invite the person who made the identification to sit in your office and answer any questions they may have.
9. Some funeral homes present a flower or other small token to the person making the identification.

Some funeral homes provide attention to the body prior to identification. Your state may have laws or statutes governing what may or may not be done to a body for this purpose. The circumstances as well as the condition of the body can vary and the attention rendered may involve some or all of the following:

1. Unwrap or undress the remains and inspect the physical condition, noting the condition on the embalming case report.
2. Be certain the *funeral home identification tag* is securely attached to the body and that all forms of identification *are the same.*
3. Inventory and record valuables, personal belongings, or other items on the deceased.
4. Document the presence of any medical or mechanical devices or equipment on the body. Inform the family of devices that must be removed, such as pacemakers, when cremation is chosen.
5. Position the deceased with arms and legs straight, when possible.
6. Comb and brush the hair.
7. Clean the face, close the eyelids, and deodorize the body with a topical disinfectant spray.
8. Cover the deceased with undergarments or an apron and wrap the deceased in a clean sheet.
9. Refrigerate the body. If the body is placed in a pouch, ensure that another identification tag is securely attached to the exterior of the pouch.

We must also consider what to do when the body is decomposed or the death was due to violence. Both of these conditions can create a problem for the funeral director regarding identification. In both instances, people who do not understand our liability in disposing of a body, especially by cremation, can accuse us of adding to a family's emotional stress or being insensitive. Yet, for our peace of mind and that of the family, we must be assured of the identity of the body before proceeding. When conventional viewing is impossible, identification can also be accomplished by alternative methods that can include photographs, scars or tattoos, physical deformities, or dental records. Advanced decomposition and violent deaths can render identification almost impossible. Often, the coroner or another agency is involved in these instances, and they generally establish the identity of the remains before releasing them to the family or funeral home. *Make it a practice to ask the coroner for written acknowledgment of the identity of the remains.* On your letterhead, have the next of kin sign a statement acknowledging that identity was established by the coroner or other agency, that the remains are in such a condition that renders them not viewable, and that the funeral home is held harmless from any claims relating to the failure or inability to identify the remains at the funeral home.

When the next of kin or legal representative declines to verify the identity, some funeral homes have them sign a waiver. To the funeral home, a waiver may provide a sense of ease in reducing liability and a way of helping the family by not having them visually identify the body. However, it can also provide the funeral home with a false sense of security. A waiver can be useless unless *all of the next of kin* sign it or if your funeral home operates in a state whose laws permit fewer than all of the next of kin to waive each person's rights. Using a waiver raises numerous questions and is not the "cure all" that some funeral directors want it to be. No matter how assuring such a form may appear on paper, even when properly executed by all of the next of kin, legally *it will not protect your funeral home from the other family whose loved one has been mistakenly cremated, buried, or shipped.* All courts may not recognize waivers. It is suggested that you seek counsel from an attorney before using any type of waiver.

Today, we deal with a skeptical and demanding consumer. With cremation, you only get one chance to do it right. As we know and as the courts have stated, cremation is final and irreversible. The funeral home is normally the last in a line of those who can ensure the identity of the deceased person. This responsibility does not end with the identification at the funeral home. Identification is not just an event but is a *continuous process throughout the entire sequence of disposition.* Our obligation to the family and the resultant liability extends to outside contractors and agents as well. Funeral directors will be held accountable for everything their employees and organizations did or failed to do while serving a bereaved family. Our practices, procedures, and policies are now held to higher standards than ever before. Just because we never employed certain professional practices in the past is no excuse. Standards of care change and we must adapt to change. Verifying the identity of decedents in our care prior to any form of disposition is a standard of care. Funeral service can no longer give excuses. Risk management and risk reduction must be a part of our professional practice in 2005 and beyond. *It makes good sense for all concerned and is an essential part of what we do.*

About the author: Michael Kubasak has a life-long career in funeral service and formerly owned his own funeral home for 30 years. He is a licensed funeral director, embalmer, and certified crematory operator and is the author of the book *Cremation and the Funeral Director: Successfully Meeting the Challenge.* In addition to providing frequent presentations and workshops throughout the United States on leadership, management, customer service, operational topic, and consultation to funeral cremation providers, Mr. Kubasak serves as an expert witness in litigation cases. Known as "the funeral director's coach," he is President of Kubasak Associates and can be reached at 702.250.6856 or *mkubasak@aol.com.*

### The Mathematics of Embalming Chemistry*: Part I. A Critical Evaluation of "One-Bottle" Embalming Chemical Claims

*Jerome F. Frederick, PhD*
*Director of Chemical Research, Dodge Chemical Company.*

Few concepts can be more misleading and destructive to the professional future of the modern embalmer than the belief that "one-bottle embalming" is technically possible or even ethically admissible. The faulty reasoning behind this kind of wishful thinking is predicated on the premise that one single 16-oz bottle of embalming chemical can be made to contain *all* of the essential chemical components required for the complete embalming of the "average" case, regardless of the condition variables present in such a case.

Certain unscrupulous "fluid merchants," who are actually not bona fide embalming chemical manufacturers at all, have good reason to foster this misleading and unrealistic view. They do so with an obvious ulterior motive in mind. To put it plainly, they hope to win favor in the profession on the strength of a sensational economy appeal by claiming that embalming can be accomplished far more inexpensively with just one bottle of their super-duper elixir. Nothing could be further from the truth. To those who really understand the science of tissue preservation, such a claim smacks strongly of the chicanery and flimflam of the old-time "medicine men" who in earlier days ranged the frontiers in their flashy horse-drawn vans and sold cure-alls "good for man or beast" to the trusting pioneer folk in the far-flung outposts of expanding America. Times have changed, but credulity, it seems, remains a dominant factor of human nature even in this enlightened day and age. Although stemming more from trustfulness than ignorance, unquestioning belief in the impossible and impractical still threatens the success of the misguided individual, but even more important, tends to undermine the very foundation of funeral service itself.

Misleading, illogical, and technically faulty, the "one-bottle" concept must be explored in depth before its pitfalls can be made clear to all ethical embalming practitioners, for if allowed to gain momentum unopposed, such a trend can only give the critics and detractors of funeral service valid evidence to win public support for their destructive efforts.

In order to guide our readers toward a true and realistic evaluation of the hazards inherent in the "onebottle" concept, we will divide the discussion of the subject into two parts. In the first portion, we will center our analysis upon a hypothetically "perfect case"—one in which no type of chemotherapy had been administered prior to death and where no problems other than those met within the normal course of tissue preservation face the embalmer. We must realize, of course, that no such case actually exists. But it gives us the unbiased starting point needed to expose the fallacies of the "one-bottle" embalming chemical concept and so reveal its hidden threat to the profession.

In cases where modern chemotherapy has been brought into play prior to death—and this encompasses some 90% of the cases treated by embalmers nowadays—the calculations for the analysis and critical evaluation must be revised. For here, the hazards of "one-bottle embalming" take a sharp upward turn—and its inadequacy becomes greatly intensified.

We know, for instance, that cases in which the new antibiotic *kanamycin* has been used for some time prior to death require a much greater concentration of the arterial chemical than that indicated for cases that have not been treated with this drug. Expressed in its simplest terms, this requirement stems from the fact that the antibiotic causes changes in the kidneys. In consequence, the kidney tissues accumulate large concentrations of nitrogenous and ammoniacal wastes. And, as every embalmer knows, there is no more effective way to neutralize formaldehyde than reacting it with ammonia.

---

*Reprinted from the *De-Ce-Co Magazine* 1968;60(5), with permission. Copyright: The Dodge Company.

We shall take this part of our discussion, however, later and for the present confine ourselves to an analysis of the "perfect case," keeping in mind that it is purely hypothetical—for nowhere in our present chemotherapeutic era will the professional embalmer ever encounter such a case! Remember also that in any discussion concerning a topic such as this one, it is necessary to establish and accept certain basic scientific assumptions. While these may not apply directly to 100% of our cases in actual practice—"perfect" or otherwise—they do take into consideration the most common variables and so hypothesize a truly realistic and typical "specimen" case. For example, an *average* adult cadaver weighing 65.3 kg (or 65,300 g) has been shown to contain a *total protein* content of 10.7 kg (or 10,700 g of protein), by Brozek et al. (*Annals of the New York Academy of Sciences* 1963;110:123).

When formaldehyde reacts with protein, and *only* protein—and here again, we simplify the discussion by deliberately overlooking the fact that formaldehyde will also react with *other* components of the human body besides protein—it requires about 4.0–4.8 g (or 4.4 g average) of formaldehyde to totally react with and fix exactly *100 g of a soluble protein*. Nonsoluble proteins require even more preservative.

Now, as pointed out by J. F. Walker in his treatise (*Formaldehyde*, 2nd ed. New York: Reinhold, 1953, 315), the 4.4 g of formaldehyde is required to totally fix and preserve, for "all times," the 100 g of soluble protein.

The average cadaver has about 10,700 g of protein. To totally and "forever" preserve *all* the protein present in this average cadaver, we would need

$$10{,}700/100 \times 4.4 = 470.8 \text{ g of formaldehyde}$$

Let us consider, then, an average 16-oz bottle of arterial fluid. If it contains only 30% formaldehyde (most modern arterials contain other preservatives in addition to formaldehyde), it would be technically defined as a "firming" or "high-index" fluid. Its formaldehyde content is computed as follows:

1 U.S. fl oz = 29.6 mL

16 fl oz = 473.6 mL of fluid, of which 30% is formaldehyde,

hence $0.30 \times 473.6 = 142.08$ g of formaldehyde.

If we require 470.8 g of formaldehyde to totally preserve all the protein in an average body, then that amount of this chemical in a 30% fluid will contain only enough formaldehyde to preserve

$$142.08/470.8 = 0.3 \text{ or } 30\% \text{ of all the protein in that average cadaver.}$$

These calculations, as we pointed out earlier in this article, are necessarily predicated upon assumptions that must be accepted to establish a basis for computation. But even allowing the most liberal margin of error, it can be readily seen that *no single 16-oz bottle of fluid* could possibly deliver the minimal acceptable degree of preservation—even in a "high-index" formulation! And this, remember, is calculated on the conditions of an *average* case!

Yet, as theoretical figures, these must not be construed as applicable to every like instance. There are many truly capable and excellent embalmers whose professional standards demand the most critical technical perfection who can point to instances where they have achieved adequate preservation with as little as $1\frac{1}{2}$ or 2 bottles of arterial fluid.

But none among them would rightfully claim that he uses *only one* bottle of arterial per case as *standard operating procedure*, for to do so would reflect unfavorably upon his professional judgment. Even the most ingenious and careful practitioners must admit that they are compelled to vary the concentrations of arterial chemical to meet the exigencies and special conditions present in each specific case. Most conscientious embalmers, in fact, use the full complement of "adjunct" chemical when the need for them is indicated—restorative humectants when there is evidence of emaciation or dehydration, water conditioners to neutralize chemical conflict in their solutions, modifiers, pre-injections, co-injections, and vascular conditioning expedients. It is their familiarity with these "tools of the trade" that sets them apart as an elite professional class, where attitude and course of action are closely patterned on that of the medical man who employs every pharmaceutical and surgical expedient available to him as the need becomes apparent and modifies his treatment according to the conditional factors present in the case at hand. Imagine, if you can, a doctor who would be content to use the *same drug* in the *same concentration* on every case he treats! The analogy is very close to "one-bottle embalming."

But even if it were possible to produce a reasonably acceptable, if not perfect, embalming result with the "one-bottle" tactic, the embalmer who chose to place such paltry economy above the true objectives of his profession would indeed be asking for trouble. For the value of his reputation can scarcely be counted in fluid ounces of arterial chemical. Sensibly enough, few are ready to risk so much for so little in return—and the profession can well spare those who fall by the wayside with "one-bottle embalming."

Now, back to the hard facts of embalming chemistry. Even if it were technically possible to increase the amount of formaldehyde in a 16-oz bottle of arterial chemical to an absolute 100%, we would have barely enough to "fix" the total protein present in the "average perfect case." This, of course, is not feasible because of the intrinsic chemical–physical nature of formaldehyde. But mere "fixation" or stabilization of the body proteins does not constitute total embalming. The result of using such an arterial would be a rock-hard, ghastly gray cadaver—a far cry indeed from the lofty standards of modern embalming! And where would we put our diffusion stimulating constituents in a 100% formaldehyde fluid? Or the cosmetic modifiers, blood solvents, and vascular conditioning components? Without these, could this super-duper 100% formaldehyde arterial do the job we want it to do? Could it penetrate and preserve *all* the proteins in our hypothetical "average" case? Could it get past the "average" number of circulatory obstacles we would be almost certain to encounter in such a case? Lacking its normal complement of supporting constituents, it is hardly likely that this 100% formaldehyde fluid would win any applause from experienced professionals.

It should be plainly apparent at this point in our discussion that the "one-bottle" technique offers more danger to embalming results and professional reputation than the earnest, ethical embalmer is willing to risk. But our analysis and evaluation would not be quite complete if we did not take a moment to quiet the suspicion that "one-bottle" embalming might become valid through technical advances in injection equipment. We refer specifically to the use of high-pressure embalming. Although embalming under such pressures may *appear* to use only one bottle of arterial chemical to achieve preservation, the technique merits the most critical scientific scrutiny. There is now evidence that high-pressure embalming actually causes the preservation to be "blown" to the superficial areas of the body. The result is a "taut skin" appearance that gives the *impression* of true preservative firming, but actually fails to embalm the deep underlying tissues, creating a condition that can obviously cause the embalmer a great deal of trouble.

In any event—no matter which technique is employed—we must face the incontrovertible mathematical truths of embalming. Knowing the way proteins react with preservatives leaves no illusions that one-bottle embalming will ever become a practical reality. Claims to the contrary should be viewed with cautious skepticism, for there is every indication that they will prove wholly false and unworthy of acceptance by the ethical professional.

---

**The Measurement of Formaldehyde Retention in the Tissues of Embalmed Bodies**[*]

*John Kroshus • Joseph McConnell • Jay Bardole*
*Editor's Note: John Kroshus is Chairman of the Funeral Service*
*Education Program and Jay Bardole is Chairman of the Chemistry Department at Vincennes University. Joseph McConnell is an Evansville (Indiana) Funeral Director.*

---

## INTRODUCTION

As a result of tests conducted jointly by the Funeral Service Education Program and Chemistry Department at Vincennes (Indiana) University, a procedure has been developed by which the amount of formaldehyde retained in the tissues of a dead human body can be measured. It appears as though this project, which can provide a quantitative analysis of formaldehyde retention, might be used to evaluate the efficiency of new embalming techniques or products and thereby create the possibility of reducing the material expenditures in embalming.

In addition, improved techniques may also upgrade the quality of embalming results. Reducing material expenditures means that costs can be reduced, and if this can be accomplished without sacrificing results, it will constitute a significant advance for funeral service.

Embalmers have long suspected that a substantial amount of chemicals injected into a body during arterial embalming simply pass through the blood vascular system and are lost with the other fluids that drain from the body. Other tests have indicated that this was perhaps true. Now it is possible to measure quite accurately just how much chemical is lost and how much remains in the body.

The research project has indicated that approximately 50–55% of the arterial fluid injected into a body is lost along with the venous drainage. It seems evident that funeral service needs to examine ways by which embalming can be made more efficient and thereby reduce the waste of arterial fluid. Again, this procedure can be used to evaluate the efficiency with which embalmers are operating.

The procedure for measuring formaldehyde retention in the tissue of embalmed bodies has been adopted from a quantitative analysis experiment used to determine the amount of formaldehyde in pesticides.[1] Basically, the formaldehyde retention experiment involves reacting a sample of the venous drainage with sodium hydroxide and hydrogen peroxide.

The ratio of sodium hydroxide to formaldehyde is one to one in the reaction. This means that for every mole of formaldehyde present, 1 mole of sodium hydroxide will be used up in the reaction. Thus, by determining how much sodium hydroxide is used, the amount of formaldehyde present in the venous drainage can be calculated. That amount is then subtracted from the amount of formaldehyde originally injected into the body, and the amount of formaldehyde retained in the body is known.

The hydrogen peroxide is reduced during the reaction and provides hydroxide ions to the formaldehyde, which oxidizes to formic acid. The formic acid reacts with the sodium hydroxide to produce a sodium salt and water.

That solution is then titrated with sulfuric acid, and the data gathered are used to calculate how much sodium hydroxide reacted with the formaldehyde in the venous drainage sample.

## METHODOLOGY OF THE STUDY

### Standardization of Chemicals.

The sodium hydroxide and sulfuric acid used in the experiment must be standardized before being used. The procedure for the standardization of these chemicals is similar to that used in most elementary chemistry courses, and in this instance, the object is to make solutions that have a normality of one. What this means basically is that the acid and the base will react in such a way that they will neutralize one another if mixed in equal amounts.

### Practice Titration.

Once the chemicals have been standardized, it is also necessary to test them in laboratory conditions. For this reason, the solutions of sodium hydroxide and sulfuric acid were tested against a solution where the amount of formaldehyde was known. This allowed for a comparison of the calculations based on data gathered by titrations with predictable results.

**PROCEDURE.** Embalming chemicals were mixed with water to produce 150 mL of 1% formaldehyde solution. This was possible because of the standard "index" of arterial fluids, which states that index is the amount of formaldehyde present in 100 mL of solution. By using the formula, volume one times concentration one is equal to volume two times concentration two, the formaldehyde solution was mixed to contain 1% formaldehyde. Since the experiment used a 30-index fluid, 5 mL of the arterial fluid was mixed with 145 mL of water to produce the solution.

Using a volumetric flask, the 150 mL of formaldehyde solution was divided into three 50-mL portions, each of which was poured into separate 500-mL flasks.

---

[*]Reprinted from the Director, Vol. 54, No. 3, Milwaukee, WI: National Funeral Directors Association, NFDA Publications Inc., 1983, with permission.

Fifty milliliters of the sodium hydroxide was then added to each of the flasks.

Fifty milliliters of hydrogen peroxide was then added to each of the flasks.

Heat was then added to each of the 500-mL flasks to stimulate the reaction. The heat was continued until the bubbles of the reaction stopped and then for about 10 minutes longer.

When the reaction was completed, the flasks were cooled.

Next, a 50-mL burette was thoroughly cleaned and rinsed and filled with sulfuric acid. The amount was recorded on a data sheet.

Indicator was then added to the now cool "basic" solution, and the titration was begun. This procedure was repeated for each of the 50-mL portions of the formaldehyde solution with the initial and final burette readings recorded on the data sheet.

**OBSERVATION.** The titration is a back titration. The amount of acid delivered to reach the point of equilibrium was inversely proportional to the amount of formaldehyde that was present in the original solution. Therefore, the greater the amount of sulfuric acid delivered, the less the amount of formaldehyde present.

At the end point of the titration, the equivalents of the base and the equivalents of the acid should be equal. The difference between the equivalents in the calculations indicates that a certain amount of the sodium hydroxide was used up as formaldehyde was oxidized. As previously mentioned, the formaldehyde and the sodium hydroxide react on a one-to-one basis. The amount of sodium hydroxide absent from the original 50 mL is therefore directly proportional to the amount of formaldehyde that is in the drainage taken from a body, or in this case, to the amount of formaldehyde mixed to create the 1% solution.

**TITRATION DATA.** The burette readings indicate the amount of acid delivered in the titrations. The amounts are averaged, and the average is used to calculate the amount of base that reacted with formaldehyde.

**CALCULATIONS.** The difference of the equivalents of acid and base will determine the amount of base equivalents that react with formaldehyde. That figure is then multiplied by the formula weight of formaldehyde (which equals one equivalent of formaldehyde) that has as its product the grams of formaldehyde that reacted with the sodium hydroxide.

### The Embalming Procedure.

The embalming procedure in the experiment was done using the legs of a dead human body as subjects in obtaining samples. This was done for two main reasons. One, to ensure that there were no adverse effects from the embalming that would distort the normally exposed portions of the body, namely, the face, neck, and hands. Two, it allowed the experimenter to strike a comparison on tissue that was very similar in nature.

The researcher made every effort to keep the procedures identical for the injection of each limb. It should also be pointed out there is no deviation from normal embalming procedure.

Femoral arteries and veins were raised and ligated on both the left and right legs of the deceased.

Two gallons of pre-injection was then mixed in 1-gallon quantities. Six ounces to the gallon of a formaldehyde-free pre-injection chemical was added to each gallon. The embalming machines were then filled and set for pressure and rate of flow.

One machine was set to a pressure gauge reading of 6 pounds per square inch, with a rate of flow of 1 gallon per 5 minutes. The other machine was set to a pressure gauge reading of 60 pounds per square inch, with pulsation, and a rate of flow of 1 gallon per 5 minutes.

Arterial injection tubes and venous drain tubes were then inserted into the arteries and veins, respectively.

The embalming machines were then started and the legs were injected simultaneously.

During the pre-injection, the drainage was not saved. The object of the pre-injection was to "flush" out the vascular system and replace the blood and tissue fluids with the pre-injection solution. This is a very important point because the pre-injection solution was composed of known elements, while the embalmer could not be sure what was in the blood and tissue fluids of the body.

Once the pre-injection was completed, hoses were placed on the venous drain tubes, and collection containers were installed to collect the drainage from the preservative injection.

The preservative solution was mixed in a 1-gallon container with a dilution of 6 oz of arterial fluid per gallon. The arterial fluid used was 30 index. The solution was then divided into 1.5-gallon portions, and each machine was filled with 0.5 gallon of the arterial solution.

Again the limbs were injected simultaneously, and this time the drainage was saved from the beginning to the end of the injection of the 0.5-gallon portions. By saving the drainage throughout the injection, it was felt that the samples saved constituted a representative sample of the drainage total.

It should be pointed out that the independent variable in this experiment was a variation in pressure gauge readings on the embalming machines being used. As mentioned previously, the independent variable could be changed to include a new technique, new product, or new solution mixture. Whatever the independent variable being tested happens to be, the remainder of the experiment stays the same.

### Titration of Drainage Samples.

The drainage samples saved from the embalming were kept in separate containers. Care was taken throughout the titration to make sure the samples were not mixed.

A 150-mL portion of the "low-pressure" sample was divided into three 50-mL portions and placed into three 500-mL flasks.

To each flask, 50 mL of sodium hydroxide was added.

To each flask, 50 mL of hydrogen peroxide was added.

The flasks were then placed over heat. The heat served to speed up the reaction and was maintained until the tiny bubbles of the reaction ceased. As the reaction was in full progress during heating, the mixture in the flasks tended to foam over. Toward the end of the reaction, the foam would gradually disappear.

The same procedure was then followed for a 150-mL portion of the "high-pressure" sample.

All flasks were carefully labeled and observed during the course of the reaction. It should be pointed out that heat has no adverse effect on the final results. The solutions cannot be overheated.

When all reactions were complete, the flasks were placed in an ice bath until they were cool.

The contents of a flask were then placed into a clean 250-mL beaker. A magnetic stirring rod was placed in the beaker, and the beaker was placed on an automatic magnetic stirring device.

An electrode was then placed into the beaker, and the pH of the solution was registered on a pH meter connected to the electrode. The pH reading was recorded on a graph sheet. The graph sheet was contained in a grapher that was connected to the pH meter. The grapher would make a graph of the pH changes during the titration.

To begin the titration, an Automatic Constant Rate Burette and the grapher were turned on simultaneously. The Automatic Burette would deliver sulfuric acid into the 250-mL beaker of drainage sample. The automatic stirring device would mix the solution as the titration progressed.

The researcher was able to monitor the titration through the end point and until it could be determined that the basic solution present at the outset of the titration had become an acid solution.

The final pH reading was recorded on the end of the graph, and the amount of sulfuric acid delivered by the Automatic Burette was also recorded on the end of the graph. The initial and final pH and burette readings were used to calculate the amount of sulfuric acid needed to reach equilibrium in the solution.

That amount would help determine the amount of sodium hydroxide, which had reacted with formaldehyde in the solution. That figure, in turn, was used to determine the amount of formaldehyde in the drainage sample. The difference of the amount of formaldehyde in the drainage sample and the amount of formaldehyde injected was the amount of formaldehyde retained in the tissues.

This entire experiment was repeated over 10 times during the course of about 2 and 1.5 years. The object was to find a pattern that would indicate proof of the superiority of either "high" or "low" pressure in embalming. At no time was any direct comparison made between bodies. Direct comparisons were made between legs of the same body until an overall pattern was established. In this case, the experiment showed that there was very little difference in formaldehyde retention in bodies embalmed with "high" pressure as compared to bodies embalmed with "low" pressure. It has already been pointed out that an independent variable of pressure could be switched for any number of variables that would warrant testing.

The procedure is precise and accurate. It would seem to open countless possibilities for improvement of presently accepted arterial embalming techniques as well as for the testing of newly developed techniques. It may also provide definitive answers to questions about the value of the multitude of pre-injections, coinjections, water correctives, and supplemental chemicals on the market today.

## REFERENCE

1. Welcher FJ, ed. *Standard Methods of Chemical Analysis*, 6th ed., Volume Two—Industrial and Natural Products and Non-instrumental Methods. Part B. Princeton, NJ: D. Van Nostrand Company, Inc., 1963:1878–1879.

### The Two-Year Fix: Long-Term Preservation for Delayed Viewing[*]

*by Kerry Don Peterson*

This article is taken from excerpts of a workshop presented at NFDA's 1991 annual convention by Kerry Don Peterson, Director of the Body Donor Program—University of Utah School of Medicine.

Operating a body donor program is in many ways an enlightening experience, and I have found a number of similarities exist between funeral service and anatomic science. Just one of these similarities is the practice of embalming.

The history of funeral service and anatomic science merged for a brief period at the close of the Civil War as a result of the work of Anatomist Thomas Holmes who developed a method to preserve dead human bodies to elongate and enhance the dissection process. Holmes capitalized on the idea after the war by offering his embalming services to Washington, D.C., funeral homes and from this embalming evolved into what it is today.

Anatomic embalming is unique when compared to mortuary embalming as we in the anatomic sciences have the opportunity to view our embalming successes or failures over a period of 2 years. As a result, we must learn the necessary techniques for long-term preservation or suffer the consequences.

One of the last cases I embalmed while a full-time employee of a funeral home 8 years ago was the body of a 39-year-old woman who had been stabbed 109 times. The family desired a traditional funeral with embalming followed by cremation. Being a homicide, the body was autopsied and could not be cremated until the county attorney cleared the case because cremation would have destroyed potential unfound evidence. It was going to be 6–9 months until the cremation could be performed; yet, the family indicated a desire to see the body just prior to cremation for a final goodbye. So here I was, presented with an autopsied body carrying 109 stab wounds on every part of the body, including the face. It was the beginning of summer and the family wanted a final viewing in 6–9 months.

I embalmed the woman as thoroughly as I knew possible by using a higher volume of more concentrated arterial fluid, hypoed the autopsy flaps, quadruple bagged the viscera and treated it with three bottles of cavity chemical, packed pledgets of cotton soaked in insecticide and cavity chemical in the body's orifices, and used an inordinate amount of drying compound in the abdominal and thoracic cavities. At the time of the funeral, the body looked great. Afterward, it was stored in the coolest room in the funeral home, which usually stayed between 60 and 70 degrees Fahrenheit. Stone oil and lanolin cream were applied to the face and hands throughout this time. Over the storage period of 7 months, the body manifested increasing signs of dehydration and tissue shrinkage, some graying and darkening of the tissues, and development of a slight odor.

All in all, I did not feel too bad about the results given the circumstances. With deodorant powder in the casket and some opaque makeup and wax, the body looked okay. The family did

---

[*]Reprinted from the Director, Vol. 63, No. 4, Milwaukee, WI: National Funeral Directors Association, NFDA Publication Inc., 1992, with permission.

not sing praises at the final viewing, but they seemed happy. Again, this all took place about 8 years ago, and since then, I found I could have done a much better job.

Over the last 5 years, I have experimented with normal mortuary supplies and chemicals on 135 cadavers (these cadavers exhibited a full complement of physical and pathologic conditions, including edema, ascites, jaundice, chemotherapy, obesity, and skin-slip; there were even a few "normal" cases) and through trial and error have devised what I consider to be the best method to preserve and store a body for extended periods of time. Each of these 135 cadavers was held and observed for 2 years. The majority of them exhibited minute dehydration, no discoloration, no blebs, no odor, and no mold. Using this method, I have also reinjected cases that were embalmed a week prior and it has not affected the end result, provided cavity work was not performed. I would like to mention the method was derived on the prep room table, not on a computer or through chemical equations on paper.

I have arbitrarily broken the long-term preservation process into three steps: (1) pre-injection details, (2) application of chemicals, and (3) method of storage. Most of the steps covered are no doubt part and parcel of your normal routine, but it is the sum of all these steps that leads to long-term embalming success. Negligence in one or two of the procedures can lead to partial or total embalming failure.

## PRE-INJECTION

To achieve long-term preservation, the embalmer must employ all known and accepted techniques of thorough embalming; shortcuts will cause future headaches. The body should be thoroughly disinfected using a reputable disinfectant and warm water, and the body's orifices should be sprayed or swabbed. *Rigor mortis* should be relieved. Elevate the body above the preparation table with positioning devices under the buttocks, shoulders, and ankle bones. This will take the weight off of most tissues on the back of the body, allowing for better fluid distribution to the area. Prior to the use of positioning devices, I had some bodies exhibit fluid distribution failure on only the weight-bearing posterior portions of the body. Once positioned, the face can be shaved and the facial and body features posed. In setting the facial features, I suggest you restore as much natural contour to the cheeks and eyelids as possible because the arterial fluid recommended will set the facial features firmer than you may be used to. Hypoing of tissue builder will still be an option after the injection of the arterial chemical but, once again, the tissues will be more rigid and less susceptible to tissue builder distension.

An embalmed body is like a petri dish for mold to grow on when stored for long periods of time. Since cotton and absorbent paper products (tissues and paper towels) are likely to harbor mold spores, they should be treated with a sporicide, such as phenol, prior to contact with the body during all three steps of the process.

## APPLICATION OF CHEMICALS

To begin step two, select the vessel to be raised. I have had success with both the femoral artery and the carotid arteries, although I personally prefer the latter because it allows for better draining of the internal jugular vein. Most important is that you use the vessel you are most familiar working with. Be advised that venous drainage is of the utmost importance for cosmetic effect but is of no consequence for preservation; in fact, many medical schools do not drain a drop of blood when injecting their cadavers.

After you have raised the selected vessel, make a "T" incision in the artery with the base of the "T" pointing the direction of cannula (arterial tube) insertion. This should be part of your normal embalming routine. When a cannula is inserted in the "T" incision, it is less likely that the tunica intima or tunica media will separate from the tunica adventitia. Ligature compression will also do less damage to the arterial layers when the "T" incision is used, which is very important in those cases you reinject. I generally insert a closing drain tube in the vein as it seems a superior way to regulate venous drainage and resistance, when it works! About 60% of the time I replace the drain tube with drainage forceps at some point during the injection process.

Chemical selection and storage techniques are the crux of long-term preservation. In mixing your chemicals, you want a sufficient amount of preservatives, antidehydrants, mold retardants, and accessory chemicals to break up clots, lubricate the vessels, and reduce surface tension. Water has none of these qualities. If you only have arterial and cavity chemicals on your shelves, your success will be no better than what I had with the stab victim. Every reputable manufacturer of embalming chemicals has an array of chemicals that preserve, break up clots, lubricate vessels, reduce surface tension, act as an antidehydrant, and contain phenol or specific retardants. The truth of the matter is you *do not* need most of these chemicals to inject the average case, but you *do* need all of them to inject a case you are going to keep around the funeral home for a couple of years unless you want to deal with dehydration, blebs, mold, odor, discoloration, and so on.

The minimum amount of chemical I have injected with 100% satisfactory results is two tanks of the following:

### *First Injection.*

*Formaldehyde:* Sixty-four ounces (four 16oz bottles) with an index range of 21–27%. I have tried using less, but some of those cases failed.

*Water corrective:* Use 64 oz, even if your morgue has soft water. Water corrective has an array of qualities that enhance the injection process, some of which include (1) it inactivates the minerals in body fluids just as it inactivates minerals in the water supply, (2) it extracts inert gases from the water supply and the body, (3) it defibrinates the blood, (4) it maintains a proper acid–base relationship between chemicals and the body, (5) it intensifies permeability of arterial solutions, and (6) it maintains the potency of formaldehyde and coinjectants against the body's natural chemical barriers.

*Vascular lubricant/clot dispenser:* Sixty-four ounces, which not only aids in drainage but also protects the capillaries from searing when using harsher chemicals and makes the tissues more receptive.

*Mold retardant:* Thirty-two ounces of mold retardant or 8 oz of phenol-containing cauterant *or* 16 oz of phenol-containing cavity fluid. *Note*: To avoid jelling, this chemical is usually best when premixed with your vascular lubricant or clot disperser before adding it to the embalming machine tank. When mixing new chemicals, it is a good idea to test mix a small batch.

*Dye:* More or less than normally added, but the amount of time you hold a body will be the main factor in determining how much dye to use if you choose to dye at all. *Note the use of phenol-containing products in the embalming machine may void the manufacturer's warranty.*

*Water:* Add enough water to make a solution totaling no more than 16 oz over 2 gallons.

### Second Injection.

The second injection is the same as the first *unless* you are using an arterial formaldehyde that does not contain a humectant or if one of the accessory chemicals does not contain a glycol (such as ethylene or propylene glycol), which acts as a humectant. If you have not injected a humectant in the first injection, add humectant to the second injection by reducing the water corrective and vascular lubricant by 16 oz each (a total of 32 oz) and replacing it with 32 oz of humectant.

Usually two injections of this chemical mixture will suffice, but at times, I have had to mix and inject subsequent batches. Do not be tempted to shortcut chemicals on subsequent batches and remember that other rules of embalming apply, so do what you always do when you successfully embalm a case. Sometimes you will need to inject multiple points, and sometimes you will need to hypo an area to get adequate fluid to the tissues. Contrary to what I was told in mortuary science school, I have found hypoing to be a very effective treatment for any tissues not receptive to arterial injection. Hypoing the flaps of an autopsy with the same chemical is a must. Also on autopsy, a liberal application of external preservation cream on the underside of the scalp is warranted.

I do not recommend a pre-injection before the injection of this arterial formula. Pre-injection was part of my normal routine in the funeral home, and I tried to incorporate it into the anatomical routine, but my results were less than satisfactory. Tissues only have the capacity to absorb limited amounts of fluid, and when embalming for long-term preservation, you want the more stringent fluid absorbed by the tissues.

Particular items to be aware of during the injection procedure include:

- *Manifestations of the chemical:* While embalming, you may note the skin manifesting what I call an orange peel demarcation. The skin sometimes takes on the color and texture of a dehydrated orange peel. This demarcation is normal and passes in 24–48 hours. When using phenol, you might also note 1/8th- to 1/4th-inch white patches; this is also normal and goes away shortly after embalming.
- *Drainage:* When phenol is used, your drainage may become gritty. But regardless of whether or not phenol is used, the more stringent chemicals inherently lead to poor drainage late in the embalming process. It is also a good practice to tie off the vein while injecting the last quart or two of chemicals.
- *Swelling considerations:* Weigh the variables. If you see swelling of facial features occurring and the body is well perfused except the feet, stop injecting and hypo the feet. If the face starts swelling and the body is a long way from being embalmed, lower the pressure or flow, raise and clamp both carotids, and open the jugulars. Be aware that when the body is in storage, swelling diminishes to near normal contours naturally within a month's period of time.
- *Purge:* The more stringent fluids often lead to copious purge. This purge is often the same color as the fluid you are injecting and seems to run out as fast as it is injected, but most of the time, fluid distribution is unaffected.
- *Pressure and flow considerations:* I find the pressure versus flow debate to be one of the most confusing issues of embalming science. With the flow closed on my machine, I set the pressure gauge at 25 pounds and open the flow until the pressure drops to 18–20 pounds; on my machine, this is an unencumbered rate of flow of 22 oz per minute. I do adjust the pressure down when injecting those bodies that appear prone to swell and often increase the rate of flow later in the embalming process when the body is taking fluid well and not swelling. If your normal pressure and flow settings give you good results, I advise you to continue using these settings. **Always use the pulse**—studies prove the slight pause in fluid movement increases the amount of fluid absorbed into the tissues. If your machine does not have a pulse feature, turn the machine off for 5 minutes at each quarter tank interval; also wait 10 minutes between the first and the second injection as the rest periods give the tissues a chance to absorb the fluid and offer you a chance to evaluate your progress.
- *Bright dye effect:* The accessory chemicals you mix in this arterial formula not only make the tissues more receptive to formaldehyde but also make the tissues more receptive to dyes. The catch here, however, is that over a period of 2 months the dye starts to bleach or wash out. When embalming, if you know how long you will have to hold the body, add dye accordingly. What appears bright red at the conclusion of embalming will be very light red in a year. Take this into consideration.
- *Monitor body features for displacement during embalming.*
- *Chemistry:* Provided you have injected two tanks of formula and feel you have adequately preserved the body, you have actually injected twice as much formaldehyde as embalming chemistry tells us it is necessary to react with and preserve the soluble proteins of a 160-pound person. Considering you lose arterial formula during drainage and that there are other factors to consider when embalming besides soluble proteins, it should become apparent that this dilution of fluid is in line with the accepted chemical principles of embalming.

When the body has received enough fluid, ligate the arteries and veins, treat the internal incision, suture, and apply incision sealer to the outside of the incision.

Using a 30-cc syringe and your longest hypo needle, inject the brain. Direct the needle through the medial canthus of the eye (pretty much straight back, but you may have to feel around a bit to locate the superior orbital fissure), through the superior orbital fissure, and into the cranial cavity. Inject 30 cc of formaldehyde slowly through each eye socket into the cranial cavity, drawing the needle outward. Avoid swelling the eye sockets by injecting the bulk of fluid well within the cranial cavity.

At this point, I suggest you do any hypo tissue building or restorative work necessary. Then apply a liberal amount of cream to the face, neck, hands, and wrists.

If the body does not warrant immediate cavity treatment, delay cavity work for 12–24 hours and then perform the work in the usual manner followed by an injection of 16–32 oz of cavity chemical.

## METHOD OF STORAGE

In storage you want to create an environment for the body that (1) maintains an osmotic balance of moisture between the body and its environment to prevent dehydration, (2) protects the body from mold growth, and (3) provides a preservative buffer between the body and its external environment. The storage technique is easily accomplished and requires 5 minutes a week, at most, to maintain. The required supplies include the following:

1. A thick, plastic sheet large enough to loosely wrap the body with excess to tuck beneath.
2. A hospital gown or cloth shroud.
3. A spray bottle.
4. A chemical wetting agent consisting of two-thirds of a gallon of humectant (glycol or antifreeze), 4 oz of mold retardant (thymol or phenol), and 1 gallon of water.
5. A body rest or wooden two-by-fours or four-by-fours.

## PROCEDURE

1. Lay the large plastic sheet on a table surface.
2. Place the body rest or cut wood on the plastic sheet (body rests should be high enough to keep all parts of the body off of the table surface).
3. Semisaturate the hospital gown or shroud with the wetting agent. Dress or wrap the body in the gown or shroud but do not cover the face or feet. Put the rest of the wetting agent in a spray bottle.
4. Place the draped body on the body rests and wrap the plastic sheet loosely around the body. Tuck the free ends of the plastic snugly under the body, trapping a moderate amount of air in with the body (do not wrap the body tightly in the plastic sheet).
5. Place the body in a cool spot. Refrigeration is not necessary but it does help.

Check the body every 3 or 4 days for the first couple of weeks. Aspirate or sponge out free liquids in the bag (it is quite normal for some bodies to precipitate 2 gallons of fluid), keep the cloth shroud moist with the spray bottle, and apply cream to the face and the hands as necessary. The plastic wrapping normally creates a rain garden environment.

After the first 2 weeks have passed, weekly maintenance consisting of spraying the shroud with wetting agent, draining pooled liquids, and reapplying cream to the face and hands is more than sufficient to maintain the body in its environment. Mix more wetting agents when necessary. If a part of the body seems to be going soft (which I have never had happen), hypo treatment is still an option.

Before final viewing, remove the body from the wraps, wash thoroughly with an ample amount of soap, and proceed with the normal cosmetic routines.

I do not suggest this method of preparation for every case as the method is costly and time consuming. As embalmers, we know it is not our charge to preserve artifacts for future centuries, but to disinfect and prepare bodies of the dead for therapeutic funeralization of the presently living. I do, however, suggest this method for long-term preservation or when a firm base is required for reconstruction or restoration.

> **Occupational Exposure to Formaldehyde in Mortuaries**[*]
>
> *L. Lamont Moore, CIH CSP*
> *Safety Sciences Department, Indiana University of Pennsylvania, Indiana, Pennsylvania*
>
> *Eugene C. Ogrodnik, MS*
> *Dean, Pittsburgh Institute of Mortuary Science, Pittsburgh, Pennsylvania*

*A short-term project was conducted to evaluate occupational exposure to formaldehyde in mortuaries. The study group consisted of 23 mortuaries located in Allegheny County, Pennsylvania. These establishments had business volumes ranging from 35 to 500 embalmings per year. On-site surveys were conducted at each location to examine ventilation systems and review work practices. Breathing zone and room air samples were subsequently collected during actual embalming procedures in a number of the smaller facilities with less well-designed ventilation systems. One of the primary objectives of the project was to educate participating mortuary directors about the potential health hazards associated with occupational exposure to formaldehyde. An extensive literature review was completed to summarize related epidemiological and environmental studies for participants. Additionally, the monitoring data were compared to previous observations and exposure estimates. Results of this study did not reveal employee exposures that approached existing limits established by the Occupational Safety and Health Administration (OSHA).*

Formaldehyde is a colorless, pungent, irritant gas that is water soluble and most frequently marketed as 37–56% aqueous solutions, commonly known as *formalin*. Formaldehyde vapor is very irritating to the respiratory tract, eyes, and exposed surfaces of the skin. Inhalation of high concentrations can cause laryngitis, bronchitis, and bronchopneumonia. Liquid formaldehyde solutions may cause severe burns on contact with the eye. Formaldehyde will act as a primary skin irritant, causing an erythematous or eczematous dermatitis reaction.

Formaldehyde solutions do not have a high degree of systemic toxicity, and acute and chronic exposures generally result in varying degrees of irritation, which are usually localized. Symptoms commonly experienced by the general population are nonspecific, transient, exposure dependent, and usually mild. In some cases, however, formaldehyde may act as an allergic (immunologically mediated) skin sensitizer, and it may also exacerbate respiratory distress in individuals with preexisting or formaldehyde-induced bronchial hyperactivity. It may not be feasible for sensitized persons to work in an area where there is any possibility of exposure, even at very low levels.

---

[*]Reprinted from the *Journal of Environmental Health* 1986;49(1), with permission.

Formaldehyde has an odor threshold far below 1 part per million (ppm). Stern[1] reported the lower limit for odor detection to be 0.05 ppm with throat irritation first occurring at 0.5 ppm. Bourne and Seferman[2] established the threshold for eye irritation at 0.13–0.45 ppm. The experience of numerous investigators has been that rapid inurement to such concentrations develops and there is a general absence of complaints from most workers exposed below 2 or 3 ppm.[3] According to existing OSHA regulations, the permissible limit for 8-hour time-weighted average exposure to formaldehyde is 3 ppm. The acceptable ceiling concentration is 5 ppm and the acceptable maximum peak is 10 ppm for 30 minutes. This standard was adopted in the mid-70s based on the irritant properties of formaldehyde.

The American Conference of Governmental Industrial Hygienists[3] has listed formaldehyde as a substance suspect of carcinogenic potential for man. In 1983, they proposed an 8-hour time-weighted average exposure limit of 1 ppm with a short-term exposure limit of 2 ppm for a maximum of 15 minutes. They point out that these concentrations may not be sufficient to prevent sensitized persons from suffering irritation but should be adequate to avoid development of persistent adverse effects.

In 1976, the National Institute for Occupational Safety and Health[4] recommended to OSHA that occupational exposure to formaldehyde be limited so that no employee is exposed at concentrations that exceed 1 ppm during any 30-minute period. This recommendation presumably was designed to protect the health of employees over their working lifetime, but may not be adequate to protect sensitized or hypersensitive individuals.

Plunkett and Barbela[5] completed a mail survey of 57 embalmers in 20 California funeral homes during 1976. Nine had symptoms compatible with acute bronchitis, and 17 were considered to have chronic bronchitis. No data on formaldehyde exposure levels, work practices, ventilation, or frequency of exposure were gathered. Nevertheless, there was enough evidence to suggest that more in-depth studies of this profession should be considered.

Levine et al.[6] studied nearly 100 West Virginia morticians who were attending an educational program during 1978. Standardized respiratory disease questionnaires and pulmonary function tests were administered to the group. The pulmonary function of morticians compared favorably with that of residential populations in Oregon and Michigan. Among the study group, those who had presumably embalmed the largest number of bodies did not demonstrate a higher than expected incidence of chronic bronchitis or pulmonary function deficits. The authors concluded that long-term intermittent exposure to low levels of formaldehyde had exerted no meaningful chronic effect on respiratory health. No actual data on formaldehyde exposures, ventilation, or work practices were gathered as part of this study.

Williams et al.[7] recently published the results of exposure studies conducted in seven West Virginia funeral homes. Area and personal samples were used to evaluate the embalmers' exposure to formaldehyde, phenol, and 23 organic solvents and particulates. Twenty-five personal samples revealed time-weighted average formaldehyde concentrations that ranged from 0.1 to 0.4 ppm during the embalming of intact bodies, and ranging between 0.5 and 1.2 ppm during preparation of autopsied cases. The overall average exposures were 0.3 ppm and 0.9 ppm, respectively. Concentrations of other airborne chemicals and of particulates were negligible. Time-weighted averages were calculated over the length of time actually required for the embalming. Embalming technique and condition of the body appeared to be the major determinants of formaldehyde exposure in preparing autopsied bodies. The importance of room air exchange rate could not be determined from this study. Overall, exhaust ventilation appeared to reduce formaldehyde concentrations in general room air but had little effect on the embalmer's personal exposure.

Kerfoot and Mooney[8] completed an extensive study of six funeral homes in the Detroit area, collecting 187 air samples under various conditions. The vapor concentrations encompassed a range between 0.09 and 5.26 ppm. The average formaldehyde concentrations ranged between 0.25 and 1.30 ppm under normal working conditions with an overall average of 0.74 ppm.

It was not clear whether personal or area samples were obtained. Ventilation systems were evaluated in terms of air changes per hour and compared with average concentrations of formaldehyde found in each facility. The largest number of air changes did not always correspond to the lowest concentration of vapors. The authors concluded that the location of the fan and size of the room were also significant factors. They also pointed out that all six establishments were above average facilities and inferred that formaldehyde concentrations in smaller, less well-designed funeral homes might be markedly higher.

In 1979, NIOSH[9] conducted a health hazard evaluation of the embalming laboratory at the Cincinnati College of Mortuary Science. The request had been prompted by the early disability retirement of an embalming instructor who had developed asthmatic bronchitis after 5 years of laboratory exposure. Air samples were collected via general area and personal breathing zone sampling during actual work conditions and simulated accidents involving spillage of embalming fluids. Formaldehyde concentrations exceeded the proposed ACGIH threshold limit value of 1 ppm in 7 of 13 samples collected. All of the excessive concentrations were detected during simulated (worst case) situations, or during one afternoon when the ventilation system was inoperable.

A study of mortality among undertakers licensed in Ontario, Canada, was completed by R. J. Levine[10] in late 1982. He selected a cohort of 1477 embalmers licensed between 1928 and 1957 and examined the cause of death in 337 men who had died before 1978. The ratio of observed to expected deaths from each cause was expressed as a percentage or standard mortality ratio. No significant increase in mortality was detected for any form of cancer. Deaths from cancers at sites of potential contact with formaldehyde—skin, nose, oropharynx, larynx, and esophagus—were less than expected, as were deaths from cancer of the lung.

Walrath and Fraumeni[11] of the National Cancer Institute published a study in 1983, which investigated whether embalmers in New York State, compared with the general population, had a greater proportion of cancer deaths that might be associated with exposure to formaldehyde. The study group consisted of approximately 1132 deceased embalmers who had been licensed to practice in New York State between 1902 and 1979. The difference between observed and expected numbers of deaths from malignant neoplasms was elevated, but not significantly. Skin cancer mortality was significantly elevated, primarily among those licensed for more than 35 years. Mortality was slightly elevated for kidney cancer, leukemia, and brain cancer. No excess mortality was observed for cancers of the respiratory tract and no deaths ascribed to nasal cancer.

Walrath and Fraumeni[12] published the results of a similar study of California embalmers in 1984. The authors examined the death certificates of 1007 embalmers and calculated proportionate mortality ratios for the major causes of death. Mortality was significantly elevated for total cancer, arteriosclerotic heart disease, leukemia, and cancers of the colon, brain, and prostate. There were no deaths from nasal cancer, and the pattern of lung cancer mortality was unremarkable. One of the inherent weaknesses of both the California and the New York studies is that sample sizes were of insufficient size to detect rare conditions such as nasal cancer. Although the respiratory tract would presumably be the prime target site for formaldehyde carcinogenicity, the authors conclude that available epidemiological evidence suggests attention should be given to possible cancer risks at other sites, including the brain, bone marrow, and colon. It may be of significance to note that the Ontario study[10] did not indicate an elevated risk of cancer based on a study of 300+ death certificates. However, larger studies performed in New York[11] and California[12] both showed excess deaths from leukemia and brain cancer.

Patty's text[13] suggests that aldehydes cannot be regarded as potent carcinogens. The irritant properties of the compounds preclude substantial worker exposure under normal conditions. The extreme reactivity of formaldehyde, acrolein, and chloroacetaldehyde, for example, produces reactions at epithelial surfaces that tend to limit their absorption into the body. The rapid metabolic conversion to innocuous materials also may limit those critical reactions necessary to initiate systemic tumorigenesis. However, formaldehyde induced tissue irritation may promote tumor formation initiated by another compound. Therefore, caution is warranted, and certainly, further epidemiologic studies must be performed to define any hazard that may exist.

Since 1979, there have been several research reports linking formaldehyde exposure to cancer. These studies were based on exposure of rats and mice to concentrations of 2, 6, and 15 ppm for 30 hours per week over a period exceeding 2 years.[14] On the basis of these findings, NIOSH recommended in 1981 that as a prudent measure, occupational exposure be reduced to the lowest feasible limit.

## MATERIALS AND METHODS

On-site surveys were conducted at each facility to interview the funeral director about work procedures, evaluate the overall floor plan, calculate room volume, and record airflow measurements where appropriate. Subsequently, air sampling was conducted in a number of the funeral homes with poorly designed ventilation systems. Where feasible, samples were collected from the breathing zone of the embalmer during the entire period required for the embalming, usually 45–75 minutes.

Air was drawn through a liquid sampling medium using MSA Model G pumps set at a flow rate of 500 cc per minute. Calibration was accomplished prior to the surveys using a primary standard (soap-bubble meter) as suggested by the manufacturer. Pumps were adjusted as necessary to maintain the desired flow rate throughout the sampling period. A midget impinger with fitted glass bubbler containing 15 mL of a 10% aqueous methanol solution was used to collect air samples to be analyzed for formaldehyde. At the conclusion of the sampling period, samples were transferred to polyethylene bottles, sealed, labeled, and shipped to an approved industrial hygiene laboratory.

At the laboratory, samples are reacted with hydrazine reagent to form a hydrazone derivative, then analyzed by differential pulses polarography. This sampling and analytical technique (ID-102) was developed at OSHA's Analytical Laboratory in Salt Lake City, Utah. The coefficient of variation ($CY_T$) for the total sampling and analytical technique is 0.08. This value corresponds to a standard deviation of 1 mg/m$^3$ at the OSHA permissible exposure limit of 3 ppm.

## RESULTS AND DISCUSSION

The embalming rooms examined as part of this study varied significantly in terms of their size, layout, and the effectiveness of the ventilation system. Preparation rooms were equipped with ventilation systems that produced from 0 to 20 air changes per hour with a mean of 7.6 air changes per hour. Three facilities had exhaust systems that produced no measurable air movement at all. Only 17% of these rooms had an exhaust grate or fan that was positioned to prevent fumes from being drawn through the breathing zone of the employee.

The size of embalming rooms ranged from 735 to 5000 ft$^3$ with a mean of 1950 ft$^3$. Less than 10% of the establishments had any provisions for the introduction of makeup air into the work area. The only source of makeup air would have been leakage around doors or windows throughout the structure.

Eight personal samples were collected from the breathing zone of funeral directors during separate embalming procedures in six different funeral homes. None of these establishments had ventilation systems that would be considered above the norm described above. Exposure concentrations summarized in **Table 1** show a range of 0.03–3.15 ppm with an overall average of 1.1 ppm during the period required for the embalming. Embalming procedures typically last 45–75 minutes depending on the condition of the subject. When we assumed zero exposure during the unsampled portion of the shift, 8-hour time-weighted average exposures ranged from 0.01 to 0.49 ppm, with an overall mean of 0.16 ppm.

The data summarized in **Table 2** provide a comparison of our limited data with that of more extensive studies by Kerfoot and Mooney[8] and Williams et al.[7] Allegheny County exposure estimates reflect slightly higher formaldehyde concentrations that may be associated with the smaller, poorly designed preparation rooms where sampling was conducted. Plans for a longer-term study were abandoned when our initial monitoring revealed 8-hour time-weighted average exposures to be well below the OSHA permissible exposure limit of 3 ppm.

| TABLE 1. Summary of Formaldehyde Exposure Measurements Based on Personal Sampling | | | |
|---|---|---|---|
| | Low (ppm) | High (ppm) | Average (ppm) |
| Time-weighted average exposure during the period required for the embalming procedure | 0.03 | 3.15 | 1.1 |
| Exposure estimate for the full work-shift, an 8-hour time-weighted average | 0.01 | 0.49 | 0.16 |

*Note*: Calculation of 8-hour time-weighted averages was completed making the assumption that exposure would have been zero during the unsampled portion workshift.

Six area samples were also collected from general workroom air in proximity to preparation tables, usually in conjunction with personal sampling. Results summarized in **Table 3** suggest that area sampling is not representative of the embalmers' actual exposure. Where concurrent sampling was carried out, concentrations found in the employee's breathing zone were up to twice as high as measurements taken from general workroom air several feet away.

There are a number of conclusions to be drawn from this study, despite its limited scope. First, the authors found many funeral directors to be largely unaware or poorly informed about the continuing controversy over the carcinogenic potential of long-term exposure to formaldehyde. Second, it was clear that most funeral homes in this study had ventilation systems or floor plans that were largely ineffective in controlling exposure during embalming procedures. The position of the exhaust grate commonly draws contaminants through the embalmer's breathing zone. Third, the authors' data suggest that personal breathing zone samples are likely to provide the most accurate indicator of employee exposure in the embalming room.

Occupational exposure to formaldehyde in funeral homes should rarely exceed permissible exposure limits established by OSHA. These limits were adopted in the early 1970s to protect employees against the irritant properties of formaldehyde and may not be sufficiently stringent in view of the chemical's suspected carcinogenic potential. It is reasonable to assume, however, that there are regular occasions where embalmers' exposures exceed the short-term exposure limits of 2 ppm during any 15-minute period recommended by ACGIH in 1983 and the NIOSH recommendation of 1981, which suggests exposure be kept at the lowest feasible limit.

| TABLE 2. Comparison of Allegheny County Exposure Data with Previous Studies | | | |
|---|---|---|---|
| **Estimated Formaldehyde Exposure During Embalming (in ppm)** | | | |
| | Low (ppm) | High (ppm) | Average (ppm) |
| Kerfoot/Mooney (1975)[8] | 0.25 | 1.39 | 0.74 |
| Williams/Levine/Blunden (1984)[7] | | | |
| Intact cases | 0.10 | 0.40 | 0.30 |
| Autopsied cases | 0.50 | 1.20 | 0.90 |
| Allegheny County (1984) | 0.03 | 3.15 | 1.10 |

| TABLE 3. Comparison of Formaldehyde Concentrations Detected in Workroom Air During Embalming Procedures—Area Versus Personal Sampling | | | |
|---|---|---|---|
| | Low (ppm) | High (ppm) | Average (ppm) |
| Area samples taken in proximity to preparation tables | N.D.[a] | 0.84 | 0.45 |
| Personal samples collected from the breathing zone of embalmers | 0.03 | 3.15 | 1.1 |

[a]N.D. signifies "not detected."

More extensive epidemiological and laboratory studies will be carried out before the issue of formaldehyde carcinogenicity is resolved. Funeral directors or embalmers represent a profession that should be of continuing interest to epidemiological researchers studying the long-term exposure to formaldehyde. Should more definitive evidence be developed with regard to the carcinogenic effects of formaldehyde, large-scale education efforts and installation of improved engineering controls will become priority within the funeral home industry.

## REFERENCES

1. Stern AC. *Air Pollution*. New York: Academic Press, 1968; Vol. 1, p. 484.
2. Bourne HG, Seferman S. Wrinkle proofed clothing may liberate toxic quantities of formaldehyde. *Industrial Medicine & Surgery* 1959;28:232.
3. American Conference of Governmental Industrial Hygienists. *Documentation of the Threshold Limit Values*. Cincinnati, OH: ACGIH, 1983:197.1.
4. National Institute of Occupational Safety and Health. *Criteria for a Recommended Standard.... Occupational Exposure to Formaldehyde*. Baltimore, MD: NIOSH, 1976:P.B. 76-273805.
5. Plunkett ER, Barbela T. Are embalmers at risk? *American Industrial Hygiene Association Journal* 1977;38:61–62.
6. Levine RJ, DalCorso RD, Blunder PB, Battigelli MC. The effects of occupational exposure on the respiratory health of West Virginia morticians. *Journal of Occupational Medicine* 1984;26:91–98.
7. Williams TM, Levine RJ, Blunden RB. Exposure of embalmers to formaldehyde and other chemicals. *American Industrial Hygiene Association Journal* 1984;45:172–176.
8. Kerfoot EJ, Mooney TF. Formaldehyde and paraformaldehyde study in funeral homes. *American Industrial Hygiene Association Journal* 1975;36:533–537.
9. National Institute of Occupational Safety and Health. *Health Hazard Evaluation*. Cincinnati: College of Mortuary Science Embalming Laboratory; 1980:HHE 79-146-670, NTIS Pub. PB80-192099.
10. Levine RJ. Mortality of Ontario undertakers. In: *C.I.I.T. Activities*. Research Triangle Park, NC: Chemical Industry Institute of Toxicology, 1982.
11. Walrath J, Fraumeni JF. Mortality patterns among New York embalmers. *International Journal of Cancer* 1983;31:407–411.
12. Walrath J, Fraumeni JF. Cancer and other causes of death among California embalmers. *Cancer Research* 1984;44:4638–4641.
13. Clayton GD, Clayton FE, eds. *Patty's Industrial Hygiene and Toxicology*, 3rd ed. New York: John Wiley & Sons, 1981: Vol 2A.
14. National Institute of Occupational Safety and Health. *Intelligence Bulletin 34: Formaldehyde: Evidence of Carcinogenicity*, Baltimore, MD: NIOSH, 1981.

> **The Strange Case of Dr. Jekyll and Formaldehyde (Is It Good or Is It Evil?)**
>
> by Maureen Robinson

## FORMALDEHYDE'S SPLIT PERSONALITY

Formaldehyde, is it good or is it evil? It is a carcinogen, it is not a carcinogen, it is a probably carcinogen, it is not. . . . I think you get the picture. There is a lot of uncertainty in the data. Where there is no uncertainty is in the benefits formaldehyde provides an as an embalming agent. Where there has been some misguided information, is in the reporting to the public that there is enough formaldehyde put in the ground each year in the United States to fill eight Olympic size swimming pools, and that the dead human body poses no health risks to those that come in direct contact with the body. Individuals making these claims are not scientists. Information is being taken out of context from extremely reputable sources and being inaccurately presented to the public.

There is a social movement, which seems to imply that, as a group, funeral service professionals (FSPs) are not concerned about the environment. Are funeral directors that are using formaldehyde saying that there is no need for us as an industry to look at being more "green" and more responsible with our environment? I would hope that this is absolutely not a true statement. FSPs should be looking at ways to make changes that can benefit our planet earth. How that is presented and marketed to the public should be done in a responsible way. The use of formaldehyde is not a major environmental issue. Its misuse can, however, potentially create very serious health issues. It is true that going out in the sun unprotected could cause skin cancer. There are, however, billions of people outside enjoying that sun each day. The informed individual will reduce their risk of skin cancer by wearing protective sunscreen. The responsible embalmer will use personal protective equipment (PPE) and ventilation to minimize formaldehyde exposure.

In an effort to help the environment, each funeral home and funeral service professional should identify things they can do differently at their place of business and in their homes that would help sustain our planet for our children, our children's children, and so on. The current track we are on, in which the burning of fossil fuels is our primary energy source, is not sustainable. Projections indicate that if we continue burning fossil fuels at this current rate, we will deplete this natural resource in the next 5 to 100 years. Fossil fuel prices cannot remain artificially low, nor can government continue to subsidize their producers.

In the United States, we are approximately 95% dependent on these nonrenewable resources. We need to see a paradigm shift from the use of conventional oil, coal, and natural gas to alternative fuel sources that do not contribute to global warming. Solar energy, wind energy, and geothermal energy need to take the forefront. This shift will not occur without our pressure on local, state, and national politicians.

Our world population cannot continue to grow at its current rate. How about the issue of trying to sustain 8.9 billion people on this planet by 2050: If as a country or a world we do not start addressing some of these bigger environmental and social issues, soon the debate on a choice of an arterial fluid will be laughable at best. As FSPs and responsible stewards of our planet earth, we can work together in developing a lifestyle that is more environmentally sustainable. There will be "an environmental corner" in this publication each quarter to aid in communicating our strategies within our profession and our daily lives. We can learn from one another and show that in solving large-scale environmental problems, individuals do matter.

This is not to imply that we should disregard any potential health effects or safety issues. It is just to state that the use of formaldehyde in funeral service cannot even begin to make its way onto the list of top environmental global issues. If current scientific studies reveal that formaldehyde is a known carcinogen and poses a threat of nasopharyngeal cancer in embalmers, then appropriate measures should be taken to better protect embalmers from this threat. The National Funeral Directors Association (NFDA) has already started to address this issue. In the face of renewed worldwide focus on formaldehyde and its risks, they have issued formaldehyde-specific best management practices (BMPs).

## BEST MANAGEMENT PRACTICES

NFDA formed a panel to draft the BMPs that then underwent a peer review by funeral directors, educators, and leading chemical suppliers to make sure that the BMPs were protective, workable, and sensible. The Funeral Service Environmental Working Group also reviewed the BMPs, which were then approved by the NJDA Executive Board in January 2009. Brining in the Environmental Working Group for part of the peer-review process is another positive indication that FSPs are concerned about the environment. The BMPs have been designed as a dynamic tool that can change to reflect any new evaluations of formaldehyde by domestic and international organizations, including the current study released by the National Cancer Institute (NCI).

The first BMP addresses preparation room ventilation. Preparation room ventilation is the single most important factor in reducing health risks associated with formaldehyde exposure. The BMPs state that there should be no fewer than 10–15 air changes per hour supplied to the preparation room for each active embalming table. Jack Adams, in his November 2004 *Dodge Magazine* article, "The Preparation Room: Ventilation," recommends 20 air changes per hour. A properly functioning HVAC system aids in reducing the risk of formaldehyde exposure in the workplace. This seems to indicate that it would be prudent to shoot for a range of 10–20 air changes per hour. To ensure use of the ventilation system, wire the ventilation system's activation to the preparation room's light switch. Monitor the effectiveness of the preparation room HVAC system no less than annually. Jack also emphasizes the importance of having the preparation room under negative pressure. That is, more air is exhausted than is taken into the room. This keeps the other parts of the building from being contaminated with air from the preparation room.

The second BMP states that in addition to a properly ventilated preparation room, a thorough case analysis of the condition of the remains should be made before embalming. When performing the embalming, only use the amount of formaldehyde necessary to achieve a quality result. I think this is supportive of the overall environmental strategy of "reduce, reuse, and recycle," as well as an excellent strategy to reduce potential formaldehyde exposure to the embalmer.

Which actually moves us to the third BMP, which indicates the importance of taking precautions in the preparation room to limit formaldehyde exposure and emissions during routine embalming. A simple strategy to greatly reduce the embalmer's exposure to formaldehyde would be to always add the arterial fluid to the water in the embalming machine. A sign should be posted near each embalming machine as a constant reminder to employees of this simple procedure. At Worsham College of Mortuary Science, where I teach microbiology, chemistry, and anatomy, my students have assured me that this procedure is taught in their embalming labs. Hopefully, they will continue this work practice long after leaving Worsham College.

Formaldehyde exposure to the embalmer will be greatest when a formaldehyde spill occurs. Sit down as a staff and brainstorm a list of your specific work practices that could help to minimize the potential for formaldehyde spills. Post the list and institute the work practices. Conduct short training sessions with new employees and refresher training sessions for current employees. If you are the boss, lead by example. If you teach embalming laboratories, this would be an excellent team exercise to conduct in your laboratories. Feel free to e-mail your results, and I will be sure to share them with others.

Even with these work practices in place, formaldehyde spills will occasionally occur in the workplace. Formaldehyde spills should be cleaned up immediately. There are spill kits available; however, an ammonia solution can be used as an inexpensive and effective formaldehyde neutralizer: When formaldehyde and ammonia react, a compound called *urotropin* is formed. Urotropin is an organic nitrogen compound. The formation of urotropin demonstrates the affinity of formaldehyde for nitrogen. Any source of nitrogen can bring about a similar neutralization reaction. Many decomposition products are derivatives of ammonia ($NH_3$) and would therefore neutralize the effects of formaldehyde. Therefore, embalming the body as soon after death as is possible can limit the concentration of formaldehyde necessary for a successful embalming, which in turn is an effective way to limit the formaldehyde exposure to the embalmer.

There are many other simple ways to limit formaldehyde exposure. Always keep the lid on the embalming machine, always use a sink cover to limit splashing and exposure, and use all appropriate PPE to avoid skin and eye contact with formaldehyde. Another good recommendation is to switch from latex gloves to nitrile gloves. The BMPs point out that nitrile has high chemical resistance against formaldehyde without the failure rate of latex. These recommendations, and others, are all easy and inexpensive to incorporate into your work practices. Posting friendly reminders for personnel will help to minimize bad habits from creeping into daily work routines.

One of the most effective strategies in limiting formaldehyde exposure to the embalmer would be to capture the formaldehyde emissions before those emissions enter the breathing zone of the embalmer. This can be accomplished by utilizing a local exhaust ventilation (LEV) system. Employees may choose to wear a properly fitted respirator. The key here is wearing a *properly fitted* respirator. Respirators should not be interchanged between employees. Each employee must be properly fitted, and they should then store their respirator where they store their other personal belongings, so that others do not inadvertently grab their personal protective gear. An improperly fitted respirator is not effective. Respirators should be worn when cleaning up a formaldehyde spill.

The fourth BMP reminds us that special cases such as embalming organ procurement cases and autopsied remains can increase the embalmer's formaldehyde exposure risk. It becomes even more imperative that embalmers follow the above-mentioned strategies when dealing with these types of cases.

The fifth BMP requires embalmers to be familiar with and follow federal, state, and local environmental, OSHA and health requirements that apply when an embalming is performed. Unfortunately, the longer we are at a job, the less familiar we become with these requirements. To keep formaldehyde in a good light, we need to change this strategy. I think it is also a natural progression that the longer we work at a job, the more shortcuts we tend to take, and the more complacent we can become in regard to personal safety and protection. I caution embalmers to keep this thought in the back of their minds.

Here is a true story. I was performing a test in an organic testing laboratory, a test I had performed safely and without incident thousands of times. One of the safety precautions was to bring down the glass sash on the ventilated hood in which I was performing my tests. During the test, the glassware that I was using exploded. The material in the glassware at the time was boiling. An additional safety precaution that took me less than 10 seconds most likely saved me from serious injury or a potentially fatal accident. After the accident, we reevaluated the entire laboratory procedure and found an additional step that could be added to hopefully avoid this incident from happening again in the future. This type of strategy could be incorporated when an accident occurs in the preparation room as well.

## FORMALDEHYDE COUNCIL IS HOLDING CONSTANT VIGIL

The Formaldehyde Council is a nonprofit organization that represents the leading producers and users of formaldehyde in the United States. The National Funeral Directors Association is one of its many members. The Formaldehyde Council is dedicated to promoting the responsible use and benefits of formaldehyde and ensuring its scientific evaluation. Their organization is focused on the relationship between formaldehyde and the public health and assuring that the utilization of formaldehyde and the public policies governing its use are based on sound science. Sound science is science that has undergone the rigors of a scientific community peer review. Junk science has not undergone the rigors of a scientific peer review. Social movements often present junk science as sound science and in the process often do more damage to the case they are trying to make. Some of the current articles and advertisements that are being published about formaldehyde and FSPs are perfect examples of why environmental science and other forms of sound science should be driving regulatory change, and not emotionalism, social movements, marketing schemes, or media hype based on junk science.

## WHAT IS FORMALDEHYDE?

Let us take a closer look at the chemical that has drawn so much attention at the national and international level and has provided a full-time job for both those defending its use and those proposing a ban of its use. Here is an age-old question: what is formaldehyde? Formaldehyde is a simple molecule made of hydrogen, oxygen, and carbon and is a natural part of our world and the product of many natural processes. Lots of organisms use formaldehyde for the carbon it contains. It is made by our bodies and occurs naturally in the air that we breathe. In fact, metabolic processes break it down to simple carbon dioxide and water. Plants and animals also produce formaldehyde. If organisms that live in soil and water do not break down the formaldehyde, sunlight breaks it down through a process known as photo degradation. It is even emitted as a by-product of certain vegetables such as Brussel sprouts and cabbage when they are cooked. Beware, there may be a proposal banning farmers' markets!

Formaldehyde is soluble in water, so it does not accumulate in the fatty tissues of terrestrial or aquatic organisms. Processes like bioaccumulation and biomagnifications are not a primary concern. Certain pesticides, for example, may bioaccumulate in organisms and then biomagnify in the environment. DDT is an example of a persistent organic chemical, which, due to its fat solubility, will accumulate in the fatty tissues of aquatic and terrestrial organisms. This sets up the potential for biomagnifications through simple food chains and complex food webs. Chemicals such as DDT can be found as a pollutant in water in the parts per trillion level be consumed by plankton, small fish, large fish, and by the time a bird consumes that large fish, be present in the parts per million level. This was the primary drive behind the ban of the use of this pesticide in the United States. Rachel Carson feared that without a ban on DDT, we would one day have a "Silent Spring" without the voices of birds in spring. Unlike DDT, formaldehyde is water soluble and will not bioaccumulate in the fatty tissues.

## THE CHEMISTRY OF FORMALDEHYDE AND ITS ACTION IN FIRMING PROTEINS

The molecular formula for formaldehyde is HCHO of $CH_2O$. Formaldehyde is a colorless gas. It is very soluble in water. Formaldehyde is generally available as formalin, an aqueous solution containing 37% formaldehyde gas by weight of 40% by volume. This expresses the limits of the solubility of formaldehyde in water. To increase the solubility above this level, ethanol can be added to the solution.

Formaldehyde can polymerize to form paraformaldehyde. The more $CH_2O$ units that add into the structure, the heavier the molecule becomes, until it precipitates out of solution in the form of waxy-like flakes. If the arterial solution on your shelf has exceeded its shelf life, you may observe these flakes in the bottom of the bottle. This precipitation also occurs in acidic solutions. Methanol is generally added to arterial fluids as an antipolymerizing agent for formaldehyde. Remember if the formaldehyde in your arterial has formed paraformaldehyde, the available formaldehyde for an embalming has been reduced.

In a very alkaline solution, formaldehyde is unstable. Formaldehyde has a very limited pH range. If the surrounding medium becomes too acidic, it polymerizes; if it becomes too alkaline, it breaks down. Again, if the formaldehyde breaks down, there will be less formaldehyde available for an embalming. The breakdown of proteins as the body decomposes will form organic nitrogen compounds, such as amino acids, which further break down to produce amines and ammonia. Each of these products contributes to producing an alkaline environment and may contribute to the formation of foul odors. Therefore, the more advanced the decomposition, the more nitrogen is available to neutralize the formaldehyde, hence a greater formaldehyde demand on the need for a higher index solution to adequately embalm and firm the tissues of the body. Uremic poisoning can also increase formaldehyde demand. When someone has died as a result of kidney failure, the potential of urea (an organic nitrogen compound) in the blood is greatly increased. Hence, the importance of completely flushing this contaminated blood from the system. Again, increased nitrogen content would call for increased formaldehyde demand, thus increasing the risk of formaldehyde exposure to the embalmer.

The chemistry between formaldehyde and the proteins of the body is very fascinating. When formaldehyde reacts with water, it forms methylene glycol. There is very little free formaldehyde in a formalin solution. The methylene glycol forms methylene bridges between the nitrogen atoms of adjacent proteins. In the process of this reaction, water is lost. Cross-linking of protein removes one molecule of water for every cross-link that is formed. As water is lost, the proteins become more viscous or firm. In other words, the main chemical action of formaldehyde in embalming is the coagulation of protein. The protein's resistance to digestive enzymes is also increased. The proteins also become less susceptible to hydrolysis. An abundance of water could reverse the embalming results. Hence, cases of edema would increase the formaldehyde demand. Any process that can reduce the amount of excess tissue fluid prior to embalming would again decrease the need for a higher index fluid and would protect the embalmer from increased formaldehyde exposure.

## BESIDES AS AN EMBALMING AGENT, HOW IS FORMALDEHYDE USED?

According to the Formaldehyde Council, formaldehyde is used in thousands of products. Chemistry has allowed the responsible use of formaldehyde in personal hygiene products, vaccines, film used in x-rays, soaps, detergents, cosmetics, plastics, carpeting, clothing, resins, glues, and medicines, to name a few. **Table 1** lists many products that depend on formaldehyde in their manufacture.

Did you know that funeral service only accounts for approximately 1% of the total usage of formaldehyde in the United States? Imagine the number of jobs that would be eliminated with a ban on formaldehyde if funeral service only accounts

## TABLE 1. Formaldehyde's Many Uses

| Home Construction Applications | Home Interiors | Aerospace Applications | Automotive Applications |
|---|---|---|---|
| Asphalt shingles, sheathing, cladding, and roofs<br>Walls, wall panels, and floors | Electrical boxes and outlets<br>Furniture, countertops, cabinets, and cabinet doors Bedding, seating, and carpet underlay<br>Appliances: Washers, dryers, and dishwashers<br>Plumbing: Faucets, showerheads, and valve mechanisms<br>Paints and varnishes | Brake pads, landing gear, lubricants<br>Tire cord adhesives<br>Seats, seatbelt buckles<br>Insulation of doors and windows, and interior walls and floors | *Fuel System Components* Pump housings and filters Impellers, reservoirs, senders, and gas caps<br>*Under the Hood*<br>Molded components and engine and metallic parts, automatic transmission parts, and carburetor floats<br>*Exterior*<br>Exterior primer, clear coat, and trim<br>Tire cord adhesive, bumper<br>*Interior*<br>Seats, steering wheel, and interior trim<br>Brake pads, dashboard, and fascias<br>Instrument knobs, hooks, fasteners, and clips, locks, speaker grilles<br>Trunk release levers<br>Door handles, door panels, and window cranks<br>Seatbelt buckles Windshield wiper parts<br>Cup holders and head rests |

for 1% of the usage of formaldehyde in the United States. With these types of economic ramifications, decisions on formaldehyde must be based on sound science, not junk science, media-hype, or the "flim-flam" of marketers. Our economy is already fragile, unemployment rates are very high, and government spending must be wise and prudent.

Interestingly enough, formaldehyde is instrumental in the manufacture of many products, but often little or no formaldehyde is present in the final product. Also, glues and adhesives that are made with formaldehyde are exceptional bonding agents. Formaldehyde-based products are key to the manufacture of automobiles, including the paint, as well as the production of dollar bills, the ink used in books, magazines, and newspapers, wood products, and agricultural products including fertilizers. In textiles, formaldehyde-based material helps bind dyes to fabrics and improves a fabric's resistance to wrinkles.

In many instances, because of formaldehyde's unique physical and chemical properties, few compounds can replace it as a raw material without reducing performance and making the final product more expensive. Whether it is plywood for home construction, fuel system components for automobiles, or components of heart valves and pacemakers, using formaldehyde translates into enormous health and safety benefits, more affordable housing and automobiles, and many products with a consistent quality.

## EVERYDAY MEDICAL APPLICATIONS

The microbiologist and anatomist in me found the following applications very fascinating. Urinary tract infections can be treated using a derivative of formaldehyde. Using formaldehyde-based drugs to treat UTIs eliminates the creation of bacterial resistance to antibiotics. We are seeing the emergence of many drug-resistant strains of bacteria, caused by the use, misuse, and overuse of antibiotics and other antimicrobials. Bacteria are incapable of developing resistance to formaldehyde. Formaldehyde is used to create the hard capsules of many time-released drugs. The formaldehyde-based pill coatings allow the capsule to dissolve slowly and promote maximum absorption of the medicine. In both of these instances, the body's metabolic processes would naturally break down any small residual amounts of formaldehyde. Formaldehyde is used to make plastics used in artificial heart valves, pacemakers, and artificial limbs. More than 10 types of vaccines are made each year that use formaldehyde as the delivery system.

## THE LIFE SCIENCES

Formaldehyde provides many benefits to the life sciences. Formaldehyde is used in research laboratories throughout the world as tissue preservative. It has been used for more than 100 years in embalming for its preservative and disinfecting qualities. Being able to adequately preserve tissue samples allows researchers to identify proteins, DNA, and RNA. The ability to preserve tissues has benefited those in the field of medicine, the pharmaceutical industry, the field of forensics, funeral service, and those involved in the training of these esteemed professionals.

## CONSUMER AND OCCUPATIONAL SAFETY

The fact has been established that formaldehyde and formaldehyde-based products are used to manufacture thousands of products that are purchased daily in the United States. It should make American consumers more comfortable about purchasing these products, knowing that three agencies, the United States Environmental Protection Agency (US EPA), the Consumer Product Safety Commission (CPSC), and the United States Department of Housing and Urban Development (HUD), have addressed indoor air exposure to formaldehyde. With the combination of governmental regulation and voluntary product emission standards, indoor formaldehyde emissions have declined significantly. Formaldehyde is an extensively regulated material. Mandatory government regulations set standards to protect health and the environment. These requirements allow for the safe production, storage, handling, and use of formaldehyde.

Governmental regulations that help to protect consumers and the environment, the United States Department of Labor's Occupational Safety and Health Administration (OSHA) sets standards for workplace exposures to formaldehyde. These comprehensive health standards include limits on permissible exposures, requirements for monitoring employee exposures in the workplace, protective measures including engineering controls, medical surveillance, and communication and training about hazards. OSHA provides comprehensive health standards for formaldehyde exposure by embalmers in their Formaldehyde Standard. The permissible exposure limit (PEL) is 0.75 ppm (parts of formaldehyde per million parts air) measured as a time-weighted average (TWA). ATWA is the level of formaldehyde gas present in the air, averaged over a 9-hour time period. The short-term exposure limit (STEL) is a high formaldehyde gas limit to which employees may be safely exposed for a short time; the limit is 2 ppm for a time not to exceed 15 minutes; the employee may not be exposed to this higher limit for this limited amount of time more than 4 times per 8-hour work day. The STEL was included in the standard mainly to allow for autopsy procedures.

## FORMALDEHYDE UNDER FIRE IS NOTHING NEW

Formaldehyde has been under continuous fire for close to 40 years. In March of 1972, Dr. Jerome F. Fredrick published the first in a new series, "Ecological Factors in Embalming." Here were some of his comments as they applied to the public's growing concern over embalming and air pollution:

1. Even if the embalmer were to inject the body with chemically required quantities that would ensure the thorough conversion of all protein, the fumes emanating from such a cadaver would be nonexistent.
2. The embalmer should also be mindful of pathogenic organism release, which is much more important insofar as the public health goes.
    a. Limit the manipulations of a cadaver.
    b. Thorough disinfection of the skin surfaces prior to arterial embalming.
    c. Another very important source of bacterial air pollution is via the forced expiration of entrapped air in the lungs of a cadaver. Airborne diseases such as tuberculosis and some of the fungal lung diseases can be guarded against if the embalmer, during the course of his embalming procedures, is on his/her guard to avoid pressures on the thoracic cavity of the case he/she is working on. In support of Dr. Fredrick, I would point to the documented case in *Mortuary Management*, 2000, where an embalmer acquired tuberculosis from the deceased that he had embalmed. The John Hopkins School of Medicine verified this with DNA analysis. Yet, we still hear that the "dead human body poses no health threat to the public or the embalmer."
    d. The thorough disinfection of the cadaver is the most important way in which the professional embalmer can contribute to the public health, and to the ecology, at the same time. I would say Dr. Fredrick was ahead of his time.

In November, 1982, Margaret S. Boothe, then the Director of the Dodge Cambridge Research Laboratories, published a three-part article "Formaldehyde: Friend of Foe?" Ms. Boothe, also an analytical chemist, reported on many interesting findings on formaldehyde:

1. She described a cancer study that was conducted by the Chemical Industry Institute of Technology (CIIT) in 1979, in which laboratory rats exposed to formaldehyde vapor developed nasal cancer. Here is a summary of the study:
    a. It indicated that for exposures of 15 ppm for 6 hours/day, 5 days/week, for 16 months, formaldehyde is carcinogenic. At this level after 16 months, 3 rats out of 120 animals had developed nasal cancer.
    b. Up to 18 months, no cancer had developed in rats exposed to 2 and 6 ppm.
    c. Also, mice that were exposed at 2, 6, and 15 ppm formaldehyde over the same time period of time showed no occurrences of cancer.
    d. At 15 ppm, a human being would run screaming from the room the instant of first exposure. A man would be blind from tearing and unable to stand the pain of breathing at 15 ppm.
2. Formaldehyde manufacturers, EPA, TSCA, NIOSH, Formaldehyde Institute (now called the Formaldehyde Council), and other research facilities are constantly collecting, reviewing, and publishing data on the effect of formaldehyde on laboratory animals and upon people who are in contact with it in the workplace. The information coming out of these studies so far has been the foundation for the decision by the EPA not to include formaldehyde in its list of carcinogens at this time. I would add that since the time of Ms. Boothe's work, the EPA has classified formaldehyde as a probable carcinogen, but has not succumbed to pressures by the Sierra Club, or others, to upgrade this classification, or pose a ban on formaldehyde. It is my hope that the EPA would not make such a ruling without a thorough review of all the scientific and historical data currently available on formaldehyde by the National Academy of Sciences, as per the recommendation of the Formaldehyde Council.
3. Again it is well to warn that, as with all chemicals, care and good management practices should be the watch words of the day. Despite the date this article was written by Ms. Boothe, this is still excellent advice. Please refer again to the best management practices (BMPs) developed by the NFDA.

In 1991, Dr. Fredrick, published an article "Formaldehyde-Phobia: Friend or Foe?" Dr. Fredrick begins his article, "Probably no chemical has ever had the publicity and reputation that formaldehyde has acquired over the last 20 years." Some of his findings can be summarized as follows:

1. It has been publicized as the basic chemical responsible for all life in the universe.
2. It has been found by spectroscopic analysis in the huge clouds that occupy interstellar space.
3. It is probably the first step in synthesis of sugars during the process of photosynthesis in green plants.

4. This primeval chemical is one of the building blocks of all life on the earth.
5. Formaldehyde is a carcinogen; formaldehyde is not a carcinogen. Formaldehyde is an irritant; it is not an irritant. The upshot was to make the public really formaldehyde phobic!
6. The nonscientific sector of the public became wary of whether formaldehyde would leak out of the embalmed bodies. All of the formaldehyde is reacted with the excess proteins in the body. And hence, there is none left over to leak out. In other words, what Dr. Fredrick would say today is that there are not eight Olympic-sized swimming pools full of formaldehyde in the ground. There are not even eight Olympic-sized bathing suits full of formaldehyde in the ground as a result of the embalming process.
7. Even if the modern embalmer were to use enough formaldehyde to "over embalm" and the excess leaked out, it would immediately react with the nitrogenous components contained in all soils to form innocuous urotropin. Any small amount of the chemical that theoretically could "leak" into the atmosphere would be rapidly broken down to water and carbon dioxide by ultraviolet light or by heat from the sun. Remember back to my earlier discussion on the neutralization of formaldehyde by nitrogen compounds. This is the primary reason OSHA does recommend the use of ammonia ($NH_3$) in a formaldehyde spill. It will neutralize the formaldehyde. Likewise, with an advance case of decomposition, there will be more organic nitrogen compounds and a greater demand for formaldehyde.
8. At the time of Dr. Fredrick's article, the State of New Jersey's Department of Environmental Protection, Division of Hazardous Waste considered formaldehyde that has been used to embalm a body no longer a "generically hazardous waste" under the state's listing of chemical hazards. In other words, the formaldehyde is not present as such (in leakages from embalmed bodies), but rather as the spent reaction products (which are not hazardous wastes). Leakage of formaldehyde from embalmed cadavers in our cemeteries does not constitute any possible threat to soils and/or potable waters in the area. Any research that I conducted in this area also supports Dr. Fredrick's findings.

## SCIENTIFIC STUDIES ON HEALTH EFFECTS

Since we have established that formaldehyde does not bioaccumulate in the environment, let us discuss its health effect from a purely scientific standpoint. There has been much work done in this area both past and present. There have been irritation studies, exposures studies, and cancer studies. Epidemiologists, oncologists, and toxicologists have devoted careers to studying formaldehyde. Scientific endeavors with no promise of fame and fortune. Pure science. No gimmicks, no marketing schemes. Just sound science on which environmental regulation can be based. The following is a summary of some of the findings from these studies.

### Irritation Studies

Formaldehyde can be irritating to the eyes, nose, and throat, but for most people, the irritation appears to be highly subjective. An expert panel review of over 150 published studies found that eye irritation does not become significant until around 1 ppm (part per million), and moderate to severe eye, nose, and throat irritation occurs at 2–3 ppm. The expert panels found that a level of 1 ppm would not cause eye irritation in 75–95% of all people exposed. In any case, normal environmental exposures and embalming occupational exposures are less than these levels.

### Cancer Studies

In the area of evaluating the cancer risk associated with formaldehyde, the Formaldehyde Council brought in experts in the field to evaluate the many studies that have been conducted. One such expert, Dr. Gary Marsh, since 1978 has conducted more than 25 occupational epidemiology studies of health effects from various workplace exposures. A major focus of his research has been the evaluation of human health effects from formaldehyde exposure.

Dr. Marsh reports that most of the epidemiology evidence for assessing human cancer risk from formaldehyde exposure comes from three large cohort studies of industrial workers: one in Britain and two in the United States by the National Institute of Occupational Safety and Health (NIOSH) and the National Cancer Institute (NCI). In 2004, the International Agency for Research on Cancer or IARC reclassified formaldehyde as carcinogenic in humans based largely on evidence from the NCI study that formaldehyde causes nasopharyngeal cancer. The NCI finding was based on only eight nasopharyngeal deaths among exposed workers, an increase of only two nasopharyngeal deaths from IARC's 1995 classification of formaldehyde as a probable carcinogen. Only one nasopharyngeal cancer death was observed in the other two cohort studies combined. The evidence that formaldehyde causes other cancers, such as leukemia, was deemed nonsufficient by IARC.

Recent literature reviews and reanalysis of the NCI cohort data conducted by Dr. Marsh's research group have cast considerable doubt on the validity of NCI's findings and IARC's reclassification. For example, his research group showed that NCI's findings for nasopharyngeal cancer were driven entirely by an anomalous finding in 1 of 10 study plants, termed Plant 1. Six of the eight nasopharyngeal cancer deaths occurred among exposed workers in this single plant, resulting in a statistically significant 10-fold excess in nasopharyngeal cancer with a 35% deficit in nasopharyngeal cancer deaths among exposed workers in the remaining 9 plants.

Dr. Marsh's group also conducted an independent and expanded cohort study of Plant 1. They concluded in their latest published report that the anomalous finding of the nasopharyngeal cancer in Plant 1 may be related to previous work in the extensive local metal industry. These jobs entailed possible exposures to several risk factors for nasopharyngeal cancer, including sulfuric acid mists, mineral acid, metal dust, and heat.

In summary, Dr. Marsh's group concluded that their analysis of the NCI cohort data did not support NCI's suggestion of a causal association with formaldehyde and nasopharyngeal cancer. They believe that the 2004 decision by IARC to reclassify formaldehyde as a Group 1 substance was premature, considering the small number of nasopharyngeal cancer deaths, the missing evidence from the British and NIOSH cohort studies, the anomalous finding for nasopharyngeal cancer in Plant 1, and their new evidence that the nasopharyngeal cancer risk in the influential Plant 1 may be related to previous work in the metal industry.

On November 27, 2005, the Formaldehyde Council was encouraged that the U.S. Environmental Protection Agency intended to wait until it had the benefit of enhanced scientific data from the National Cancer Institute (NCI) before updating its carcinogenic classification for formaldehyde under its Integrated Risk Information System (IRIS) program. EPA currently classifies formaldehyde as "probably carcinogenic to humans" under the IRIS program. As was stated earlier in this article, there still seems to be a lot of uncertainty in the data, again warranting an extensive study by the National Academy of Sciences.

In August 2008, the EPA denied a Sierra Club petition to promulgate national formaldehyde regulations similar to those adopted in California by the California Air Resource Board (BCARB). The EPA ruled that there was insufficient data to assess the risk proposed by formaldehyde or to identify the least burdensome means of protecting against such a risk. Instead, the EPA said it would initiate a proceeding to investigate whether and what type of regulatory or other action might be appropriate. The Formaldehyde Council brought in experts that support the current stance taken by the EPA. Here is a summary of Dr. F. J. Murray of San Jose, California, in regard to the CARB proposal to lower formaldehyde emissions:

"The health benefits of CARB's proposal to lower formaldehyde emissions have been over-estimated by a cancer risk assessment that does not use the most current peer-reviewed scientific information. Importantly, more recent and sophisticated risk assessments of formaldehyde by other respected regulatory agencies, including US EPA, Health Canada, and the World Health Organization (WHO), predict the cancer risk is as much as 36,000 times lower than the estimate relied upon by the CARB study. These assessments indicate that the proposed reductions in formaldehyde emissions will not produce any meaningful reduction in cancer cases in California.

CARB should carefully evaluate the proposal to reduce exposure to formaldehyde, particularly the extremely low limits proposed in Phase 2, in light of the tenuous public health benefits represented by the estimated reduction in cancer cases in California. If reducing exposure to formaldehyde will not result in any meaningful reduction in cancer risk in California, the proposed action must be questioned. Given the fact that over 100,000 Californians are expected to die annually from cancer, it is especially important to focus the state's resources on actions that will result in cancer and improvement in public health."

On May 12, 2009, the Formaldehyde Council was kept busy responding to the latest article on formaldehyde that was published in the *Journal of the National Cancer Institute*. The NCI article was entitled, "Mortality From Lymphohematopoietic Malignancies Among Workers in Formaldehyde Industries: The National cancer Institute Cohort." This study was a continuation of a study that followed through December 31, 1979, and updated through December 31, 1994, in which formaldehyde exposure was associated with an increased risk of leukemia. NCI extended the follow-up through December 31, 2004. Evaluation of risks over time suggests a possible link between formaldehyde exposure and leukemia. The NCI reported that observed patterns could be due to chance or could be consistent with a causal association within the relatively short induction-incubation period, characteristic of leukemogenesis. The NCI conclusion was that further epidemiological study and exploration of potential molecular mechanisms are warranted.

The Formaldehyde Council believes that the significant disparity between the author's conclusions and the actual data underscores the need for reevaluation of this latest report in conjunction with the broader body of existing formaldehyde research. The Formaldehyde Council supports the commission of a scientific peer review of formaldehyde by the prestigious National Academy of Sciences (NAS). This intensive scientific peer review would consider all existing research data on formaldehyde. The Formaldehyde Council is hopeful that NAS will produce a scientifically sound interpretation of all current research on formaldehyde and that our government will use the NAS analysis as the basis for developing appropriate formaldehyde policies and regulations to enhance public health. This recommendation of the use of sound science to make policy decisions with large-scale ramifications makes good environmental and economic sense and is a very responsible and ethical approach.

## SUMMARY

Since the 1990s, the National Cancer Institute studies have shown that effective ventilation is the single most important factor in protecting embalmers exposed to formaldehyde from harm. NFDA is considering conducting a study that will investigate strategies for keeping the air in the prep room formaldehyde free. The study would ultimately lead to the design of a cost-effective prep room ventilation system.

As always, consumers need to be careful that some products may be presented as better for the environment and truly are not. Sometimes, the only thing green about the product you are buying is the container it comes in or the cash ending up in the marketer's pocket. The good news is we already know that, based on current information available, formaldehyde use in funeral service is not a serious environmental issue. So let us work together to follow BMPs in funeral service that could help protect the health and safety of FSPs. As professionals, we can band together to promote the strict implementation of the BMPs in our funeral homes and businesses. In doing so, we can cast a shadow over the evil personality of formaldehyde and let the good personality shine brightly.

## REFERENCES

Bastionon D, Matos BS, Aquino WF, Pacheo A, Mendes JMB. Geophysical surveying to Investigate Groundwater Contamination by a Cemetery. Proceedings of the Symposium on the Application of Geophysics to Engineering and Environmental Problems: The Annual Meeting of the Environmental and Engineering Geophysical Society: February 20–24, 2000:709–718.

Bean LE, Blair A, Leubin JH, Stewart PA, Hayes RB, Hoover RN, Hauptmann M. Mortality from lymphohematopoietic malignancies among workers in formaldehyde industries: The National Cancer Institute Cohort. *Journal of the National Cancer Institute* 2009;101:751–761.

Boothe MS. Formaldehyde: friend or foe? Parts I-III *The Dodge Magazine*, November 1982:4+

Chan GS, Scafe M, Emami S. *Cemeteries and Groundwater: An Examination of the Potential Contamination of Groundwater Preservatives Containing Formaldehyde.* Queen's Printer for Ontario, 1992.

Corley C. Burials and cemeteries go green. *NPR*, April 26, 2009.

Dempsey PA. The future of formaldehyde. *The Forum*, January 2009:22–28.

Dent BB. Cemetery Decay Product Profiles: Two Cases in Australia, Unconsolidated, Sandy Aquifers. Searching for Sustainable Future: 15th Australian Geological Convention, July 3–7, 2000; Sydney:130.

Dorn JM. *Thanatochemistry*, 2nd ed. Upper Saddle River, NJ: Prentice Hall, 1998.

"FCI Fact Sheet on JNCI Study on Occupational Exposure to Formaldehyde." May 12, 2009. May 18, 2009.

"FCI JNCI Talking Points." Formaldehyde Council, 12 May 2009. 18 May 2009 http://www.formaldehyde.org. Formaldehyde Council. "Formaldehyde Industry Disputes Findings of JNCI Report." Press release. Formaldehyde Council. 12 May 2009. Formaldehyde Council. 18 May 2009 http://www.formaldehyde.org.

"Formaldehyde: Hazard Recognition." January 27, 2009.

"Formaldehyde." January 27, 2009.

Fredrick JF. Ecological factors in embalming: Parts I-IV. *The Dodge Magazine*, March 1972: 20+.

Fredrick JF. "Formaldehyde-phobia: Friend or foe. *The Dodge Magazine*, June 1991: 11+.

Green CL, Fitch JH. Death Knell for Formaldehyde. *The Director*, May 2009: 48–51.

Hayes R. Mortality of U.S. embalmers and funeral directors. *American Journal of Industrial Medicine* 1990;18:641–652.

Hopkins DW, Wiltshire PEJ, Turner BD. Microbial characteristics of soils from graves: An investigation at the interface of soil microbiology and forensic science. *Applied Soil Ecology* 2000;14:238–288.

Levine R. The mortality of Ontario undertakers and a review of formaldehyde-related mortality studies. *Journal of Occupational Medicine* 1984;26:740–746.

Loh, MM, Levy JI, Spengler JD, Houseman EA, Bennett DH. Ranking cancer risks of organic hazardous air pollutants in the United States. *Environmental Health Perspectives* 2007;115:1160–1168.

Marsh G. Reevaluation of mortality risks from leukemia in the formaldehyde Cohort Study of the National Cancer Institute. *Regulatory Toxicology and Pharmacology* 2004;40:113–124.

Mayer RG. *Embalming: History, Theory, and Practice*, 4th ed. New York: McGraw-Hill, 2006.

Miller GT. *Environmental Science*, 11th ed. Belmont, CA: Thomson, 2006.

National Funeral Directors Association. Formaldehyde best management practices. *The Director*, May 2009: 52–56.

National Funeral Directors Association. NFDA green funeral service Q&A. The Director, February 2009: 32–36.

Q&A on JNCI. *Formaldehyde Council*. May 12, 2009. May 18, 2009.

United Nations Environment Publications. OECD SIDS. Formaldehyde. Paris, France, 2002.

Untitled. The Australian Institute of Embalming (December 2008).

Walrath J. Mortality patterns among embalmers. *International Journal of Cancer* 1983;31:407–411.

Walrath J, Fraumeni JF, Jr. Cancer and other causes of death among embalmers. *Cancer Research* 1984;44:4638–4641.

What Will Be Formaldehyde's Fate? Funeral Service Insider 24 Nov. 2008. World Health Organization. Concise International Chemical Assessment Document 40: Formaldehyde. Geneva, 2002.

World Health Organization. *Environmental Health Criteria for Formaldehyde.* Geneva, 1989.

---

**The Preparation Room: Ventilation***

*Jack Adams, CFSP*

Care and custody for the dead human body is and will always be the most important activity a funeral home does. The work done in the preparation room is the foundation for the funeral home. The preparation room itself needs to provide a comfortable and safe work environment. A room of adequate size, with proper ventilation and lighting, and furnished with the necessary working equipment will often result in higher-quality work results.

With OSHA and public health concerns, there is greater interest in preparation room safety and design. In addition to having properly sized doors, sanitary flooring and walls, and lighting and environmental controls, the room needs to reflect comfort and safety measures that do not interfere with but rather enhance the work routines of the embalmer.

The size and location of the prep room is important when building a new funeral home or remodeling. If possible, the room should be large enough to accommodate three remains and have private access, with doors of sufficient size, opening into hallways that lead to casket storage rooms, chapels, and garage reception areas. As call volume goes over 150 per year, the preparation room needs to be larger to accommodate the greater volume.

An enclosed garage for delivering remains and loading vehicles should be near or adjacent to the prep room. The garage entry and exit into the preparation room needs to be private and away from any public visibility.

The ventilation system is a safety as well as a comfort factor for employees using the preparation room. New and remodeled preparation rooms need to comply with local building codes and OSHA standards. Ideally, the room should have its own independent heating, cooling, and ventilation system. Unfortunately, this type of independent system is rare, especially in older funeral homes. Air from the prep room should not be recirculated to other parts of the building. Once the size and space of a room has been determined, a proper ventilation system can be designed.

Embalmers know the effects, such as watery eyes and coughing spells, brought about by inadequate ventilation in the preparation area. In addition to formaldehyde, even common cleaning chemicals such as ammonia, household bleach, and many of the disinfectants employed will have irritating side effects.

Proper ventilation is the most important factor in any prep room. Too many prep rooms are designed without input from an embalmer. Eight-inch-diameter kitchen exhaust fans seemed to be the normal ventilation for preparation rooms in older funeral homes. Of course, this fan does not come close to supplying proper ventilation for the prep room. A properly ventilated embalming room must be able to handle any aerosol pathogen or chemical concerns, including a chemical spill, as well as the odors associated with decomposition.

Certain infections are circulated by the airborne route including varicella, measles, and tuberculosis. The usual mode

---

*Reprinted by permission from *The Dodge Magazine*, Nov.–Dec., Vol. 96, No. 5, 2004. Copyright: The Dodge Company.

of contaminating the air is breathing, coughing, and sneezing. When death occurs, these functions stop, so why the concern? During removals and embalming, tasks like transferring bodies to cots and tables, washing and embalming remains, and aspirating are common ways to create aerosols. Even unwrapping or undressing remains can cause potentially dangerous breath-like aerosol action in a preparation room. Gentle unwrapping or removing remains from a transfer pouch can reduce aerosols dramatically.

These potential aerosol exposures and exposures to blood and body fluids are the reasons that embalmers are required to use universal precautions and personal protection equipment. Physicians are aware of airflow patterns to limit transmission of airborne pathogens. The duration of time that airborne viruses remain in a room depend on the rate of air exchanges. The CDC recommends that patients requiring isolation for infectious diseases such as TB be placed in rooms having negative airflow. These rooms should have frequent air changes. The air should be exhausted directly outside without recirculation.

The American Society of Heating, Refrigeration and Air Conditioning Engineers (ASHRAE) design airflow systems for health control within hospitals and industries using chemicals in their everyday operation.

The Centers for Disease Control and Prevention (CDC), the National Institute for Occupational Safety (NIOSH), and the American National Standard Institute (ANSI) are all active in recommending guidelines for proper ventilation for health facilities and the workplace. Because of that, we have used them for part of our sources for this article. The two most common reasons for controlling ventilation would be for infection control and control of chemical contaminants.

The armed forces are presented with unique situations because of their exposure to medical isolation, pathology, and chemical exposure. The Navy for instance has ventilation requirements for their ships that give us a good source for recommended air changes per hour. For instance, acid store rooms aboard ship are required to have 15 air changes per hour. Chlorine gas cylinder rooms are required to have 30 air changes per hour. Paint lockers on ships are required to have 15 air changes per hour.

The Air Force requirements on Heating, Ventilation, and Air Conditioning (HVAC) systems are geared to infection control. Contaminated areas, such as infectious isolations areas and autopsy rooms, should maintain a negative air pressure relative to adjoining rooms and corridors. Air from these rooms should not be recirculated through a cold air return back through the central air system. The negative air pressure ensures that other rooms in the building will not be contaminated from the isolation or autopsy room. This principle should be the same for our prep rooms.

Some of the Air Force requirements for ventilation in medical facility rooms by air changes per hour (ACH) are as follows:

| Location | Outdoor Air (ACH) | Total Air (ACH) | Exhaust Air to Outside |
|---|---|---|---|
| Trauma room | 5 | 12 | Optional |
| Nursery suite | 5 | 12 | Optional |
| Infectious isolation | 2 | 12 | Yes |
| Autopsy rooms | 2 | 12 | Yes |

You can see that the infectious disease rooms and the autopsy rooms are considered to be high risk and require air to be exhausted outside without any recirculation. Preparation rooms certainly should be considered high risk, and these are rooms where potential chemical exposure is possible. So now that we realize that we work in areas that are potentially hazardous to us, how many air changes per hour would be adequate for our preparation room?

While researching this topic and contacting NIOSH, AIA, ASHRAE, ANSI, and various other sources for ventilation information, it was made obvious that preparation room ventilation was not covered under any existing guidelines or standards. As long as an embalming room passes a Formaldehyde Monitor test, it is considered safe. Because it is relatively easy to stay within the acceptable limits for formaldehyde, too many prep rooms still have the older ventilation systems, and this might consist of only a 14-inch exhaust fan.

Just because a preparation room can pass a monitoring test, it does not mean that it is a comfortable place to work. It could be a room that is recirculating pathogens and chemical fumes into other parts of the building. Autopsy rooms are considered high risk and are recommended to have 12 air changes per hour, and two of those changes should consist of outside air.

So, once again we are in a position to use our own common sense for the safety of our own workers. Because a preparation room presents a greater degree of chemical exposure than an autopsy room, this embalmer would like to work in a room with 20 air changes per hour. I have personally recommended 20 air changes per hour (ACH) to funeral homes, and those that have complied are the best ventilated and most comfortable preparation rooms that I have ever worked in. The room should be under negative pressure. That is, more air is exhausted than is taken into the room. This keeps the other parts of the building from being contaminated with air from the preparation room. If the funeral home does not have an independent heating and ventilation system for the prep room, a one-pass system can be utilized when remodeling. This means that any air going into the preparation room will not be allowed to reenter or recirculate into any part of the funeral home.

## FIGURING AIRFLOW IN AIR CHANGES PER HOUR

Fans are usually rated in CFMs (cubic feet per minute). In order to relate these "per minute" ratings to our ACHs (air changes per hour), we must divide ACH by 60 (the number of minutes in an hour). So the formula for determining the CFMs of the fan to purchase is:

Divide the number of air changes per hour you desire by 60 and then multiply that figure by

room size in cubic feet

Calculate the volume of the preparation room by multiplying length, width, and height of the room in feet, or

$$\text{length in feet} \times \text{width in feet} \times \text{height in feet} = \text{volume in cubic feet}$$

(feet × feet × feet = cubic feet)

For example, a room 20 ft. × 10 ft. and 10 ft. high will have a volume of 2000 CF (cubic feet). If one wants 20 air changes per hour, then they will have to simply calculate the volume in cubic feet, divide by 20/60, and you will have the minimum required CFM rating of an exhaust, which could achieve the 20 air changes per hour (667 CFM, in this case). Once the funeral director knows the volume of the preparation room area and calculates the exhaust requirement, then the equipment supplier or installer can easily help.

To achieve a desired 20 air changes per hour, you could use the following chart to help choose the proper size of exhaust fan;

| (Cubic Ft. Per Minutes) | |
| --- | --- |
| Room Size | Volume – Divided by 3 = CFM |
| (a) 10 × 15 and 10 ft. high: | 10 × 15 × 10 = 1500 cubic ft./3 = 500 CFM |
| (b) 10 × 20 and 10 ft. high: | 10 × 20 × 10 = 2000 cubic ft./3 = 667 CFM |
| (c) 20 × 20 and 10 ft. high: | 20 × 20 × 10 = 4000 cubic ft./3 = 1333 CFM |

### Risk of Infection and Tracking of Work-Related Infectious Diseases in the Funeral Industry

*Susan Salter Davidson, MS, MT (ASCP) and William H. Benjamin, Jr. PhD*
*Birmingham Alabama*

The routine tasks carried out by FSPs would seem to put them at significant risk of exposure to several infectious agents. Exposure by way of splashes to the mucus membranes, inhalation of aerosolized body fluids, and direct inoculation can result in infectious diseases caused by multiple species of bacteria, viruses, and prions. The purpose of this review is to determine what is known of the risk of exposure to infectious agents that FSPs experience in the workplace, identify prevention and postexposure strategies utilized in the funeral business, and determine occupationally acquired infection rates among this group.

## METHODS

A literature search was carried out using the PubMed service of the National Library of Medicine (April, 2006). Abstracts were reviewed, and applicable articles were obtained. Internet sources included the Web sites of the Centers for Disease Control and Prevention (CDC), the United States Department of Labor, the U.S. Census Bureau, the National Funeral Directors Association (NFDA), and the American Board of Funeral Service Education.

## RESULTS

### Risk of Exposure

The risk of exposure to infectious agents in the health care setting is well documented; however, one occupational group that appears to be underrepresented in the infectious disease literature is FSPs. A recent literature review sponsored by the British Institute of Embalmers found that the risk of exposure is well documented but that there is a need for additional studies focusing on the suggested link between reported infections and the embalming procedure.[1] That review, as well as this one, also found a lack of studies in the literature focusing on the implementation of effectiveness of infection control practices in the funeral business.[1]

There were 2,448,288 reported deaths in the United States during 2003, the majority of which was followed by embalming according to the NFDA.[2,3] An infectious disease was the reported cause in 99,232 of these individuals and is recognized as a frequent contributor to mortality, even when not documented as the primary cause of death.[2] The infectious nature of cadavers, regardless of their cause of death, has been documented.[1,4–8] The routine transport and embalming of cadavers place the FSP in a position to be exposed to multiple infectious agents that are transmissible by mucocutaneous contamination, aerosolization, and direct inoculation.[1,8–15]

Two common bacterial pathogens that may be contracted through mucocutaneous contamination are methicillin-resistant *Staphylococcus aureus* (MRSA) and *Streptococcus pyogenes*. Long recognized as a nosocomial pathogen, MRSA is establishing itself as a community-acquired infectious agent with increasing frequency.[10,16,17] Because of the prevalence of MRSA in the population both as a commensal and as a pathogen, the FSP has a potential exposure risk from the remains of individuals who expired in health care facilities and those who died in other settings.[18,19] Group A streptococcus has been shown to survive on the cadavers of victims of invasive disease, presenting a serious infectious risk to the FSP because it may be transmitted by direct contact and as a result of direct inoculation following even minor nicks to the skin during autopsy.[8,12,17,20–22]

FSPs may be exposed to gastrointestinal organisms through direct contact with leaking fecal material when manipulating corpses, which can lead to transmission via the fecal–oral route.[8] The two microorganisms of greatest concern for transmission are non-typhi *Salmonella* and hepatitis A, whereas *Salmonella typhi*, *Shigella* species, Cryptosporidia, *Helicobacter pylori*, and other microorganisms are less of a risk in the developed world.[12,23–25] Another group of Enterobacteriaceae that have the potential to present a risk to FSPs are the extended-spectrum β-lactamase producers (ESBLs) because of their growing prevalence and refractoriness to treatment, resulting in higher mortality rates when responsible for bacteremia.[26,28]

Infectious agents transmitted primarily by the airborne route that should be of concern for the FSP include *Mycobacterium tuberculosis* and the virus responsible for severe acute respiratory syndrome (SARS).[1,8,13,29,30] Tuberculosis is a leading cause of disease and death, with more than one-third of the global population being infected. Attempts to control the infections are complicated by the high prevalence of multiple drug-resistant strains, which are common in some populations.[31] The risk of exposure to *M. tuberculosis* experienced by FSPs is documented for airborne transmission and through direct inoculation.[1,6–8,10,32,34]

SARS is a newly recognized infection disease, and there are no published reports of transmission from cadavers to FSPs. Moore et al. analyzed the data available on SARS and published guidelines for infection control in the health care setting, which were tested in Toronto.[30] Others have also published reviews of the infection control literature concerning SARS, and the WHO has released guidelines addressing management of known or suspected cases.[29,30,35,36] Because of the virulent and contagious nature of the SARS virus, it is of special concern to both the health care worker (HCW) and the FSP.[29]

The three most common blood-borne pathogenic viruses FSPs are at risk of exposure to are the hepatitis B virus (HBV), the hepatitis C virus (HCV), and the human immunodeficiency virus (HIV).[1,8,9,11,12,15,37–42] The risk of exposure to blood and other body fluids for this occupational group has been the subject of a limited number of studies.[9,11,37,42,43] Studies focusing on the occurrence of HBV among FSPs show that members of this occupational group have a higher rate of infection than control groups.[1,6,9,12,37] However, widespread implementation of vaccination programs has dramatically lowered the infection rate among HCWs and FSPs.[39,41,44]

HCV is the most prevalent blood-borne pathogen in health care settings, with many chronically infected individuals being asymptomatic. Currently, there is no HCV vaccine available.[12,45–48] The long-term viability of HIV in cadaver tissue is recognized, and the literature reports a documented case of seroconversion in a pathologist following necropsy, along with two possible and one documented seroconversions in FSPs.[12,38,49–54] Thus, the importance of the prevention of transmission of HCV and HIV during the embalming procedure is clear, especially in light of these documented cases of transmission of HIV.

The Marburg and Ebola hemorrhagic fever viruses are not endemic in the United States, but the continuing sporadic outbreaks on the African continent, the previous occurrence of infection in European countries, the ease and speed of international travel, and their classification as category A bioterrorism agents warrant their inclusion in a discussion of potential exposure risks for FSPs.[7,55–57] Secondary transmission of these two viruses is known to occur following unprotected exposure to patients and cadavers through mucocutaneous contact and blood and body fluid exposure.[7,58,59] Aerosolization cannot be definitively excluded as a mode of transmission.[58,60] Guidelines have been published for the management of suspected or confirmed cases of these viral infections and include postmortem instructions.[7,56–58,61]

Another important group of infectious diseases of concern to FSPs is the transmissible spongiform encephalopathies (TSEs) or Creutzfeldt–Jakob disease (CJD) in humans, including kuru, iatrogenic, and new variant CJD (vCJD).[62–64] The mode of transmission of prions is not completely understood, with 85% of patients showing no recognizable pattern of transmission, but it is known that iatrogenic CJD has been passed from cadavers to recipients of human growth hormone, dura mater, and corneal grafts as well as between living patients following use of contaminated neurosurgical equipment.[62–64] Blood-borne transmission has been implicated in two cases of secondary vCJD infections in the United Kingdom, prompting concern that the blood supply could be contaminated with the responsible prion because of asymptomatic donor contributions.[63–68] Because prions are not destroyed by formaldehyde or embalming is not recommended for autopsied or traumatized bodies, but, if the procedure is necessary, the CDC suggests following the WHO guidelines.[62,69]

Although most cases of TSE have been located in countries other than the United States, the government is vigilant in monitoring CJD and vCJD cases and has taken steps to prevent an outbreak.[64] Transmission of TSE between patients, to HCW, and to FSP is a major concern because supportive treatment is all that can be done for victims because these diseases are invariably fatal.[63,64]

The potential for transmission of multiple infections agents while engaging in the routine tasks of FSPs has been demonstrated. The nation's primary source of occupational information is the Occupational Information Network (O*NET) sponsored by the U.S. Department of Labor Employment and Training Administration, and their Summary Report for Embalmers and Funeral Directors provides a detailed description of the tasks performed by FSPs that place them at risk.[70] There have been a limited number of published studies documenting actually exposure events.[1,9,11,42,55] The use of sharp implements during the embalming procedure places the FSP at risk of blood-borne pathogen exposure via needlestick, cuts, and splashes. The routine aspiration of blood and other body fluids carries the risk of aerosolization of droplet nuclei. The collection of fluid in the chest cavity of the deceased because of putrefaction of tissue can lead to frothing and gurgling through the nose and mouth of the corpse.[1,9,11]

## Exposure Prevention and Management Strategies

Evaluation of exposure prevention and postexposure strategies utilized in the funeral business is difficult. There are few published references focusing on infection control in this setting.[1,9–11,37,42] Funeral homes fall under the mandates of the Occupational Safety Hazard Association's Bloodborne Pathogens Standard (number 1910.13100), which requires that employers have a written exposure control plan and meet the methods of compliance.[71] These methods include the practice of universal precautions, the implementation of engineering and work practice controls, and the provision of PPE. There does not appear to be a monitoring system in place to determine the effectiveness of adherence to the standard by tabulating exposure events or infection rates among FSPs.[71] The CDC maintains the National Surveillance System for Health Care Workers, which is a voluntary program that monitors exposure events among hospital-based HCWs to HIV, HBV, HCV, and *M. tuberculosis* to assess trends, prevention strategies, and postexposure prophylaxis, but funeral homes are not part of this surveillance program.[72]

A further reason evaluation is difficult is the absence of infection control activities in funeral homes analogous to those found in most health care facilities. These activities are implemented to analyze policies and procedures to control infectious disease transmission. Although compliance among FSPs has not been studied to the degree that it has for HCWs, much of the data from the HCWs can be applied to the funeral business. It is known that compliance is greater if employees feel that their organization is interested in safety, if they have current and correct knowledge of the availability of PPE, and if they perceive that compliance is mandatory.[30] There has been speculation concerning the usefulness of disclosing to FSPs the specific infectious nature of particular cadavers, but it has been shown that this knowledge does not affect compliance in a significant percentage of employees.[10] The autonomous nature of the work performed by FSPs might be a factor contributing to noncompliance issues. Postexposure actions followed by the FSP might be less than those of the HCW because of the expectation and relative ease of reporting exposure events and receiving postexposure care in most health care settings.

The role continuing education plays in compliance among FSPs is another area that appears not to have been evaluated fully. The American Board of Funeral Service Education, the accrediting agency for schools offering degrees in funeral service, requires students to complete successfully the basic science courses, including microbiology and pathophysiology, and the examinations for licensure administered by each state include sections covering these subjects.[73,74] More than 30 states require annual continuing education credits for licensed funeral directors and embalmers, but there are no specific requirements for infection control subject matter.[73,74] Studies have suggested a need for continuing education to ensure adherence to infection control policies.[29,30,75]

## Occupationally Acquired Infection Rates

It is difficult to determine the occupationally acquired infection rate among FSPs. One possible explanation for the apparent underrepresentation of FSP in the infection control literature could be that embalmers and funeral directors are placed under the Personal Care and Service Occupations group rather than being included in the Healthcare Practitioners and Technical Occupations or Healthcare Support Occupations groups in the Bureau of Labor Standard Occupational Classification (SOC) system.[76] This SOC system is consistent with the Census 2000 Alphabetical Indexes of Industries and Occupations used in coding information gathered by governmental and private agencies for statistical reporting programs.[76,77] Another contributing factor is the lack of standardized coding on death certificates for the occupation of the decedent, although multiple governmental agencies are working together to make improvements in the coding system to standardize this data.[78] Underreporting of exposure events by individual employees along with the lack of infection control oversight programs in the funeral business could also be factors making this determination difficult.

An additional topic that is worthy of mention is the exposure risk experienced in countries other than the United States and Canada, which are the only two countries that routinely embalm the deceased. Other countries have various types of funeral services available, but embalming is reserved for cases requiring a prolonged viewing period or for shipment of the corpse. In most areas, family members wash the dead and prepare them for internment, and only rudimentary steps are taken to prevent the spread of communicable disease if it is known to be present.[79] According to the WHO mortality records, worldwide, there were 10,903,977 deaths attributed to infectious and parasitic diseases in 2002, and the majority of these deaths occurred in areas other than the United States and Canada.[80] Thus, as with many issues related to infectious diseases, the developing world could benefit from better surveillance as well as implementation of controls to prevent transmission related to handling of the dead.

## DISCUSSION

This review of published literature demonstrates that FSPs have a risk of exposure to bacterial and viral pathogens as well as to prion-mediated diseases. It reveals a lack of published studies focusing on the implementation and effectiveness of infection control policies for this occupational group as well as the difficulty involved in determining actual infection rates related to workplace exposure events. Questions that should be the focus of future studies include determining the level of employee compliance with existing infection control policies, accessing factors that influence compliance, and evaluating the effectiveness of existing policies in preventing exposure events and actual infections as well as implementing better systems to determine the infection rates of the various agents in this occupational group.

## REFERENCES

1. Creely KS. Infection risks and embalming. Institute of Occupational Medicine. 2004. Available at http://www.iom-World.org/pubs/IOMTMO401.pdf. Accessed April 1, 2005.
2. National Center for Health Statistics. Death: final data for 2003. National Vital Statistics Reports 2006. Available at http://www.cec.gov/nchs/data/hestat/finaldeaths03 tables.pdf#2. Accessed January 28, 2006.
3. National Funeral Directors Association. National Funeral Directors Association fact sheet 2005. Available at htt:www.nfda.org/nfdafactsheets/php. Accessed July 27, 2005.
4. Rose GW, Hockett RN. The microbiologic evaluation and enumeration of postmortem species from human remains. *Health Laboratory Science* 1971;8:75–78.
5. Hinson MR. Final report on literature search on the infectious nature of dead bodies for the Embalming Chemical Manufacturers Association. Embalming Chemical Manufacturers Association 1968. In: Mayer RG, ed. *Embalming History, Theory, and Practice*, 3rd ed. New York: McGraw-Hill, 2000:649–652.
6. Rendon LR. Dangers of infection. In: Mayer RG, ed. *Embalming History, Theory, and Practice*, 3rd ed., New York: McGraw-Hill, 2000:652–654.
7. Nolte KB, Taylor DG, Richmond JY. Biosafety considerations for autopsy. *The American Journal of Forensic Medicine and Pathology* 2002;23:107–122.
8. Healting TD, Hoffman PN, Young SE. The infection hazards of human cadavers. Communicable Disease Report. *CDR Review* 1995;5:R61–R68.
9. Gershon RR, Vlahov D, Farzadegan H, et al. Occupational risk of human immunodeficiency virus, hepatitis B virus, and hepatitis C virus infections among funeral service practitioners in Maryland. *Infection Control and Hospital Epidemiology* 1995;16:194–197.
10. Gershon RR, Vlahov D, Edsamilla-Cejudo JA, et al. Tuberculosis risk in funeral home employees. *Journal of Occupational and Environmental Medicine* 1998;40:497–503.
11. Nwanyanwu OC, Tabasuri TH, Harris GR. Exposure to and precautions for blood and body fluids among workers in the funeral home franchises of Fort Worth, Texas. *American Journal of Infection Control* 1989;17:208–212.
12. Burton JL. Health and safety at necropsy. *Journal of Clinical Pathology* 2003;56:254–260.
13. Morgan O. Infectious disease risks from dead bodies following natural disasters. *Revista Panamericana de Salud Publica* 2004;15:307–312.

14. Hanzlick R. Embalming, body preparation, burial, and disinterment: An overview for forensic pathologists. *American Journal of Forensic Medicine and Pathology* 1994;15:122–131.
15. Claydon SM. The high-risk autopsy: Recognition and protection. *American Journal of Forensic Medicine and Pathology* 1993;14:253–256.
16. Fridkin SK, Hagerman JC, Morrison M, et al. Methicillin-resistant *Staphylococcus aureus* disease in three communities. *The New England Journal of Medicine* 2005;352:1436–1444.
17. O'Brien KL, Beall B, Barrett NL, et al. Epidemiology of invasive group A streptococcus disease in the United States, 1995-1999. *Clinical Infectious Disease* 2002;35:268–276.
18. Kuehnert MJ, Hill HA, Kupronis BA, et al. Methicillin-resistant-*Staphylococcus aureus* hospitalizations, United States. *Emerging Infectious Diseases* 2005;11:868–872.
19. Lowy FD. Staphylococcus aureus infections. *The New England Journal of Medicine* 1998;339:520–532.
20. Greene CM, Van Beneden CA, Javadi M, et al. Cluster of deaths from group A streptococcus in a long-term care facility-Georgia, 2001. *American Journal of Infection Control* 2005;33:108–113.
21. Centers for Disease Control and Prevention. Active Bacterial Core Surveillance (ABCs) Report Emerging Infections Program Network: Group A streptococcus, 2004-provisional. 2005. Available at http://www.cec.gov/ncidod/dbmd/abcs/survreports/gas04prelim.pdf. Accessed January 28, 2006.
22. Hawkey PM, Pedler SJ, Southall PJ. *Streptococcus pyogenes*: A forgotten occupational hazard in the mortuary. *British Medical Journal* 1980;281:1058.
23. Sepkowitz KA. Occupationally acquired infections in health care workers. Part II. *Annals of Internal Medicine* 1996;125:917–928.
24. Swaminathan B, Barrett TJ, Fields P. Surveillance for human Salmonella infections in the United States. *Journal of AOAC International* 2006;89:553–559.
25. Niyogi SK. Shigellosis. *Journal of Microbiology* 2005; 43:133–143. of anatomy. *The New England Journal of Medicine* 1994;331:1315.
26. Schwaber MJ, Navon-Venezia S, Kaye KS, et al. Clinical and economic impact of bacteremia with extended spectrum-β-lactamase-producing Enterobacteriaceae. *Antimicrobial Agents and Chemotherapy* 2006;50:1257–1262.
27. Tumbarello M, Spanu T, Sanguinetti M, et al. Bloodstream infections caused by extended-spectrum-β-lactamase-producing *Klebsiella pneumonia*. Risk factors, molecular epidemiology, and clinical outcome. *Antimicrobial Agents and Chemotherapy* 2006;50:498–504.
28. Moolman GJ, Jankowits CE, Bezuidenhout S, et al. Beta-lactamases in Enterobacteriaceae-an ever-present threat. *South African Medical Journal* 2006;96:331–334.
29. Gamage B, Moore D, Copes R, et al. Protecting health care workers from SARS and other respiratory pathogens: A review of the infection control literature. *American Journal of Infection Control* 2005;33:114–121.
30. Moore D, Gamage B, Bryce E, et al. Protecting health care workers from SARS and other respiratory pathogens: Organizational and individual factors that affect adherence to infection control guidelines. *American Journal of Infection Control* 2005;33: 88–96.
31. Centers for Disease Control and Prevention. Tuberculosis in the United States. 2004. Available at http://www.cec.gov?nchstp/tb/surv/surv2004/default.htm. Accessed October 1, 2005.
32. Lauzardo M, Lee P, Duncan H, et al. Transmission of *Mycobacterium tuberculosis* to a funeral director during routine embalming. *Chest* 2001;119:640–642.
33. Sterling TR, Pope DS, Bishai WR, et al. *Transmission of Mycobacterium tuberculosis* from a cadaver to an embalmer. *The New England Journal of Medicine* 2000;342:246–248.
34. Demiryurek D, Bayramoglu A, Ustacelebi S. Infective agents in fixed human cadavers: A brief review and suggested guidelines. *Anatomical Record* 2002;269:194–197.
35. World Health Organization. Hospital infection control guidance for severe acute respiratory syndrome (SARS). 2003. Available at http://www.who.int/csr/sara/infectioncontrol/en/. Accessed October 1, 2005.
36. World Health Organization. Consensus document on the epidemiology of severe acute respiratory syndrome (SARS). 2003. Available at http://www.who. int/csr/sars/en/WHOconsensus.pdf. Accessed October 1, 2005.
37. Turner SB, Kunches LM, Gordon KF, et al. Occupational exposure to human immunodeficiency virus (HIV) and hepatitis B virus (HBV) among embalmers: A pilot seroprevalence study. *American Journal of Public Health* 1989;79:1425–1426.
38. Douceron H, Deforges L, Gherardi R, et al. Long-lasting postmortem viability of human immunodeficiency virus: A potential risk in forensic medicine practice. *Forensic Science International* 1993;60:61–66.
39. Beltrami EM, Williams IT, Shapiro CN, et al. Risk and management of blood-borne infections in health care workers. *Clinical Microbiology Reviews* 2000;13:385–407.
40. Riddell LA, Sherrard J. Blood-borne virus infection: The occupational risks. *International Journal of STD & AIDS* 2000;11:632–639.
41. Twitchell KT. Bloodborne pathogens: What you need to know. Part II. *AAOHN Journal* 2003;51:89–97.
42. Beck-Sague CM, Jarvis WR, Fruehling JA, et al. Universal precautions and mortuary practitioners influence on practices and risk of occupationally acquired infection. *Journal of Occupational Medicine* 1991;33:874–878.
43. McDonald L. Blood exposure and protection in funeral homes. *American Journal of Infection Control* 1989;17:193–195.
44. Mahoney FJ, Stewart K, Hu H, et al. Progress toward the elimination of hepatitis B virus transmission among health care workers in the United States. *Archives of Internal Medicine* 1997;157:2601–2605.
45. Memon MI, Memon MA. Hepatitis C: An epidemiological review. *Journal of Viral Hepatitis* 2002;9:84–100.
46. Williams I. Epidemiology of hepatitis C in the United States. *The American Journal of Medicine* 999;107:52–59.
47. Alter MJ, Kruszon-Moran D, Nainan OV, et al. The prevalence of hepatitis C virus infection in the United States, 1988 through 1994. *The New England Journal of Medicine* 1999;341:556–562.
48. Lanphear BP. Transmission and control of bloodborne viral hepatitis in health care workers. *Occupational Medicine* 1997;12: 717–730.
49. Henry K, Dexter D, Sannerud K, Jackson B, Balfour H, Jr. Recovery of HIV at autopsy. *The New England Journal of Medicine* 1989;321:1833–1834.
50. deCraemer D. Postmortem viability of human immunodeficiency virus-implications for teaching of anatomy. *The New England Journal of Medicine* 1994;331:1315.
51. Johnson MD, Schaffner W, Atkinson J, et al. Autopsy risk and acquisition of human immunodeficiency virus infection: A case report and reappraisal. *Archives of Pathology & Laboratory Medicine* 1997;121:64–66.
52. Bankowski MJ, Landa AL, States B, et al. Postmortem recovery of human immunodeficiency virus type I from plasma and mononuclear cells: Implications for occupational exposure. *Archives of Pathology & Laboratory Medicine* 1992;116:1124–1127.

53. Nyberg M, Suni J, Haltia M. Isolation of human immunodeficiency virus (HIV) at autopsy one to six days postmortem. *American Journal of Clinical Pathology* 1990;94:422–425.
54. Do AN, Ciesielski CA, Metler RP, et al. Occupationally acquired human immunodeficiency virus (HIV) infection: National case surveillance data during 20 years of the HIV epidemic in the United States. *Infection Control and Hospital Epidemiology* 2003;24:86–96.
55. Centers for Disease Control and Prevention. Brief report: Outbreak of Marburg virus hemorrhagic fever–Angola. October 1, 2004–March 29, 2005. *MMWR* 2005;54:308–309.
56. Centers for Disease Control and Prevention. A guidebook for surveillance medical examiners, coroners, and biologic terrorism and case management. *MMWR* 2004;53:RR08.
57. Ligon BL. Outbreak of Marburg hemorrhagic fever in Angola: A review of the history of the disease and its biological aspects. *Seminars in Pediatric Infectious Diseases* 2005;16:219–224.
58. Borio L, Inglesby T, Peters CJ, et al. Hemorrhagic fever viruses as biological weapons: Medical and public health managements. *Journal of American Medical Association* 2002;287:2391–2405.
59. Peters CJ. Marburg and Ebola-arming ourselves against the deadly filoviruses. *The New England Journal of Medicine* 2005;352:2571–2573.
60. Leffel EK, Reed DS. Marburg and Ebola viruses as aerosol threats. *Biosecurity and Bioterrorism* 2004;2:186–191.
61. Centers for Disease Control and Prevention. Management of patients with suspected viral hemorrhagic fever. *MMWR* 1988;37:1–16.
62. Centers for Disease Control and Prevention. CEC. Questions and answers: Creutzfeldt-Jakob disease infection control practices. 2005. Available at http://wwwcec.gov/ncidod/dvrd/cjc/infectioncontrolcjd.htm. Accessed October 1, 2005.
63. Chesebro B. Introduction to the transmissible spongiform encephalopathies or prion diseases. *British Medical Bulletin* 2003;66:1–20.
64. Belay ED, Schonberger LB. The public health impact on prion diseases. *Annual Review of Public Health* 2005;26:191–212.
65. Brown P, Will RG, Bradley R, et al. Bovine spongiform encephalopathy and variant Creutzfeldt-Jakob disease: Background, evolution, and current concerns. *Emerging Infectious Diseases* 2001;7:6–16.
66. Llewelyn CA, Hewitt PE, Knight RS, et al. Possible transmission of variant Creutzfeldt-Jakob disease by blood transfusion. *Lancet* 2004;363:417–421.
67. Peden AH, Head MW, Ritchie DL, et al. Preclinical vCJD after blood transfusion in a PRNP codon 129 heterozygous patient. *Lancet* 2004;364:527–529.
68. Brown P. Pathogenesis and transfusion risk of transmissible spongiform encephalopathies. *Developmental Biology (Basel)* 2005;120:27–33.
69. World health Organization. WHO infection control guidelines for transmissible spongiform encephalopathies: Report of a WHO consultation. Geneva, Switzerland, 23–26 March 1999. Available at http://www.who.int/csr/resources/publications/bse/WHO CDS CSR APH 2000 3/en/. Accessed October 1, 2005.
70. Occupational Information Network. Summary report for: 11-9061.00 Funeral Directors. 2004. Available at http://online.onetcenter.org/link/summary/11.9061.00. Accessed October 1, 2005.
71. Occupational exposure to bloodborne pathogens—OSHA; final rule. *Federal Register* 1991;56:64004–182.
72. *Centers for Disease Control and Prevention. Surveillance system for hospital health care workers*. 2005. Available at http://www.cec.gov/niosh/docs/chartbook/. Accessed October 1, 2005.
73. National Funeral Directors Association. Careers in funeral service. 2005. Available at http://www.nfda.org/careers.php. Accessed April 6, 2005.
74. Bureau of Labor Statistic. US Department of Labor Occupational outlook handbook. 2004-05 edition. Available at http:/www.bls.govioco/acos011.htm. Accessed May 21, 2005.
75. Berhe M, Edmond MB, Bearman GM. Practices and an assessment of health care workers' perceptions of compliance with infection control knowledge of nosocomial infections. *American Journal of Infection Control* 2005;33:55–57.
76. US Department of Labor Standard Occupational Classification System. Available at http://www.bls.gov/soc/home.htm. Accessed May 21, 2005.
77. US Census Bureau. Housing and Household Economics Statistics Division. 2004. Available at gov/hhes/www/ioindex.overview.html. Accessed May 13, 2005.
78. Department of Health and Human Services. Mortality by occupation, industry, and cause of death: 24 reporting states (1984-1988). 1997. Available at http://www.cdc.gov/niosh/bk97114.html. Accessed March 25, 2005.
79. Habenstein RW, Lamers WM. *Funeral customs the world over*, 4th ed. Milwaukee, WI: Bulfin Printers, Inc, 1994.
80. WHO. Burden of disease estimates by region in 2002. World Health Report: 2004.

---

**Creutzfeldt–Jakob Disease: A Comprehensive Guide for Healthcare Personnel Section 3—Information for Embalmers**[*]

*Curtis D. Rostad, CFSP*

## FOREWORD

CJD is a baffling disease. Not only because there is so much we do not know, but even what we do know has been misunderstood, exaggerated or understated, misrepresented, and miscommunicated.

On the one hand, CJD is a fatal disease; yet, we know little of its transmission. Its threat to our health is often minimized to the public to avoid undue panic; yet, health care workers are given specific cautions to protect themselves.

In our attempts to avoid unnecessary fear of the disease, we sometimes fail to separate the differences in exposure that exist between living with a person with CJD, caring for a patient in the hospital setting, handling lab and pathology samples, and caring for the body after death—especially when an autopsy has been performed.

This section includes what the funeral director and the embalmer need to know about CJD. While the exposure to CJD is limited when the person is alive, mortuary care increases that exposure. Even then, we can say little about what risk that exposure presents other than that it appears to be small.

Still, we must present the facts (as we know them today), issue our cautions, and offer our suggestions as to how to care for the remains in a safe, yet professional manner.

---

[*]Ruth Carrico, PhD, RN, CIC, Christian Davis Furman, MD, MSPH, Curtis D. Rostad, CFSP, Dorothy Cannan Hyde, MSW, Med. Chicago Spectrum Press, Louisville, KY., 2005. *Reprinted with permission of the author.*

**Admittedly, the extent of care the funeral director feels is prudent to offer is a matter of professional evaluation and personal decision.**

**We hope we have presented in this section the information they need to make those decisions and the tools to complete their tasks in as safe a manner as possible.**

*Curtis Rostad, CFSP.*

## INTRODUCTION

Throughout the 130 plus years of modern embalming, funeral service has faced many infectious and potentially fatal diseases and has still found ways to serve families and protect the public health.

We have survived the emergence of TB, polio, hepatitis, and HIV/AIDS because we have formaldehyde and other embalming chemicals that effectively kill the bacteria and viruses that cause these diseases and we have learned to protect ourselves from infection during the embalming process.

As long as we never encounter an organism that is resistant to formaldehyde and other embalming chemicals, and as long as we have the means to protect ourselves, we will always be able to serve the public with our skills.

But *what if*, in the future, an organism comes along that we cannot destroy through embalming? What then?

Well, the future is now. *Such a disease exists.*

- There is no diagnostic test for it.
- You can have it for up to 25 years and not know it.
- There is no vaccine.
- There is no cure.
- There is no treatment.
- It is infectious.
- It is always fatal.
- Formaldehyde does not touch it.
- There are no embalming chemicals that will kill it.
- Common methods of disinfection and sterilization will not kill it.

It is called *Creutzfeldt–Jakob disease.*

## WHAT IS CREUTZFELDT–JAKOB DISEASE?

Creutzfeldt–Jakob disease, or CJD, is a one of a family of diseases known as transmissible spongiform encephalopathies (TSEs). It was first identified and described by both Creutzfeldt and Jakob in the 1920s.

It is a fatal neurological disease for which there is no treatment and no cure.

There is no vaccine available.

Other TSEs include kuru (a disease associated with cannibalism in New Guinea) and Gerstmann–Straussler–Scheinker syndrome.[1]

There are also similar diseases among animals. In sheep and goats, it is called scrapie. In deer and elk, it is known as chronic wasting disease. In cows, it is called bovine spongiform encephalopathy (BSE) or "mad cow disease." An outbreak of this disease in Great Britain in 1995 caused worldwide concern over whether or not this disease could be transferred from animal to human through the eating of contaminated meat or other animal products.[2] As a result, shipment of cattle or meat products into the United States was halted.

The first case of BSE in the United States was discovered in a single cow in Washington state in December of 2003. The cow reportedly came from Canada where mad cow disease had been found earlier.

A new variant of CJD called nvCJD has been identified in Britain and has been proven to be associated with BSE. Humans apparently contract the disease from eating beef from cows with BSE. The new variant kills younger people (average age 28), and unlike classic CJD, the incubation period appears to be months (7–24) rather than years in length. As of this writing, no cases of nvCJD have been diagnosed in the United States.[3,4]

## WHO GETS CJD?

Creutzfeldt–Jakob disease affects both men and women worldwide usually between the ages of 50 and 75.

## WHAT CAUSES IT?

CJD results when abnormal protein accumulates in the brain cells. Scientists do not know what triggers the conversion of protein from the normal to the abnormal form, although a genetic defect has been identified that might provide a clue.[5,6] Some believe the conversion is caused by a spontaneous mutation of the normal protein itself, whereas other scientists believe a virus or viruslike entity may be involved.[7]

This abnormal protein, believed to be the causative agent of CJD, is known as a *prion* (pronounced "pryon"),[8] a protein-based molecule with no RNA or DNA that is smaller than a virus.[9]

Actually, because the prion disease we see today differs in many respects from the original description of CJD, some scientists question whether or not the disease we see today is indeed the same disease described by Creutzfeldt and Jakob some 70 years ago.[10]

## WHAT ARE THE SYMPTOMS OF CJD?

The initial symptoms are subtle and can include insomnia, depression, confusion, personality/behavioral changes, strange physical sensations, balance and coordination disorders, loss of memory, and visual problems.

Rapidly the patient deteriorates with progressive dementia and usually myoclonus (involuntary irregular jerking motions) as the disease progresses. Language, sight, muscular weakness, and coordination problems worsen.

The patient finally loses all mental and physical functions. Coma follows and death is usually due to pneumonia precipitated by the bedridden, unconscious state.

The duration of CJD from the onset of symptoms to death is usually 1 year or less, most commonly 2–6 months.[11]

## HOW COMMON IS IT?

The official mortality rate is approximately 1 death per million population worldwide per year.[12] CJD is still classified as a rare disease (although the National Center for Infectious Diseases considers it an "emerging infectious disease").[13] This figure appears to be understated because CJD is often misdiagnosed. Because of the dementia it causes, it is often confused with Alzheimer.

One study done by Yale University showed that 13% of patients with Alzheimer were found upon autopsy to actually have CJD.[14]

Approximately 80% of deaths were among persons aged 60 or older. Among this age group, the death rate from CJD is 4.5 per million persons.[15]

## HOW IS IT DIAGNOSED?

There is no definitive diagnostic test for CJD. The disease is suspected when a patient develops a rapid dementia and myoclonus. A 14-3-3 spinal test is 95% effective in supporting a clinical diagnosis of CJD. Unfortunately, the only 100% effective diagnostic tool available is an autopsy with appropriate tests.[16]

The postmortem finding of a coarse spongy-like surface of the brain (and the underlying microscopic cellular changes) is characteristic of CJD, thus the term, spongiform.

## HOW LONG DOES IT TAKE FOR SYMPTOMS TO DEVELOP?

A person can become infected with CJD and have no symptoms for typically 12–25 years, although the disease can run its course and result in death in less than 3 years from the time of infection.

## HOW DO YOU GET IT?

Three epidemiologic forms of CJD are well recognized. The familiar (genetic) form (5–10% of cases) results from a genetic mutation.

Approximately 1% of cases are iatrogenic (resulting from a medical procedure), including neurological procedures using contaminated instruments, corneal transplant, from electroencephalographic electrodes, cadaveric dura mater grafts, and pituitary hormone administration.[17]

Sporadic CJD accounts for 80–85% of all cases. These cases result from the mutation of the protein by some unknown cause.[18]

## SO IT IS INFECTIOUS?

Yes. Although CJD was first described in the 1920s, it was not considered a transmissible disease until 1966.[19]

In 1974, a case of CJD transmission as the result of a corneal transplant was reported.[20]

In 1977, CJD transmission caused by silver electroencephalograph electrodes previously used in the brain of a person with CJD was reported. The transmission occurred despite decontamination of the electrodes between patients.[21]

In 1985, there were a series of case reports showing that cadaver-extracted pituitary human growth hormone could transmit CJD.[22] Shortly thereafter, it was shown that human gonadotropin administered by injection could also transmit CJD from person to person.[23]

CJD was first reported in a recipient of a dura mater transplant in 1987.[24]

## IS CJD A DANGER TO HEALTH CARE AND MORTUARY STAFF?

As of today, over two dozen cases of CJD exist among health care workers, including physicians, neurologists, pathologists, and laboratory technicians exposed to CJD. There are as yet no documented cases of transfer of the disease from a deceased patient to mortuary staff.

However, the cause of 80–85% of the cases of CJD is unknown and because it can take up to 25 years for symptoms of CJD to develop, it could be decades before we find out the true number of infections of CJD in health care workers exposed to patients with the disease.

## WHAT BODY FLUIDS AND ORGANS ARE INFECTIOUS?

Since this is a neurological disease, the cerebrospinal fluid is highly infectious. The transmissible agent has also been shown to be present in the brain, spleen, liver, lymph nodes, lungs, spinal cord, kidneys, cornea and lens, bone, and to a much lesser degree, blood.

It is not found in tears, nasal mucous, saliva, urine, or feces. Therefore, there is little risk involved in becoming infected by casual contact or by living with a person with CJD.[25]

It is important to understand this when dealing with the family of the deceased. During life, they were able to have normal contact with their family member with no adverse health consequences or risk of infection.

Now that the person is dead, they may not be able to understand why you hesitate to care for the person they loved.

This is simply because during life, the points of contact with a CJD patient are not infectious. It is after death, when invasive procedures are done, when contact with the prion is possible.

## CAN YOU GET CJD FROM BLOOD?

That is the question being debated and researched at the present time. Although there have been no documented cases of CJD resulting from blood or blood transfusion, consider the following.

The Red Cross will not accept blood from a person with CJD symptoms or family history of CJD. A history of CJD disqualifies a patient from being an organ donor.

Human CJD has been reported to have been transmitted to mice by the injection of infected blood from human patients into mouse brain.[26]

Studies of experimental CJD in guinea pigs and mice have shown that the infectious agent is present in the blood before clinical disease develops.[27]

Sufficient evidence of animal transmission suggests that the disease has the potential to be transmitted through blood. Human epidemiological evidence only indicates that if blood transmission occurs, it is likely rare.[28]

Cases of CJD have been found among persons who have received blood transfusions, but the link between the disease and the transfusion has not been proven. Four Australians have been reported with CJD following transfusion. However, the source of the blood transfusions was undocumented.[29] There is a recent report in the western United States of three patients contracting CJD and dying after receiving a transfusion from a person who had CJD. This has not been confirmed.

Several cases of CJD following a blood component (albumin) transfusion have been reported. Two cases have been confirmed to have come from a person who died of CJD.[30]

The members of the Special Emphasis Panel on Creutzfeldt–Jakob disease, National Heart, Lung, and Blood Institute, have agreed that "an unqualified and irreducible risk of exposure to CJD through blood and blood products does exist...."[31]

Since there is no definitive direct evidence of infection from blood *transfusions*, there obviously can be no answer to whether or not CJD can be contracted by other blood *contact*. However, the absence of evidence is not evidence of the absence of transmission of CJD through blood.[32]

So there is as yet no definitive answer to the question, but the evidence would suggest that extreme caution in exposure to blood is warranted.

## IS IT AIRBORNE? CAN YOU GET CJD BY BREATHING IT?

The risk of infection from aerosols, droplets, and exposure to intact skin, gastric, and mucous membranes is not known.

Nevertheless, the National Institutes of Health strongly cautions laboratory workers to avoid the generation of aerosols and droplets during the manipulation of tissues or fluids known or suspected to be contaminated with CJD.[33]

## AND CJD IS HARD TO KILL?

Yes, the organism is not destroyed by formaldehyde, phenol, glutaraldehyde, alcohol, dry heat, boiling, hydrogen peroxide, ultraviolet radiation, or standard gravity sterilization.

The only effective sterilization technique is steam pressure sterilization (a process not commonly available to most funeral homes). However, even this method is not foolproof. In 2001, a major hospital in Denver reported the exposure of CJD to six patients who had undergone neurosurgery, as a result of the use of CJD contaminated surgical instruments *after* autoclaving. As a result, they have changed their procedure to include disposal of all surgical instruments used on a known or suspected CJD patient. Other medical centers are known to double autoclave these surgical instruments. Incineration is also effective but obviously destroys equipment along with the organism.

The use of sodium hypochlorite (household bleach) is often mentioned as a potential disinfectant, but its results are inconsistent. It is highly corrosive to metal instruments, gives off irritating fumes, and cannot be used as an embalming agent.[34] For maximum effectiveness, soaking for 2 hours is recommended. Wiping floors or countertops with bleach therefore would not produce this level of disinfection.

Sodium hydroxide (lye) is also mentioned as a disinfectant but has also shown inconsistent results and is also corrosive. In addition, it is a hazardous substance itself, which must be neutralized prior to disposal, thus raising OSHA and EPA concerns for handling and disposal. Finally, it deteriorates with age, so it loses whatever effectiveness it may have while in storage.[35]

Finally, it has been shown that the disease organism has long-term survivability. It is still viable and can be transmitted after an inactive period of a year or more.[36,37]

## EMBALMING CONSIDERATIONS

First of all, a basic review of some embalming fundamentals. Embalming is defined by the following three terms:
1. Disinfection
2. Preservation
3. Restoration

A person who dies from CJD will not present any particular challenges to preservation. The selection of embalming fluid, fluid strength, and fluid volume will be the same as a similar body deceased from any other cause.

Similarly, the appearance of the body will be no different than that of a similar body deceased from any other cause. No special restorative techniques will be necessary.

However, CJD is resistant to formaldehyde and every other embalming fluid component or disinfecting chemical, including glutaraldehyde, phenol, and alcohol. Nothing you can do with the body will render it disinfected.

Therefore, *by definition*, you cannot technically embalm a person who is deceased from CJD.[38]

You can produce tissue firmness and preservation. You can produce a pleasant cosmetic effect. But you have not really embalmed the body.

When you have completed the arterial injection, the disease organism is just as much alive as it was when you began.

## PERSONAL PROTECTION MEASURES

While there are no industry-specific standards of protection for mortuary staff when discussing CJD, we can emulate what is done in the medical field.

Most pathology departments have additional guidelines for handling patients deceased from CJD.

Typically, this includes wearing two or three pairs of disposable gloves (rubber or latex, never vinyl), protective eye covering and face shield, mask, cap, jumpsuit, waterproof apron, and shoe coverings. (Hospital guidelines go beyond what is normally considered "standard" universal precautions when dealing with CJD.)

Avoid causing aerosol distribution of contaminants. Avoid contact with all tissues and body fluids.

All solid waste should be placed in a leak-proof container and disposed of by incineration.

Instruments should be disinfected by autoclave or incinerated. They can also be containerized and disposed of as medical waste.

All surfaces should be wiped with sodium hypochlorite. Despite its shortcomings, the use of ordinary household bleach is recommended for general disinfective use in the embalming room and especially when dealing with CJD. Surfaces that may be contaminated should be wiped with a .5% solution (1:10 dilution) of bleach.[39,40]

Since the organism has also been isolated in several internal organs, aspiration of the body should not be attempted.[41] Minute pieces of the internal organs can be aspirated into the trocar, exposing the embalmer to the organism, and the trocar will remain contaminated after the process is completed.

Like other diseases, we are going to be exposed to CJD unknowingly. But when we know or suspect the presence of CJD, we can take steps to protect ourselves. We cannot totally eliminate the risk of exposure to any disease, but when we know it is present, special care is warranted.

Finally, you would be well advised to consult with local public health authorities before attempting preparation to see if special handling of the case is required. Most states and counties have regulations concerning the handling of infectious disease cases. Whether or not it is specifically named in the regulations, CJD is an infectious disease. There may be restrictions on shipping, public viewing, or other exposure to the general public.

## ADDITIONAL CONCERNS FOLLOWING AUTOPSY

The CJD organism is concentrated in the brain and the spinal column. While we might assume that exposure to the CJD organism is rather limited when handling the "normal" case, the embalmer is fully exposed to the organism when an autopsy has been performed, when death follows neurosurgery, or when death is due to head trauma.

The embalmer is well advised to request that the body be placed in a body pouch following autopsy to minimize contamination of the cot and removal vehicle or exposure of the removal personnel.

If restoration of the remains is attempted, all instruments, the embalming table, embalming room, and embalming room personnel are exposed to the organism, and there are no procedures available that will guarantee rendering the organism harmless. The organism can remain viable for over a year.

Limit the number of people who are exposed to the body by limiting admission to the preparation room during the preparation process. Exposure to others after the body has been repaired should also be limited. This would include other embalmers, hairdressers, cosmetologists, and so on.

## WHAT SHOULD BE THE FINAL DISPOSITION?

There have been no specific tests done to determine if the prion is destroyed during the cremation process. This has led some to speculate that the prion is some type of superbug that cannot be destroyed. Incineration has been shown to destroy the prion at 1000 degrees Fahrenheit. Therefore, it is reasonable to assume that cremation, which is also essentially incineration, also destroys the prion. Also, since the prion is normally destroyed during autoclaving, which is steam under pressure at 130+ degrees Celsius, we can safely assume that the 1660+ degree Fahrenheit crematory will also destroy it.

Likewise, there have been no specific tests as to what happens to the prion when it is buried. Since we know that the prion can live for a year under normal conditions, there is no reason to believe that it can survive any longer than that underground. Assuming that the body remains intact inside the casket or casket and vault for at least a year, the interred body should pose no threat to the environment or underground water sources.

## SHOULD PREPARATION BE ATTEMPTED?

Knowing what we know about CJD (and probably more importantly, what we *do not* know), the question as following must be asked:

Should an embalmer attempt to embalm a body with CJD?

Some funeral directors who have been called on to serve a family where CJD is the cause of death have had this question answered for them. The family physician has already told the family that they cannot expect to have the body embalmed, have a public viewing, or a funeral. Some families have been told that the body should be cremated immediately upon death.

There is no reason for a family to feel obligated to choose cremation. By use of a body pouch and/or a sealing-type casket, there is no reason why an unprepared body with CJD cannot have a public funeral and an earth burial.

While we may not agree with the conclusion reached by the physician, we should at least note the seriousness he attaches to this disease.

We must also note, however, that misinformation within the medical community has also led some physicians to tell families that the disease cannot be easily transmitted and there should be no concerns on the part of the funeral home. Even the medical community has a long way to go in educating its members about CJD.

Whether or not an embalmer agrees to prepare the body is a personal decision that should be weighed carefully.

It is quite different from the questions we faced years ago when AIDS was first identified. Even though we did not know much about AIDS initially, we had an effective embalming technique and the chemicals available to render it harmless if we were careful in our procedures.

While the Americans with Disabilities Act (The ADA) has made AIDS a disability and requires embalmers to embalm AIDS cases or risk civil liability, the refusal to attempt to do what is impossible is an entirely different matter.

Since neither the Department of Justice nor the courts have ruled on the issue of handling CJD, a funeral home refusing to attempt preparation may indeed have to defend their decision if an ADA enforcement action is brought against it.

The case will hinge on whether this risk of CJD can be eliminated by "reasonable modifications" to the embalming process.[42]

Since no embalming fluid exists that will render the prion harmless, it would be argued that there is no "reasonable modification" to be made.

The threat of defending oneself from an ADA complaint must be weighed against the personal health risks involved.

The other difference that we can note between the history of AIDS and the history of CJD is that within months of its discovery, we knew a lot about AIDS, what it was, how it was transmitted, and so on. CJD was identified over 70 years ago and still we know very little about it.

With CJD, the question of preparation can only be answered after carefully considering the facts and weighing the consequences.

- We are being confronted with a 100% fatal disease.
- There is no cure; there is no treatment. There is no vaccine.

- The mode of transmission of this disease in humans is largely unknown.[43]
- There is no effective embalming treatment.
- There is no effective disinfecting technique for instruments, equipment, or the preparation room itself.
- The organism can survive and remain viable for over a year, possibly infecting others during that time.
- You may become infected with this disease and not know it for decades.

It would appear that CJD is not a vicious, rampant, killer organism intent on wiping the human race from the face of the planet. The numbers indicate something far less than a worldwide epidemic, to say the least. There is no need for panic or hysteria. We are not facing Black plague or Ebola.

However, it is a fatal illness and we cannot take that lightly. And it is not a disease we can do much with, either by way of protective measures or by embalming technique.

Universal precautions coupled with cautious, deliberate work practices, and a dose of plain common sense will do much to reduce the exposure risk.

But the risk cannot be eliminated and the full extent of that risk is unknown. Is it worth it?

How much risk are you willing to take?

If you determine that the risk of infection is minimal in the "normal" case and attempt preparation, do you still refuse to attempt preparation of the autopsied case where the highly infectious brain, spinal column, and cerebrospinal fluid are exposed?

Should you refuse to attempt preparation when there is no concrete evidence that you can be infected with CJD in the preparation process? What happens if it is proven that there is no risk of CJD infection from a dead human body? What happens if it is proven that infection *is* possible?

If you refuse to prepare the body, will the family choose another funeral home? What effect could this refusal have on your reputation of service within the community? What liability might a funeral home face if they refuse to attempt preparation?

What liability might your funeral home face if it is shown that an employee contracted CJD from a body that they prepared in your funeral home?

What moral obligation do you have to protect your employees versus your moral obligation to serve the public?

Although not specifically addressed by OSHA, the "General Duty Clause" of the Blood-borne Pathogen Standard would require the employer to protect employees from a known hazard. Since CJD is certainly a known hazard, employers would be required to protect their employees from this hazard.

It would appear that CJD would require steps beyond that of "universal precautions" and indeed the question is—can the employer adequately protect their employees from CJD if preparation is attempted?

Some surgeons have refused to operate on a person known to be infected with CJD. Some pathologists have refused to perform an autopsy on a deceased patient who is known or suspected to harbor the CJD organism. Can you base your own decision on theirs?

Indeed knowledgeable authorities within the medical community flatly advise against embalming, including the National CJD Surveillance Unit in the United Kingdom.[44]

Can you justify embalming a CJD case for what you charge knowing that equipment may have to be destroyed after use and additional precautions must be taken? (Which might illustrate the fact that embalming *any* case is worth a lot more than what you might presently charge?)

These are questions that funeral home staff members should discuss before accepting a person deceased from CJD or suspected CJD.

The embalmer deserves to be fully informed about CJD before they make that decision. That decision should be respected and there should be no thought that there is a shirking of "professional responsibility" by electing not to attempt preparation.

## CONCLUSIONS

Ideally, there would be definitive answers. Unfortunately, science has not yet provided them.

Ideally, we would have all of the answers. Unfortunately, such is not the case. We simply do not have definitive answers to many of our questions.

Even knowledgeable people within funeral service have honest points of disagreement. Some see little risk, at least in the nonautopsied case. Some flatly refuse to touch a CJD case, autopsied or not.

Add to that the complications of OSHA obligations to protect employees and ADA requirements to provide services as a "public accommodation" and we can see that the situation becomes even more complicated.

Too many in funeral service know nothing at all about CJD. Too many have never even heard of it.

Some will attempt embalming only because that is what embalmers do. Anything less might appear cowardly, especially when the foe is unseen.

That means that too many are going to be exposed to CJD without ever having considered the long-term effects of their decision to handle or not handle a CJD case.

While we may not have definitive answers, what we do have are cautions.

What we do have are warnings.

Someday we should have more.

Someday this report will be outdated.

Until then . . .

## PROCEDURAL GUIDELINES FOR MORTUARY CARE OF CRUETZFELDT–JAKOB DISEASE

. . . And that is where the original manuscript ended in 1998.

Since that time, we really have not learned that much more about CJD, but as more and more embalmers become aware of it and the potential danger it presents, it becomes obvious that we as a profession need some guidelines or protocols on the handling of a known or suspected case of CJD.

What follows then is what we hope is a reasonable set of procedural guidelines for the embalmer based on what we know today.

Before using them, read the entire article on CJD so that you better understand the disease and its risks to you and other employees. You also need to know the legal and business risks of not preparing the body. We recommend that you read the other material available listed in Appendix A to make a fully informed decision.

> **NOTICE AND DISCLAIMER**
> These CJD preparation guidelines are based on the knowledge available to the industry at the date of writing. These procedures may become outdated based on more current information. The embalmer must keep apprised of the latest information available.
>
> The procedures outlined are, in the professional opinion of the author, a reasonable response to the potential risks posed by CJD. The individual funeral home owner and embalmer must make their own independent decisions based on the risks presented by preparing or not preparing a person with known or suspected CJD and be responsible for them.
>
> The decision then to proceed or not to proceed is purely the decision of the funeral home and/or the individual embalmer. The author cannot be held responsible for the consequences or results of either decision.

The **"exposure level"** rating of 1 (low) to 5 (high) indicates the level of potential exposure to the prion. Basically, no exposure to blood or cerebrospinal fluid creates a negligible or very low potential exposure level. Exposure to blood or certain other body fluids produces a medium potential exposure level, since the causative agent for CJD is found in the blood, although in small amounts. Exposure to the brain and/or cerebrospinal fluid produces a high potential exposure level because these (and to a lesser degree, other internal organs) are the primary reservoirs for the prion.

It does not in any way imply a risk of developing CJD, because the chances of contracting the disease from exposure to blood, body fluids, brain, and spinal fluid, and so on are not known, but are admittedly low.

It simply makes sense, however, that the lower the exposure to the prion, the lower the chances of contracting CJD. But even maximum exposure to the prion is no indicator that a person will eventually contract CJD.

The term **"intact"** as used here is defined as a body that has not been autopsied, has no brain or spinal column injury, and does not display any excessive blood or body fluid leakage.

Since we maintain that a person deceased with CJD cannot technically be "embalmed" (since the body cannot be disinfected, which defines embalming) we will use the words "prepare" or "inject" to refer to the procedures that on any other body would be considered "embalming."

**"Universal Precautions"** refers to an approach to infection control that considers all deceased human bodies to be infectious and must be handled as such. OSHA regulations require that universal precautions be practiced. This requires the proper use of **personal protective clothing and equipment (PPE)**. In the case of a CJD case, universal precautions must also take into consideration the possibility that the deceased could have other diseases of concern to the embalmer. Therefore, recommendations concerning universal precautions will be based on other diseases also and indeed should be utilized on every case regardless of any assumed cause of death. For instance, we recommend the use of face masks not because CJD is an airborne disease (there is no evidence to suggest that) but because TB is an airborne disease and the principle of universal precautions says we assume the person may have this and other diseases also and we must protect ourselves accordingly.

### CJD GUIDELINES

**TASK:**
Removal of remains

**BODY CONDITION:**
Intact

**EXPOSURE LEVEL:**
0–1 (Negligible/very low)

**RECOMMENDATION:**
The body can be removed and transported with little if any risk to mortuary personnel.

**UNIVERSAL PRECAUTIONS/PRERECOMMENDED:**
Minimum: Gloves
   Face mask or barrier cloth over face of the deceased.
   Additional protective clothing and equipment as indicated.

**PROCEDURE:**
Follow basic sanitary procedures that should be utilized on any removal.
   Cover the cot surface with a protective plastic such as a casket cover.
   Transfer remains to cot. Wrap body completely in protective plastic to eliminate contact with the cot.
   Place used gloves and other PPE in sealed plastic bag for later disposal.
   Wash hands with disinfectant soap. Transport.
   If the body exhibits any bleeding, open wounds, or other leakage, a body pouch is recommended.
   Leave body wrapped until disposition is determined.
   Disinfect cot with Clorox.

### CJD GUIDELINES

**TASK:**
Removal of remains

**BODY CONDITION:**
Nonintact (autopsied)

**EXPOSURE LEVEL:**
2 (low) if body is pouched to 4 (high) if mortuary personnel must directly handle remains.

**RECOMMENDATION:**
The body can be removed and transported, but extra precautions are warranted.

**UNIVERSAL PRECAUTIONS/PRE-RECOMMENDED:**
Minimum: Gloves
Face mask or barrier cloth over face of the deceased.
Additional protective clothing and equipment as indicated.

**PROCEDURE:**
The hospital or autopsy facility should be asked to place the remains in a body pouch taking care not to contaminate the outside of the pouch. The removal personnel should monitor this task to observe any contamination of the outside of the pouch.
Hospital or autopsy facility should retain all organs removed, especially the brain.
This pouch should then be placed in an outer pouch to further insure no contamination of the cot.
Place used gloves and other PPE in sealed plastic bag for later disposal.
Wash hands with disinfectant soap. Transport.
Leave body pouched until disposition is determined. Disinfect cot with Clorox.

### CJD GUIDELINES

**TASK:**
Preparation (injection) of remains

**BODY CONDITION:**
Intact

**EXPOSURE LEVEL:**
3 (Medium)

**RECOMMENDATION:**
We recommend the body not be prepared by arterial injection.

**UNIVERSAL PRECAUTIONS/PRE-RECOMMENDED:**
Minimum: Gloves, gown, face mask/eye shield, head, and shoe covers.

**PROCEDURE:** (If injection is attempted)
Restrict embalming room access to necessary personnel only.
Follow preparation procedures as indicated by body condition.
Fluid strength, quantity, and dilution will be determined by overall condition of the body, because this will have no effect on the CJD prion.
Use drain hose to sewer system to minimize exposure to blood.
Minimize the number of instruments used. Do not aspirate body.
Containerize and dispose of all instruments, tubes, hoses, needles, and so on.
Place all gloves and other PPE in sealed plastic bag for disposal.
Clean table and other embalming room surfaces with Clorox.
Wash hands with disinfectant soap.

*NOTE: There are no practical procedures available to ensure destruction of the prion once it has contaminated the preparation room.*

### CJD GUIDELINES

**TASK:**
Preparation (injection) of remains using "no drainage" method*

**BODY CONDITION:**
Intact

**EXPOSURE LEVEL:**
2 (Low)

**RECOMMENDATION:**
We recommend the body not be prepared by arterial injection. This method reduces the level of exposure if injection is attempted.

**UNIVERSAL PRECAUTIONS/PRE-RECOMMENDED:**
Minimum: Gloves, gown, face mask/eye shield, and shoe covers.

**PROCEDURE:** (If injection is attempted)
Restrict embalming room access to essential personnel only.
Inject body with no drainage.*
Do not aspirate body.
Minimize the number of instruments used. Containerize and dispose of all instruments,
tubes, needles, and so on.
Clean table and other embalming room surfaces with Clorox.
Place all gloves and other PPE in sealed plastic bag for disposal.

*NOTE: There are no practical procedures available to ensure destruction of the prion once it has contaminated the preparation room.*

### CJD GUIDELINES

**TASK:**
Preparation of remains

**BODY CONDITION:**
Nonintact (autopsied)

**EXPOSURE LEVEL:**
5 (Full exposure to the causative agent)

**RECOMMENDATION:**
Preparation and/or restoration of the body should not be attempted and is strongly discouraged.

---

*See Appendix B for "nodrainage" injection method.

**UNIVERSAL PRECAUTIONS/PRERECOMMENDED:**
Minimum: Gloves, gown, face mask/eye shield, and shoe covers.

**PROCEDURE:** (If injection is attempted)

Restrict embalming room access to essential personnel only.

Minimize the number of instruments used.

Follow preparation procedures as indicated by body condition.

Fluid strength, quantity, and dilution will be determined by overall condition of the body, because this will have no effect on the CJD prion.

Use extreme care in not contaminating embalming room with blood.

Containerize and dispose of all instruments, tubes, needles, and so on.

Clean table and other embalming room surfaces with Clorox.

Place all gloves and other PPE in sealed plastic bag for disposal. Wash hands with disinfectant soap.

*NOTE: There are no practical procedures available to ensure destruction of the prion once it has contaminated the preparation room.*

## CJD GUIDELINES

**DISPOSITION AND OTHER HANDLING:**

**Refrigeration**—Body should remain wrapped in plastic or body pouch while under refrigeration.

**Viewing**—Viewing the unembalmed intact remains does not present a particular hazard beyond that of any other disease.

Utilizing universal precautions, body can be sanitized (body surfaces) and features can be set.

To avoid unnecessary manipulation of the body and exposure to body fluids, body should remain wrapped in plastic and clothing should be draped over remains after casketing or placement on viewing table.

This may be an acceptable alternative for the family that desires a viewing.

If viewing is requested after cranial restoration, exposure to the prion is present, especially in the hair. A hairdresser would be exposed, if the hair is to be done before viewing as would those who touch the body during viewing. Since the risks here are unknown, we strongly caution the funeral home against restoration or viewing of autopsied remains.

**Cremation**—Body should already be wrapped in plastic or placed in a body pouch. Body should also be in a rigid alternative cremation container or casket. With no direct contact with the body, no special precautions are required by crematory personnel.

While there have been no specific studies to definitively determine that the CJD prion is destroyed during the cremation process, it is normally destroyed by routine autoclave procedures (>130 degrees Celsius for 15 minutes), which is done at a much lower temperature. Indeed the preheating of the retort alone is likely to be sufficient to destroy the prion.

Incineration at a temperature of 1000 degrees Fahrenheit is considered effective against the CJD prion.

Therefore, we can safely assume that the prion is destroyed during the cremation process (1600+ degrees Fahrenheit) and the handling of the cremated remains (ashes) poses no threat to crematory personnel.

**Entombment**—Body should already be placed in a body pouch. Using appropriate universal precautions, body should be treated with external embalming powder to minimize odors. Body should be placed in an inner sealer case or sealer-type casket. (Note: Mausoleum regulations may require embalming or have regulations concerning communicable diseases. Check mausoleum requirements before assuring family that entombment will be allowed.)

Since the CJD prion can survive under normal conditions for up to a year, we assume that it will also survive for that long within the mausoleum. Assuming that the casket remains intact for at least a year, it should present no further health hazard if later removed. Even then, the casket should not be opened for any reason.

**Burial**—Body should already be wrapped in plastic or be in a body pouch before casketing. Body should be placed in an inner sealer case or sealer-type casket.

Since the CJD prion can survive under normal conditions for up to a year, we assume that it will also survive for that long underground. To assure that the casket remains intact for at least a year, a vault or graveline should also be used.

**Disinterment**—Since the CJD prion can survive under normal conditions for up to a year, we assume that it will also survive for that long underground or in a mausoleum. We recommend that no disinterment be made for at least the first year following interment. Even prior to that time, if the casket is intact and sealed, the body should not present any appreciable risk. Even then, the casket and/or vault should not be reopened during the disinterment and reinterment.

**Disposal of liquid waste (drainage)**—If injection with drainage is attempted, it presents the additional problem of what to do with the drainage. Since formaldehyde has no effect on the prion, normal disposal into the sewer system means introducing an unknown quantity of the prion into the sewer system.

As an alternative, some have proposed treating the drainage with a chemical known to have some effectiveness against the prion, such as sodium hydroxide (lye) or sodium hypochlorite (bleach).

This presents further complications however.

Formaldehyde, which would also be in the drainage, should never be mixed with bleach.

Lye mixed with water produces heat and presents its own handling and disposal hazards.

Any attempts at treating the drainage further expose the embalmer to the prion as well as additional chemical hazards.

Therefore, although it may not seem to be an adequate solution, the most logical answer is to dispose of the drainage directly into the sewer system with a minimum of exposure to the embalmer.

This situation alone should be further justification for not attempting arterial injection of the body.

**Disposal of solid waste (PPE, etc.)**—All solid waste including gloves, gowns, and sheets that have been used or that may have come into contact with the CJD case should be sealed in plastic and disposed of as hazardous waste.

**Treatment of instruments**—Disposable instruments should be used and also disposed of as hazardous waste or sharps. Nondisposable instruments should likewise be disposed of and not reused. Since the CJD prion has been shown to survive autoclaving if not done at proper temperature (and since most funeral homes do not have access to an autoclave), attempts at sterilization are not recommended.

# Appendix A
## Additional Recommended Reading

"A CJD Primer"
    James F. Burnside, CFSP
    Curtis D. Rostad, CFSP
    Kurt Soffe, CFSP
    *The Director*, July 2000

"ADA vs. CJD"
    T. Scott Gilligan, Esq.
    *The Director*, August 2000

"CJD and OSHA"
    Edward M. Ranier, Esq.
    *The Director*, September 2000

"CJD and the Environment"
    Carol Green, Esq.
    *The Director*, April 2001

"Should Funeral Homes Embalm CJD Cases"
    James F. Burnside, CFSP
    *The Director*, May 2001

# Appendix B

## "No Drainage" Injection Method

While injection of a known or suspected CJD case is not recommended, the exposure level can be greatly reduced if injection of the intact body is done with no drainage.

With this method, exposure is limited to incidental leakage at the injection site.

Restrict embalming room access to essential personnel only.

Minimize the number of instruments used.

Use universal precautions as with all embalming procedures, that is, gloves, gown, face mask and eye shield, and head and shoe covers.

Prepare remains for injection like any other case, that is, position body, wash remains, set features, and so on.

Cover table with disposable plastic sheet or place small disposal emesis basin under incision site to catch incidental leakage and avoid contamination of table.

Soak up any incidental leakage and dispose of towel or cotton in sealed plastic bag.

INJECTION POINT: Single injection point of the embalmer's preference. Carotid injection is recommended to eliminate need to reverse tube to inject lower leg and ease in controlling incidental leakage.

FLUID: Standard arterial fluid chosen based on overall condition of body.

CONCENTRATED FLUID: Same as would be used if this were a normal injection based on overall body condition.

DILUTED FLUID SOLUTION: No more than 2 gallons total. A "normal" body can easily retain this amount of fluid in the arterial/venous system without swelling. For a small or emaciated case, this amount may be reduced to 1–1.5 gallons. Mix total amount of concentrated fluid to be used to make this amount of solution.

That is, if you would normally use 16 oz of arterial to 2 gallons of fluid to embalm this body and then use another 16 oz in a final 2 gallon injection—in this case, you would mix the entire 32 oz of fluid into 2 gallons (or less) of diluted solution.

PRESSURE: Use same injection pressure as if this were a normal injection based on overall body condition.

RATE OF FLOW: Use minimum rate of flow. This is the secret to success. Monitor body closely for signs of swelling. If distention or swelling occurs, it is because of too high a rate of flow, not too much pressure or too much fluid.

Note that some older machines are incapable of operating at a rate of flow low enough to prevent distention or swelling.

Do not aspirate body. If abdominal gases must be relieved, use a large bore needle into the intestinal spaces taking care not to produce leakage or puncture of internal organs that may house the prion.

Containerize and dispose of all instruments, tubes, needles, and so on.

Clean table and other embalming room surfaces with Clorox.

Place all gloves and other PPE in sealed plastic bag for disposal.

Wash hands with disinfectant soap.

### ABOUT THE AUTHOR

Curtis D. Rostad, CFSP, is a licensed funeral director and embalmer with over 30 years experience as an employee, manager, funeral home owner, and consultant.

He also serves as executive director of the Wyoming Funeral Directors Association, a position he has held since 1987, and served as the executive director of the Colorado Funeral Directors Association from 1988 to 1992. He is a member of the American Society of Association Executives (ASAE), the Colorado Society of Association Executives (CSAE), and the Council of Funeral Association Executives.

He has an extensive background in forensics and death investigation with 7 years of serving as a county coroner. He is a member of the American College of Forensic Examiners and is a Board Certified Forensic Examiner with a specialty in death investigation through the American Board of Forensic Examiners.

Curtis D. Rostad, CFSP
6138 Trailhead Rd.
Highlands Ranch, CO 80130
1 (303) 471-6072
email crostad@aol.com

---

**Hepatitis from A to G**[*]

*Kim Collison*

---

Viral hepatitis is a worldwide health problem. It is estimated that 300 million people throughout the world carry the hepatitis B virus, whereas over 4 million Americans have hepatitis C. Considering the frequency of contact with blood and body fluids when working in funeral service, it is important to understand how the hepatitis viruses are transmitted and what precautions you need to follow to protect yourself.

Hepatitis is defined as an inflammation of the liver that can damage this organ and even cause death. While there are several etiologic agents that may be responsible for liver inflammation, the term "hepatitis" is most commonly associated with

---

[*]Reprinted with permission from *The Dodge Magazine*, Jan.–Feb., Vol. 91, No. 1, 1999. Copyright: The Dodge Company.

several distinct viruses. Hepatitis has been documented for centuries including accounts of human hepatitis appearing in Babylonian texts and Hippocrates' works. However, it has only been in the last 40 years that the hepatitis viruses have been discovered and identified. The signs and symptoms of all types of hepatitis are similar, so blood tests are necessary to determine which of the nine known viruses is causing the disease.

Viral hepatitis can be separated into two basic groups based on their mode of transmission. Hepatitis A and E are transmitted via the fecal–oral route, while hepatitis B, C, D, G, and GBV are blood-borne. The blood-borne viruses are spread whenever there is the possibility of the exchange of blood or body fluids.

## HEPATITIS A

Hepatitis A, formerly called infectious hepatitis, is caused by the enterically transmitted hepatitis A virus. The Centers for Disease Control and Prevention (CDC) estimate that over 140,000 cases of acute hepatitis A occur in the United States each year, accounting for approximately 80 deaths. Worldwide, the incidence of hepatitis A (HAV) infection exceeds 1.5 million cases. HAV is especially common in parts of Asia, Africa, South America, and Mexico. HAV enters the body through the digestive system, when one eats food or drinks water that has been contaminated with fecal material. Hepatitis A can also be spread via fresh fruits, salads, or vegetables washed in contaminated water.

The virus can be transmitted between family members, within institutions, by food handlers, and through sexual contact. An HAV positive person can spread the disease even if he or she has no symptoms. Hepatitis A generally produces a mild infection that lasts 6–10 weeks. Children and young adults account for 50–60% of the reported cases of HAV. Once you have the infection, you develop a natural immunity, so you never become infected again. Being vaccinated or just following good hand washing practices will protect you from acquiring hepatitis A in the prep room.

## HEPATITIS E

In 1990, the virus that is responsible for enterically transmitted non-A, non-B hepatitis was discovered. Hepatitis E (HEV) is prevalent in Asia, Africa, and the Middle East and has caused epidemics in Mexico. Like hepatitis A, hepatitis E is transmitted in water contaminated with infectious human waste. HEV generally produces a mild infection with an overall fatality rate of 1–3%. However, this disease does pose a serious risk to pregnant women, causing a fatality rate of 15–25%. There is not a blood test available for diagnosing hepatitis E, and researchers are currently testing a possible vaccine. Because there is the potential for contamination with fecal material in the prep room, strict adherence to universal precautions should protect you from both hepatitis A and E.

## HEPATITIS D

Hepatitis D, or delta hepatitis, is a blood-borne virus that only exists in combination with the hepatitis B virus. The prevalence of hepatitis D in the United States is low, except in IV drug users and multiple transfused individuals. The coinfection of hepatitis B and D results in a severe disease state and often results in severe chronic liver disease. There is no vaccine available for hepatitis D. However, because it can only exist with hepatitis B, the hepatitis vaccine will therefore offer protection against hepatitis D.

## HEPATITIS G

Hepatitis G virus (HGV) is spread in the same manner as other conventional blood-borne viruses. The risk factors for HGV are similar to those of hepatits B and C—namely, IV drug use, multiple blood transfusions, and accidental sharps injuries. Chronic infection develops in 90–100% of individuals infected with HGV.

## HEPATITIS GBV

In June 1995, hepatitis GBV was discovered. It also appears to be transmissible through contaminated blood and body fluids. Extensive hepatitis research is still necessary, since approximately 20% of cases of acute and chronic hepatitis cannot be attributed to any of the known viruses.

## HEPATITIS C

Most hepatitis cases that were once referred to as blood-borne non-A, non-B are now known to be due to the hepatitis C virus (HCV). The recent identification of HCV and the development of screening tests for it have brought to light the enormity of the worldwide health problem. According to the American Liver Foundation, over 4 million people in the United States have chronic hepatitis C. In addition, each year an estimated 150,000 people are infected with HCV, and about 10,000 die of hepatitis C. The CDC now predicts that over the next 10 years, the hepatitis C death toll will triple. Hepatitis C has been responsible for most cases of transfusion-related hepatitis. However, since 1989, blood products have been screened for hepatitis C, and no longer pose a risk. Today, one of the leading causes for liver transplantation is the presence of cirrhosis and/or liver cancer due to hepatitis C.

Hepatitis C is transmitted in many of the same ways as hepatitis B, and therefore, they share many of the same risk factors. Essentially any activity that results in the transfer of contaminated blood or body fluids can result in the transmission of HCV. Common risk factors are IV drug use, chronic hemodialysis, accidental sharps injuries, tattooing, body piercing, being the offspring of HCV-positive mothers, and intranasal cocaine use. Studies show that the incidence of household (nonsexual) transmission of HCV range from 0% to 11%. They also estimate that the risk of hepatitis C transmission from a single needlestick involving HCV-positive blood is 3–10%.

An average of 6- to 7-week incubation period follows infection with the hepatitis C virus. The early stage of HCV infection is termed acute hepatitis, and it may be mild or severe. Unlike the illness that occurs following infection with hepatitis A or B, many people with HCV will initially suffer flulike symptoms, while the virus quietly damages the liver. According to recent studies, up to 80% of people with acute hepatitis will develop chronic hepatitis—that is, hepatitis that continues beyond a

6-month period—and they may remain infected for several years or life. Up to 25% of these patients will progress to hepatic cirrhosis. Also, hepatitis C is a known predisposing factor in the development of liver cancer.

In 1992, the FDA approved the use of interferon-alpha 2b for treating selected cases of chronic hepatitis C. Although studies have shown that this treatment can lead to significant improvement in liver function tests, it has some major drawbacks. First of all, it is expensive and has numerous side effects. Also, fewer than half of HCV-infected individuals respond to treatment, and most trials report at least a 50% relapse rate within 6 months of completing therapy. In October 1997, the FDA approved the use of Infergen, a biologically engineered version of interferon. Unfortunately, Infergen is about as effective as interferon against the hepatitis C virus.

Any accidental sharps injury or mucous membrane exposure to blood or body fluids in the prep room should be immediately documented and reported. Because postexposure testing of the source will be difficult, you should assume the source is positive for HCV. You should have a blood test to check for anti-HCV immediately following the exposure and you should be tested again for anti-HCV and for the liver enzyme ALT. There is no established postexposure prophylaxis for hepatitis C.

## HEPATITIS B

It is estimated that 300 million people throughout the world carry the hepatitis B virus (HBV). In China, Southeast Asia, and Africa, up to 12% of the population carries the hepatitis B virus. In this country, approximately 200,000–300,000 people become infected with HBV each year. On the basis of estimates from the CDC, there are approximately 1.25 million chronic carriers, or people with ongoing hepatitis B infection, in the United States alone. Of these people, nearly 5000 die from cirrhosis or liver cancer each year. The CDC reports that almost 12,000 health care workers become infected with HBV each year, with about 200 dying from the disease.

The hepatitis B virus can be found in blood, saliva, semen, vaginal secretions, cerebrospinal fluid, peritoneal fluid, pericardial fluid, and basically any other body fluid contaminated with blood. Blood is the single most important source of hepatitis B and other blood-borne pathogens in the occupational setting. Often overshadowed by the fear of AIDS, hepatitis B is a greater threat in terms of infection, sickness, and death—mainly because it is a much hardier virus.

The hepatitis B virus is passed either directly from an infected individual by contact with his or her body fluid or indirectly, by contact with dried blood or body fluids on clothing or other surfaces. HBV is acquired through the skin by way of cuts, scrapes, hangnails, or needle sharing. Other means are by tattooing, by ear or body piercing, or by sharing razors, pierced earrings, toothbrushes, or nail clippers. It is also acquired through the mucous membranes such as the eyes, nose, or mouth by exposure to infected blood or body fluids, through sexual contact, and through contact between an infected mother and her newborn child. Also, hemophiliacs are a high-risk group due to their need for numerous blood products, many of which were not screened for HBV before 1975.

Needlesticks continue to be the main source of occupational exposure. More than 800,000 needlesticks and sharps injuries are reported each year, although the number of actual injuries is believed to be much higher. Because there can be 500 million hepatitis B viral particles in 1 cc of carrier's blood, the risk of acquiring HBV from a needlestick ranges from 6% to 30%. After an exposure and an incubation period of 60–180 days, symptoms such as fatigue, enlarged liver, and jaundice will appear. The short-term consequences of an HBV infection include an average 8–12 weeks off work and risk of permanent liver damage. Long-term effects include chronic active hepatitis, cirrhosis, liver cancer, and death.

The best methods for protection against HBV are strict adherence to universal precautions and the hepatitis B vaccine. The first hepatitis B vaccine was derived from human plasma and became available in 1982. In 1986, a genetically engineered vaccine was licensed by the FCA. When given in the deltoid muscle, the hepatitis B vaccine produces protective antibody in more than 90% of healthy individuals. A blood test to check for the development of protective antibodies can be done 1–6 months after completing the three-injection vaccine series. Currently, there are different theories regarding the need for booster doses and how to treat those individuals who fail to produce protective antibodies following the vaccination series.

Should an exposure occur in the prep room, testing and treatment should be initiated within 72 hours. The exposure source should be assumed to be positive. You will require blood tests and should also receive one dose of hepatitis B immune globulin and one dose of the hepatitis B vaccine. Follow-up testing is generally done 6 months postexposure.

Hepatitis is a worldwide health problem and a major occupational hazard in funeral service. It is important that you understand how these different viruses are transmitted, because you are most likely embalming undiagnosed hepatitis positive remains. Your best protection against hepatitis B is the hepatitis B vaccine. Your best protection against all forms of hepatitis is following universal precautions.

## BIBLIOGRAPHY

Department of Labor, Occupational Safety and Health Administration, 29CFR Part 1920.1030, Occupational exposure to bloodborne pathogens, final rule. *Federal Register.* 1991;56:64004–64182.

Hepatitis C: Improved Options Available for Diagnosis and Treatment. *Mayo Clinic Update* 1993;9:7–8.

Kuhns MC. Viral hepatitis. *Laboratory Medicine* 1995;26:650–659.

Larsen JT, Larsen HS. Viral hepatitis: An overview. *Clinical Laboratory Science* 1995;8:169–173.

Mordechai E, Belmont M. The pivotal role of serum hepatitis C viral load in disease progression. *Advance for Medical Laboratory Professionals* 1998;10:17–19.

Pallatroni L. Needlesticks: Who pays the price when the costs are cut on safety? *Medical Laboratory Observer* 1998;30–36, 88–91.

Protection Against Viral Hepatitis: Recommendations of the Immunization Practices Advisory Committee. *MMWR* 1990;39:1–23.

Shute N. Hepatitis C: A silent killer. *U.S. New and World Report,* June 22, 1998;60–66.

Witthaus D. New federal guidelines for HCV lookback. *Medical Laboratory Observer.* September 1998;22–26.

Zuckerman AJ. The new GB hepatitis virus. *Lancet* 1995;345:1453–1454.

> **The Increase in MRSA and VRE***
> *Mike Cloud, Jr.*

## ABOUT THE AUTHOR

Mike Cloud is a licensed embalmer and funeral director from Newnan, GA. He has been an OSHA coordinator for 4 years. Mike graduated with honors from Gupton-Jones, and is a member of the Academy of Graduate Embalmers of Georgia.

Let us take a few moments to explain the pathogens of MRSA, VRE, and VRSA. Then, I will make some recommendations as to the disinfection and preparation of a deceased body with these conditions.

*S. aureus* (also referred to as Staph aureus and abbreviated *S. aureus*) is one of the most common causes of nosocomial (hospital-acquired) and community-acquired infections worldwide. In 1992, the 19,000 deaths directly caused by nosocomial infections made them the 11th leading cause of death in the US population.[1] In 1998, Dr. William Jarvis of the CDC stated, "We estimate that today two million patients develop a hospital-acquired infection in the United States each year. Of that number, 90,000 die as a result of those infections."[2]

These Staph pathogens are mutating so as to become resistant to a series of drugs, including penicillin and methicillin. Until recently, doctors were treating *S. aureus* with methicillin. Some of these Staph organisms have become resistant to methicillin (and so are called methicillin-resistant *Staphylococcus aureus* or MRSA). The antibiotic vancomycin is effective against MRSA pathogens, but is considered a last ditch defense. As time passes, these pathogens may become resistant not only to a single type of antibiotic but even perhaps to two or more antibiotics in combination. The initials MRSA can also be an acronym for a similar but different set of words: multiple-resistant Staph aureus.

Of course, each of you can see that these Staph aureus pathogens that are methicillin resistant could become VRSA (vancomycin-resistant Staph aureus). Sad to say, that has happened. At the beginning of 1999, the third reported case of VRSA killed a middle-aged Hong Kong woman. Many people naturally carry the Staph aureus organism as part of their normal flora with no sign of illness. These people are said to be colonized with the bacteria.

The growth of VRE, MRSA, and VRSA may be attributed to more invasive procedures, using breathing tubes and intravenous catheters, for example. *The Surgical Infection Society Position of Vancomycin-Resistant Enterococcus* (October, 1996), a publication of the American Medical Association, stated, "Presumably much of this spread occurs as a result of carriage of enterococci on the hands of health care workers and through interhospital transfers of patients colonized with these enterococci." Later in their report, they note, "This problem is growing rapidly; the incidence of VRE infections has increased 20fold in the United States between 1989 and 1993, and 34fold in intensive care units."[3]

Even at the removal site, one should use universal precautions. We should not guess whether the deceased has VRE, MRSA, or even HIV. Remember, if we are to err, let us err on the side of caution. All bodies should be treated as if they are contagious. Rectal swabs were taken from 30 patients known to be harboring VRE. All were tested, but only 14 showed positive for the disease. Even our best tests are imperfect. Of secondary but real concern should be the professional image we convey to the family and others who see us in the performance of our work. Certainly we cannot allow ourselves to become passive carriers who might infect others because of our lack of appropriate procedures.

After the body has been transferred to the cot, hand washing and disinfection are imperative. The paper by the AMA that I have been quoting stated, "The CDC has since published guidelines establishing hand washing as the most important procedure for preventing nosocomial infections." The publication further states, "The institution of universal precautions to protect health care workers from human immunodeficiency virus and other virus, by promoting the use of gloves, may have given workers a false sense of security, with neglect of hand washing."[3]

Upon returning to the preparation room, we should spray a topical disinfectant such as Dis-Spray over the entire sheet covering the deceased before transferring the body from the cot to the embalming table or before removing the sheet. Fold the sheet back from the face while liberally spraying the face with topical disinfectant. Remember that Staph aureus is part of the normal flora of the nasal tract and even the mouth. Therefore, I recommend the use of a swab saturated with Dis-Spray along the walls and the opening of the oral and nasal cavities. Continue to topically disinfect the surface of the body before positioning on the table.

Once the body is on the embalming table, spray the remaining linen on the cot before placing it in the linen disposal. Next, liberally spray the cot and pillow. I have noticed that many times we fail to completely disinfect the cot. One must be mindful to allow the disinfectant to remain on the area long enough to do its job.

Continue with the arterial embalming procedure as usual. During aspiration and cavity fluid injection, I suggest that specific attention be given to the digestive tract. Also use a cavity fluid that has additional disinfectant properties such as Metafix. At the end of the embalming process and prior to final disinfection of the preparation room, it is advisable to pack the vagina, rectum, and any other areas that have folds with a cotton pack saturated with formaldehyde-based chemical.

It is vital for embalmers to remember that organisms that have become resistant to antibiotics inside the living human body do not become in any way more resistant to the disinfecting chemicals such as formaldehyde, which we use in our embalming procedures. If we achieve thorough distribution, we will achieve disinfection, and families viewing the body will not be at any greater risk than from nonresistant (equally disinfected) bacteria. Moreover, if we follow universal precautions properly, embalmers should not become infected while performing their work (before the chemicals have had a chance to disinfect).

---

*Reprinted with permission from *The Dodge Magazine*, September–October 1999, Volume 91, No. 4. Copyright: The Dodge Company.

## REFERENCES

1. Reuters-May 14, 1998.
2. Reuters-Mike Cooper-March 11, 1998.
3. AMA, *Surgical Infection Society Position on Vancomycin-Resistant Entero*, October 1996.

---

### The Antimicrobial Activity of Embalming Chemicals and Topical Disinfectants on the Microbial Flora of Human Remains*

*Peter A. Burke and A. L. Sheffner*
*Department of Microbiology, Foster D. Snell, Inc., Florham Park, New Jersey*

---

*The antimicrobial activity of embalming chemicals and topical disinfectants was evaluated to determine the degree of disinfection achieved during the embalming of human remains. The administration of arterial and cavity embalming chemicals resulted in a 99% reduction of the postmortem microbial population after 2 hours of contact. This level of disinfection was maintained for the 24-hour test period. Topical disinfection of the body orifices was also observed. Therefore, it is probable that present embalming practices reduce the hazard from transmission of potentially infectious microbial agents within the immediate environment of embalmed human remains.*

## INTRODUCTION

For many years, embalming chemicals have been utilized to preserve and disinfect biological tissues for anatomical studies, environmental storage, and hygienic safety. The majority of these embalming chemicals are formaldehyde-based products, whose disinfectant properties have been described by Walker,[1] Lawrence and Block,[2] and Spaulding.[3] It has been reported that pathogenic organisms, such as *K. pneumoniae*, *H. influenzae*, *M. tuberculosis*, and *H. capsulatum*, are recoverable from embalmed human remains.[4-6] Thus, conceivably, infection could occur from contact with post-embalming microbial fluids and swabs of areas around orifices from cadavers to determine if commercially available embalming chemicals produce a significant reduction in the microbial flora.

## MATERIALS AND METHODS

Samples of biological fluids and swabs of the area around orifices were taken from eight cadavers to determine the antimicrobial activity of embalming fluids in vivo as a function of time. Four of the bodies were embalmed, whereas the other four cadavers were not and served as controls. The primary cause of death of the subjects was diagnosed to be other than an infectious disease (i.e., coronary thrombosis, cerebrovascular accident, and arteriosclerosis).

*Embalming Procedure.* The bodies were embalmed by a professional licensed mortician using the following procedure. The body was washed with an antiseptic soap containing 0.75% hexachlorophene and thoroughly rinsed. The cadaver was sprayed with a topical embalming disinfectant and the orifices swabbed with the same disinfectant. This disinfectant was a solution of 1.0% (w/v) formaldehyde and 0.5% (w/v) quaternary ammonium compounds in a base of isopropanol and ethylene dichloride.

Prior to dilution of the arterial embalming chemical, the tap water was treated with a water conditioning mixture formulated specifically for embalming use. This conditioner is a complexing agent that removes chemical constituents found in municipal water supplies, which could interfere with the preservative and disinfecting properties of the arterial solutions. This conditioner is basically a mixture of trisodium ethylenediaminetetraacetate and polyvinylpyrrolidone in a base of various glycols.

The arterial embalming chemical consisted of 29.8% (w/v) formaldehyde, 3.8% (w/v) anionic detergents, 4.0% (w/v) borate and germicides, 9.6% (w/v) alcohol, and various inert ingredients in a water base. The arterial embalming chemical was then diluted 6 oz to ½ gallon of water. An equal amount of co-injection chemical for the purpose of stimulating drainage and inducing penetration was added to the solution. This chemical consisted of 8.9% (w/v) chelating agents, 0.1% (w/v) reducing agents, 0.7% (w/v) preservatives, 2.0% (w/v) plasticizers, 9.9% (w/v) humectants, and various inert ingredients in a water base.

The total amount of solution injected into the body was approximately 2 to 3½ gallons, depending on the body size and weight. Two pints of cavity embalming chemical (24–28% [w/v] formaldehyde) were injected into each subject, one into the thoracic cavity and the other into the abdominal cavity. All products used in the study were commercially available embalming chemicals.

*Sample Collection.* Samples were drawn from superior and inferior anatomical sites, with sterile 18-gauge needles and 30 mL syringes. Needle puncture sites were topically disinfected with 95% ethanol. Swab samples were taken with sterile polyester swabs, which just before swabbing were immersed in sterile phosphate-buffered saline.* Biological fluids and swab cultures were taken from the following areas.

## FLUID SAMPLES

- **Lung:** The needle was inserted 3 inches to the right of the midline, through the fifth intercostal space. Pulmonary fluids or aspirates were extracted from the middle lobe of the right lung.
- **Heart blood:** The needle was inserted 1 inch to the left of the midline, through the fifth intercostal space.
- **Descending colon:** A longitudinal incision 3 inches long was made midway between the tip to the 12th rib and the anterior iliac spine; the descending colon was identified and the fecal extracted from the lumen of the colon.
- **Urinary bladder:** The needle was inserted through the external urethral orifice and the urine extracted from the lumen of the bladder.

---

*Reprinted from *Health Lab Sci* 1976;13(2):267–270, with permission from the American Public Health Association.

*Phosphate-buffered saline prepared by diluting 0.25M phosphate buffer 1/1000 in physiological saline (0.9% NaCl).

Dehydrated or coagulated sample sites were injected with sterile phosphate-buffered saline.

## Swabs of Orifices

- **Oral cavity:** Samples were taken from the buccal furrow between the mucous membrane of the upper lip and the gingiva.
- **Nasal cavity:** Swabs were made from the vestibule of the left half of the nasal cavity.
- **Anus:** Swabs were taken from the terminal inch of the anal canal.

Immediately after taking samples, the swabs were placed in Stuart's transport medium.

Samples were taken before embalming and then 2, 4, 8, and 24 hours after embalming. The bodies were covered with plastic sheeting while sampling procedure was not in process. All samples were packed in dry ice during transportation to the laboratories of Foster D. Snell, Inc., where they were immediately plated.

*Quantitative Measurement of Microbiological Flora.* Immediately following receipt in the laboratory, the biological fluids were serially diluted in thiotone peptone water blanks and subsequently plated on MacConkey and Heart Infusion Agar with 5% defribrinated sheep blood. Into both agar preparations, 0.5% Tween 80 and 0.1% lecithin were incorporated to neutralize residual microbial activity from the embalming fluids. The plates were incubated at 35–37°C for 48 hours following which a colony count was performed.

*Microbial Identification.* Isolates were identified using standard morphological and biochemical tests with the general outline utilized for identification as defined in *Bergey's Manual of Determinative Bacteriology*, eighth edition,[7] and Skerman's *Identification of the Genera of Bacteria*, second edition.[8]

## RESULTS AND DISCUSSION

In vitro, germicidal activity of formaldehyde has been established and documented for many years.[2] However, the amount of microbiological data concerning the in vivo efficacy of embalming chemicals on human remains is scant. In the present study, formaldehyde-based embalming fluids were found to be highly active in reducing the microbial flora in human remains. The microbial population was reduced greater than 99% at every site 2 hours after embalming; with control bodies, as anticipated, a continuous microbial growth pattern was observed (**Table 1**). The antimicrobial action of formaldehyde-based embalming chemicals was apparently not limited or adversely affected by the proteinaceous material or other macromolecules present in the biological fluids and tissues.

Following topical disinfection of the areas around the orifices, no growth or limited growth could be detected after 24 hours of exposure. Disinfection of the orifices occurred within 2 hours of contact. Random positive results after disinfection, however, were seen because the bodies were not protected from the environment with the exception of a nonsterile plastic cloth.

Differential monitoring of the microbial population revealed that microorganisms translocate across anatomical barriers, which during life prevent penetration and translocation. These body defenses are as follows: epithelial and mucous membrane coverings, reticuloendothelial system, blood drainer barrier.

**TABLE 1.** Antimicrobial Activity of Embalming Chemicals and Topical Disinfectants on Microflora of Human Remains

| Treatment | Anatomical Site | Pre-embalming | Treatment Period (hours) | | | | % Reduction After 24 Hours |
| | | | 2 | 4 | 8 | 24 | |
| | | | Mean Microbial Populations[a] | | | | |
|---|---|---|---|---|---|---|---|
| Embalmed | Heart | $8.0 \times 10^5$ | $1.8 \times 10^2$ | $1.6 \times 10^2$ | $2.0 \times 10^2$ | 70 | >99 |
| Embalmed | Lung | $2.5 \times 10^1$ | <10 | <10 | <10 | <10 | >99 |
| Embalmed | Colon | $7.4 \times 10^1$ | 80 | <10 | <10 | <10 | >99 |
| Embalmed | Bladder | $1.3 \times 10^5$ | $3.8 \times 10^2$ | <10 | <10 | <10 | >99 |
| Embalmed | Oral cavity | ++[b] | 0 | 0 | 0 | 0 | – |
| Embalmed | Nasal cavity | + | 0 | 0 | 0 | 0 | – |
| Embalmed | Anus | +++ | 0 | + | 0 | 0 | – |
| Unembalmed | Heart | $2.8 \times 10^5$ | $7.2 \times 10^5$ | $7.8 \times 10^5$ | $7.5 \times 10^5$ | $9.0 \times 10^5$ | – |
| Unembalmed | Lung | $2.5 \times 10^5$ | $3.2 \times 10^5$ | $3.0 \times 10^5$ | $2.4 \times 10^5$ | $3.8 \times 10^5$ | – |
| Unembalmed | Colon | $1.5 \times 10^6$ | $1.6 \times 10^6$ | $1.7 \times 10^6$ | $1.5 \times 10^6$ | $2.2 \times 10^6$ | – |
| Unembalmed | Bladder | $2.9 \times 10^6$ | $2.3 \times 10^6$ | $2.3 \times 10^6$ | $2.4 \times 10^6$ | $2.5 \times 10^6$ | – |
| Unembalmed | Oral cavity | + | + | + | + | + | – |
| Unembalmed | Nasal cavity | + | + | + | + | + | – |
| Unembalmed | Anus | +++ | +++ | ++ | ++ | +++ | – |

[a] Organisms (mL) (mean of four subjects per group).
[b] Scale of growth from swab cultures: 0 = none, + = slight, ++ = moderate, +++ = heavy.

| TABLE 2. Isolation and Distribution of Microflora Associated with Human Remains: Anatomical Sites | | | |
|---|---|---|---|
| Heart | Lung | Colon | Bladder |
| Proteus mirabilis | Escherichia coli | Escherichia coli | Escherichia coli |
| Pseudomonas sp. | Pseudomonas aeruginosa | Micrococcus sp. | Klebsiella aerogenes |
| Staphylococcus aureus | Staphylococcus aureus | Proteus mirabilis | Proteus vulgaris |
| Staphylococcus epidermidis | Staphylococcus epidermidis | Proteus vulgaris | Proteus morganii |
| Streptococcus | Streptococcus sp. | Pseudomonas aeruginosa | Pseudomonas aeruginosa |
| Bacillus sp. | Alcaligenes faecalis | Staphylococcus aureus | Staphylococcus aureus |
| Escherichia coli | | Staphylococcus epidermidis | Staphylococcus epidermidis |
| | | Streptococcus sp. | Bacillus sp. |
| | | Bacillus sp. | |
| | | Klebsiella aerogenes | |

The organisms that were isolated from the human remains are listed in **Table 2**.

Comparison of the microbial flora before and after embalming produced no pattern or general trend. Specific microbial resistance to the antimicrobial action of formaldehyde-based embalming chemicals was not observed. No pathogenic bacteria were found following embalming.

In conclusion, it was found that the use of formaldehyde-based embalming chemicals is a satisfactory disinfectant when applied as a public health measure to reduce microbial hazards when human remains are handled.

## ACKNOWLEDGMENTS

We thank J. B. Christensen of the George Washington School of Medicine, Department of Anatomy, Washington, D.C., and R. Swaminathan, Foster D. Snell, Inc., for their professional assistance. This study was supported by the Embalming Chemical Manufacturers Association.

## REFERENCES

1. Walker JF. *Formaldehyde*. American Chemical Society Monograph Series, 3rd ed. New York: Reinhold, 1964.
2. Lawrence CA, Block SS. *Disinfection, Sterilization, and Preservation*. Philadelphia: Lea & Febiger, 1968.
3. Spaulding EH. Role of chemical disinfection in the prevention of nosocomial infection. In: *Proceedings of the International Conference on Nosocomial Infections*. Atlanta: Centers for Disease Control and Prevention; 1970.
4. Meade GM, Steenken W. Viability of tubercle bacilli in embalmed human lung tissue. *American Review of Tuberculosis* 1949;59:429.
5. Weed LA, Baggerstoss AH. The isolation of pathogens from tissues of embalmed human bodies. *American Journal of Clinical Pathology* 1951;21:1114.
6. Weed LA, Baggerstoss AH. The isolation of pathogens from embalmed tissues. *Proceedings of the Staff Meetings. Mayo Clinic* 1952;27:124.
7. Buchanan RE, Gibbons NE, eds. *Bergey's Manual of Determinative Bacteriology*, 8th ed. 1974.
8. Skerman VK. *Identification of the Genera of Bacteria*, 2nd ed. 1967.

---

### The Microbiologic Evaluation and Enumeration of Postmortem Specimens from Human Remains*

*Gordon W. Rose, PhD*
*Associate Director, Department of Mortuary Science, Wayne State University, Detroit, Michigan*

*Robert N. Hockett, MS*
*Research Associate, School of Dentistry, University of Michigan, Ann Arbor, Michigan*

Several recognized and potential pathogens, both bacterial and mycotic, were recovered consistently from body fluids and/or aspirates withdrawn from human cases certified to have died from causes other than an infectious disease. Samples were taken from five anatomic sites of varying postmortem time intervals. Filter membrane culture techniques were used for primary isolation and enumeration. Some isolates seemed to imitate classical growth curve indications of exponential increase at the 6-hour to 8-hour postmortem interval. Densities reached a level of 3.0–3.5 million organisms per milliliter or gram of sample at the 12- to 14-hour interval, the time period of maximal microbiologic translocation and proliferation. These studies indicate that unembalmed human remains are capable of contributing a multitude of infectious doses of microbial agents to a body handler, the body storage area, or to the environment adjacent to the body storage area.

## INTRODUCTION

Research in postmortem microbiology is not new; Achard and Phulpin presented data on the recovery of microorganisms from human remains in 1895.[1] Sampling has generally followed the opening of body cavities.[2-4] One improvement in technique was the use of animal model systems[5] as an investigational tool. The amount of scientific data originating from this area of microbiologic investigation remains scant. The bibliography of

---

*Reprinted from *Health Lab Sci* 971; 8(2), with permission from the American Public Health Association. Presented before the laboratory section at the Ninety-Eighth Annual Meeting of the American Public Health Association, Houston, TX, Oct. 29, 1970.

the Embalming Chemical Manufacturers Association[6] is to be recommended for background.

The study utilized the application of the relatively new technique of membrane filtration (MF) to the qualitative and quantitative microbiological evaluation of body fluids and/or aspirates. Winn et al. reported the use of this technique in postmortem studies in 1966.[7] They described two advantages of the MF technique: (1) the MF method provides a three-dimensional approach to the cultivation of microorganisms and (2) it yields more accurate and reproducible quantitative results.

## METHOD

Death certifications on all human remains sampled indicated the primary cause of death to be other than an infectious disease (e.g., coronary thrombosis, cerebrovascular accident, and arteriosclerotic disease). Samples were secured from refrigerated cases over a postmortem period of 72 hours for temporal profile purposes. Samples were withdrawn from upper or superior to lower or inferior anatomic sites, with 18 gauge needles and 25 mL Luer syringes. Dehydration or coagulation of some samplings required aspirates of injected sterile phosphate-buffered saline (PBS). Topical disinfection of needle puncture sites was effected with an iodophore (Hi-Sine (R), Huntington Laboratories, Huntington, IN). The sampling needle was directed into the cisterna magna (cisterna cerebellomedullaris) at the base of the cerebellum via the foramen magnum for the withdrawal of cerebrospinal fluid. Heart blood samples were taken from the left ventricle by directing the needle to the upper border of the fifth rib just to the left of the sternum. Pulmonary fluids and/or aspirates were taken from the lungs for the third sampling. The needle was directed into the transverse colon at the level of the umbilicus to sample the lumen contents. Finally, urinary bladder needle taps were made from a site marking the intersection of the median line and the pubic bone.

All samples were initially diluted 1:3 or 1:4 in PBS, and 0.1 mL of each diluted sample impinged on 0.45em MF, and then washed with 10.0 mL of PBS. The MFs with impinged organisms were rolled onto primary isolation agar plates of MacConkey, phenylethyl alcohol/blood, and chocolate blood. Aerobic incubation at 35–37°C for 24–48 hours and preliminary picking of isolates were routinely practiced. Isolates were characterized by pertinent methods.[8,9]

## RESULTS AND DISCUSSION

**Table 1** lists the bacterial isolates from the five anatomical areas sampled.

The selection of sampling sites was based on anatomic considerations of the normal microbial flora associated with specific anatomic areas during life. The epithelial and mucous membrane coverings and linings are normally during life intact anatomic barriers to bacterial penetration and translocation. The reticuloendothelial system is a second nonselective barrier that helps to deter translocation during life. The blood–brain barrier is probably the last line of anatomic defense against many potential microbial invaders. The cerebrospinal fluid, a filtrate of circulating blood, maintains its biologic integrity in a closed system of circulation.

All of the selected sampling sites were easily accessible and, with the exception of the colon, yielded essentially liquid specimens. The colon contents occasionally required a presampling

**TABLE 1. Bacterial Isolates from Five Anatomical Sites**

| Organism | Cerebrospinal Fluid | Lung | Heart Blood | Transverse Colon | Bladder Urine |
|---|---|---|---|---|---|
| *Alcaligenes faecalis* | x | x | | x | x |
| *Bacillus sp.* | | | x | x | |
| *Corynebacterium diphtheriae*[a] | x | x | | x | |
| *Escherichia coli* | x | x | x | x | |
| *E. coli* (A–D) × | | | | | x |
| *Klebsiella aerogenes* | x | x | x | x | x |
| *Micrococcus sp.* | x | x | x | x | x |
| *Proteus mirabilis* | | | x | x | x |
| *Proteus vulgaris* | | | | x | |
| *Providencia* | | | | x | |
| *Pseudomonas aeruginosa* | x | x | x | x | x |
| *Shigella flexneri* | | | | x | |
| *Staphylococcus aureus* | x | x | x | x | x |
| *Staphylococcus epidermidis* | x | x | x | x | x |
| *Streptococcus* (Group D) | x | x | x | x | x |
| *Streptococcus pneumoniae* | | x | | x | x |

[a]Not a typical isolate.

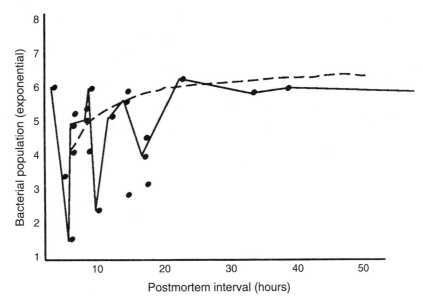

**Figure 1.** Bacterial population versus postmortem interval.

injection of sterile PBS. Needle penetration of the selected sites involved minimal manipulation of the body areas and permitted the rapid procurement of specimens in a state best suited for MF processing.

Thorough washing of each impinged MF reduced or removed the possible effects of specific and nonspecific inhibitors that might have been associated with the specimens. Each MF was quickly transferred to the basic group of primary isolation agars. The direct rolling of the MFs onto the agar surfaces facilitated contact between the matrix and surface-oriented microorganisms and growth substrates.

The MF allowed the impingement of a standardized volume (0.1 mL) of diluted specimen that gave total plate colony counts that were mathematically referable to densities per milliliter or per gram of original sample. Gridded MFs improved the accuracy of colony counting; plate counts in excess of 200 per plate were not recorded. Processed MFs were sterilized with ethylene oxide and stored for possible future serotaxonomic or other studies.

Bacteria *normally* associated with the transverse colon during life, with the exception of clinically opportunistic conditions, do not translocate. They are, by description of the U.S. Public Health Service Ad Hoc Committee on the Safe Shipment and Handling of Etiological Agents,[10] "Agents of no... [to] ordinary potential hazard." This general statement assumes a knowledge of infectious disease and immunology. There might well be logical disagreement originating from those who have attempted the treatment of infections from enteric "commensals."

The colon was chosen as the translocation reference baseline for indicator organisms isolated from other sampling sites. The brain, lung, and heart samples frequently yielded recognized pathogens in addition to the indicator commensals and opportunists. Many of the same indicator organisms were isolated from all five sampling sites. This is indicative of the extent to which bacteria, both pathogenic and nonpathogenic, can be translocated within a period of 6–8 hours after death.

The quantitative results (**Fig. 1**) of the study indicate that a postmortem multiplication of the isolates begins approximately 4 hours after death and assumes a logarithmic-like increase between 6 and 8 hours after death. The bacterial cell densities reach a peak of approximately 3 to 3½ million organisms/mL or gram of fluid or tissue within 24–30 hours after death.

Within a postmortem interval of 4–6 hours, there is a body-wide redistribution of endogenous flora. Postmortem chemical changes in and manual manipulation of human remains may cause these organisms to exit from any of the body orifices and contribute contamination to adjacent environments. This places the body handlers and other personnel in or near the body storage area at higher risk.

## ACKNOWLEDGMENT

Support for this study was received from the National Funeral Directors Association.

## REFERENCES

1. Achard C, Phulpin E. Contribution a l'etude de l'envahissement des organes par les microbes pendant l'agonie et apres le mort. *Archives of Medical Expert Anatomical Pathology* 1895;7:25–47.
2. Burn CG. Experimental studies of postmortem bacterial invasion in animals. *The Journal of Infectious Diseases* 1934;54:388–394.
3. Carpenter HM, Wilkins RM. Autopsy bacteriology: Review of 2,033 cases. *Archives of Pathology* 1964;77:73–81.
4. De Jongh D, Lottis JW, Green GS, et al. Postmortem bacteriology. *American Journal of Clinical Pathology* 1968;49:424–428.
5. Burn CG. Postmortem bacteriology. *Journal of Infectious Diseases* 1934;54:395–403.
6. Hinson MR. Final report on literature search on the infectious nature of dead bodies for the Embalming Chemical Manufacturers Association. Mimeo, 1968.
7. Winn WR, White ML, Carter WT, et al. Rapid diagnosis of bacteremia with quantitative differential membrane filtration culture. *Journal of American Medical Association* 1966;197:539–548.
8. Cowan ST, Steel KJ. *Manual for the Identification of Medical Bacteria*. London: Cambridge University Press, 1966.
9. Harris AH, Coleman MB. *Diagnostic Procedures and Reagents*. Washington, DC: American Public Health Association, 1963.
10. Anonymous. *Classification of Etiologic Agents on the Basis of Hazard*. Atlanta: Centers for Disease Control (US DHEW, USPHS), 1970.

> **Professional Hair Care for Human Remains**
> Darla A. Tripoli, CO, LFD, CFSP

When the words restoration or restorative art are mentioned in the funeral profession, one usually thinks of a trauma case where extensive restoration skills are needed to repair damaged head and facial features. However, embalmers practice the art of restoration on each and every case in the embalming room. Sometimes, dramatic restoration is needed, but most often, it is the smaller details of care of human remains, which demonstrate our skills in restoration and professionalism in body preparation.

Attention to detail when caring for the hair of human remains is essential for authenticity of the decedent's appearance and a pleasing visual experience for the family members and the public.

The task of grooming the hair and the application of tastefully chosen cosmetics can have a dramatic impact on the final appearance of the deceased. Perhaps, the smaller details of restoration, like professional hair care, are considered secondary because they are not perceived to be true "restoration." This is an incorrect assumption. When it comes to hair care, sometimes trained professionals are hired by the funeral home to care for the deceased's hair. From a business perspective, this can become quite costly to the funeral home. With basic knowledge of hair, techniques, and products, a funeral professional can begin to take responsibility for more of the hair care and grooming themselves. Not only can this raise the level of professionalism of the worker, but it can also prevent valuable service dollars being lost at the funeral home by hiring an outside source. In some cases, it is wise to hire a professional, but oftentimes with the right knowledge and the right skills, a funeral professional can achieve quality and professional hair care results.

## HAIR BASICS

Hair strands are primarily made up of a protein called *keratin*. Keratin is a tough, water insoluble type of protein that is also found in skin, fingernails, and toenails. Individual hair strands are made up of three layers. The outer layer, called the *cuticle*, is microscopically demonstrated as clear cells that appear flat and tight to the hair strand giving them the appearance of "shingles." The inner layer is called the *cortex*. The medulla is found inside the cortex.

With undamaged hair, the outer layer, the cuticle, which has the appearance of scales or shingles, appears flat, tight, and imbricate on this strand of hair. This gives us many clues to the condition of the hair. This hair is, most likely, virgin hair. Virgin hair has never been chemically altered by perms or colors and will visually demonstrate a shiny, healthy appearance. This type of hair is easy to identify because virgin hair will be easy to comb, easy to style, and have superior shine. This is not the type of hair we often see in the preparation room.

With damaged hair, the cuticle of this hair strand is not smooth. The cuticle is damaged, rough, broken, and does not imbricate. This indicates that the hair has been damaged in some way, either by hair color, bleach, permanent waves, or the misuse of heating devices used on the hair. This hair will be difficult to comb or brush, is usually very dry, tangles very easily, and is visually dull and flat with little or no luster. This is often the type of hair observed in the preparation room.

## HAIR CLEANSING

There are many types of hair care products available on the market. Purchasing professional shampoos and conditioners in a beauty supply store will ensure the best products at reasonable prices. Oftentimes, employees are trained licensed cosmetologists who can answer any questions about which products to purchase. A 32-oz bottle with a pump for one-handed efficiency in the preparation room is ideal.

Step one is properly cleansing the hair. There are three basic types of shampoo that are recommended in the preparation room. They are described in the following paragraphs.

*Stripping Shampoo*—These shampoos have a high alkaline content. They range from 7.5 to 8.5 on the pH scale. These shampoos are considered a deep cleansing type. This shampoo will rid hair of grease, dirt, blood, medication, and styling product buildup (gels and hairsprays) on hair strands. Depending on the cleansing needs, one application of this type of shampoo is generally effective in cleansing the hair.

*Medicated*—May be used to rid hair of obvious dandruff flakes on the hair/scalp.

*Acid Balanced*—These shampoos are used for color-treated or permanently waved hair. Typically, these types of shampoo have a pH of 4.5–5.5. This type of shampoo is considered nonstripping and will not dull, strip, or harm hair color. It will remove dirt effectively without harming the hair or dulling hair that has been artificially colored. It is also recommended to have a pediculicide available to treat pediculosis capitis (commonly known as *head lice*). Pediculosis capitis is a communicable disorder and can be contagious to the embalmer. Proper use of PPE at all times, which includes a head covering, will help keep the embalmer protected. If infestations on the scalp of the human remains are found, it is wise to check the eyebrows, eyelashes, and any facial hair for infestation as well, and treat accordingly. Sometimes, cases seen with a severe infestation of pediculosis capitis must be treated more than one time.

### Hair Cleansing Procedures

Wet the hair with water. While the hair is wet, pump a small amount of the selected shampoo into a gloved hand, rub your hands together, and then evenly apply the shampoo, beginning at the scalp and then throughout the hair to the ends. Lather, rinse well, and repeat if necessary. Rinse the hair thoroughly.

If a buildup of styling products is observed in the hair, do not comb or brush the hair first. This can break the hair or tear it from the root. Saturate the hair with water and then shampoo as indicated above.

## HAIR CONDITIONING/INSTANT DRAMATIC RESTORATION

Hair that is damaged is matte, nonreflective, dry, drab, dull, and difficult to comb or brush. Application of a hair conditioner can dramatically change the appearance of the hair, adding shine, luster, and manageability. Hair conditioner can help to correct any physical or chemical damage observed in the hair.

The main ingredients in hair conditioners are moisturizers, surfactants, glossers, fatty oils, polymers, lubricants, detanglers, and thermal protectors. Conditioners are frequently acidic with a low pH. Hair conditioners work on the outside of the hair strand (where the cuticle is found) to help close or "fill in" the damaged spaces on the cuticle. This will smooth the hair strand and change the appearance of the hair. By utilizing this product, the hair will better reflect light, be easier to comb, and it will give the hair a healthy, sleek, and shiny appearance.

### Conditioning Procedures

After the hair is cleansed and rinsed properly, pump a small amount of conditioner into the palm of a gloved hand and work the conditioner from the scalp to the ends of the hair strands. Follow by using a wide-tooth hair pick to evenly distribute the conditioner throughout the hair. Start from the scalp and comb the conditioner to the ends of the hair strands. Leave the conditioner on the hair strands for a few minutes and then rinse thoroughly. Typically, only one application of hair conditioner is necessary. Sometimes if the hair is badly damaged, the conditioner can be left on for a longer period of time and then rinsed thoroughly. This product dramatically restores shine and luster and positively changes the appearance of the hair. Visually this is an important restorative step that must not be omitted.

## CRANIAL INCISIONS

If the body has been autopsied and the decedent has long, thick, and/or extremely tangled hair, care is essential as to not to pull or tear the hair from the scalp when embalming/suturing the cranium. Hair conditioner and a wide-tooth hair pick can help alleviate frustration for the embalmer in this situation. This also will prevent damage to the hair caused by pulling or tearing hair from the scalp.

### Procedure

With your hands, apply a small amount of hair conditioner to the hair, working from the scalp to the ends of the hair strands. Using a wide-tooth hair pick, comb through the hair until the hair is tangle-free. Part the hair along the cranial incision. Gather half the hair on the top of the head and secure it with a clamp. Keep the bottom half of the hair secure with a clamp at the nape of the neck. After embalming, shave or cut the hair to the scalp 1/8′ above and below the incision. This will help prevent the hair from becoming tangled when suturing. Suture the incision, take the hair out of the clamp(s), shampoo the hair properly again, and then condition the hair again, if needed.

## SCALP DISORDERS

The most common scalp disorders observed in the preparation room are pityriasis steatoides and pityriasis capitis simplex. Pityriasis capitis simplex is dry, scaly dandruff. Pityriasis steatoides disorder is often seen as a greasy, waxy, thick scaly type of dandruff commonly seen in the elderly. This is often caused by an excess of sebum production that causes flaking skin to stick together and form scales over the scalp. It is common to see scratch marks or gouge marks on the scalp as this disorder can itch and can be quite uncomfortable during life. These types of scales can be difficult to remove without causing the appearance of brown marks visible on the skin, called *demarcation marks*. However, they can be unsightly if left untreated and present on the scalp. It is wise to attempt to gently remove these thick scales before the embalming process begins.

### Procedure

For the disorder pityriasis capitis simplex, a medicated shampoo can be used to cleanse the hair and the scalp. For the disorder pityriasis steatoides, another method can be utilized. Treat pityriasis steatoides observed on the scalp before the embalming process. Pump a generous amount of creamy hair conditioner into a gloved hand and, using fingertips, work the conditioner directly onto the scalp **only**. Allow the conditioner to penetrate the scales until the scales start to loosen and dissolve. Then, carefully comb through the hair until all the scales are removed from the scalp. Using a proper shampoo, shampoo the hair thoroughly until the scales are removed from the hair strands and the hair appears clean. Rinse and repeat until all the scales are removed. Use hair conditioner again this time working a small amount through the hair strands to help close the cuticle and to restore health and shine. Rinse thoroughly.

## CURLY HAIR

Curly hair tends to have a coarser texture than straight hair and has greater tensile strength than fine hair. It is typically drier and more brittle and has a tendency to frizz.

Shampoos/conditioners that have a cream base work best with curly hair. Before drying or styling, apply a small amount of serum, a thick honey-like substance that is used to combat frizz. It is best to let curly hair dry naturally. By letting hair air-dry, the curls will be more natural and there will be less chance of frizz.

If time is of the essence, it is possible to speed up drying time. Blot excess moisture from curly hair with paper towels. Do not rub curly hair vigorously with a towel to remove moisture. A diffuser can be used to dry curly hair quickly. Diffusers can be purchased at a beauty supply store or drugstore and are relatively inexpensive. A diffuser diffuses air onto the hair through the hair dryer to remove moisture but retains the curl. Attach a diffuser on the end of a standard hair dryer. While drying curly hair with a diffuser, use a low-temperature setting and a low airflow setting and try not to touch the hair with your hands or fingers as this will cause the hair to frizz. When drying curly hair with a diffuser, begin at the root level and work in circular motions until the hair is dry.

## BLOW DRYING

It is always best to let hair air-dry, especially if the hair is damaged or fragile. Fragile hair has less tensile strength and has a tendency to break easily. Great care and caution must be taken when caring for this type of hair.

If the hair is in a good condition, and time is a factor, utilizing a blow-dryer will help remove moisture from the hair quickly. It is wise to have a variety of brushes to dry/style hair. A round brush, a vent brush, and a natural bristle brush will work on most hair types. A round brush is used for styling and volume, a vent brush for hairstyles that lay flat against the head, and a natural bristle brush for ethnic hair or straight hair.

Be sure to keep the blow-dryer moving at all times and on a medium to low-temperature setting. Begin at the nape of the neck and move forward, drying the roots first and then the ends of the hair strand. Be sure to thoroughly dry the nape of the neck, as this is a common place for mold growth.

## PROFESSIONALLY FINISHED HAIR

Embalmers can enhance any final hairstyle with professional finishing products. One product that works well on most hair types is a glosser or finishing spray. These coat the hair with silicone polymers that reflect light and give the hair a shiny, finished appearance. A spray that lists, among its ingredients, mica, is a superb choice. This mica spray is highly reflective and gives a professional looking shine to any hairstyle. It can be used on any hair type, including male facial hair, creating extraordinary shine and the appearance of healthy hair. This type of spray is nonsticky and is the finishing touch to a professional appearance. It can be applied without buildup on the hair. It especially works very well with overhead lighting seen in viewing rooms. This product is reflective, eye catching, and positively enhances any finished hairstyle.

## TRIMMING HAIR BASICS

Many times, especially in the final stages of an illness, personal grooming is not a priority. It is important to communicate with the family the possibility of hair cutting or trimming. If the remains need a bit of hair trimming or grooming, here are a few tips to achieve professional results.

Begin by securing the proper tools. It is wise to have hair-trimming shears. These can be purchased in a beauty supply store. Shears are balanced, sharp, and specific for hair cutting. A balance comb is a wise purchase. These inexpensive plastic combs have units of measure on the comb, which makes it easier to have accurate measurements when cutting hair. A few hair clips or butterfly clamps will help keep the hair manageable while trimming.

### Basic Hair-Trimming Procedure

Before beginning, ensure that the hair is clean, conditioned, and tangle-free. Trim hair when the hair is wet (unless it is a hair replacement, then trim when dry). When hair is wet, it appears longer than it will when it is dry. Hair will appear shorter when dry. This is called the "drying factor." Take into consideration the "drying factor," especially when trimming or cutting curly hair and/or bangs.

Part the hair in small sections at a time, securing the hair with a hair clamp. Make parts approximately a half-inch wide and less than a quarter of an inch thick. Ensure the parts are very straight. When trimming, use the index finger and the middle finger to hold the section of hair securely between them and cut the hair straight across. Use fingers as a guide to cut along the fingers in a straight line. While cutting or trimming hair, only move the thumb up and down while trimming for maximum control. Hair has elasticity and can easily stretch when wet and pulled. Do not pull or tug on the hair when holding the hair to trim. When possible, lay hair flat on the skin when trimming. Use the nose, ears, and/or the mandible as measurement guides to keep both sides even. When trimming or cutting, start conservatively. It is possible to go back and trim more hair if necessary.

## BALD SCALP

For a finished, professional appearance for bald scalps, it is essential to follow a few simple steps. First, exfoliate any dry skin flakes seen on the scalp. For mild flakes, use generous amounts of massage cream before, during, and after embalming. Before cosmetics are applied, remove the massage cream with a lint free gauze pad to gently remove all visible dry skin flakes from the scalp. The preferred method of applying cosmetics to a bald scalp is by airbrushing the cosmetics onto the skin. Airbrush cosmetics are highly pigmented and water based. These cosmetics dry to a matte finish and are rub-resistant. Airbrushing cosmetics on the scalp will minimize the chance of soiling the pillow or the interior of the casket with cosmetic.

## WIG CARE/SECURING TO SCALP

Sometimes, a family will bring in a wig that their loved one wore in life to be attached to the scalp for an authentic look of the deceased. With a little knowledge about wigs and wig care, we can be confident that the appearance will be pleasing to the family.

There are two types of hair used when making wigs: human hair and synthetic hair. Both need to be treated with care.

Before securing the wig to the scalp, a little preparation is needed. If the natural hair is long, secure the hair tightly to the head with bobby pins. Then identify which is the front of the wig and which is the back. The label is always in the back of the wig. There are usually two tabs (one on either side) that should line up with the ears. Before putting the wig on the decedent, give the wig a shake to fluff the style. Stand at the end of the embalming table where the head is. Grab the wig by each tab (on the side) and slip the wig over the head with the label toward the back. Line up the front of the wig with the hairline. Lift the head from the neck block and gently pull the wig down toward the nape of the neck. In some wigs, there are Velcro tabs to adjust the tightness of the wig to the scalp. Once the wig is placed properly, lined up with the hairline and secure at the nape, then adjust tightness using the Velcro tabs. Style the wig with fingers or comb.

### Soiled Wigs

Dirty or soiled wigs should be properly cleansed before placing on the decent. First, gently brush through the wig with a wide-tooth comb or brush. Fill a sink with cold water and add a capful of gentle shampoo (baby shampoo works well). Immerse the wig in the cold water for a few minutes and agitate gently. Rinse the wig in cold water until the shampoo is completely removed. Allow the wig to air-dry naturally. Do not brush the wig when wet, as this will damage or remove the wig fibers. Heat will damage the wig and so do not use a blow-dryer or heated appliances on the wig hair. Blot any excess moisture with a towel. Allow the wig to air-dry on an empty plastic bottle covered by a towel. A Styrofoam head should be avoided as they can possibly stretch the wig.

## FACIAL HAIR

When trimming or shaping facial hair on the deceased, clear, concise communication with the families is essential. Examining close-up photos of the facial hair and asking good questions regarding shape and styling will ensure the family is satisfied with the end result.

Begin by shampooing and conditioning facial hair. Dry gently with a towel and comb the hairs into place so that the hairs are all in the same direction.

## Beards

Secure the proper tools before beginning. Choose a wider-toothed comb for trimming beards. Either scissors or clippers can be used to trim the hair. This is generally the personal preference of the embalmer. Begin by an ear and then clip the upper edges of the beard, cheeks, the jaw line (work top to bottom), and then lastly, the neckline. Reduce facial hair length slowly and conservatively as to not remove too much, working one side and then the other, and check for balance and symmetry on both sides.

Rechargeable cordless clippers work best in the prep room. These offer more control and precision. When determining length, choose the proper attachments and place on the end of the clippers. Double-check that the attachment is securely and firmly attached to the clippers before beginning. While choosing to trim without attachments, use a balance comb for length and control. Comb through the beard hairs and run the clippers along the length of the comb.

Scissors can also be used to trim beards. The scissor over comb technique takes practice and skill to get the beard uniform in length and shape. The tools chosen to trim beards are a personal preference.

## Moustaches

For trimming moustaches, a small mustache comb and scissors or clippers are needed. Begin by combing the moustache hairs straight down toward the upper lip. Start trimming in the middle and trim toward one side of the mouth and then the other. Use a fluff brush to remove hair clippings from the skin. Finish with a small amount of pomade or petroleum jelly to hold the hair in place. Set the facial hair with hair spray and finishing spray with mica for luster and shine.

## CONCLUSION

Learning new skills and techniques, and incorporating them in body preparation, will lead to a higher level of professional care of human remains. Understanding basic fundamentals of hair care will allow embalmers to take a more active role in hair care of the deceased. This will prevent valuable service dollars being lost, while still providing exceptional care to the deceased, resulting in a positive lasting memory image for family members.

---

### Restricted Cervical Injection as a Primary Injection Method

*Ben Whitworth, CFSP*

---

There is much debate as to what embalming fluid we mix and subsequently inject when preparing the dead human body during the embalming process. There is also much debate as to how this fluid is injected and this is backed up by a range of embalming machines. Some machines offer low rates of injection pressure and high rates of flow, some offer higher rates of pressure and lower rates of flow and others cover all bases. There is also much debate as to the best site or sites of injection, when one is injecting embalming fluid into the dead human body.

During my career so far, I have been honoured to provide educational seminars to a wide range of embalmers across the world and have been further privileged to write for numerous embalming and funeral service publications. One thing that has been a constant in all these seminars and articles is the need to listen to what the body in front of us is saying. I don't of course mean a spoken conversation, but our professional interpretation of what we observe of the remains. The forensic pathologist is skilled in such observations when it comes to assessing time, manner, mode and cause of death. The embalmer must be skilled in their own observation and assessment of the case in hand. No two cases are ever the same and it would be foolish to apply the same treatment in every case and hope for different or unique outcomes.

As a working embalmer in the United Kingdom, I face many different challenges. There are long delays between death, viewings, funeral services and final disposition taking place. Autopsies are rarely sympathetic to the embalmer and the bereaved may have unrealistic expectations when it comes to viewing the deceased (an issue not helped by a variety of television dramas and social media influencers). As a rule, 99% of the deceased human bodies in my care will have been refrigerated for several days, may have been kept in such cold storage without proper positioning devices or protection from dehydration thanks to a suitable emollient cream. Medical Science is advancing dramatically and we are seeing more and more cases of Oedema, Jaundice and bodies that are more challenging to embalm and preserve thanks to drug therapies. We also see the effects of addictions and dependencies on a range of drugs.

Overcoming these challenges will test all embalmers and there is not one single silver bullet that can be used in all these cases, however Restricted Cervical Injection {RCI} is one tool at the disposal of the embalmer to ensure the best possible outcome in all cases. Restricted Cervical Injection allows the embalmer to effectively separate the head from the rest of the body so that the arterial solution injected can be tempered to meet the exact needs of the body and the head. An example of this may be the oedematous case, where oedema is present in the body or limbs, but not the head. The strong solution needed to successful treat the body may not be suitable for the head and could cause over fixation of the facial tissues or dehydration, leading to additional procedures and heavier cosmetic application to achieve an acceptable viewing experience.

When using Restricted Cervical Injection, the embalmer will typically raise both the left and right Common Carotid Arteries. The right Internal Jugular vein is also raised as this provides an ideal site for venous drainage. The distal portion of the left Common Carotid Artery will be ligated closed, and the proximal portion will be opened to allow for the insertion of an arterial tube which is then ligated in place. With a drainage tube or suitable drainage instrument placed in the right Internal Jugular Vein, ligatures are placed proximally and distally around the right Common Carotid Artery, which is then opened to allow for arterial tubes to be placed. Some embalmers may place artery tubes that are fitted with stopcocks while others may leave the proximal aspects of both carotids open to allow arterial fluid to bypass the head and facial tissues while injecting the rest of the body. Restricted Cervical Injection will not stop arterial fluid from reaching the head while the rest of the body is injected. Fluid entering the left and right Subclavian Arteries will enter the left and right Vertebral Arteries and travel up into the head, through the Basilar Artery and ultimately leave the head via the internal Carotid Arteries which become the Common Carotid Arteries. This wordy explanation highlights one of many anastomoses found within the human body and as embalmers we rely on these heavily to ensure full and complete distribution of the arterial solution we are injecting. Exploiting this system, and basic fluid mechanics (fluid will always take the path of least resistance) we can at least restrict the amount of fluid that reached the tissues of the head before we are ready to inject them directly.

At this point, I would mention that I use Restricted Cervical Injection on around 90% of the non-autopsy cases that I embalm. As previously mentioned, in the UK embalmer face long delays before embalming can be performed and this creates many problems. The use of Restricted Cervical Injection helps to overcome many of these issues. Over time I have adjusted my approach and would seek to share my own adjustments as far as possible with other embalmers.

The first concerns venous drainage. Use of the right Internal Jugular Vein is recommended as this is the closest point to the centre of circulation within the body and deoxygenated blood is returned to the right Atrium of the Heart before being pumped to the lungs and then around the body. Through the right Internal Jugular, the embalmer can access the right Brachiocephalic vein which feeds into the Superior Vena Cava and the right Atrium of the Heart. On the left side, the left Internal Jugular Vein runs into the Left Brachiocephalic vein and then into the Superior Vena Cava. Thorough clearance of blood from the tissues will always enhance the cosmetic effect of embalming but there is a second consideration. Excess blood in the tissues can react with formaldehyde to form methyl-haemoglobin, one of many causes of 'embalmers grey'! There are of course other causes of this tiresome problem, however poor venous drainage can exacerbate this situation. As Restricted Cervical Injection requires the embalmer to raise both the left and right Common Carotid Arteries, I would recommend that both left and right Internal Jugular Veins are raised as well. The distal aspect of the left Internal Jugular Vein can be ligated closed, however by opening the proximal aspect of the left Internal Jugular Vein, the embalmer increases the potential for effective venous drainage of the head and facial features helping to clear discolorations and reduce the risk of post embalming greying of the tissues. If venous drainage from the right Internal Jugular Vein is poor, the embalmer can always open the distal aspect of the left Internal Jugular Vein and insert a pair of drainage forceps. In the past, I have used this to clear clots from the left Brachiocephalic Vein, which has improved drainage from the left upper limb, in turn, increasing the cosmetic appearance of the left hand post arterial injection.

The second alteration to the Restricted Cervical Injection method is the site of injection for the treatment of the body. It is usual in most textbooks and guides that injection distally into the body is achieved from injection into the right Common Carotid Artery. For the past 15 years or so, I have always injected the body from the left Common Carotid Artery. My decision to do this is based on the anatomy of the Aortic Arch and my observations of cases and results. If we look at the Aorta, we can split it into three parts. The Ascending Aorta, the Aortic Arch and the Descending Aorta. Focusing on the Aortic Arch we have the right Brachiocephalic or Innominate Artery. This bifurcates to become the right Subclavian Artery and the right Common Carotid Artery. Next to this is the left Common Carotid Artery and then further along is the left Subclavian Artery. In raising the right Common Carotid Artery, depending on where it is raised from and what type of arterial type is used, there is a risk of placing the arterial tube in such a way as to occlude the right Subclavian Artery or direct the flow of fluid from the arterial tube directly into the right Subclavian Artery. This could mean that either the right arm is embalmed before the rest of the body or it receives very little fluid during the injection, leading the embalmer to raise a different artery and inject the arm directly. By injecting the body via the left Common Carotid Artery the Aorta should fill more evenly and there should be a more even distribution of arterial solution between the left and right upper limbs as well as the rest of the body. Personally, I find that injecting the body via the left Common Carotid Artery reduces the need to raise additional arteries to complete the embalming. I have also in the past, passed a flexible arterial injection tube, based on a blind ended urinary catheter into the left Common Carotid Artery and fed this down the descending Aorta. This has allowed a stronger arterial solution to be injected more directly into the lower body and limbs to help overcome oedema, before mixing a less concentrated solution for the treatment of the upper body and head.

The control of the arterial solution entering the tissues of the head gives the embalmer exceptional control over how the embalming progresses and the final result. As mentioned initially, when treating an oedematous case, the embalmer can use a stronger solution for the treatment of the body and then make chemical adjustments before embalming the head. This can also work in reverse if one is presented with a case where there is swelling to one side of the head or other, owing to the positioning or lack of it, of the body, whilst in cold storage for an extended period of time. When presented with a subject where there is facial swelling to one side or other, the use of Restricted Cervical Injection allows for a stronger solution to be used to help reduce swelling. I have in the past injected one side of the face with a much stronger solution than the opposite side.

With jaundice cases, the use of Restricted Cervical Injection not only allows the embalmer control over fluid reaching the head of the deceased but allows the embalmer to try and balance as far as possible the arterial solution received in the tissues of the head. When treating jaundice, there is much debate on fluid mixes to use, but one thing always remains, the tissues of the body must be thoroughly saturated with arterial solution and well preserved. When confronted with a jaundice case, providing there is no generalise oedema present, I will use a Restricted Cervical Injection and will pre-inject the head first, followed by the body. Mixing a pre-injection solution that consists of equal parts of vascular conditioner, water corrective and water, I will drain from both left and right Internal Juglar Veins and try to remove as much blood from the tissues as possible. Once the head and then the body have received the pre-injection, I will continue with cleansing and grooming of the body and setting the facial features. I will then inject the body with the selected preservative solution followed by the head. The injection of the head is always done with as higher pressure as the embalming machine will produce and a very low rate of flow, typically around 6oz per minute. This has always produced excellent results with excellent clearing and colouration of the tissues and no darkening or greening post embalming.

The Restricted Cervical Injection method is also highly useful when dealing with cases where there is decomposition of the facial tissues, tissue gas is present or suspected, there is emaciation, enucleation has taken place, if the deceased is to be held for an extended period of time or if there is facial trauma or abnormalities requiring the use of instant tissue fixation. Whatever the situation, Restricted Cervical Injection assures the embalmer of achieving full tissue saturation in the most controlled way possible. Two common causes of post embalming dehydration are the injection of too little arterial fluid and arterial fluid not distributing to all areas. When it comes to the facial tissues, Restricted Cervical Injection when used properly will help to avoid these problems and reduce the need for additional treatments and cosmetic application.

The embalmer is charged with caring for and preparing the deceased human body so that the bereaved may have a positive funeral experience that meets their needs and expectations. Restricted Cervical Injection is one technique at the disposal of the embalmer that will help to ensure a thorough, balanced and pleasing result. It adds relatively little additional time to the whole embalming process and the incisions in the neck line can very easily be hidden by the use of a subcutaneous suture or the application of cosmetic wax after suturing. I know many embalmers who had made Restricted Cervical Injection part of the majority of their embalming as the results are superior to other techniques used.

### Enhance Emaciated Features Arterially Using Split Injection and Restricted Drainage

*by Sharon L. Gee*

If you poll the ranks of embalmers, the majority conduct feature enhancement or "tissue building" following embalming, prior to cosmetic application, dressing, and casketing. Therefore, academically, feature enhancement is a post-embalming treatment, separate, and distinct from arterial injection. The instrument of choice for this application is the needle and syringe. Consider the challenges of uniformly addressing the entire facial terrain in this manner while maintaining the integrity of natural and acquired facial markings. Consider eliminating this post-embalming treatment in favor of enhancing features DURING the arterial embalming.

Split injection, one-point injection, and restricted cervical injection are all injection methods that utilize the blood vascular system to deliver preservative chemicals. The split injection method (using the femoral artery as an injection site) affords the embalmer the most control in yielding uniform fluid distribution and symmetry in the facial tissues. The result can parallel a natural weight gain and present a healthy appearance. Feature enhancement through arterial injection can allow the embalmer to improve rather than change the decedent's appearance.

Split injection requires two vessel sites, one for injection and the other for drainage. It is understood that embalming fluid is more readily assimilated in the tissues nearest the site of injection and in the highest concentrations. Distance matters. To achieve symmetry of facial enhancement, the femoral (or common Iliac) vessel is raised for injection. A large volume of well-coordinated solution is injected toward the face without fear of overembalming these viewable features. The femoral vessel should be injected first distally to observe for fluid distribution, diffusion, and cosmetic coloring in the leg and to allow for adjustments of pressure and rate of flow before injecting superiorly. The benefit of distance from the femoral injection site to the head affords higher pressure and rate of flow settings to overcome vascular obstructions or resistances.

The most copious drainage is taken from the center of venous drainage in the dead human body, the heart. The site of drainage is the right atrium of the heart via a drainage instrument inserted into the right internal jugular vein. Blood, body fluids, and coagula are evacuated directly from the heart to reduce the opportunity for unwanted facial swelling. In facially emaciated decedents, the technique of restricting drainage (intermittent or alternate drainage) creates intravascular pressure so that large volumes of solution enter and remain in the facial tissues. Drainage restriction gives the embalmer the most control over fluid retention in the face and in combination with distance injection, which is the secret to enhancing contour uniformly.

While injecting, note the expansion of the intact right common carotid artery. Engorgement of this vessel is evidence of arterial preservative traveling to the head and of the intravascular pressure necessary to perfuse the preservative into the deep tissues. Pressure filtration is the passive transport mechanism chiefly responsible for preservative distribution and is created by the centrifugal embalming machine. The success of pressure filtration relies directly on the embalmer's ability to set the controls on the machine accordingly to overcome vascular resistances. Two other mechanisms, osmosis and dialysis, work concurrently with the force of the embalming machine to deliver and perfuse the tissues with preservative.

The embalmer optimizes the performance of the arterial chemical with the addition of co-injection and specialty chemicals. These additive chemicals boost the ability of the arterial preservative to distribute within the vascular system, to diffuse the deeper tissues to bind ultimately, with the protein molecules, and to create a necessary moisture balance within the tissues. Because large volumes of solution are injected toward the delicate facial tissues, the arterial formulation must not be too harsh. Hypertonic solutions may sear the capillary beds, hindering further distribution. Co-injections temper the harshness of formaldehyde, adjust pH, soften coagula, and condition the vascular system to readily accept the preservative. Co-injections act as a substitute for water. Water has no benefit to the embalmer save its function to dilute the chemicals. Lanolin-based specialty chemicals promote moisture retention to yield natural skin contour and pliability for the best and most natural presentation of the decedent. Humectant fluids also hydrate the tissues to prevent shrinking, wrinkling, and discoloration and reduce the surface evaporation that will occur over the course of the visitation and funeral. A word of caution, excessive humectant will yield the reverse effect; moisture is drawn from the tissues and dehydration is accelerated.

It is important that during injection of the last portion of the arterial solution, attempt to fully restrict drainage so that a very positive pressure is built within the vascular system. Once the embalmer is satisfied that a sufficient volume of solution has reached all tissues of the body and there has been a noted improvement of the sunken facial features, injection can be stopped. Carefully remove instruments and immediately tie off the vessels so that a positive pressure is maintained in the vascular system. Delay aspiration as long as possible giving tissues a time to fully firm and react to the arterial chemicals.

The embalmer of today faces new challenges brought forth by medical science advancements that extend the life span. Terminal patients are actively dying over longer intervals of time. Extended agonal periods create numerous embalming complications. One-point injections are a luxury and not the standard. Embalmers no longer believe multiple incisions symbolize defeat, rather the use of multiple sites for injection and drainage yields optimal value.[1]

## Embalming—United Kingdom and European
*Peter J. Ball, FBIE*
*Secretary, The European Association of Embalmers*

The subject of this discussion is embalming or, as it is often called in Europe—thanatopraxy. The European name of thanatopraxy was created to distinguish between the perception that embalming was in some way similar to mummification as practiced by the ancient Egyptians (among others): it is likely that the word embalming does not translate readily into non-English languages without attracting this inference. This is further underlined in some countries where embalming is forbidden by law, whereas thanatopraxy is a legitimate practice.

There is often a distinction between what is perceived as embalming by the medical profession and that practiced by the funeral business in the United Kingdom and other countries of similar funeral customs. It is as much a question of custom and purpose that serves to define the difference between the two types; for the sake of clarity, I intend to use the term "thanatopraxy" to differentiate between "funeral" embalming and "medical" embalming. Medical embalming is concerned only with preservation; thanatopraxy is concerned with preservation and presentation because of the practice of viewing the body by relations and friends of the bereaved. Thanatologists will argue the psychological benefits of this practice, but I do not propose to dwell on this subject that in itself provokes lengthy discussion. It has been part of funeral customs for many years within the United Kingdom and other countries to view the deceased, before the final disposal of the body; I am aware that this is not the case with many other countries where different cultures and therefore differing customs prevail. However, there does seem to be a common psychological need for some form of ceremony surrounding the disposal of the dead human body, and in many countries, a need to view the body is part of that ceremonial.

Medical embalming of the nonautopsied subject is achieved by the injection of a preservative mixture containing formaldehyde as the basic chemical—usually into the common carotid artery. This is supplemented by the injection of strong preservative into the thoracic and abdominal cavities. Drainage of blood is not often attempted, and the final appearance of the deceased is not an important consideration, preservation is the objective. High volumes of chemical are injected, which causes swelling of tissues in the face and limbs, and these tissues also tend to turn a gray color because of the reaction to formaldehyde. If the body has been the subject of an autopsy, medical embalming techniques vary. Some procedures involve the injection of preservative into the common carotid, subclavian, and femoral arteries supplemented by hypodermic injection into trunk tissues; others may simply inject straight into the tissues without use of the blood vessels. These techniques are not designed to accommodate viewing of the body and were never intended for this purpose. Modern usage outside of medical school subjects is more concerned with the safe and hygienic transport of deceased persons over long distances for the benefit of the transporting agent and the hygiene laws of any country or state who authorize entry of the body.

Thanatopraxy is concerned with the preservation, hygiene, and appearance of the dead human body, and in that sense shares two of the same objectives achieved by medical embalming, that is, those of preservation and hygiene. However, the crucial difference of rendering the remains fit for viewing demands a different approach. The chemicals used for injection into the arterial system are made from carefully compiled formulae with the end of achieving a natural appearance. Of necessity, these are stable compounds designed to overcome or, at worst, neutralize the effects of morbid conditions within the body to be treated, it is not surprising therefore that there are specialized formulations for some of the more common conditions such as jaundice, edema, and tissue gas.

In its simplest form, thanatopraxy is the injection of preservative chemical under pressure into the arterial system, which is then forced out into the capillaries to reach the tissue cell. Protein is coagulated by reaction with the embalming chemical, and blood is forced back toward the heart. In the nonautopsied subject, it is a matter of the introduction of a canula into a major artery, the injection of preservative chemical under pressure, and the removal of the blood via a vein drainage tube inserted into the internal jugular vein to reach the right atrium of the heart. The major arteries in normal use for adults are the common carotid, axillary, or femoral artery; the veins normally used are the internal jugular or the axillary vein. The technique is to inject through the artery until sufficient pressure is present in the vascular system, which is then relieved by opening a tap on the vein drainage tube; the blood flows through the tube and connects into a collecting jar for ultimate disposal. The vein tube is then closed, and injection is continued to build up pressure before opening the vein tube again to drain more blood, this alternation continues until the operator is satisfied that preservative has been distributed to all parts of the body.

If for any reason drainage through a vein is not possible, the introduction of a trocar into the right atrium of the heart is an effective means of blood drainage, the blood being drawn through the trocar into a closed container under a vacuum. On completion of injection, the trocar and aspiration apparatus is employed for removal of body fluids within the trunk cavities. As well as achieving preservation and disinfection, the effect of the injection is to restore normal color to the tissues and remove postmortem discoloration.

If the body has been the subject of an autopsy, a different technique is necessary and is dependent very much on the extent of the examination. Where there has been the complete removal of the organs in the trunk cavities during autopsy, these are again removed by the operator and treated, allowing access to the major arteries. Where they are intact, it is normal to inject distally into the common carotid, subclavian, and common iliac arteries; where there is damage to these, injection commences from the point distally beyond the damage. The blood drainage flows back into the cavities and is subsequently removed by aspiration. It is normally with the arteries of the head that the majority of difficulties occur, often as a result of careless removal of the tongue. I am fortunate in the area where I work to have a skilled postmortem technician who is able to remove the tongue, trachea, and esophagus without excising the common carotid arteries. In many instances, the damage is severe, and injection may only be possible via the external carotid, internal carotid, and external maxillary or facial arteries, and even these are often sufficiently damaged as to be of no practical use. The face is the most important area for viewing with the hands next in order of visual importance and it seems at times that some of the persons engaged in autopsy work are not aware of the consequences of their actions. For example and again in my area, some forensic pathologists are removing the facial tissues from the bones of the face, to leave the face held in place only by the tissues around the nose and eyes. This almost eliminates the possibility of arterial injection and removal of discoloration's caused by blood remaining in the blood vessels and significantly reduces the chance of viewing without signs of putrefaction. Further difficulties can be caused by the nature of the incision used for opening the trunk and head. The "V" incision causes the most damage to the neck and facial tissues, this consists of an incision from the pubes to the sternal notch and from that point across the neck on each side behind the ears and across the skull; the line of the incision is continuous. The incision causing the least damage extends from the sternal notch to the pubes, and the incision for cranial examination extends from behind one ear across the back part of the skull to a point behind the other ear.

These, briefly, are the methods employed by the qualified practitioner; there are many other complications and variations to the basic injection techniques described today. On completion of the injection, all tissues should be restored to a natural color with discoloration removed. The operator then washes and disinfects the body, cleaning all orifices and placing the features in an attitude of repose. Dressing of the body may be by the use of the deceased's own clothes or of funeral clothing as supplied by the funeral director. Injuries are treated and covered with cosmetics; the use of these varies according to the customs and beliefs of the deceased. The end result is that the deceased is presented with a more acceptable appearance than that of a person with the more obvious signs of death, so providing a more pleasant memory of the last time that it is possible to see them. This then defines the major objective of thanatopraxy—to render the experience of viewing the deceased less of an ordeal to those who are taking their final leave. Clearly, the appearance can only remain acceptable if preservation is achieved, equally disinfection is a vital feature because of the need for some mourners to touch and even kiss their loved one.

Thanatopraxy does not set out to achieve permanent preservation; there are many additional factors that influence this as I feel sure this assembly is already aware, and additional or even different techniques would be employed to achieve that objective. It is concerned only with the delay of putrefactive changes until after final disposal of the body.

There have always been difficulties with the transport of people who die many miles away from their home; the numbers of these have increased dramatically with the advent of ease of travel. On an international scale, a significant number of people die abroad and repatriation is required. In most of these cases, embalming or thantopraxy is a requirement by the transporting agency or the receiving country itself. In those countries where viewing is part of the funeral customs, it is often the case that this is impossible because of either poor quality treatment or the deceased has become unrecognizable. The latter instance arises from medical embalming because embalming by anybody other than members of the medical profession is forbidden in the country where the death has occurred. Unless the individual concerned has undergone training in modern embalming techniques, at best, it is unlikely that anything more than preservation will be achieved. This causes genuine distress to the bereaved, and if they insist upon viewing will leave only an unpleasant memory. I make no comment on the many examples of poor quality embalming received in some international transports, as professionals yourselves you would not condone incompetence. The worst examples of incompetent treatment seem to occur where the remains have been hermetically sealed and the coffin reopened for viewing on arrival at its destination. It may be that opening the coffin again was not considered to be a possibility; however, embalming has been paid for and should be carried out efficiently.

In conclusion, I would like to refer to the modern operator who may not be a qualified doctor. In Europe, it is only in France that a state qualification is required to practice thanatopraxy although other European countries are starting to legislate at local government level. In some cantons in Switzerland, it is now permissible for qualified operators to treat bodies for international transport, where until recently only doctors were permitted to do this. This is welcomed because there is a need for a qualified operator, properly trained for the care of the dead as a service to the bereaved person at a difficult time. In general, the interest of the medical profession is not concerned with the disposal of the deceased after life has become extinct. In some European countries, there is no prohibition against the use of unqualified persons. Suffice it to say that knowledge of disease, hygiene, anatomy and physiology, and other disciplines are an essential background to an efficient performance of the work in the modern scenario, and these form the basis of study for the modern embalmer or thanatopractitioner.

> ### The Art of Embalming and its Purpose
> Ron Hast
> From Mortuary Management, October 2006

Whenever I am asked to explain embalming, my response has been "Embalming is the best known method of presenting a deceased person in a state that will last well through the memorial event." If more information is requested, I say, "Blood is replaced with preservative chemicals, similar to a transfusion."

It is the privilege of any funeral director to decide whether an unembalmed body will be publically viewed, but to say the reason for requiring embalming is "to protect the public health" is not substantiated by any known scientific study. It is fair to expect anyone making such a claim would also enforce strict universal precautions from the instant mortuary personnel touch an unembalmed decedent, which is often not practiced, nor is it practiced in most health care institutions. If any health issues exist, they relate to those who handle, transport, and embalm bodies. Occupational hazards are not family or public risks. Handling an unembalmed body from initial care, refrigeration, casketing, and final cosmetic details can be more difficult than handling an embalmed body. But public presentation without embalming has been successfully and safely accomplished.

We know of the formal traditions and practices in Japan, England, and Jewish and Muslim communities, where refrigeration and frozen gel packs are routinely used throughout their services for stabilization and presentation, including those for large public audiences. For generations, these procedures have been practiced.

There are some who go so far as to claim that I am "anti-funeral" and opposed to the principles of proper funeral services. This is not true. I recognize the art of embalming, but also recognize the fact that bodies are often effectively and cosmetically presented throughout the world, including the United States, without embalming and health issues. I have observed this technique and results on numerous occasions. There are certainly instances and circumstances where embalming may be the best choice for temporary preservation and cosmetic enhancement. But it is not mandatory; it is a choice. If laws requiring embalming in certain states exit "for public health reasons," it is possible they are unfounded or politically based.

It is sad to note that certain death care "professionals" openly admit that if a family insists on viewing an unembalmed body, they make little attempt to enhance its appearance. If a client complains, their ready answer is that permission to embalm was denied and therefore appearance may be unsatisfactory.

With this topic coming to the forefront, several credentialed individuals were interviewed and contributed statements.

Dr. Lakshmanan Sathyavagiswaran, M.D., pathologist and chief medical examiner for the Los Angeles County for the past 15 years—well respected, appreciated, and honored by the medical profession and funeral service—says, "there is no reason that an unembalmed dead human body should be infectious to anyone attending visitation or public services. Persons transporting and handling bodies or cutting into them may be vulnerable in rare instances, with little or no risk if proper precautions are taken. To refuse to present a body unembalmed because of public health risk is unfounded. On rare occasions of certain deaths resulting from contagious disease, our office may encourage placing a face mask on the decedent before and during transportation and containment, and disposing without embalming or viewing. In the event, however, it becomes necessary to hold a body for an extended period of time before public services can be held, arterial embalming is recommended. Riding on an airplane or a bus may be a public health risk; the presence of an unembalmed body is not."

"The fact that dead bodies are a potential cause of epidemics after a disaster is almost always broadcast after major disasters. This 'fact' is a myth, and depriving survivors of appropriate burial ceremonies for their relatives may administer yet another blow to already injured or weakened persons. The only situation in which handling corpses is a risk is during epidemics of infectious diseases such as cholera. Even in these situations, no reason exists to totally deprive families from honoring their dead if they follow certain precautions. We have not at any point prescribed embalming as a method of protecting public health," says Bernadette Burden, Centers for Disease Control and Prevention (CDC), Atlanta, Georgia.

The question posed to the Dodge Company is whether they believe that a dead human body is a potential health risk. Their answer is "yes," because disease organisms do not die when a body dies. Rather, the lack of an immune system allows many of these organisms to reproduce very quickly. "We are not saying that a body, properly handled, is a health risk in every situation; rather, that it should be treated with care and that the person handling the body should use universal precautions as required by OSHA."

Should embalming be required in every situation if there is to be a viewing? Their answer is "no, we do not feel that embalming should be required as a condition to view unless the individual died from an infectious disease. We are of threat opinion only if the viewing family or individual is made aware of the natural process of decomposition, of how the body may look and of the time constraints placed on planning and holding a service when there is no embalming. Everyone has a different level of expectation and what one family or individual may find acceptable, another may find totally unacceptable. In today's litigious society (even with signed legal agreement indicating awareness of potential health risks and other potential problems) these issues need to play an important role in whether or not a business owner requires embalming if there is to be a public viewing," according to Debbie Dodge, The Dodge Chemical Company, Cambridge, Massachusetts.

"Representing that something, such as embalming, is legally required when that isn't the case is a violation of the FTC Funeral Rule and may give rise to liability under state laws as well," says Douglas O. Meyer, attorney and death care specialist, Woodland Hills, California.

"The art of embalming raises far above the clinical descriptions and opinions of direct handling of a human dead body. We must acknowledge that in many cultures, families take hold of a deceased person and intimately relate to the body from the moment of death to final disposition. It is unprofessional to primarily claim embalming is to protect public health. Our talents and artistry have proven to comfort survivors, giving them the best opportunity to embrace their dead without offensive natural occurrences. We do our work with pride, confidence and our contribution to the dignity of life through the death experience. It is the highest level of care through the death experience. It is the highest level of care and support to those who appreciate its values," notes Robert G. Mayer, author of *Embalming: History, Theory and Practice* (four editions), Pittsburgh, Pennsylvania.

Two long-term professors of accredited colleges of mortuary science were asked the following questions and gave the following answers (indicated as A1 and A2).

**Q:** Do the Schools teach methods and techniques of care for unembalmed bodies to be viewed?
**A1:** Yes, for identification purposes.
**A2:** Yes, briefly mentioned, but more on the subject is in order.

**Q:** Are students taught that embalming protects public health?
**A1:** Yes.
**A2:** Yes, and we test on that.

**Q:** Do students who graduate from your program understand that embalming protects public health?
**A1:** Yes.
**A2:** Yes.

**Q:** If a friend died and the spouse requested the unembalmed body to be present and viewed for a large public service, would you refuse to accommodate?
**A1:** No.
**A2:** No.

**Q:** Would you warn the family of public health exposure risks?
**A1:** No.
**A2:** No.

The content of what they are teaching is inconsistent with the facts. One admitted, "Your information is indefensible. Changes need to be made to the curriculum." Their candid comments and open discussion on the subject were impressive, and one instructor expressed willingness to change what he teaches in light of professional opinions and scientific conclusions.

The American Board of Funeral Service Education defines embalming as "The process of chemically treating the dead human body to reduce the presence and growth of microorganisms—to temporarily inhibit organic decomposition and to restore an acceptable physical appearance."

If a reason for embalming is to slow decomposition (and provide a base for cosmetic enhancement), refrigeration must also be acknowledged as a method of temporary preservation that yields similar stabilizing results. Is there some reason that many funeral directors do not have refrigeration facilities?

I emphasize that this information is not an attempt to promote death care without embalming. The values of embalming are well known. But firsthand knowledge of many who believe and claim to their clientele (when asking permission to embalm) if viewing is planned, embalming is required to protect the public health is misleading. To say embalming is a requirement of your firm to present the body for visitation and funeral services may be closer to the truth.

All said, here is a thoughtful way to request permission to embalm: "Trusting us to provide care and services includes certain choices and authorizations. If you intend to have formal viewing and public services, embalming is proper to control natural changes that may occur. May we have your authorizations to proceed?" If further information is requested about embalming, it may be said that "Natural discoloration, gasses, fluids and odors may occur. Embalming controls these and other concerns."

### Embalming COVID-19: Infection Control and Storage*

Jzyk S. Ennis, PhD

Early 2020, global embalmers faced a pandemic caused by a new, infectious version of the coronavirus (SARS-COv-2); more commonly known as COVID-19. Scientists and infectious control physicians classified COVID-19 as a highly infectious and transmitted disease. "*Risk of Infection and Tracking of Work-related Infectious Disease in the Funeral Industry*," a study published by Susan Davidson and Dr. William Benjamin appears in the Selected Readings section of this textbook. The study contains the statement: "The infectious nature of cadavers, regardless of their cause of death, has been documented. The routine transport and embalming of cadavers place Funeral Service Personnel (FSP) in a position to be exposed to multiple infectious agents that are transmissible by mucocutaneous contamination, aerosolization, and direct inoculation." Embalmers are trained to approach every case as potentially infectious (Universal Precautions). Infectious protocols were instituted immediately for the embalming of COVID-19 cases. PPE supplies were found to be woefully lacking worldwide; becoming virtually impossible to obtain new surpluses for funeral home use. Most funeral homes faced insufficient quantities of PPE needed for the pandemic.

A reverse look at another coronavirus, Severe Acute Respiratory Syndrome (SARS) brings a valuable comparison. SARS bears a close resemblance to COVID-19. Another close consideration is *M. tuberculosis* (TB). In the study, "*Protecting health care workers from SARS and other respiratory pathogens: A review of the infection control literature,*" findings support the proper selection of PPE, reduction of procedures that can cause aerosolization of particles, and environmental disinfection as critically important to reduce the potential of infection of health care workers, like embalmers. Furthermore, the study found medical procedures, like intubation, could actually cause

---
*The original version of this article appeared in *The Texas Director*, April 2020.

smaller droplets of infectious materials to travel greater distances than coughing or sneezing.

The following procedures practiced during embalming can cause aerosolization of particles: aspirating, cleaning, and packing of nasal and oral orifices and cavity aspiration of the lungs and structures in the throat. Davidson and Benjamin found that, "The routine aspiration of blood and other body fluids carries the risks of aerosolization of droplets nuclei." Great care should be taken in each of these procedures, and only the licensed embalmer should be exposed during the embalming process. Limiting the number of people performing embalming procedures to reduce the potential for exposure and infection is highly recommended. Covering the face of the decedent with a damp cloth during transport and pre-embalming procedures is highly recommended. COVID-19 is known to be a respiratory illness. The virus can also be detected in the blood by serum testing. While not considered a blood-borne infection, a prudent step to reduce risk is the use of closed drainage during embalming. A venous drain tube is preferred to the angular spring forceps. A generous length of tubing sufficient to reach the drain is connected to the device to contain blood drainage along its route toward disposal. Furthermore, cover the drainage sink or water control unit to prevent aerosolized particles from becoming airborne; plexiglass or plastic film is suggested. Clean and sanitize disposal units and sink surfaces after use.

## Best Practices for the Embalming of Bodies with COVID-19:

- Follow protocols of the CDC and reputable health authorities.
- Properly don (put on) all required and appropriate PPE.
- Minimize aerosolization of infected materials.
- Carefully disinfect nasal and oral cavities with a mortuary-grade disinfectant. Firmly pack orifices after cleaning; oral and nasal purge during embalming can aerosolize infectious materials.
- Use a high index arterial fluid to mix a high strength arterial solution concentration (see below).
- Use a slow rate of flow. A high rate of flow can cause distention of internal organs, lead to purge, and the aerosolization of infectious materials.
- Use approved hospital/mortuary-grade disinfectants that kill coronavirus and other infectious agents. Follow the required surface contact time for maximum efficiency. Failure to follow guidelines can result in improper and inadequate disinfection.
- Properly doff (remove) and dispose of all PPE in an approved biohazard waste container.
- Perform embalmer hygiene after doffing PPE: immediately wash hands; a minimum of 20 seconds is advised to reduce microbial contaminants.
- Conduct periodic post-embalming monitoring of the remains until final disposition; make necessary corrections.

SARS-CoV-2 is a new virus and embalmers question arterial fluid selection and solution concentration. Embalming standards of care provide guidance to the embalmer. COVID-19 impacts the respiratory system similar to diseases like tuberculosis (TB). Organ and tissue damage is commonly observed in COVID-19 patients. High-strength concentrations near 5.75% were required during and immediately following the influenza pandemics of 1918 and 1919. Early embalming chemicals lacked the advancements of current products; formaldehyde gray was expected using the harsh formulations of the time. Modern standards indicate a **minimum** arterial solution strength of 2.0% for effective tissue preservation and sanitizing. The infectious nature of COVID-19 coupled with expected time delays between embalming and final disposition, necessitates a strong, well-coordinated solution. Chemical selection is based upon the pre-embalming analysis and professional judgment of the embalmer. Mortuary care standards for the preparation of armed forces service members in the United States require no less than 5.0% concentration, by volume, of formaldehyde; the total volume injected not less than 1 gallon per 50 pounds of body weight. A reference to embalming concentration, in the Selected Reading section (*Summary of Guidelines Submitted to OSHA from the National Funeral Directors Association Committee on Infectious Disease (NFDA)*) suggests a 3.0% concentration for infectious disease cases. These guidelines offer realistic starting points for the embalmer facing a COVID-19 embalming case.

Cavity aspiration and treatment must be performed so as to reduce aerosolization of infectious materials during the process. Aspiration of the cavities should be performed immediately after arterial injection. Following aspiration, introduce 32–48 ounces of a high index cavity fluid. Perform cavity re-aspiration and re-injection of cavity chemical as needed. Topically apply a mold inhibiting chemical when a lengthy interval before final disposition is anticipated and also when the deceased is placed into mortuary refrigeration or a holding area that may be prone to climate dampness. Inspect the embalmed remains periodically for signs of tissue softening, purge, odors, leakage, insect infestation, tissue gas, dehydration, and other conditions that require corrective embalming treatments.

In cases of autopsy, the structures of the respiratory system are customarily removed along with the visceral organs. Additional consideration should be given to the body cavities. Use a hospital/mortuary grade disinfectant to liberally spray the body cavities of the autopsied case. Treat the bag containing the viscera with liberal cavity chemical. Follow CDC recommendations and infectious protocols for disposal of body bags and other contaminated items.

In conclusion, short of any directive from the CDC or other governmental agency preventing embalming of a COVID-19-related deaths, embalming can continue to be performed as long as standards of care for infectious embalming are observed. Embalming reduces risk and allows physical memorialization of the dead at a later date when delays in disposition are inevitable. Mortuary refrigeration after embalming may provide an extra layer of security until the time of memorialization and final disposition. Similar to military combat training, embalmers are trained for combat with an invisible pathogen and tasked with caring for those who have died from it. Embalmers that stay informed, follow CDC guidelines, professional standards of care, wear appropriate PPE, and consider experience and good common-sense practices will continue to safely embalming those who have died from COVID-19 complications. The families, friends, and communities will have the meaningful closure they need.

## Cosmetic Airbrushing of Un-embalmed Decedents*

*By Daryl M. Hammond*

As an increasing number of families consider cremation as the final method of disposition, funeral directors are faced with more requests for private family viewing of their loved one prior to cremation. When this service does not involve arterial embalming, several challenges exist for the embalmer to successfully present un-embalmed remains.

The main challenge for the embalmer is to compensate for the physical condition of the body. A preliminary case analysis should be done before the arrangement conference, whenever possible, in order to direct the family as to when a viewing time is most feasible. Sometimes the deceased body will present a near-perfect scenario for successful viewing, even when viewing cannot happen until several days after death. Sometimes this can be accomplished with minimal effort on the part of the embalmer. More often, the deceased is not in near-perfect condition. Refrigeration, if available, may slow the cycle of decomposition and "purchase" needed time.

Some difficult situations include emaciation, edema, swelling, purge, discoloration of the face or hands, trauma, autopsy or tissue donation, gas accumulation and advanced decomposition of the body. While treatments exist to temporarily stabilize the body from further decomposition changes occurring during the viewing, the family can't appreciate the effort required by the embalmer. The result is noticeable, but the effort required to achieve those results is not. More than anything, the family will notice the cosmetics. Successful cosmetic application that erases intense discolorations or trauma will provide a comforting and lasting memory picture.

The application of airbrush cosmetics is ideal for concealing intense discolorations on un-embalmed tissues of the face and hands.

A few specific preparations must be made *before* applying airbrush cosmetics to any remains, but especially un-embalmed remains. The body should be bathed, the hair shampooed and fingernails cleaned and groomed before cosmetic application. Shave the face as necessary, women and children too. Cosmetic will stick to fine facial hair and produce an unsatisfactory appearance. Pay particular attention to the removal of hair in the nostrils, ears and on the neck.

The skin of the face and hands must be clean, free from oils and fully dry before applying airbrush cosmetics. Lanolin-based massage creams and sprays leave an oily residue that will interfere with the adhesion of airbrush cosmetics. To ensure the best adhesion of the cosmetic to resist rub-off when the skin surface is touched or kissed during viewing, perform a preliminary cleansing of oily skin.

The use of pure acetone (propanone) on a cotton pad is a highly effective solvent for removing oily creams and sprays as well as deposits of dead skin cells and sebaceous oils on the skin's surface. A thorough cleansing of oils from the facial terrain includes any facial crevices, especially alongside the wings of the nose and in the furrows of the forehead, and along the hairline, in the eyebrows and the eyelashes. Acetone will also remove the stubborn residue left behind from bandage adhesives.

Feature setting is critical for satisfactory results. The use of eye caps, mouth closures, tissue filler and cotton may be necessary to achieve optimal appearance. Eyelids and lips must be properly aligned and secured with an adhesive prior to airbrushing. The force of air expelled from the tip of the airbrush can re-open the eyes and mouth when the adhesive bond is weak. Cotton strips should be placed as deeply as possible into the nasal cavities. Air flow from the airbrush may enter the nostrils and force out any fluids that have collected in the nasal passages. Once the above preparations have been addressed, airbrush cosmetics can be successfully applied.

First, select an airbrush system that will generate steady air pressure (in a range from 20–40 psi). The component separate from the "gun", is called the air compressor. The compressor sets the force of the air flow and air pressure. A lower air flow and pressure lets the operator get closer to the surface for covering smaller areas, will use less cosmetics, and produces less overspray onto areas, like a styled hairline. A higher flow and pressure will provide broader and faster coverage but will use more volume of cosmetic quickly. The potential for overspray of cosmetics is also greater under higher pressures.

Next, select a water-based airbrushing cosmetic for easy cleanup without the need for solvents. A small piece of cotton, dry foam rubber or your fingers work great for stripping water-based foundation from the hairline. Cosmetic lines offer everything from foundation to blush, eyeshadow, eyebrow and eyelash color, and lip color. Personal preference dictates. You may prefer to apply only the foundation cosmetic using the airbrush to conceal difficult discolorations or cover any wax work. Then follow with application of your choice of traditional cosmetics overtop the airbrushed foundation. Water-based airbrush cosmetics will dry very quickly, however be certain. Perform a touch test first to ensure dryness before applying ornamental cosmetics. If you accidentally apply the wrong color or too much of it, you don't need to remove it and start all over again. Simply spray overtop with the airbrush cosmetic and reapply the traditional cosmetic.

When ornamental nail polish is not an option, the fingernails may also be treated with a light dusting of airbrushed cosmetic for a very natural look.

At the completion of all cosmetic application, apply a light coat of clear finishing spray, such as hairspray or artist lacquer, to the face, neck, and hands to seal against rub-off and cosmetic transfer. The deceased is now ready for the final viewing.

One final note. We are the true experts when it comes to caring for the deceased. The additional time and attention you have given to the deceased will translate into going that extra mile for the family! They will notice.

Daryl M. Hammond is a licensed Funeral Director and Embalmer in north Georgia. In 1993, Daryl developed a line of cosmetics, *DMH Airbrush Foundation*, for his personal use. Soon after, he began marketing his complete airbrushing kit to local funeral homes. To advance the restorative art skills of his fellow embalmers, Daryl created a series of *Restorative Art Training Heads* (*RATH*). RATH training models are used by numerous mortuary and university programs across the country.

---

*Originally published in Michigan Funeral Directors Association Journal. Volume 79(4), Fall 2019. © Copyright 2019, MFDA Services Corporation. All rights reserved. Used with permission.

## REFERENCES

1. Mayer R. *Embalming History Theory and Practice.* 5th ed. New York: McGraw Hill Medical, 2012.
2. Davidson S., Benjamin W. Risk of infection and tracking of work-related infectious diseases in the funeral industry. Selected reading. In: *Embalming History, Theory and Practice,* 5th ed. New York: McGraw Hill Medical, 2012, p. 647.
3. Gammage B., Moore D., Copes R., et al. Protecting health care workers From SARS and other respiratory pathogens: A review of the infection control literature. *American Journal of Infection Control* 2005;33:114–121.
4. Davidson S., Benjamin W. *Risk of infection and tracking of work-related infectious diseases in the funeral industry.* Selected reading. In: *Embalming: History, Theory, and Practice,* 5th ed., New York: McGraw Hill Medical, 2012, p. 648.
5. Mayer R. *Embalming: History, Theory, and Practice,* 5th ed. McGraw Hill Medical: New York, 2012, p. 126.
6. Mayer R. *Embalming: History, Theory, and Practice,* 5th ed. McGraw Hill Medical: New York, 2012.
7. Ennis J. *Embalming Standards of Care.* KDP Publishing, 2016.
8. Ennis J. *Embalming and Renal Failure: A Silent Danger for Embalmers.* KDP Publishing, 2018.
9. Mayer R. *Embalming: History, Theory, and Practice,* 5th ed., New York: McGraw Hill Medical, 2012, pp. 611–612.
10. Mayer R. *Embalming: History, Theory, and Practice,* 5th ed. New York: McGraw Hill Medical, 2012, pp. 610–611.

## FOOTNOTES FOR SELECTED READINGS

[1] Ricketts, Maura, et al. Emerging Infectious Diseases, Volume 3, Number 2, 1997. National Center for Infectious Diseases, CDC.

[2] Division of Viral and Rickettsial Diseases, National Center for Infectious Diseases, CDC.

[3] Ibid.

[4] Brown P. The human spongiform encephalopathies: Kuru, Creutzfeldt-Jakob Disease, and the Gerstmann-Straussler-Scheinker. *Current Topics in Microbiology and Immunology* 1991;172:1–20.

[5] The gene is known as the scrapie amyloid precursor gene and is located on chromosome 20.

[6] Brown P. National Institute of Neurological Disorders and Strokes.

[7] Manuelidis L. The dimensions of Creutzfeldt-Jakob disease. *Transfusion* 1994;34:915–928.

[8] Sanders et al. *Dorland's Medical Dictionary,* 28th ed., 1998.

[9] Ozel M. Small viruslike structure in fractions from scrapie hamster brain. *Lancet* 1994;343:894–895.

[10] Adams RD, et al. *Principles of Neurology,* 6th ed., 1998:771–773.

[11] De Silva R. Human spongiform encephalopathy: clinical presentations and diagnostic tests. In: *Methods in Molecular Medicine: Prion Diseases;* 1996:15–33.

[12] Masters CL, et al. Creutzfeldt-Jakob disease: patterns of worldwide occurrence and the significance of familiar and sporadic clustering. *Annals of Neurology* 1979;5:177–188.

[13] Holman R, et al. Creutzfeldt-Jakob Disease in the United States, 1979–1994. *Emerging Infectious Diseases* 1996;2(4):333–337.

[14] Campbell D, et al. CJD Fact Sheet, *CJD Voice.*

[15] Ibid.

[16] Gibbs CJ. National Institutes of Health.

[17] Collinge J, et al. Genetic predisposition to iatrogenic Creutzfeldt-Jakob disease. *Lancet* 1991;337:1441–1442.

[18] Lasmezas CI, et al. Transmission of the BSE agent in mice in the absence of abnormal prion protein. *Science* 1997;275:402–405.

[19] Will RG, et al. A new variant of Creutzfeldt-Jakob disease in the UK. *Lancet* 1996;347:921–925.

[20] Gibbs CJ, et al. Creutzfeldt-Jakob disease: transmission to the chimpanzee. *Science* 1968;161:388–391.

[21] Brown P. Environmental causes of human spongiform encephalopathy. Methods in molecular medicine: prion diseases. Humana Press, 1996:139–154.

[22] Esmonde T, et al. Creutzfeldt-Jakob disease and lyophilised dura mater grafts. *Journal of Neurology, Neurosurgery and Psychiatry* 1994;56:999–1000.

[23] Centers for Disease Control. *Morbidity and Mortality Weekly Report* 1985;34:359–60, 365–366.

[24] Nevin S, et al. Subacute spongiform encephalopathy: A subacute form attributable to vascular dysfunction. *Brain* 1960;83:519–564.

[25] National Institutes of Health, Biomedical Laboratory Safety, Section VII, Viral Agents.

[26] Manuelidis EE, et al. Transmission to animals of Creutzfeldt-Jakob disease from human blood. *Lancet* 1985;2:896–897.

[27] Lavelle GC, et al. Isolation from mouse spleen of cell populations with high specific infectivity from scrapie virus. *Infection and Immunity* 1972;5:319–323.

[28] Heye N, et al. Creutzfeldt-Jakob disease and blood transfusion. *Lancet* 1994;343:298–299.

[29] Creange A, et al. Creutzfeldt-Jakob disease after liver transplantation. *Annals of Neurology* 1995;38:269–272.

[30] Patry D. Neurology, 1998, June. Dept. of Medicine, University of Calgary.

[31] Minutes of the Special Emphasis panel on Creutzfeldt-Jakob Disease and Blood Transfusion. September 24–25, 1997.

[32] Ricketts M, et al. Is Creutzfeldt-Jakob disease transmitted in blood? *Emerging Infectious Diseases* 1997;3(2):155–163.

[33] National Institutes of Health, Biomedical Laboratory Safety, Section VII, Viral Agents.

[34] Brown P. Guidelines for High Risk Autopsy Cases: Special Precautions for Creutzfeldt-Jakob Disease. College of American Pathologists, Autopsy Performance and Reporting, 1990.

[35] Ibid.

[36] Adams RD, et al. *Principles of Neurology,* 6th ed., pp. 771–773.

[37] Bernoulli C, et al. Danger of accidental person to person transmission of Creutzfeldt-Jakob disease by surgery. *Lancet* 1977;1.

[38] Strub CG, Frederick LG. *The Principles and Practice of Embalming.* LG Frederick, Dallas Texas, 1967.

[39] Guidelines for Control of Infections in Hospital Pathology, University of Washington Medical Center, 1998.

[40] Dilution of bleach should be done at the time of use. Bleach diluted with water loses its effectiveness within hours of being diluted. Maximum effectiveness of bleach takes at least 10–30 minutes of contact. In the case of CJD, 2 hours of soaking is recommended.

[41] National Institutes of Health, Biomedical Laboratory Safety, Section VII, Viral Agents.

[42] Gilligan TS. ADA vs CJD, The Director, 2000.

[43] National Center for Infectious Diseases, Hospital Infections Program. Creutzfeldt-Jakob Disease: Epidemiology, Risk Factors and De-contamination.

[44] Will RG. Professor, National CJD Surveillance Unit, West General Hospital, Edinburgh, 2000.

# Glossary

## Embalming, Restorative Art and Mortuary Cosmetology Terms*

**Abdominal anatomical regions.** (1) Nine regions of the abdomen as demarcated by four imaginary planes, two of which are horizontal (indicated by lines drawn across the right and left tenth ribs and across the right and left anterior superior iliac spines) and two sagittal (indicated by lines drawn from the midpoint of inguinal ligament to the nipples on the chest and right and left sides). Upper row: right hypochondriac, epigastric, left hypochondriac. Middle row: right lateral, umbilical, left lateral. Lower row: right inguinal, pubic, left inguinal. (2) Four regions of the abdomen as demarcated by two imaginary planes, one horizontal and the other midsagittal: upper right quadrant, upper left quadrant, lower right quadrant, and lower left quadrant.

**Abrasion.** Antemortem injuries resulting from friction of the skin against a firm object and causing removal of the epidermis.

**Abscess.** Localized accumulation of pus.

**Abut.** To touch or contact, as with the tarsal plates of the closed eyelids.

**Accessory chemicals.** Chemicals used in addition to vascular (arterial) and cavity embalming fluids. Include but are not limited to hardening compounds, preservative powders, sealing agents, mold preventive agents, and compress application agents.

**Acetone.** Dimethyl ketone; a colorless liquid used to soften and remove scabs; a solvent for restorative wax; a stain remover.

**Acquired facial markings.** Facial markings that develop during one's lifetime, primarily as a result of repetitious use of certain muscles.

**Acquired immunodeficiency syndrome (AIDS).** Specific group of diseases or conditions that are indicative of severe immunosuppression related to infection with the human immunodeficiency virus (HIV).

**Action level (AL).** Exposure limit usually one half of the Occupational Safety and Health Administration (OSHA) legal limit for a regulated substance. This level is established to ensure adequate protection of employees at exposures below the OSHA limits, but to minimize the compliance burdens for employers whose employees have exposures below the 8-hour permissible exposure limit (PEL). The AL for formaldehyde is 0.5 ppm.

**Actual pressure.** See Pressure.

**Adipocere/Grave wax.** Soft, grayish-white to brown, wax-like material composed of oleic, palmitic, and steric (fatty) acids. Formed by the postmortem hydrolysis and hydrogenation of body fats. Most prominent in the subcutaneous tissue but can occur wherever fat is present. Recent research indicates bacterial enzymes may be primarily responsible by converting unsaturated liquid fats (oleic acid) to saturated liquid fats.

**Aerobic.** In the presence of free oxygen.

**Aerosol.** Colloidal solution dispensed as a mist.

**Aerosolization.** Dispersal as an aerosol. Minute particles of blood and water become atomized and suspended in air when water under pressure meets the blood drainage or when flushing an uncovered flush sink.

**Agglutination.** Intravascular: increase in viscosity of blood brought about by the clumping of particulate formed elements in the blood vessels.

**Agonal algor.** Decrease in body temperature immediately before death.

**Agonal coagulation.** In reference to blood, a change from fluid to thickened mass.

**Agonal dehydration.** Loss of moisture from the living body during the agonal state.

**Agonal edema.** Escape of blood serum from an intravascular to an extravascular location immediately before death.

**Agonal fever.** Increase in body temperature immediately before death.

**Agonal period.** Period immediately before somatic death.

**Agonal translocation.** See Translocation.

**Airbrush.** Pressured atomizer used for spraying liquid paint or cosmetic on a surface.

**Algor mortis.** Postmortem cooling of the body to the surrounding temperature.

**Alkaline hydrolysis.** A method of disposition for human and pet remains using heat and lye. Also called aquamation, biocremation, resomation, flameless cremation, or water cremation.

**Alopecia.** Absence or loss of hair.

**Alternate drainage.** Method of injection-drainage in which embalming solution is injected and then injection is stopped while drainage is open.

**Alveolar process.** Bony ridge found on the inferior surface of the maxilla and the superior surface of the mandible that contains the sockets for the teeth.

**American Congress of Governmental Industrial Hygienists (ACGIH).** An organization of professional personnel in government agencies or educational institutions who are employed in occupational safety and health programs.

**Amino acids.** Building blocks of which proteins are constructed and the end products of protein digestion or hydrolysis. The basic formula is $NH_2$–CHR–COOH–amino group, an alpha carbon, any aliphatic or aromatic radical, and a carboxyl group.

**Anaerobic.** In the absence of free oxygen.

**Anasarca.** Severe generalized edema.

**Anatomical guides.** Descriptive references for locating arteries and veins by means of the anatomical structures that are known.

**Anatomical limits.** Points of origin and points of termination in relation to adjacent structures. Used to designate the boundaries of arteries.

**Anatomical position.** The body is erect, feet together, palms facing forward, and thumbs pointed away from body.

---

*Portions prepared by the Embalming (2016) and Restorative Art (2014) Syllabus committees of the American Board of Funeral Service Education.

**Anchor.** Material or technique employed to secure tissues or restorative materials in a fixed position; an armature.
**Aneurysm.** Localized abnormal dilation or outpocketing of a blood vessel resulting from a congenital defect or a weakness of the vessel wall.
**Aneurysm hook.** Embalming instrument used primarily for blunt dissection and raising vessels.
**Aneurysm needle.** Embalming instrument used primarily for blunt dissection and raising vessels; the "eye" in the hook of the aneurysm needle is for passing ligature beneath vessels.
**Angle of the mandible.** Body angle formed by the junction of the posterior edge of the ramus of the mandible and the inferior surface of the body of the mandible.
**Angular spring forceps.** Multipurpose instrument (size can vary) used in the embalming process (e.g., as a drainage instrument).
**Angulus oris eminence.** Small, convex prominence found lateral to the end of the line of closure of the mouth; a natural facial marking.
**Angulus oris sulcus.** Groove found at each end of the line of closure of the mouth; a natural facial marking.
**Anomaly.** Deviation from the normal.
**Antecubital.** In front of the elbow/in the bend of the elbow.
**Antemortem.** Before death.
**Antemortem subcutaneous emphysema.** A distension of the body tissues by the presence of gas or air beneath the skin; an antemortem condition brought about by a surgical procedure, trauma, or by a puncture or tear in the pleural sac or the lung tissue.
**Anterior.** Before or in front of; an anatomical term of position and direction, which denotes the front or forward part.
**Anterior nares.** External nostril openings.
**Anterior superior iliac spine.** A bony protuberance that can be palpated topographically, found on the ilium, the superior broad portion of the hip bone; the origin of the inguinal ligament and the sartorius muscle.
**Anticoagulant fluid.** Ingredient of embalming fluids that retards the natural postmortem tendency of blood to become more viscous or prevents adverse reactions between blood and other embalming chemicals.
**Apparent death.** Condition in which the manifestations of life are feebly maintained.
**Aqueous.** Watery; prepared with water as a solvent.
**Aqueous humor.** Clear, thin, alkaline fluid that fills the anterior chamber of the eyeball.
**Armature.** Framework; a material, commonly of pliable metal or wood, employed to provide support for a wax restoration.
**Arterial (solution) delivery.** Movement of the vascular solution from its source (e.g., embalming machine tank) through the machine apparatus, connective tubing and arterial tube into an artery.
**Arterial (vascular) fluid.** Concentrated, preservative, embalming chemical that is diluted with water to form the arterial solution for injection into the arterial system during vascular embalming. Its purpose is to inactivate saprophytic bacteria and render the body tissues less susceptible to decomposition.
**Arterial solution.** Mixture of arterial (vascular) fluid and water used for the arterial injection. May include supplemental fluids.
**Arterial tube.** Tube used to inject embalming solution into the blood vascular system.
**Arteriosclerosis.** Term applied to a number of pathological conditions causing a thickening, hardening, and loss of elasticity of the walls of the arteries.
**Articulation.** Place of union between two or more bones.
**Ascites.** Accumulation of serous fluids in the peritoneal cavity.
**Asepsis.** Freedom from infection and from any form of life. Sterility.
**Asphyxia.** Insufficient intake of oxygen. Numerous causes.
**Aspiration.** Withdrawal of gas, fluids, and semisolids from body cavities and hollow viscera by means of suction with an aspirator and a trocar.
**Asymmetry.** Lack of symmetry, balance, or proportion.
**Atheroma.** Fatty degeneration or thickening of the walls of the larger arteries occurring in atherosclerosis.
**Autoclave.** Apparatus used for sterilization by steam pressure, usually at 250°F (121°C) for a specific time.
**Autolysis.** Self-destruction of cells. Decomposition of all tissues by enzymes that form without microbial assistance.
**Autolytic enzyme.** The body's own digestive enzymes that are capable of destroying body cells (autolytic decomposition).
**Autopsy.** Postmortem examination of the organs and tissues of a body to determine cause of death or pathological condition. Necropsy.
**Bactericidal agent.** Agent that destroys bacteria.
**Bacteriostatic agent.** Agent that has the ability to inhibit or retard bacterial growth. No destruction of viability is implied.
**Balsamic substance.** Resin combined with oil. A fragrant, resinous, oily exudate from various trees and plants.
**Base.** (1) In cosmetology, the vehicle in a cosmetic (oil base); the initial application of cream or cosmetics. (2) The lower part of anything, the supporting part.
**Base of the axillary space.** Armpit.
- **Anterior boundary.** Established by drawing a line along the fold of skin that envelops the lateral border of the pectoralis major muscle.
- **Lateral boundary.** Established by drawing a line that connects the two points where the pectoralis major and latissimus dorsi muscles blend into the arm.
- **Medial boundary.** Established by drawing a line that connects the two points where the pectoralis major and latissimus dorsi muscles blend into the chest wall.
- **Posterior boundary.** Established by drawing a line along the fold of skin that envelops the lateral border of the latissimus dorsi muscle.

**Basket weave suture.** (Cross-stitch) Network of stitches that cross the borders of a cavity or excision to anchor fillers and sustain tissues in their proper position.
**Bilateral.** Having two sides.
**Bilateral differences.** Dissimilarities existing in the two sides or halves of an object.
**Bilateral silhouette.** The bilateral view; an inferior or superior viewpoint that permits the comparison of the two sides or halves of an object or facial feature.
**Biohazard.** Biological agent or condition that constitutes a hazard to humans.
**Biological death.** Irreversible somatic death.
**Bischloromethyl ether (BCME).** A carcinogen potentially produced when formaldehyde and sodium hypochlorite come into contact with each other. Normally occurs only in a controlled laboratory setting and requires a catalyst.
**Bleach.** Chemical that lightens or blanches skin discoloration.
**Bleaching.** Act of lightening a discoloration by hypodermic means or by surface compress.
**Bleaching agent.** A chemical that lightens a skin discoloration.
**Blister.** Thin vesicle on the skin containing liquid matter.
**Blood.** Cell-containing fluid that circulates through the blood vascular system and is composed of approximately 22% solids and 78% water.
**Bloodborne pathogens.** See Bloodborne Pathogens Standard.
**Bloodborne Pathogens Standard (29 CFR 1910.1030).** Occupational Safety and Health Administration (OSHA) regulation concerning exposure of employees to blood and other body fluids. The following are OSHA definitions.
- **Blood.** Human blood, human blood components, and products made from human blood.

- **Bloodborne pathogens.** Pathogenic microorganisms that are present in human blood and can cause disease in humans. These pathogens include, but are not limited to, hepatitis B virus (HBV) and human immunodeficiency virus (HIV).
- **Contaminated.** Marked by the presence or reasonably anticipated presence of blood or other potentially infectious materials on an item or surface.
- **Contaminated laundry.** Laundry that has been soiled with blood or other potentially infectious materials or may contain sharps.
- **Contaminated sharps.** Any contaminated object that can penetrate the skin including, but not limited to, needles, scalpels, broken glass, and exposed ends of dental wires.
- **Engineering controls.** Eliminate or reduce exposure to a chemical or physical hazard through the use or substitution of equipment or engineered machinery. Examples: room ventilation and air exchange; backflow preventers and vacuum breakers.
- **Exposure incident.** Specific eye, mouth, other mucous membrane, nonintact skin, or parenteral contact with blood or other potentially infectious materials that results from the performance of an employee's duties.
- **Occupational exposure.** Reasonably anticipated skin, eye, mucous membrane, or parenteral contact with blood or other potentially infectious materials that may result from the performance of an employee's duties.
- **Parenteral.** Introduced into the body by way of piercing the mucous membranes or the skin barrier, for example, by needlesticks, human bites, cuts, and abrasions.
- **Personal protective equipment (PPE).** Clothing and equipment worn by an employee for protection against a hazard.
- **Universal Precautions.** An approach to infection control in which all human blood and certain human body fluids are treated as if they are contaminated with HIV, hepatitis B virus (HBV), and other bloodborne pathogens.
- **Work practice controls.** Controls that reduce the likelihood of exposure by altering the manner in which a task is performed (e.g., prohibiting recapping of needles, not allowing blood splatter or aerosolization of blood while draining during the embalming process).

**Blood discoloration.** Discolorations, intravascular or extravascular, resulting from changes in blood composition, content, or location.

**Blood pressure.** Pressure exerted by the blood on the arterial wall in the living body and measured in millimeters of mercury.

**Blood vascular system.** Circulatory network composed of the heart, arteries, arterioles, capillaries, venules, and veins.

**Blunt dissection.** Separation and pushing aside of the superficial fascia leading to blood vessels and then the deep fascia surrounding blood vessels, using manual techniques or round-ended instruments that separate rather than cut the protective tissues.

**Body of the mandible.** Horizontal portion of the lower jaw.

**Boil.** Acute, deep-seated inflammation in the skin. Usually begins as a subcutaneous swelling in a hair follicle.

**Bridge.** Raised support; the arched portion of the nose, which is supported by the nasal bones; a structure or span connecting two parts of a mutilated bone.

**Bridge suture.** (Interrupted suture) A temporary suture consisting of individually cut and tied stitches employed to sustain the proper position of tissues.

**Bruise.** (Ecchymosis) An injury caused by a blow without laceration; a contusion.

**Buccal cavity.** The space between the lips and the gums and teeth; the vestibule of the oral cavity.

**Buccal depressions.** Natural, shallow concavities of the cheeks that extend obliquely downward from the medial or lateral margins of the cheekbones.

**Buccinator.** Principle muscle of the cheek that compresses the cheeks and forms the lateral wall of the mouth.

**Bucco-facial sulcus.** Vertical furrow of the cheek; an acquired facial marking.

**Buffer.** Embalming chemical that effects the stabilization of acid–base balance within embalming solutions and in embalmed tissues.

**Bulb syringe.** Self-contained, soft rubber manual pump designed to create pressure to deliver fluid as it passes through one-way valves located within the bulb. It is used only to deliver fluids; it cannot be used for aspiration.

**Burn.** To oxidize or to cause to be oxidized by fire or equivalent means; a tissue reaction or injury resulting from the application of heat, extreme cold, caustic material, radiation, friction, or electricity.

**Cadaver.** Dead human body used for medical purposes, including transplantation, anatomical dissection, research, and study.

**Cadaveric lividity.** Postmortem intravascular red–blue discoloration resulting from hypostasis of blood (livor mortis).

**Cadaveric spasm.** Prolongation of the last violent contraction of the muscles into the rigidity of death.

**Calvarium.** Domelike superior portion of the cranium. That portion removed during cranial autopsy.

**Calvarium clamp.** Device used to fasten the calvarium to the cranium after a cranial autopsy.

**Canalization.** Formation of new channels in a tissue.

**Cancer.** Any malignant neoplasm marked by uncontrolled growth and spread of abnormal cells.

**Capillaries.** Minute blood vessels, the walls of which comprise a single layer of endothelial cells. Capillaries connect the smallest arteries (arteriole) with the smallest veins (venule) and are where pressure filtration occurs.

**Capillary permeability.** Ability of substances to diffuse through capillary walls into the tissue spaces.

**Capri garment.** Plastic protective garment designed to cover the legs, buttocks, and abdomen. A combination of pants and stockings.

**Carbohydrate.** Compound containing hydrogen, carbon, and oxygen. Sugars, starches, and glycogen are carbohydrates.

**Carbuncle.** Circumscribed inflammation of the skin and deeper tissues that ends in suppuration and is accompanied by systemic symptoms such as fever and leukocytosis.

**Carcinogen.** Cancer-causing chemical or material.

**Carmine.** (Crimson) Purple-red in coloration.

**Carotene.** The yellow pigment of the skin.

**Cartilage.** A specialized type of dense connective tissue; attached to the ends of bones and forming parts of structures, such as the nasal septum and the framework of the ear.

**Cast.** Casting; any object that has been made from a mold; the positive reproduction obtained from a negative impression.

**Cauterizing agent.** A chemical capable of drying tissues by searing; caustic.

**Cavitation.** Formation of cavities in an organ or tissue. Frequently seen in some forms of tuberculosis.

**Cavity embalming.** See Embalming.

**Cavity fluid.** Embalming chemical that is injected into a body cavity following aspiration in cavity embalming. Cavity fluid can also be used as the chemical in hypodermic and surface embalming.

**Cellular death.** Death of the individual cells of the body.

**Cement.** Substance used to promote the adhesion of two separated surfaces such as the lips, eyelids, or margins of an incision.

**Center of fluid distribution.** Ascending aorta and/or arch of the aorta.

**Center of venous drainage.** Right atrium of the heart.

**Centers for Disease Control and Prevention (CDCP, CDC).** Major agency of the Department of Health and Human Services, with headquarters in Atlanta, Georgia, concerned with all phases of control of communicable, vector borne, and occupational diseases.

**Centrifugal pump embalming machine.** Embalming machine that uses motorized force; pulsating and non-pulsating types available.

**Channeling.** Restorative treatment usually accompanied by aspiration, gravitation, or external pressure to remove gases or excess liquids from tissues; passages are made through the tissues with a scalpel, hypodermic needle, or trocar.

**Charred.** Reduced to carbon; the state of tissues destroyed by burning.

**Chelate.** Substances that bind metallic ions. Ethylenediaminetetraacetic acid (EDTA) is used as an anticoagulant in embalming solutions.

**Chemical postmortem change.** Change in the body's chemical composition that occurs after death, for example, release of heme leading to postmortem staining.

**Chemotherapy.** Application of chemical reagents in the treatment of disease in humans. May cause an elevated preservation demand.

**Chin.** The prominence overlying the mental eminence; located at the medial-inferior part of the face; mentum.

**Chin rest.** One of several methods used for mouth closure (antiquated).

**Cilia.** Eyelashes.

**Clinical death.** Phase of somatic death lasting from 5 to 6 minutes during which life may be restored.

**Closed drainage technique.** A drainage procedure that limits the exposure of the embalmer to the drainage. Tubing is attached to a drain tube allowing drainage to flow directly from a vein into a sanitary disposal system; tubing may also be attached to a trocar and aspirator allowing drainage to be taken from the right atrium of the heart to the sanitary disposal system.

*Clostridium perfringens.* Anaerobic, saprophytic, spore-forming bacterium, responsible for tissue gas. Referred to as a gas bacillus.

**Coagulating agents.** Chemical and physical agents that bring about coagulation.

**Coagulation.** Process of converting soluble protein into insoluble protein by heating or contact with a chemical such as an alcohol or an aldehyde. Solidification of a sol into a gelatinous mass. Agglutination is a specific form of coagulation.

**Co-injection fluid.** Supplemental fluid used primarily to enhance the action of vascular (arterial) solutions.

**Collodion.** Clear syrup-like liquid that evaporates, leaving a contractile, white film; a liquid sealer.

**Columna nasi.** Fleshy termination of the nasal septum at the base of the nose; located between the nostrils; the most inferior part of the mass of the nose.

**Coma.** Irreversible cessation of brain activity and loss of consciousness. Death beginning at the brain.

**Communicable disease.** Disease that may be transmitted either directly or indirectly between individuals by an infectious agent.

**Comorbidity.** The presence of one or more additional conditions or diseases co-occurring with a primary condition.

**Complexion.** Color and texture of the skin, especially that of the face.

**Compound fracture.** A broken bone piercing the skin.

**Compress.** Gauze or absorbent cotton saturated with water or an appropriate chemical and placed under or upon tissues to preserve, bleach, dry, constrict, or reduce swelling.

**Concave.** Exhibiting a depressed or hollow surface; a concavity.

**Concha.** Concave shell of the ear; the deepest depression of the ear.

**Concurrent disinfection.** Disinfection practices carried out during the embalming process.

**Concurrent drainage.** Method of drainage in which drainage occurs continuously during vascular (arterial) injection.

**Condyle.** Rounded articular process on a bone.

**Congealing.** See Coagulation and Agglutination.

**Conjunctiva.** Mucous membrane that lines the eyelid and covers the white portion of the eye.

**Constrict.** To contract or compress.

**Contagious disease.** Disease that may be transmitted between individuals, with reference to the organism that causes a disease.

**Contaminated.** See Bloodborne Pathogen Rule.

**Contour.** Outline or surface form.

**Contusion.** Bruise.

**Cords of the neck.** Vertical prominences of the neck; an acquired facial marking.

**Cornea.** Transparent part of the tunic of the eyeball that covers the iris and pupil and admits light into the interior.

**Corneal sclera button.** That portion of the cornea recovered for transplantation in situ.

**Coronavirus.** Any of a family (Coronaviridae) of large single-stranded RNA viruses that have a lipid envelope studded with club-shaped spike proteins; infect birds and many mammals including humans, and include the causative agents of MERS, SARS, and COVID-19.

**Coroner.** Official of a local community who holds inquests concerning sudden, violent, and unexplained deaths.

**Coronoid process.** The anterior, non-articulating process of the ramus of the mandible, which serves as the insertion for the temporalis muscle.

**Corpulence.** Obesity.

**Corrective shaping with cosmetics.** (Corrective shaping) Cosmetic technique consisting of highlighting those parts of the face or individual features to enlarge or bring them forward or shadowing them to reduce the appearance of size or deepen a depression.

**Corrugator.** Pyramid-shaped muscle of facial expression that draws the eyebrows inferiorly and medially.

**Cosmetic.** Preparation for beautifying the complexion and skin.

**Cosmetic base.** Initial application of a cream or paste cosmetic to skin tissues.

**Cosmetic fluid.** Embalming fluid that contains active dyes and coloring agents intended to restore a more natural skin tone through the embalming process.

**Counterstaining compound.** Dye that helps to cover internal discolorations such as jaundice or postmortem stain.

**Coverall.** Plastic garment designed to cover the body from the chest down to the upper thigh.

**Covid-19.** See coronavirus.

**Cranial embalming.** Method used to embalm the contents of the cranial cavity through aspiration and injection of the cranial chamber by passage of a trocar through the cribriform plate.

**Cranium.** That part of the human skull that encloses the brain.

**Cremated remains.** Those elements remaining after cremation of a dead human body.

**Crepitation.** Crackling sensation produced when gases trapped in tissues are palpated, as in subcutaneous emphysema or tissue gas.

**Creutzfeldt–Jakob disease (CJD).** Rare, degenerative, fatal brain disorder. CJD is a transmissible spongiform encephalopathy (TSE) or prion disease. CJD affects one person in every one million per year worldwide; approximately 350 cases annually reported in the United States.

**Cribriform plate.** Thin, medial portion of the ethmoid bone of the skull.

**Crimson.** Deep purplish-red in coloration.

**Cross-linkage of proteins.** In embalming, the chemical joining of proteins brought about by the chemical reaction of aldehydes with different forms of nitrogen. Cross-linkage results in firmness of embalmed tissue.

**Crown.** (Vertex) Topmost part of the head.

**Cuticle remover.** Commercially prepared solvent used to remove dead cuticle from the nails and obstinate scabs.

**Cyanosis.** A bluish discoloration of the skin and the mucous membranes due to inadequate oxygenation of the blood, such as anoxia and hypoxia. Cyanosis can be present at birth, referred to as a "blue baby." Classic discoloration found in asphyxiation deaths caused by carbon monoxide poisoning (CO).

**Cyst.** Closed sac, with a definite wall, that contains fluid, semifluid, or solid material.

**Death.** Irreversible cessation of all vital functions—nonlegal definition.

**Death rattle.** Noise made by a moribund person caused by air passing through a residue of mucus in the trachea and posterior oral cavity.

**Death struggle.** Semi-convulsive tremors that often occur before death.

**Decapitation.** Separation of the head from the body; to decapitate is the act of such separation.

**Decay.** Decomposition of proteins by enzymes of aerobic bacteria.

**Decomposition.** Separation of compounds into simpler substances by the action of microbial and/or autolytic enzymes.

**Deep filler.** Material used to fill cavities or excisions and to serve as a foundation for the superficial wax restoration.

**Defibrillator.** Implantable Cardioverter Defibrillator (ICD); medical device that resets the electrical state of the heart by application of an electric current. Surgically-implanted defibrillators must be removed prior to cremation. See also Pacemaker.

**Dehydration.** Loss of moisture from body tissue that may occur antemortem or postmortem (antemortem: febrile disease, diarrhea, or emesis; postmortem: injection of embalming solution or through absorption by the air).

**Denatured protein.** Protein whose structure has been changed by physical or chemical agents.

**Dental prognathism.** (Buck teeth) Oblique insertion of the teeth.

**Dental tie.** Ligature around the superior and inferior teeth employed to hold the mandible in a fixed position; antiquated method of mouth closure.

**Dentures.** Artificial teeth.

**Depression.** Hollow or concave region; the lowering of a part.

**Depressor anguli oris.** Facial expression muscle that depresses the angle of the mouth.

**Depressor labii inferioris.** Facial expression muscle that draws the lower lip inferiorly and slightly lateral.

**Derma.** (Dermis, skin) Corium, or true skin.

**Desiccation.** Process of drying out.

**Desquamation (skin-slip).** Sloughing off of the epidermis, wherein there is a separation of the epidermis from the underlying dermis.

**Dialysis.** Separation of substances in solution by the difference in their rates of diffusion through a semipermeable membrane.

**Differential pressure.** See Pressure.

**Diffusion.** Movement of molecules or other particles in solution from an area of greater concentration to an area of lesser concentration until a uniform concentration is reached.

**Diffusion (arterial solution).** Passage of some components of the injected embalming solution from an intravascular to an extravascular location. Movement of the embalming solutions from the capillaries into the interstitial fluids.

**Digastricus.** Double-bellied muscle that draws the hyoid bone superiorly.

**Digits.** Fingers and toes. The thumb is the number one digit for each hand and the large toe is the number one digit for each foot.

**Dimples.** Shallow depressions located on the cheek or chin in a rounded or vertical form; natural facial markings.

**Disarticulate.** Disjoining of bones.

**Discoloration.** Any abnormal color in or on the human body.

**Disease.** Any deviation from or interruption of the normal structure or function of a body part, organ, or system.

**Disinfectant.** An agent, usually chemical, applied to inanimate objects/surfaces to destroy disease-causing microbial agents, but usually not bacterial spores.

**Disinfection.** Destruction and/or inhibition of most pathogenic organisms and their products in or on the body.

**Dissection.** Act of cutting apart.

**Distend.** To expand or swell.

**Distortion.** State of being twisted or pushed out of natural shape or position.

**Distribution (fluid).** Movement of embalming solutions from the point of injection throughout the arterial system and into the capillaries.

**Dorsum.** Top; the anterior protruding ridge of the nose from the root to the tip of the lobe.

**Dowel.** Wooden or metal rod used as an armature.

**Drain tube.** Embalming instrument, inserted into a vein, used to aid the drainage of venous blood from the body.

**Drainage.** Discharge or withdrawal of blood, blood clots, interstitial and lymphatic fluid, and embalming solution from the body during vascular embalming, usually through a vein.

**Drench shower.** Occupational Safety and Health Administration–required safety device for release of a copious amount of water in a short time.

**Dry ice.** Carbon dioxide cooled to the point at which it becomes solid; this occurs at $-110$ degrees Fahrenheit.

**Dry gangrene.** See Gangrene.

**Dryness.** Freedom from wetness; a condition of tissues necessary for the adhesion of cement, sealer, deep filler, or wax.

**Dye.** (Coloring agent) Substances that, on being dissolved, impart a definite color to the embalming solution. Dyes are classified as to their capacity to permanently impart color to the tissue of the body into which they are injected.

**Ecchymosis.** (Bruise) Discoloration of the skin caused by the escape of blood within the tissues; generally accompanied by swelling.

**Edema.** Abnormal accumulation of fluids in tissues or body cavities.

**Electric aspirator.** Device that uses a motor to create a suction for the purpose of aspiration.

**Electric spatula.** Electrically heated blade that may be used to dry moist tissue, reduce swollen tissue, and restore contour.

**Electrocardiogram (ECG, EKG).** Record of the electrical activity of the heart.

**Electroencephalogram (EEG).** Record of the electrical activity of the brain.

**Emaciated.** (Emaciation) Excessive leanness; a wasted condition resulting in sunken surfaces of the face.

**Embalming.** Process of chemically treating the dead human body to reduce the presence and growth of microorganisms, to temporarily inhibit organic decomposition, and to restore an acceptable physical appearance (ABFSE).

- **Cavity embalming.** Direct treatment other than vascular (arterial) embalming of the contents of the body cavities and the lumina of the hollow viscera. Usually accomplished by aspiration and then injection of chemicals using a trocar.
- **Hypodermic embalming.** Injection of embalming chemicals directly into the tissues through the use of a syringe and needle or a trocar.
- **Surface embalming.** Direct contact of body tissues with embalming chemicals.
- **Vascular (arterial) embalming.** Use of the blood vascular system of the body for temporary preservation, disinfection, and restoration. Usually accomplished through injection of embalming solutions into the arteries and drainage from the veins.

**Embalming analysis.** (Case analysis) That consideration given to the dead body before, during, and after the embalming procedure is completed. Documentation is recommended.

**Embalming and Decedent Care Report.** Also called a case report. Document used for listing postmortem body conditions and recording treatments performed by funeral personnel for each body received into a facility for preparation, sheltering, transfer to, or from a different facility, or shipped in from another funeral facility.

**Embalming machine.** Centrifugal pump used for embalming; machine uses motorized force to create pressure and delivery speed for injection of embalming chemicals and solutions.

**Eminence.** Prominence or projection of a bone.
**En bloc.** As a whole; surgical or autopsy procedure in which organs or tissues are removed altogether; en masse.
**Engineering controls.** See Bloodborne Pathogens Rule.
**Enucleation.** Surgical removal of the entire eye globe (en bloc); surgical technique to remove an entire mass without preliminary cutting or dissecting.
**Environment.** Surroundings, conditions, or influences that affect an organism or the cells within an organism.
**Environmental Protection Agency (EPA).** Governmental agency with environmental protection regulatory and enforcement authority.
**Enzyme.** Organic catalyst produced by living cells and capable of autolytic decomposition.
**Epidermis.** Outermost layer of skin; cuticle or scarf skin.
**Erythema.** A reddening of the skin, caused by a dilation of the superficial blood vessels in the skin. Erythematous rash. Antemortem pathological discoloration.
**Ether.** Clear, volatile liquid used as a wax solvent or to remove grease, oil, and adhesive tape stains.
**Excise.** To remove as by cutting out.
**Excision.** Area from which tissue has been removed.
**Expert test of death.** Any procedure used to prove a sign of death, usually performed by medical personnel.
**Exposure incident.** See Bloodborne Pathogen Rule.
**External auditory meatus.** Opening or passageway of the ear.
**External pressure.** Weight applied to a surface.
**Extravascular.** Outside the blood vascular system.
**Extravascular blood discoloration.** Discoloration of the body outside the blood vascular system, for example, ecchymosis, petechia, hematoma, and postmortem stain.
**Extrinsic.** From outside the body.
**Eye cap.** Thin, domelike shell made of hardened cloth, metal, or plastic placed beneath the eyelids to restore natural curvature and to maintain the position of the closed eye.
**Eye enucleation.** Removal of the eye for tissue transplantation, research, and education.
**Eye enucleation discoloration.** Extravasation of blood as a result of eye enucleation.
**Eye socket.** (Orbit) Bony region containing the eyeball; the orbital cavity.
**Eyebrows.** (Supercilium) Also the superficial hairs covering the superciliary arches.
**Eyelids.** (Palpebrae) Two movable flaps of skin that cover and uncover each eyeball.
**Eyewash station.** Occupational Safety and Health Administration–required emergency safety device providing a steady stream of water for flushing the eye.
**Face.** Anatomically, the region from the eyes to the base of the chin; physiognomically, the region from the normal hairline to the base of the chin.
**Facial markings.** Character lines of the face and neck; wrinkles, grooves, cords, and dimples.
**Facial profiles.** Silhouettes of the face from the side view.
**Fat.** Organic compound containing carbon, hydrogen, and oxygen. Chemically, fat is a triglyceride ester composed of glycerol and fatty acids.
**Fatty acids.** Product of decomposition of fats.
**Febrile.** Characterized by high fever, causing dehydration of the body.
**Federal Trade Commission (FTC).** The agency of federal government created in 1914 to promote free and fair competition by prevention of trade restraints, price fixing, false advertising, and other unfair methods of competition.
**Fermentation.** Bacterial decomposition of carbohydrates.
**Fever blisters.** Lesions of the mucous membrane of the lip or mouth caused by herpes simplex type I or II virus or by dehydration of the mucous membrane in a febrile disease.
**Filler.** Material used to fill a large cavity (e.g., plaster of Paris and cotton; liquid sealer and cotton).
**Firming.** Rigidity of tissue due to chemical reaction.
**Firm wax.** (Wound filler) The most viscous type of wax; a puttylike material used to fill large cavities or to model features.
**First-degree burn.** (Hyperemia) Injury caused by heat that produces redness of the skin.
**Fixation.** Act of making tissue rigid. Solidification of a compound.
**Fixative.** Agent employed in the preparation of tissues, for the purpose of maintaining the existing form and structure. A large number of agents are used, the most important one being formalin.
**Floater.** A dead human body, in a body of water, which has generated sufficient decomposition gasses to float to the surface of the water (face down).
**Florid.** Flushed with red, when describing a complexion; not as vivid as ruddy.
**Fluorescent light.** Illumination produced by a tubular electric discharge lamp; the fluorescence of phosphors coating the inside of a tube.
**Flush (flushing).** Intravascular blood discoloration that occurs when arterial solution enters an area (such as the face), but due to blockage, blood and embalming solution are unable to drain from the area.
**Fold.** Elongated prominence adjoining a surface.
**Foramen magnum.** Opening in the occipital bone through which the spinal cord passes from the brain.
**Forehead.** That part of the face above the eyes.
**Formaldehyde (HCHO).** Colorless, strong-smelling gas that when used in solution is a powerful preservative and disinfectant. Potential occupational carcinogen.
**Formaldehyde gray.** Gray discoloration of the body caused by the reaction of formaldehyde from the embalming process with hemoglobin to form methyl hemoglobin (methemoglobin).
**Formaldehyde Rule.** Occupational Safety and Health Administration regulation 29 CFR 1910.1048 applies to all occupational exposures to formaldehyde; primarily requires employers to reduce and maintain employee exposures below the permissible exposure limits using engineering and work practice controls.
**Fossa.** Depression; concavity.
**Fourth-degree burn.** Total evacuation (absence) of tissue.
**Fracture.** Broken bone.
**Frenulum.** Vertical restraining fold of mucous membrane on the midline of the inside of each lip connecting the lip with the gum.
**Frontal.** Anterior; anterior view of the face or features.
**Frontal bone.** Anterior third of the cranium, forming the forehead and the anterior portion of the roof of the skull.
**Frontal eminences.** Paired, rounded, unmargined prominences of the frontal bone found approximately 1 inch beneath the normal hairline.
**Frontal process of the maxilla.** Ascending part of the upper jaw that gradually protrudes as it rises beside the nasal bone to meet the frontal bone; the ascending process of the upper jaw.
**Furrow.** (Wrinkle) Crevice in the skin accompanied by adjacent elevations.
**Furuncle.** See Boil.
**Gangrene.** Necrosis, death, of tissues of part of the body usually due to deficient or absent blood supply.
- **Dry gangrene.** (Ischemic necrosis) Condition that results when the body part that dies had little blood and remains aseptic. The arteries but not the veins are obstructed.
- **Gas gangrene.** Necrosis in a wound infected by an anaerobic gas-forming bacillus, the most common etiologic agent being *Clostridium perfringens*.

- **Moist (wet) gangrene.** Necrotic tissue that is wet as a result of inadequate venous drainage. May be accompanied by bacterial infection.

**Germicide.** Agent, usually chemical, applied either to inanimate objects/surfaces or to living tissues to destroy disease-causing microbial agents, but usually not bacterial spores.

**Glabella.** Single bony prominence of the frontal bone located between the superciliary arches in the inferior part of the frontal bone above the root of the nose.

**Glycerin.** Syrupy, colorless liquid obtained from fats or oils as a by-product of the manufacturing of soaps and fatty acids; used as a vehicle for some cosmetics.

**Gooseneck.** Rubber stopper containing two tubes, one to create vacuum or pressure and the other to deliver fluid or achieve aspiration. Possibly used in conjunction with a hand pump.

**Grave wax.** See Adipocere.

**Gravity filtration.** The settling of fluids by gravitational force to the dependent areas of the body.

**Gravity injector.** Apparatus used to inject arterial fluid during the vascular (arterial) phase of the embalming process. Relies on gravity to create the pressure required to deliver the fluid (0.43 pounds of pressure per 1 foot of elevation.).

**Green (natural) burial.** Bodies not embalmed or temporarily preserved using a non-formaldehyde biodegradable temporary preservative. All preparation of the body including the clothing worn and the casket (if used) must be biodegradable. Green cemeteries do not use traditional grave markers.

**Groove.** Elongated depression in a relatively level plane or surface.

**Grooved director.** A grooved metal instrument used to expand a vessel to guide another instrument into that vessel, such as an angular spring forceps or drain tube into a vein, or an arterial tube into an artery. The insertion end is a probe; the butterfly-shaped end is called a spoon or saddle. Vintage embalming texts refer to this instrument as a tissue needle.

**Hairline.** Outline of hair growth on the head or face; the lowest centrally located part of the hair of the cranium.

**Hand pump.** Historical instrument resembling a large hypodermic syringe attached to a bottle apparatus. Used to create either pressure for injection or vacuum for aspiration.

**Hard palate.** Anterior portion of the roof of the mouth.

**Hard water.** Water containing large amounts of mineral salts. These mineral salts must be removed from or sequestered in water (vehicle) to be used in mixing vascular embalming solutions.

**Hardening compound.** Chemical in powder form that has the ability to absorb and to disinfect. Often used in cavity treatment of autopsied cases.

**Hazard Communication Standard (Rule).** Occupational Safety and Health Administration regulation that deals with limiting exposure to occupational hazards.

**Hazardous material.** Agent or material exposing one to risk.

**Headrest.** Piece of equipment used to maintain the head in the proper position during the embalming process.

**Helix.** Outer rim of the ear.

**Hematemesis.** Blood present in vomitus. Vomiting of blood.

**Hematoma.** A swelling or mass of clotted blood caused by a ruptured blood vessel and confined to an organ or space.

**Heme.** Nonprotein portion of hemoglobin. Red pigment.

**Hemoglobin.** Red respiratory portion of the red blood cells. Iron-containing pigment of red blood cells functioning to carry oxygen to the cells.

**Hemolysis.** Destruction of red blood cells that liberates hemoglobin.

**Hepatitis.** Inflammation of the liver that may be caused by various agents, including viral infections, bacterial invasion, and physical or chemical agents. It is usually accompanied by fever, jaundice, and an enlarged liver.

**Hepatitis A virus (HAV).** Formerly called infectious hepatitis. It is caused by the enterically transmitted (oral-fecal route) hepatitis A virus.

**Hepatitis B virus (HBV).** Severe infectious bloodborne virus.

**Hepatitis C virus (HCV).** Spread by contaminated blood or body fluids.

**Hepatitis D virus (HDV).** A bloodborne virus, it can only exist in combination with the hepatitis B virus. HBV vaccine will offer protection against HDV.

**Hepatitis E virus (HEV).** Transmitted by contaminated water and human waste. Hepatitis G virus (HGV). A bloodborne virus.

**Herpes.** Inflammatory skin disease marked by small vesicles in clusters, usually restricted to diseases caused by herpes virus.

**High-index fluids.** Special vascular (arterial) fluid with a formaldehyde content of 25 to 36%.

**Holding room.** An area of a funeral home, crematory or embalming facility exclusively used for preparation of deceased human bodies by means other than embalming.

**Horseshoe curve.** Roughly U-shaped, with the front being narrower than the sweep of the curve.

**Household bleach.** Five percent sodium hypochlorite solution. Mixing 12 ounces of household bleach with 116 ounces of water yields 1 gallon of a 10% household bleach solution (5000 ppm sodium hypochlorite).

**Human composting.** See Natural organic reduction.

**Human immunodeficiency virus (HIV).** Retrovirus that causes acquired immunodeficiency syndrome (AIDS).

**Human remains.** Body of a deceased person, including cremated remains.

**Humectant.** Chemical that increases the ability of embalmed tissue to retain moisture.

**Humor.** Any liquid or semiliquid of the body, as the aqueous or vitreous humor of the eyeball.

**Hunting bow.** Shaped as a bent wood weapon with a central belly; resembling a cupid's bow. Shape of the attached margin of the upper red lip; shape of the lip line of closure.

**Hydro aspirator.** Specialized equipment connected to the water supply; creates suction for trocar aspiration of the body's cavities.

**Hydrocele.** Abnormal accumulation of fluids in a saclike structure, especially the scrotal sac.

**Hydrocephalus.** Abnormal accumulation of cerebrospinal fluids in the ventricles of the brain.

**Hydrolysis.** Reaction in which water is one of the reactants and compounds are often broken down. In the hydrolysis of proteins, the addition of water accompanied by the action of enzymes results in the breakdown of protein into amino acids.

**Hydropericardium.** Abnormal accumulation of fluid within the pericardial sac.

**Hydrothorax.** Abnormal accumulation of fluid in the thoracic cavity.

**Hygroscopic.** Absorbing moisture readily.

**Hypertonic solution.** Solution having a greater concentration of dissolved solute than the solution with which it is compared.

**Hypodermic embalming.** See Embalming.

**Hypodermic tissue building.** Injection of special creams or liquids into the tissues through the use of a syringe and needle to restore natural contour.

**Hypostasis.** Settling of blood and/or other fluids to dependent portions of the body.

**Hypotonic solution.** Solution having a lesser concentration of dissolved solute than the solution with which it is compared.

**Hypovalve trocar.** A long thin trocar used for supplemental hypodermic embalming.

**Imbibition.** Absorption of the fluid portion of blood by the tissues after death, resulting in postmortem edema. Postmortem swelling and softening of tissues and organs as a result of absorbing moisture from adjacent sources.

**Incision.** A clean cut made with a sharp instrument. In embalming, a cut made with a scalpel to raise arteries and veins.

**Incisive fossa.** Depression between the mental eminence and the inferior incisor teeth.

**Incisor teeth.** Four teeth located anteriorly from the midline on each jaw, used for cutting.

**Index.** Strength of an embalming fluid, indicated by the number of grams of pure formaldehyde gas dissolved in 100 mL of water. Index usually refers to a percentage; an embalming fluid with an index of 25 usually contains 25% formaldehyde gas.

**Infant.** Child less than 1 year of age.

**Infant trocar.** A short hollow tubular instrument with a sharp point. Used for aspiration and injection of an infant's thoracic and abdominal cavities.

**Infectious disease.** Disease caused by the growth of a pathogenic microorganism in the body.

**Infectious waste.** See Biohazard.

**Inferior.** Beneath; lower in plane or position; the undersurface of an organ or indicating a structure below another structure; toward the feet.

**Inferior nasal conchae.** Lowermost scroll-shaped bones on the sidewalls of the nasal cavity.

**Inferior palpebral sulcus.** Furrow of the lower attached border of the inferior palpebra; acquired facial marking.

**Inflammation.** Reaction of tissues to injurious agents, usually characterized by heat, redness, swelling, and pain.

**Inguinal ligament.** Anatomical structure forming the base of the femoral triangle; extends from the anterior superior iliac spine to the pubic tubercle.

**Injection.** Act or instance of forcing a fluid into the vascular system or directly into tissues.

**Injection pressure.** See Pressure.

**Inner canthus.** Eminence at the inner corner of the closed eyelids.

**Instant tissue fixation.** Embalming technique that uses a very strong arterial solution (often waterless). The solution is injected under high pressure in spurts into a body area. Very little solution is injected; the technique attempts to limit swelling; for example, in bodies with facial trauma or early decomposition.

**Instantaneous rigor mortis.** Instantaneous stiffening of the muscles of a dead human body.

**Integumentary lips.** Superiorly, the skin portion of the upper lip from the attached margin of the upper mucous membrane to the base of the nose, and inferiorly, the skin portion of the lower lip from the attached margin of the lower mucous membrane to the labiomental sulcus.

**Intercellular.** Between the cells of a structure.

**Intercellular fluid.** Fluid outside or between the cells of the body.

**Interciliary sulci.** Vertical or transverse furrows between the eyebrows; acquired facial markings.

**Intercostal space.** Space between the ribs.

**Intermittent drainage (restricted drainage).** Method of drainage in which the drainage is stopped at intervals while the injection continues.

**Interstitial fluid.** Fluid in the supporting connective tissues surrounding body cells (about one-fifth the body weight).

**Intracellular fluid.** Fluids within the cell.

**Intradermal suture.** (Hidden suture) Type of suture used to close incisions in such a manner that the ligature remains entirely under the epidermis.

**Intravascular.** Within the blood vascular system.

**Intravascular blood discoloration.** Discoloration of the body within the blood vascular system, for example, hypostasis, carbon monoxide, and capillary congestion.

**Intravascular fluid.** Fluid contained within vascular channels (about one-twentieth of the body weight).

**Intravascular pressure.** See Pressure.

**Intrinsic.** From within the body.

**Inversion.** Tissues turned in an opposite direction or folded inward.

**Inversion suture.** See Worm suture.

**Ischemic necrosis.** See Gangrene.

**Isotonic solution.** A solution having a concentration of dissolved solute equal to that of a standard of reference.

**Jaundice.** Conditions characterized by an excessive concentration of bilirubin in the skin and tissues and deposition of excessive bile pigment in the skin, cornea, body fluids, and mucous membranes with the resulting yellow appearance of the patient.

**Jaundice fluid.** Arterial fluid with special bleaching and coloring qualities for use on bodies with jaundice. Usually, formaldehyde content is low.

**Jawline.** Inferior border of the mandible.

**Jugular drain tube.** Tubular instrument of varying diameter and shape, preferably with a plunger, which is inserted into the jugular vein to aid in drainage.

**Juxtaposition.** (Simultaneous contrast) Any two hues seen together that modify each other in the direction of their complements.

**Labial sulci.** (Furrows of age) Vertical furrows of each lip extending from within the mucous membranes into the integumentary lips; acquired facial markings.

**Labiomental sulcus.** Junction of the lower integumentary lip and the superior border of the chin, which may appear as a furrow; a natural facial marking.

**Laceration.** Wound characterized by irregular tearing of tissue.

**Lanolin.** Oil from sheep wool.

**Lanugo.** (Peach fuzz) Downy hair of a fetus, child, or woman.

**Larvicide.** Substance used to kill insect larvae.

**Lateral.** Away from the midline.

**Legionnaires disease.** Severe, often fatal bacterial disease characterized by pneumonia, dry cough, and sometimes gastrointestinal symptoms (*Legionella pneumophila*).

**Lesion.** Any change in structure produced during the course of a disease or injury.

**Levator anguli oris.** Muscle of facial expression that elevates the angle of the mouth.

**Levator labii superioris.** Muscle of facial expression that elevates and extends the upper lip.

**Levator labii superioris alaeque nasi.** Muscle of facial expression that elevates the upper lip and dilates the nostril opening; the common elevator.

**Levator palpebrae superioris.** Muscle of facial expression that raises the upper eyelid.

**Ligate.** To tie off, as in ligating an artery and vein on completion of embalming or ligating the colon in autopsied bodies.

**Ligature.** Thread, cord, or wire used for tying vessels, tissues, or bones.

**Line of closure.** Line that forms between two structures such as the lips or the eyelids when in a closed position, which marks their place of contact with each other.

**Linear guide.** Line drawn or visualized on the surface of the skin to represent the approximate location of some deeper lying structure.

**Linear sulci.** Eyelid furrows that are short and broken, extending horizontally on the palpebrae themselves and that may fan from both the medial and lateral corners of the eyes.

**Lip wax.** Soft restorative wax, usually tinted, used to surface the mucous membranes or to correct lip separations.

**Lipolysis.** Decomposition of fats.

**Livor mortis.** See Cadaveric lividity.

**Loop stitch.** Single, looped suture that stands away from the skin to anchor restorative materials; to form the loop, the ligature is not pulled tautly before knotting.

**Lumen.** Cavity of a vein, artery, or intestine.

**Lysin.** Specific antibody acting destructively on cells and tissues.

**Lysosome.** Organelle that exists within a cell, but separate from the cell. Contains hydrolytic enzymes that break down proteins and certain carbohydrates.

**Maggot.** Larva of an insect, especially a flying insect.

**Major restoration.** Those restorations that require a long period of time, are extensive, require advanced technical skill, and require expressed written consent to perform.

**Mandible.** Horseshoe-shaped bone forming the inferior jaw.

**Mandibular fossa.** Glenoid fossa; the small oval depression on the zygomatic process of the temporal bone into which the condyle of the mandible articulates, just anterior to the external auditory meatus. Forms the temporal mandibular joint (TMJ).

**Mandibular sulcus.** Furrow beneath the jawline that rises vertically on the cheek; an acquired facial marking.

**Mandibular suture.** Stitch used to hold the mouth closed; placed behind the lips, one part is passed through the inferior jaw at the median plane, whereas the other part extends through the nasal septum or the superior frenulum.

**Manual aid.** Those treatments or procedures that are applied by the use of hands. Scrubbing with soap and water to remove a surface discoloration; flexing, bending, rotating, and massage of the limbs to stimulate the circulation of arterial solution and movement of blood and body fluids.

**Marbling.** A greenish-black coloration along the vessels (veins) produced by hemolysis of the blood in the vessels. Hemoglobin mixes with hydrogen sulfide to produce the discoloration observed on the skin surface when decomposition is present.

**Masking agent.** See Perfuming agents.

**Massage.** Manipulation of tissue in the course of preparation of the body.

**Massage cream.** Soft, white, oily preparation used as a protective coating for external tissues; a base for cream cosmetics and a wax softener; an emollient.

**Masseter muscles.** Muscles of mastication that close the mandible.

**Mastic compound.** Puttylike substance; an absorbent sealing adhesive that can be injected under the skin or applied to surface tissues to establish skin contour.

**Mastoid process.** The rounded projection on the inferior portion of the temporal bones just posterior to the lobe of the ear.

**Material Safety Data Sheet (MSDS). Outdated; replaced by** Safety Data Sheet (SDS)

**Matte.** Having a dull finish; as afforded by the application of loose powder, lack of sheen.

**Maxilla.** Paired bone with several processes that form the skeletal base of most of the superior face, roof of the mouth, sides of the nasal cavity, and floor of the orbit.

**Mechanical aid.** The application of treatments or procedures that utilize machines or instruments. Adjustments of pressure and rate of flow on the embalming machine; utilization of properly sized arterial tubes and/or drainage instruments. Opening and closing of drainage instruments.

**Medial.** Toward the midline.

**Medical examiner.** Official elected or appointed to investigate suspicious or unnatural deaths.

**Medium wax.** Derma surgery or restorative wax.

**Melanin.** The brown to black-brown pigment in the epidermis and hair.

**Meningitis.** Inflammation of the meninges.

**Mental eminence.** Bony triangular projection on the inferior portion of the anterior mandible.

**Mentalis muscle.** Elevates and protrudes the inferior lip, wrinkles the skin over the chin.

**Methicillin-resistant *Staphylococcus aureus* (MRSA).** Pathogenic bacterial *Staphylococcus aureus*, resistant to most drugs. A causative agent of bedsores, surgical wound infections, skin and nose infections, and pneumonia.

**Microbe (microorganism).** Minute one-celled form of life that cannot be distinguished as being of either vegetable or animal nature.

**Microbial enzyme.** The enzymes of microorganisms; a source of the enzymes that contribute to decomposition.

**Midaxillary line.** Vertical line drawn from the center of the medial border of the base of the axillary space.

**Millicurie (mCi).** That amount of radioactive material in which 37 million atoms disintegrate each second.

**Minor restoration.** Those restorations requiring a minimum effort, skill, or time to complete.

**Mixture.** Composition of two or more substances that are not chemically bound to each other.

**Modifying agents.** Chemical components of vascular fluids that control the rate and degree of tissue firmness by the fluid utilized (e.g., humectants and buffers); chemicals for which there may be greatly varying demands predicated on the type of embalming, the environment, and the embalming fluid used.

**Mold-preventive agents.** Agents that prohibit the growth of mold.

**Mortuary mastic compound.** See Mastic compound.

**Mottle.** To diversify with spots or blotches of different color (or shade).

**Moribund.** In a dying state. In the agonal period.

**Mouth former.** Device used in the mouth to shape the contour of the lips.

**Mucous membranes.** The visible red surfaces of the lips; the lining membrane of body cavities that communicate with the exterior.

**Multi-point injection (multisite).** Vascular injection that utilizes two or more injection sites.

**Musculature suture.** Method of mouth closure in which a suture is passed through the septum of the nose and through the mentalis muscle of the chin.

**Nasal bones.** Directly inferior to the glabella and forming a dome over the superior portion of the nasal cavity.

**Nasal cavity.** Space between the roof of the mouth and the floor of the cranial cavity.

**Nasal spine of the maxilla.** Sharp, bony projection located medially at the inferior margin of the nasal cavity.

**Nasal sulcus.** Angular area between the posterior margin of the wing of the nose and the nasolabial fold; a natural facial marking.

**Nasal tube aspirator.** Embalming instrument used to aspirate the throat by means of the nostrils.

**Nasolabial fold.** The eminence of the cheek and adjacent to the mouth; extending from the superior part of the posterior margin of the wing of the nose to the side of the mouth; a natural facial marking.

**Nasolabial sulcus.** Furrow originating at the superior border of the wing of the nose and extending to the side of the mouth; acquired facial marking.

**Naso-orbital fossa.** Depression superior to the medial portion of the superior palpebrae.

**Natural facial markings.** Those that are present at birth; hereditary facial markings.

**Natural organic reduction (NOR).** The contained, accelerated conversion of human remains to soil. Also called human composting.

**Necrobiosis.** Antemortem, physiological death of the cells of the body followed by their replacement.

**Necropsy.** See Autopsy.

**Necrosis.** Pathological death of a tissue still a part of the living organism.

**Needle injector.** Mechanical device used to impel specially designed metal pins into bone.

**Needlestick Safety and Prevention Act** (Pub. L. 106-430). Revision of OSHA Bloodborne Pathogens Standard (29 CFR 1910.1030);

created more specific requirements for employers to identify, evaluate, and implement safer medical devices such as needleless systems and sharps with engineered sharps protections and to maintain a sharps injury log.

**Neoplasm.** New and abnormal formation of tissue, as a tumor or growth.

**Nephritis.** Inflammation of the kidneys.

**Nevus.** Birthmark; congenital skin blemish; any congenital anomaly, including various types of birthmarks and all types of moles.

**Nitrogenous waste.** Metabolic by-products that contain nitrogen, such as urea and uric acid. These compounds have a high affinity for formaldehyde and tend to neutralize embalming chemicals.

**Noncosmetic fluid.** Type of arterial fluid that contains inactive dyes that will not impart a color change on the body tissues of the deceased.

**Nonformaldehyde fluids.** Fluids that are designed to be nontoxic and environmentally friendly. They provide a limited sanitization and preservation of the deceased body.

**Norm.** The most common characteristics of each feature; typical, common, average.

**Obese.** Having an unhealthy accumulation of fat on the body. Corpulent.

**Oblique palpebral sulcus.** Shallow, curving groove below the medial corner of the eyelids; natural facial marking.

**Occipital bone.** Lowest part of the back and base of the cranium, forming a cradle for the brain.

**Occipital protuberance.** The prominence at the center of the external surface of the occipital bone.

**Occipitofrontalis muscle.** Epicranius; draws the scalp posteriorly and anteriorly and raises the eyebrows.

**Occupational exposure.** See Bloodborne Pathogen Rule.

**Occupational Safety and Health Administration (OSHA).** A governmental agency with the responsibility for regulation and enforcement of safety and health matters for most U.S. employees. An individual state OSHA agency may supersede the U.S. Department of Labor OSHA regulations.

**One-point injection.** Injection and drainage from one location.

**Opaque.** Not transparent or translucent; not allowing light to pass through a concealing cosmetic.

**Opaque cosmetic.** A cosmetic medium able to cover or hide skin discolorations.

**Operative corrections.** Invasive treatments or procedures to correct a problem area. Examples include channeling, incisions, excisions, and wicking.

**Ophthalmoscope.** Optical instrument with an accompanying light that makes it possible to examine the retina and to explore for blood circulation.

**Optic facial sulci.** (Crow's feet) Furrows radiating from the lateral corner of the eye; acquired facial markings.

**Optimum.** Most favorable condition for functioning.

**Oral cavity.** Mouth and vestibule, or the opening to the throat.

**Orbicularis oculi muscle.** Closes the eyelids; compresses the lacrimal sacs.

**Orbicularis oris muscle.** Closes the lips.

**Orbital cavity (orbit).** Eye socket.

**Orbital pouch.** Bags under the eyes; the fullness between the inferior palpebrae and the oblique palpebral sulcus.

**Orifice.** Entrance or outlet of any body cavity; an opening.

**Ornamental.** Adornment or embellishment; a cosmetic material manufactured for street wear; the technique of cosmetic application to beautify the face.

**Osmosis.** Passage of solvent from a solution of lesser to one of greater solute concentration when the two solutions are separated by a semipermeable membrane.

**Pacemaker.** Medical device that uses electrical impulses to stimulate or steady the heartbeat. Surgically-implanted pacemakers must be removed prior to cremation. See also Defibrillator.

**Packing forceps.** Embalming instrument used in closing the external orifices of the body.

**Palatine bone.** One of the bones forming the posterior part of the hard palate and lateral nasal wall between the interior pterygoid plate of the sphenoid bone and the maxilla.

**Palpate.** To examine by touch.

**Palpebrae.** Eyelids both superior and inferior; singular palpebra.

**Parallel incision.** Incision on the surface of the skin to raise the common carotid arteries. It is made along the posterior border of the inferior one-third of the sternocleidomastoid muscle.

**Parenteral.** See Bloodborne Pathogen Rule.

**Parietal bones.** Two bones that form the roof and part of the sides of the skull.

**Parietal eminence.** Rounded peak of the external convexity of the parietal bones; determines the widest part of the cranium.

**Parts per million (ppm).** In contaminated air, the parts of vapor or gas (formaldehyde) per million parts of air by volume. In solution, the parts of chemical per million parts of solution.

**Passive transport system.** Method by which solutes and/ or solvents cross through a membrane with no energy provided by the cells of the membrane. In embalming, examples include pressure filtration, dialysis, diffusion, and osmosis.

**Pathological condition.** Diseased; due to a disease.

**Pathological discoloration.** Antemortem discoloration that occurs during the course of certain diseases such as gangrene and jaundice.

**Pediculicide.** Substance able to destroy lice.

**Penetrating wounds.** Wounds entering the interior of an organ or cavity.

**Percutaneous.** Effected through unbroken skin.

**Perfuming agents.** (Masking agents) Chemicals found in embalming arterial formulations having the capability of displacing an unpleasant odor or of altering an unpleasant odor so that it is converted to a more pleasant one.

**Perfusion.** To force a fluid through (an organ or tissue), especially by way of the blood vessels. Injection during vascular (arterial) embalming.

**Peritonitis.** Inflammation of the peritoneum, the membranous coat lining the abdominal cavity and covering the viscera.

**Permissible exposure limit (PEL).** Maximum legal limit established by the Occupational Safety and Health Administration for a regulated substance. These are based on employee exposure and are time-weighted over an 8-hour work shift. When these limits are exceeded, employers must take proper steps to reduce employee exposure. For formaldehyde, the PEL is 0.75 ppm.

**Perpendicular plate of the ethmoid bone.** Superior portion of the bony nasal septum.

**Personal protective equipment (PPE).** See Bloodborne Pathogens Standard.

**Petechia.** Antemortem, pinpoint, extravascular blood discoloration visible as purplish hemorrhages of the skin.

**Petroleum jelly.** Semisolid, yellow mixture of hydrocarbons obtained from petroleum.

**Pharmaceutical.** Drug or medicine.

**Phenol.** (Carbolic acid) Antiseptic/disinfectant employed to dry moist tissues and to bleach discolored tissues.

**Philtrum.** Vertical groove located medially on the superior lip; a natural facial marking.

**Physiognomy.** Study of the structures and surface markings of the face and features.

**Pitting edema.** Condition in which interstitial spaces contain such excessive amounts of fluid that the skin remains depressed after palpation.

**Plaster of Paris.** Calcium sulfate; a white powdery substance that forms a quick-setting paste when mixed with water.

**Platysma muscle.** Thin layer of muscle covering anterior aspect of neck.

**Platysmal sulci.** Transverse, dipping furrow of the neck; acquired facial marking.

**Pneumonia.** Acute infection or inflammation of the alveoli. The alveolar sacs fill up with fluid and dead white blood cells. Causes include bacteria, fungi, and viruses.

**Positioning devices.** Preparation room equipment for properly positioning bodies before, during, and after vascular embalming.

**Post-embalming.** That time period after the arterial injection.

**Posterior.** Toward the back.

**Postmortem.** Period that begins after somatic death.

**Postmortem caloricity.** Rise in body temperature after death due to continued cellular metabolism.

**Postmortem chemical changes.** Change in the body's chemical composition that occurs after death (e.g., decomposition, change in body pH, rigor mortis, postmortem stain, and postmortem caloricity).

**Postmortem examination.** See Autopsy.

**Postmortem physical change.** Change in the form or state of matter without any change in chemical composition, for example, algor mortis, hypostasis, dehydration, livor mortis, increase in blood viscosity, and translocation of microbes.

**Postmortem stain.** Extravascular color change that occurs when heme, released by hemolysis of red blood cells, seeps through the vessel walls and into the body tissues.

**Potential of hydrogen (pH).** Degree of acidity or alkalinity. The scale ranges from 0 to 14 with 0 being completely acid, 14 completely basic, and 7 neutral. Blood has a pH of 7.35 to 7.45.

**Potential pressure.** See Pressure.

**Precipitant.** Substance bringing about precipitation. The oxalates formerly used in water conditioning chemicals are now illegal because of their poisonous nature.

**Pre-embalming.** That period of time before the arterial injection.

**Pre-injection fluid.** Fluid injected primarily to prepare the vascular system and body tissues for the injection of the preservative vascular (arterial) solution. This solution is injected before the preservative vascular solution is injected.

**Preparation room.** Specialized area of a facility used for decedent care activities such as embalming, restoration, dressing, applying cosmetics, and other body preparations.

**Preservation.** See Temporary preservation.

**Preservative.** Chemicals that inactivate saprophytic bacteria, render unsuitable for nutrition the media upon which such bacteria thrive, and will arrest decomposition by altering enzymes and lysins of the body as well as converting the decomposable tissue to a form less susceptible to decomposition.

**Preservative demand.** Amount of preservative (formaldehyde) required to effectively preserve and disinfect remains. This amount depends on the condition of the tissues as determined in the embalming analysis.

**Preservative powder.** Chemical in powder form, typically used for surface embalming of the remains.

**Pressure.** Action of a force against an opposing force (a force applied or acting against resistance).

Types of pressure:

- **Blood pressure.** Pressure exerted by the blood on the vessel walls, measured in millimeters of mercury.
- **Injection pressure.** Amount of pressure produced by an injection device to overcome initial resistance within (intravascular) or upon (extravascular) the vascular system (arterial or venous).
- **Intravascular pressure.** Pressure developed as the flow of embalming solution is established and the elastic arterial walls expand and then contract, resulting in filling of the capillary beds and development of pressure filtration.

Types of pressure created by the embalming machine:

- **Actual pressure.** Indicates the pressure of arterial solution leaving the delivery hose and entering the body; the machine is running, the rate of flow valve is open, and fluid is being delivered.
- **Differential pressure.** The measured difference between the potential and actual pressure readings; an indicator of the rate of flow (speed of delivery).
- **Potential pressure.** Indicates the pressure existing in the delivery hose only; the machine is running but the rate of flow valve is closed, and fluid is not delivered.

**Pressure filtration.** Passage of embalming solution through the capillary wall to diffuse with the interstitial fluids by application of positive intravascular pressure. Embalming solution passes from an intravascular to an extravascular position.

**Pressure gauge.** Gauge on the embalming machine that controls the pressure of fluid delivery.

**Primary dilution.** Dilution attained as the embalming solution is mixed in the embalming machine.

**Primary disinfection.** Disinfection carried out before the embalming process.

**Prion.** A protein particle that lacks nucleic acid (smaller than a virus); implicated as the cause of various neurodegenerative diseases, for example, CJD.

**Procerus muscle.** Draws the skin of the forehead inferiorly.

**Procurement.** Recovery of organs or tissues from a cadaver for transplantation.

**Professional portrait.** Photograph or painting in which the subject has been posed and lighted flatteringly by a professional photographer or artist.

**Profile.** Side view of the human head.

**Prognathism.** Projection of the jaw or jaws that may cause problems with mouth closure and alignment of the teeth.

**Protein.** Organic compound found in plants and animals that can be broken down into amino acids.

**Proteolysis.** Decomposition of proteins.

**Ptomaine.** Any one of a group of nitrogenous organic compounds formed by the action of putrefactive bacteria on proteins, for example, indole, skatole, cadaverine, and putrescine.

**Pubic symphysis.** Fibrocartilage that joins the two pubic bones in the median plane.

**Purge.** Postmortem evacuation of any substance from an external orifice of the body as a result of pressure.

**Purpura.** An antemortem, extravascular blood discoloration. Caused by blood cells leaking into the skin or mucous membranes. Frequently seen with persons using blood thinners. Purpura lesions are larger than pin-point petechia: large purpural lesions are called ecchymosis.

**Purse-string suture.** Suture made around the circumference of a circular opening or puncture to close it or to hold the margins in position.

**Pus.** Liquid product of inflammation containing various proteins and leukocytes.

**Pustular lesion.** Characteristic pus-filled wound of a disease such as smallpox, syphilis, and acne.

**Pustule.** Small elevation of the skin with an inflamed base, containing pus.

**Putrefaction.** Decomposition of proteins by the action of enzymes from anaerobic bacteria.

**Pyramid.** Apparently solid structure having a square base and four triangular sides that meet at a central point.

**Radiate.** To spread out from a common point.

**Radiation protection officer.** Supervisor, in an institution licensed to use radionuclides, who has the responsibility to establish procedures and make recommendations in the use of all radioactive matter.

**Radionuclide.** Chemical element that is similar in chemical properties to another element, but differs in atomic weight and electric charge and emits radiation. An atom that disintegrates by emission of electromagnetic radiation.

**Ramus.** Vertical portion of the mandible.

**Rate of flow.** Speed at which fluid is injected, measured in ounces per minute.

**Rate of flow valve.** Device or setting on the embalming machine that controls the speed of fluid delivery.

**Razor burn (razor abrasion).** Mark of desiccation. A darkened, air-dried area on the skin resulting from removal of the epidermis while shaving the remains.

**Re-aspiration.** Repeated aspiration of a cavity.

**Reducing agent.** Substance that easily loses electrons and thereby causes other substances to be reduced. Formaldehyde is a strong reducing agent.

**Repose.** To lay at rest.

**Resinous substance.** Amorphous, nonvolatile solid or soft side substance, a natural exudation from plants. Any of a class of solid or soft organic compounds of natural or synthetic origin.

**Restoration.** Treatment of the deceased in the attempt to recreate natural form and color.

**Restorative art.** Care of the deceased to recreate natural form and color.

**Restorative fluid (humectant).** Supplemental fluid, used with the regular arterial solution, whose purpose is to retain body moisture and retard dehydration.

**Restricted cervical injection.** Method of injection wherein both common carotid arteries are raised.

**Restricted drainage.** See Intermittent drainage and Alternate drainage.

**Right atrium.** Chamber on the right side of the heart seen as the center of drainage. Used as a site of drainage via instruments from the right internal jugular vein and direct via the trocar or through the thoracic wall.

**Rigor mortis.** Postmortem stiffening of the body muscles by natural body processes.

**Risorius muscle.** (Laughing muscle) Narrow superficial band of muscle that pulls the angle of the mouth laterally.

**Ruddy.** Red complexion; having a healthy reddish color, said of the complexion, more vivid than florid.

**Saccharolysis.** Decomposition of sugars.

**Safety Data Sheet (SDS).** OSHA Hazard Communication Standard 29 CFR 1910.1200; requires chemical manufacturers to provide a document for each hazardous chemical to *end users* to communicate information on hazards. The document is presented in a consistent user-friendly, 16-section format. The SDS includes information, such as the properties of each chemical; the physical, health, and environmental hazards; protective measures; and safety precautions for handling, storing, and transporting the chemical. Replaced the Material Safety Data Sheet (MSDS).

**Sallow.** Yellowish, sickly color of the complexion.

**Sanitation.** Process to promote and establish conditions that minimize or eliminate biohazards.

**Saturation.** Visual aspect indicating the vividness of the hue in the degree of difference from gray of the same lightness.

**Saponification.** Process of soap formation. As related to decomposition, the conversion of fatty tissues of the body into a soapy waxy substance called adipocere or grave wax.

**Saprophytic bacteria.** Bacteria that derive their nutrition from dead organic matter.

**Scab.** Crust over a healing sore or wound.

**Scalpel.** Two-piece embalming instrument consisting of a handle and a blade used to make incisions and excisions.

**Sealer.** Quick-drying liquid that leaves a hard, thin transparent coat or layer through which moisture cannot pass.

**Sealing agents.** Agents that provide a barrier or seal against any leakage of fluid or blood.

**Sear(ing).** To cauterize tissues by heat or chemical to provide a dry foundation for restoration.

**Second-degree burn.** Those resulting in acute inflammation of the skin and blisters.

**Secondary dilution.** Dilution of the embalming fluid by the fluids in the body, both vascular and interstitial.

**Sectional hypodermic embalming.** Embalming of a large body area (e.g., hand or side of face) by the injection of embalming chemicals directly into the tissues through the use of a syringe and needle or a trocar.

**Sectional vascular embalming.** Embalming of a body area or region (e.g., arm or side of face) by the injection of an embalming solution into an artery that in life supplied blood to that particular body region.

**Semilunar incision.** Crescent shaped or flaplike incision.

**Sepsis.** Pathologic state resulting from the presence of microorganisms or their products in the blood or other tissues.

**Septicemia.** Condition characterized by the multiplication of bacteria in blood.

**Septum.** Vertical cartilage dividing nasal cavity into two chambers, responsible for asymmetry of the nose.

**Sequestering agent.** Chemical agent that can "fence off" or "tie up" metal ions so that they cannot react with other chemicals.

**Serrated.** Notched on the edge like a saw, as seen with forceps.

**Sharps.** Hypodermic needles, suture needles, injector needles, scalpel blades, razor blades, pins, and other items sharp enough to cause percutaneous injury, penetration of unbroken skin. May include other items normally not disposed of following use such as scissors, teeth, fingernails, and ribs.

**Sharps container.** Occupational Safety and Health Administration–required receptacle for proper disposal of sharps.

**Sheen.** Shine; as of the reflection of natural oils of the skin.

**Short-term exposure limit (STEL).** Legal limits established by the Occupational Health and Safety Administration to which workers can be exposed continuously for a short period without damage or injury. Exposures at the STEL should not be longer than 15 minutes and not repeated more than four times per workday.

**Sign of death.** Manifestation of death in the body.

**Simple fracture.** Fractured bone that does not pierce the skin.

**Six-point injection.** A multipoint injection in the autopsied or unautopsied body in which six areas of the body are separately injected: right and left common carotid, axillary, and femoral arteries are six arteries frequently used for a six-point injection.

**Skeletal edema.** Edema in the body appendages, trunk, and/or head as contrasted with edema of the body cavities.

**Sodium hypochlorite.** Unstable salt usually produced in an aqueous solution and used as a bleaching and disinfecting agent. See Household bleach.

**Solute.** Substance that is dissolved in a solution.

**Solution.** Liquid containing dissolved substance.

**Solvent.** Liquid holding another substance in solution.

**Somatic death.** Death of the organism as a whole.

**Spatula.** Flat, blunt, knifelike instrument used for mixing cosmetics and modeling; a palette knife.

**Split injection.** Injection from one site and drainage from a separate site.

**Sponge.** Elastic, porous mass of interlacing horny fibers that are permanently attached; remarkable for its power of absorbing water and becoming soft when wet without losing its toughness.

**Squama.** Vertical surface of the temporal bone.

**Stabilization.** Minimal decedent care procedures for temporarily suspending natural organic decomposition. Often performed for identification viewing and cultural and religious rituals such as bathing and shrouding. Cavity aspiration is performed with or without the introduction of chemical and sanitizing products. Stabilization treatment without the use of hazardous products is compatible with natural or Green burials.

**Stain removers.** Any substances or agents that will cause an external discoloration to be removed or lessened.

**Sterilization.** Process that renders a substance free of all microorganisms.

**Sterilizers.** Oven or appliance for sterilizing. An autoclave that sterilizes by steam under pressure at temperatures above 100 degree centigrade.

**Sternocleidomastoid muscle (SCM).** Muscle of the neck that is attached to the mastoid process of the temporal bone and superior nuchal line and by separate heads to the sternum and clavicle. They function together to flex the head and form the lateral boundaries of the cervical triangle and the widest part of the neck.

**Stethoscope.** Delicate instrument used to detect almost inaudible sounds produced in the body.

**Stillborn.** Dead at birth. A product of conception either expelled or extracted dead.

**Subcutaneous.** Situated or occurring beneath the skin.

**Subcutaneous emphysema.** Distension of the tissues beneath the skin by gas or air. An antemortem condition brought about by a surgical procedure or trauma.

**Submandibular.** Describing those portions that lie immediately inferior to the mandible.

**Submental sulcus.** Junction of the base of the chin and the submandibular area, which may appear as a furrow; a natural facial marking.

**Superciliary arches.** Inferior part of the forehead just superior to the median ends of the eyebrows.

**Supercilium.** Eyebrows.

**Superficial.** Toward the surface.

**Superior.** Anatomically toward the head.

**Superior palpebral sulcus.** Furrow of the superior border of the upper eyelid; acquired facial marking.

**Supine.** Lying on the back or with the face upward.

**Supplemental fluid.** A fluid the embalmer injects prior to the preservative solution (e.g., pre-injection fluid) or adds to the preservative solution to enhance certain qualities of the preservative fluid (e.g., co-injection, dye, humectant, and water conditioner).

**Supraorbital area.** Region between the supercilium and the superior palpebrae.

**Supraorbital margins.** Superior rim of the eye sockets.

**Surface compress (pack).** An absorbent material saturated with an embalming chemical and placed in direct contact with the tissue.

**Surface discoloration.** Discoloration due to the deposit of matter on the skin surface. Surface discolorations may occur antemortem or during or after embalming of the body. Examples are adhesive tape, ink, iodine, paint, and tobacco stains.

**Surface embalming.** See Embalming.

**Surfactant (surface tension reducer; wetting, penetrating, or surface-active agent).** Chemical that reduces the molecular cohesion of a liquid so that it can flow through smaller apertures.

**Surgical reduction.** Restoration to a normal position or level through surgical excision.

**Sustain.** To provide support for; to hold in a fixed position.

**Suture.** Act of sewing; also the completed stitch.

**Swab.** Bit of cotton or cloth used for removing moisture or discharges from mucous membranes as well as for applying bleaches or liquid disinfectants.

**Swarthy.** Dark-colored complexion, as a face made swarthy by the tropical sun.

**Tache noire.** A brown to black band of discolored sclera of the eye. Created by the postmortem drying of the sclera by the air.

**Taphonomy.** The scientific study of decomposition; the study of processes (such as burial, decay, and preservation) that affect remains.

**Tardieu spots.** Minute petechial hemorrhages caused by the rupture of minute vessels as blood settles into the dependent areas of organs and tissues; it is accompanied by livor mortis. Postmortem, extravascular blood discoloration. Most common in asphyxial or slow deaths.

**Temporal bones.** Inferior portion of the sides and base of the cranium, inferior to the parietal bones and anterior to the occipital bone.

**Temporal cavity.** Concave surface of the head overlying the temporal bones.

**Temporalis muscles.** Muscle of mastication that helps to close the mandible (the strongest chewing muscles).

**Temporary preservation.** Science of treating the body chemically so as to temporarily inhibit decomposition.

**Terminal disinfection.** Institution of disinfection and decontamination measures after preparation of the remains.

**Test of death.** Any procedure used to prove a sign of death.

**Thanatology.** Study of death.

**Thanatopraxy.** Embalming as practiced in European countries, it involves preservation and presentation of the body so that the body may be viewed by friends and family. This distinguishes the preparation from that of medical embalming where only preservation is a concern.

**Third-degree burns.** Burns that result in destruction of cutaneous and subcutaneous tissues (seared, charred, or roasted tissue).

**Three-quarter view.** In reference to a photograph, a view revealing the fullness of the cheeks.

**Time-weighted average (TWA).** Exposure that is time weighted over an established period. It allows the exposure levels to be averaged generally over an 8-hour period.

**Tissue builder.** Substance used to elevate sunken (emaciated) tissues to normal level by hypodermic injection.

**Tissue coagulation.** See Coagulation.

**Tissue gas.** Postmortem accumulation of gas in tissues or cavities brought about by an anaerobic gas forming bacillus, *Clostridium perfringens*.

**Tobacco tar.** Yellowish-brown discoloration of the fingernails and fingers from excessive use of cigarettes.

**Topical disinfection.** Disinfection of the surface of the body or an object.

**Tragus.** Elevation protecting the ear passage (external auditory meatus).

**Translocation.** Agonal or postmortem redistribution of host microflora on a hostwide basis.

**Transplantation.** Grafting of living tissue from its normal position to another site or of an organ or tissue from one person to another.

**Transverse.** Lying at right angles to the long axis of the body.

**Transverse frontal sulci.** Furrows that cross the forehead; acquired facial markings.

**Trauma.** Physical injury or wound caused by external force or violence.

**Trocar.** Sharply pointed surgical instrument used in cavity embalming to aspirate the cavities and inject cavity fluid. The trocar may also be used for supplemental hypodermic embalming.

**Trocar button.** Plastic threaded device used for sealing small punctures and trocar entry points.

**Trocar button applicator.** Instrument used to securely tighten the trocar button.

**Trocar guide.** Line drawn or visualized on the surface of the body or a prominent anatomic structure used to locate internal structures during cavity embalming, from a point of reference 2 inches to the left of and 2 inches superior to the umbilicus.

**Tumor.** Spontaneous new growth of tissue forming an abnormal mass.

**Undercoat.** Coloring (opaque) applied to an area, which, when dry, will be covered with wax or another colorant.

**Undercut.** Angled cut of the borders of an excision, made so that the skin surface will overhang the deeper tissues.

**Unionall.** Plastic garment designed to cover the entire body from the neck down to and including the feet.

**Universal precautions.** See Bloodborne Pathogen Rule.

**Vacuum breaker.** Apparatus that prevents the back-siphonage of contaminated liquids into potable water supply lines or plumbing cross-connections within the preparation room.

**Vasa vasorum.** Vessels on vessels (vv) are tiny blood vessels that supply the large vessel walls with nutrients.

**Vascular (arterial) embalming.** See Embalming.

**Vehicle.** Liquid that serves as a solvent for the numerous ingredients incorporated into embalming fluids.

**Vertex.** Top of the head.

**Vertical.** Perpendicular to the plane of the horizon, balanced.

**Viral hepatitis.** Inflammation of the liver caused by a virus (possibly as many as seven in number) capable of causing acute or chronic hepatitis illness. The transmission can be oral-fecal, parenteral, or sexual.

**Viscera.** Internal organs enclosed within a cavity.

**Viscosity.** Resistance to the flow of a liquid. Thickness of a liquid.

**Vitreous humor.** Semifluid, transparent substance that lies between the retina and lens of the eyeball.

**Vomer bone.** Bone of the nasal cavity situated between the nasal passages on the median plane; forms the inferior and posterior portion of the septum of the nose.

**Vancomycin-resistant enterococci (VRE).** A drug-resistant bacterium found in feces and open wounds. It can also be found associated with nasogastric tubes often in patients who have had long hospitalization.

**Vancomycin-resistant *Staphylococcus aureus* (VRSA).** *Staphylococcus aureus* pathogens that have become resistant to the drugs methicillin and vancomycin.

**Warm color areas.** Areas of the skin surface that, during life, are naturally reddened; places where cosmetics will be applied to restore the warmth that red will give.

**Water conditioner.** Complexing agent used to remove chemical constituents that could interfere with arterial formulations from municipal water supplies.

**Water hardness.** Quality of water containing certain substances, especially soluble salts of calcium and magnesium.

**Waterless embalming.** Arterial injection of an embalming solution composed of arterial fluid, humectant, and co-injection fluid. No water is added to the solution.

**Waterlogged.** Condition resulting from the use of an embalming solution containing an insufficient amount of preservative to meet the preservative demand of the tissues. The interstitial spaces are overly filled, engorged with water.

**Wax.** Restorative modeling or surfacing material composed of beeswax, spermaceti, paraffin, starch, and so on and a coloring pigment that will soften at body temperature and will reflect light in a manner similar to normal skin.

**Weather line.** Line of color change at the junction of the wet and dry portions of each mucous membrane.

**Wet gangrene.** See Gangrene.

**Wet ice.** A solid form of water; this occurs at 32 degrees Fahrenheit.

**Wetting agent.** See Surfactant.

**Wicking.** Operative aid used to hasten the removal of edematous fluids. Lengths of cotton are inserted into tissues that have undergone channeling; the cotton readily absorbs or "wicks" the edematous fluid from the area.

**Width.** Dimension of an object measured across from side to side.

**Work practice controls.** See Bloodborne Pathogen Rule.

**Worm suture.** (Inversion, draw stitch) Method of sewing an incision along the edges without entering the opening whereby the suture becomes invisible and the line of suture becomes depressed, which lends it ease of concealment by waxing.

**Zygomatic arch.** Processes on the temporal and zygomatic bones; determines the widest part of the face.

**Zygomatic arch depression.** One of the lesser concavities of the face located on the lateral portion of the cheek inferior to the zygomatic arch.

**Zygomatic bones.** Small bones of the cheeks; widest part of the cheek.

**Zygomaticofrontal process.** Lateral rim of the eye socket formed by a process of the frontal bone and a process of the zygomatic bone.

**Zygomaticus major muscles.** Muscles of the face that draw the superior lip posteriorly, superiorly, and anteriorly.

**Zygomaticus minor muscles.** Muscles of the face that draw the superior lip superiorly and anteriorly.

| ACRONYMS | |
|---|---|
| ACGIH | American Congress of Governmental Industrial Hygienists |
| AIDS | Acquired immunodeficiency syndrome |
| AL | Action level |
| ANSI | American National Standard Institute |
| BCME | Bischloromethyl ether |
| CDCP | Centers for Disease Control and Prevention |
| ECG | Electrocardiogram (also EKG) |
| EEG | Electroencephalogram |
| EPA | Environmental Protection Agency |
| FCI | The Formaldehyde Council, Inc. |
| FTC | Federal Trade Commission |
| HBV | Hepatitis B virus |
| HIV | Human immunodeficiency virus |
| IVP | Intravascular pressure |
| mCi | Millicurie |
| MRSA | Methicillin-resistant *Staphylococcus aureus* |
| NCI | U.S. National Cancer Institute |
| NIOSH | National Institute for Occupational Safety and Health |
| OPIM | Other potentially infectious material |
| OSHA | Occupational Safety and Health Administration |
| PEL | Permissible exposure limit |
| pH | Potential of hydrogen |
| PPE | Personal protective equipment |
| ppm | Parts per million |
| SDS | Safety Data Sheet |
| STEL | Short-term exposure limit |
| TLV | Threshold limit value |
| TWA | Time-weighted average |
| VRE | Vancomycin-resistant enterococci |
| VRSA | Vancomycin-resistant *Staphylococcus aureus* |

## REFERENCES

Benenson AS. *Control of Communicable Diseases in Man*, 15th ed. Baltimore, MD: Victor Graphics, 1990.

DiMaio VJ, DiMaio D. *Forensic Pathology*, 2nd ed. Boca Raton, FL: CRC Press, 2001.

Embalming Course Content Syllabus. American Board of Funeral Service Education, 2016.

Frederick LG, Strub CG. *The Principles and Practices of Embalming*, 5th ed. Dallas, TX: Professional Training Schools, 1989.

Mayer JS. *Color and Cosmetics.* Dallas, TX: Professional Training Schools, 1991.

Mayer JS. *Restorative Art*, 13th ed., Dallas, TX: Professional Training Schools, 1993.

Mayer RG. *Embalming: History, Theory and Practice*, 5th ed. New York: McGraw-Hill, 2012.

*Merriam Webster's Collegiate Dictionary*, 11th ed. Springfield, MA: Merriam-Webster, 2003.

Restorative Art Course Content Syllabus. American Board of Funeral Service Education, 2006.

Spitz WU. *Medicolegal Investigation of Death*, 3rd ed. Springfield, IL: Charles C. Thomas, 1993.

Venes D. *Taber's Cyclopedic Medical Dictionary*, 23rd ed. Philadelphia, PA: F.A. Davis, 2017.

# Index

Page numbers followed by "f" denote figures; those followed by "t" denote tables.

## A

AAMI. *See* American Academy McAllister Institute
Abdomen
 discoloration in, 283, 283f
 nine-region method of, 214, 215f
 quadrant method of, 214, 215f
 topographical divisions of, 213–216
 viscera of, 212
Abdominal aorta
 in adults, 129t, 147
 in infants, 238
Abdominal aortic aneurysm, 246, 316
Abdominal cavity
 absorbent compound placed in, 242
 aspiration of, 210f, 218
 distension of, 284f
 edema of. *See* Ascites
 partial autopsy of, 260
Abdominal feeding tube, 173, 173f
Abdominal surgery, 152
Abdominopelvic regions, 214, 215f
Abrasions, 176, 294, 296, 305
Accessory chemicals, 95
Acetone, 56, 119
*Acinetobacter baumannii*, 35
Action level, 46
Active dyes, 105, 106f
Active transport, 205
Actual pressure, 72, 200
Acute disseminated histoplasmosis, 339
Addison disease, 291
Adenosine triphosphate, 89, 279
Adipocere, 92
Adolescents, 244–245
Advanced age. *See* Elderly
*Advice for Future Corpses*, 4
Age considerations
 children. *See* Children
 elderly. *See* Elderly
 infants, 237–243, 239f–243f
Agonal algor, 84
Agonal capillary expansion, 84
Agonal coagulation, 84
Agonal dehydration, 84
Agonal edema, 84
Agonal fever, 84
Agonal hypostasis, 84

Agonal period
 changes during, 84
 definition of, 84
 length of, 83
Air passageway tubes, 171
Air pollution, 427
Air pressure machine, 72, 72f, 212
Airbrush applicator, 397–398, 398f
Albumin, 98
Alcoholism, 336–337
Alcohols, 101
Aldehydes, 99
Aleutian Islands, 354
Alexander, Joseph B., 364–365
Algor mortis, 85t, 86, 86f, 155t
Alkaline hydrolysis, 97
Alkyl dimethylbenzyl ammonium chloride, 56
Allergic reactions, 153t
ALS. *See* Amyotrophic lateral sclerosis
Alternate drainage, 190
Amaranth, 56, 106
American Academy McAllister Institute, 379
American Board of Funeral Service Education, 3, 341, 379
American Society of Embalmers Best Practice Embalming tenets, 8
*American Way of Death, The*, 4
Amines, 91
Amino acids, 100–101
Amitrole, 56
Ammonia, 56
Ammonia injection test, 94
Amyotrophic lateral sclerosis, 245
Anaerobic bacteria, 91
Anal purge, 156, 330–331, 331t
Anasarca, 306, 307t, 308
Anatomical donation to medical science, 14
Anatomical embalming, 13–14
Anatomical guide, 121
Anatomical limit, 121
Anatomical position, 121
Anemia, 246
Aneurysm, 246, 316, 317t
Aneurysm hooks, 73, 73f
Aneurysm needles, 73, 73f
Angstadt, Earle K., 396–397, 397f
Angular spring forceps, 74, 75f, 78, 143t, 144f, 190

Animals, 352
Anionic surfactants, 105
Antecubital fossa, 145
Antemortem clots, 186
Antemortem dehydration, 304–305
Antemortem period
 cellular death in, 84
 definition of, 83
Antemortem subcutaneous emphysema, 216
Anterior axillary folds, 126
Anterior cervical triangle, 121–125, 125f
Anterior horizontal incision, 140, 141f
Anterior tibial artery, 135–136, 136f, 147, 147f
Anterior triangle of neck, 121–125, 125f
Anterior vertical incision, 140, 141f
Anthropoid coffin, 351, 351f
Anthropology, physical, 396
Antibiotics, 325
Anticoagulants, 103–104
Antihypertensives, 326t
Anti-inflammatory drugs, 325
Antimetabolite drugs, 325
Aorta, 129, 129t
Aortic aneurysm, 316
Aortic arch, 129t, 201
Aortic coagulum, 196f
Aortic repair, 152
Aortic valve, 319
Armed Force Service Members, DOD mortuary standards for, 405–409
Arterial chemicals, 111t
Arterial coagula, 320, 320f
Arterial embalming
 anterior tibial artery for, 147, 147f
 axillary artery for, 144–145, 145f
 brachial artery for, 145, 145f
 as capillary embalming, 193
 cavity embalming and, 13
 common carotid artery for, 143
 definition of, 194
 dehydration effects on, 305
 description of, 12–13, 315
 external iliac artery for, 147
 facial artery for, 144, 144f
 femoral artery for, 146, 146f
 functions of, 193
 in infants, 239
 inferior vena cava for, 148

485

Arterial embalming (*Cont.*):
  internal iliac artery for, 148
  internal jugular vein for, 143–144
  popliteal artery for, 147
  posterior tibial artery for, 147, 147f
  processes involved in, 179
  radial artery for, 145, 145f
  ulnar artery for, 145, 146f
Arterial fluid
  chemical nature of, 194
  components of, 96f, 111
  definition of, 95
  density of, 115
  dilution of, 112–113
  dyes in, 103
  eco-friendly, 112
  formaldehyde-based, 112
  high-index, 116
  nonformaldehyde, 116
  packaging of, 111
  penetrating of, 223–224
  special-purpose, 112, 116
  surface embalming contraindications for, 223
  temperature of, 115
  tissue gas fluid, 116
Arterial hemostat, 73, 73f
Arterial injection
  body preparation prior to
    bathing, 161, 161f
    disinfection, 160
    external orthopedic devices, 174–175, 175f
    eye closure, 168–171, 169f–170f
    facial hair, 162f, 162–163
    four-step approach, 159
    hair care, 161–162
    lifting and transferring, 159
    lip closure, 164, 168, 169f
    medical device removal, 171–174, 172f–174f
    modesty cloth, 160, 161f
    mouth closure. *See* Mouth, closure of
    orthopedic devices, 174–175, 175f
    packing the trunk orifices, 171
    positioning of body, 163f, 163–164
    preliminary, 159
    rigor mortis, 163, 163f
    setting the features, 164–171
    shaving, 162f, 162–163
    shoulder positioning, 164
  cavity embalming after, 216
  in decomposition, 285–286
  embalming analysis of, 153, 155–156
  instant tissue fixation technique, 184–185
  multipoint injection technique, 181, 181f
  one-point injection technique, 179–181, 180f, 191
  pre-embalming treatments
    abrasions, 176
    ascites, 177
    discolorations, 175
    fractures, 175–176, 176f
    lacerations, 175–176
  purge caused by, 331
  restricted cervical injection technique, 182–184, 183f, 192, 248
  in rigor mortis, 280
  sectional, 153
  six-point injection technique, 181f, 181–182
  split injection technique, 182, 182f, 192
Arterial scissors, 74, 143t
Arterial solution
  bleaching of tissues caused by, 203
  center of distribution of, 201
  definition of, 95
  in delayed embalming, 278–279
  diffusion of
    description of, 193, 204–205, 207
    dialysis in, 206f, 206–207
    mechanisms of, 205–207
    osmosis in, 206, 206f
    pressure filtration, 205–206
    schematic diagram of, 206f
    signs of, 201–202
  distribution of, 193
    center of, 201
    improvements in, 204
    signs of, 201–203
  drainage of, 194f
  drying of tissues caused by, 203
  dyes with, 202, 202f
  "50-pound rule," 113
  gravity filtration of, 207
  guidelines for, 114
  injection of
    arterial distention before, 203–204
    combined resistance on, 197
    description of, 194–195, 195f
    extravascular resistance during, 195f, 195–197
    gases in cavities effect on, 196–197
    hollow viscera expansion during, 197
    intravascular resistance during, 195f, 195–196
    observations before, 203–204
    paths of least resistance effects on, 198–199
    rigor mortis effects on, 196
    rigor mortis relief before, 203
    vein distention before, 203–204
  at microcirculatory level, 195
  mixing of, 252
  movement of, into cells, 207, 207f
  osmosis of, 206, 206f
  osmotic qualities of, 115
  pH, 114–115
  postmortem stain effects on, 291
  quantity of, 113
  rate of flow for, 200
  retention of, 160f, 194, 194f
  signs of, 201–203
  small vessel distention caused by, 202–203, 203f
  strength of, 111–112, 156
Arterial tubes, 13, 75–76, 76f, 141f, 143t

Arteries. *See also specific artery*
  of distal leg, 135–136, 136f
  of foot, 136, 136f
  of head, 121–126, 122f–126f
  as injection point, 140
  layers of, 315, 316f
  of lower limbs, 130–136, 132f–136f
  of neck, 121–126, 122f–126f
  nerves versus, 139–140, 140t
  sclerotic, 316
  of trunk, 129, 129t–131t
  of upper limbs, 126f–129f, 126–129
  veins versus, 139–140, 140t, 316f
Arteriosclerosis, 154t, 245–246, 315–316, 317t, 319f
Arteritis, 317t
Arthritic conditions, 245
Artificial means of preservation, 347
Ascending aorta
  in adults, 129t, 201
  in infants, 238
Ascending colon, 213
Ascites, 177, 197, 292, 307t, 308, 311–312, 322, 329
Asepsis, 43
Asia, 379
Aspergillosis, 338
Asphyxiation, 317t
Aspiration. *See also* Cavity aspiration
  abdominal cavity, 210f, 218
  ascites, 312f
  cranial, 219
  definition of, 13
  pelvic cavity, 210f, 218
  thoracic cavity, 210f, 218
Astor, Jacob, 391
Atheroma, 315, 317t
ATP. *See* Adenosine triphosphate
Atrioventricular valve, 319
Attachments
  deep-link, 5
  life experiences as source of, 5
  separation of, 5
Attention Funeral Director form, 18, 24f
Auditory evoked response, 94
Australia, 379
Authorization for Minimum Care Services form, 17, 18f
Authorization for Restorative and Cosmetic Care form, 17, 17f
Authorization to Prepare Donation Cases for Viewing form, 17, 20f
Autoclaving, 42
Autolysis, 91–92, 281
Autopsy
  best practices for, 250–251
  body preparation, 252–255
  closure of cavities in, 256, 256f
  complete, 238, 239f, 250–252
  cranial cavity preparation, 256–259, 257f–259f
  definition of, 249, 250
  drainage in, 251
  facial trauma restoration, 260

final procedures in, 259, 259f
fluid dyes in, 251
fluid strength in, 251
forensic, 249–250
hospital, 249
infants, 238–239, 239f
local, 238
medical, 249
medicolegal, 249–250
outline for, 251–252
overdose death, 259
partial, 218, 238, 250, 259–260
pulmonary embolism, 259
spinal cord, 250, 251f
trunk, 252f
types of, 249–250
viscera, 255, 256f
Autopsy aspirator, 212
Autopsy compounds, 119
Autopsy gels, 118
Axilla, 126–127
Axillary artery
in adults, 127, 127f, 144–145, 145f
in infants, 238
raising of, 253–254
right, 240f
Axillary drain tube, 189f
Axillary vein, 145, 188
Aztecs, 354

**B**
Babylonians, ancient, 352
Back skin, 270f–271f
Backflow, 66
Backflow preventor, 66
Bactericidal, 43
Bacteriostatic, 43
Baillie, Matthew, 359
Bandage scissors, 74, 74f
Bandages, 197, 197f
Barnes, Carl L., 372, 376, 391f
Barrier masks, 39
Barrow, Clyde, 393
Baseball suture, 227, 227f–228f, 256, 258, 266
Basilic vein, 128, 139, 188
Bathing, of body, 161, 161f, 232
Beards, 459
Bedsore, 175
Belgium, 379–380
Bereavement, complicated, 6
Bernard, E. G., 374
BIE. *See* British Institute of Embalmers
Bilirubin, 291
Biliverdin, 292–293
Biocides Directive, 36
Biohazard symbol, 45f
Biological death, 83
Biological hazards
exposure to, 34–36
hazard communication, 41
postexposure evaluation and follow-up, 39, 41
Biological stains, 106

Bistoury knife, 73
Black eye, 290, 294. *See also* Ecchymosis
Blanchard, Stephen, 357
Bleaching fluids, 116
Blisters, 176, 296
Blood
components of, 88
discolorations of, 87t, 89
drainage of, 185, 203
hemolysis of, 89
Blood discolorations
antemortem, 288–289
ecchymosis, 290, 290f
extravascular, 289–291
hypodermic treatment for, 290
intravascular, 289
livor mortis as, 289
petechiae, 290, 290f
postmortem, 289
postmortem stain as, 291, 300f. *See also* Postmortem stain
pre-injection fluids for clearing of, 289
surface embalming for, 290
Blood thinners, 152, 289
Blood vessels. *See* Arteries; Capillaries; Embalming vessels; Veins
Blood viscosity
dehydration effects on, 305
increased, 85t, 88, 155t
livor mortis affected by, 87
Bloodborne Pathogens Standard
compliance with, 38–39
engineering controls, 38–39
Exposure Control Plan, 38
exposure determination, 38
labeling provisions required by, 41
universal precautions, 38
Bloodborne pathogens
prevention of, 403–404
record keeping about, 41–43
transmission of, 41
Blunt trauma, 297t, 300
Body. *See also* Human remains
anatomical donation to medical science, 14
bathing of, 161, 161f, 232
conditions of, embalming treatments based on, 151, 154t
final inspection of, 232
gases from, 176t, 176–177
identification tag on, 15f
plastic garments on, 232–234, 233f
positioning of, 163f, 163–164
postmortem chemical changes in, 277
postmortem cooling of, 86
refrigerated. *See* Refrigerated bodies
transfer of, 159
viewing of
after death, 6–7, 342
for identification, 342
Body bridge, 163
Body image, 5
Body lice, 160
Body lifts, 68f, 68–69
Body typing, 149

Body water, 303
Boehringer, Philip, 303
Bonding agents, 229
Bone
donation of, 270–275, 272f
en bloc removal of, 270, 272
long, 272f–274f, 272–274
Bone ossification, 242
Boniface VIII, Pope, 355
*Book of the Dead,* 349
Borates, 102–104
Bovine spongiform encephalopathy, 437
Bowsher, Ivan P., 395
Brachial artery, 127–128, 145, 145f
Brachiocephalic vein, 143
Brain death, 83
Brain purge, 211t, 331, 331t
Breakthrough duration, 109
Bridge sutures, 227, 227f
Brier, Robert, 352
British Institute of Embalmers, 378
Broken skin, 296
Brown, Charles DaCosta, 364
Bruising, postmortem, 294
BSE. *See* Bovine spongiform encephalopathy
Buffers, 102
Bulb syringe, 70
Bunnell, William J., 364
Burial
embalming and, 3–4
green, 96
Burns, 297t, 297–298, 298f, 313, 317t
Burr, Richard, 366–367
Butlerov, Alexander, 97
2-Butoxyethanol, 56
"Butterfly rash," 291

**C**
Cachexia, 247
Cadaveric spasm, 91
Cadaverine, 283
Cadavers, 14, 359–361
Callaway, C.F., 394
Caloricity, postmortem, 89, 89t, 155t, 281
Calvarium, 240, 257f
Camphor, 56
Canada, 380
Canalization, 315
Canary Islands, 353
*Candida albicans,* 338
Candidiasis, 338
Canopic urns, 350, 350f
Capillaries
description of, 13, 204
expansion of, 204, 204f
Capillary attraction, 104
Capillary embalming, 13, 193
Capillary washes, 116
Carbohydrates, 92
Carbon monoxide poisoning, 289, 297t, 298–299
Carbon tetrachloride, 56
Carbonates, 102
Cardiac disease, 247

Carmine, 105
Carotene, 287
Carotid sheath, 123, 125
Cartonage, 351
Casket, 344
*Casket and Sunnyside,* 393, 395
Casts, 174
Catalysts, 91–92
Cationic surfactants, 105
Catliff, Betty, 396
Cattell, Henry P., 364–365
Cause of death, 249
Cautery chemicals, 118
Cavity aspiration. *See also* Aspiration
    abdominal cavity, 210f, 218
    abdominal opening closure for, 220
    chemical injection, 219
    cranial, 219
    devices used for, 211–212
    in infants, 238
    pelvic cavity, 210f, 218
    reaspiration, 220–221
    thoracic cavity, 210f, 218
    trocar for, 217, 217f
Cavity embalming
    abdomen in, 212–216
    after recent surgery, 217
    arterial embalming and, 13
    aspiration. *See* Cavity aspiration
    autopsy aspirator for, 212
    chronology of, 209–211
    definition of, 13
    direct incision method, 218
    electric aspirator for, 211
    equipment for, 211–212
    hydroaspirator for, 211
    instrumentation for, 211–212
    male genitalia, 218–219
    nasal tube aspirator for, 212
    organ removal, 217
    partial autopsy, 218
    purge in, 283
    in refrigerated bodies, 282–283
    solid organs treated by, 210
    time period for, 216–217
    trocar in, 212
    tubing for, 212
    visceral anatomy in, 212–213
Cavity fluid
    bleaching properties of, 292
    definition of, 95
    fumeless, 118
    injection of, 117–118
    packaging of, 111
    re-injection of, 220–221
    volume of, 219
Cavity fluid injector, 79, 79f
Cecum, 213
Ceiling hoists, 68, 68f
Cell membrane, 206
Cellular death, postmortem, 83
Cellular edema, 307, 307t
Centers for Disease Control and Prevention
    bloodborne pathogens, 34

Central America, 354
Cerebrovascular accident, 317t
Cervicoaxillary canal, 127, 127f, 144
Chamberlain, C.B., 367
Champion Company, 393
Chelating agents, 325
Chemical(s)
    embalming uses of. *See* Embalming chemicals
    exposure to, 36
    hazardous. *See* Hazardous chemicals
    spillage of, 33
Chemical adduct system, 116
Chemotherapeutic agents, 152, 323–327, 326t
"Cherry-red" discolorations, 289, 298f
Children
    causes of death in, 244
    fluid strengths and volume in, 243–244
    pressure in, 244
    rate of flow in, 244
    vessel selection of, 243
Chin rest, 167
Chlorinated compounds, 48
Chlorine salts, 56
Chloroform, 56
Chronic disseminated histoplasmosis, 339
Chronic kidney disease-associated pruritus, 313
Chronic pulmonary histoplasmosis, 339
Cincinnati College, 370, 391, 393
Circle needle, 74
Civil War, 362–363
CJD. *See* Creutzfeldt-Jakob disease
Clarke, Joseph Henry, 370f–371f, 370–371
Clauderus, Gabriel, 357
Cleaning, 43
Clinical death, 83
*Clostridium difficile,* 35
*Clostridium perfringens,* 89, 212, 232–233, 284, 329, 335
Clots, 320f, 320–321
Coagula, 186, 317t, 320f
Coal-tar dyes, 106
Cochineal, 105
Coffin, 351
Co-injection fluids, 96, 111, 117, 291
Cold chemical sterilants, 42
Collective unconscious, 7
Collier, William, 389, 393
Colloids, 206
Colombia, 381–382
Colostomy, 173–174, 174f, 230–231, 247
Common carotid artery
    anatomical features of, 121, 125, 143
    arteriosclerosis of, 315, 319f
    branches of, 124f
    in children, 243
    elasticity of, 140f
    incisions for, 140–141, 141f
    in infants, 238
    left, 240
    one-point injection using, 179, 180f

    raising of, 143
    restricted cervical injection use of, 184
    right
        anatomy of, 125f
        one-point injection using, 179, 180f
Comorbidities, 313
Competence, in professional practice, 7
Complete autopsy, 238, 239f, 250–252
Complicated bereavement, 6
Complicated grief, 6
Compound fractures, 176, 176f
Concurrent disinfection, 43
Concurrent drainage, 190
Conditions of Participation for Hospitals, 263
Confidentiality, 7
Confluent hemorrhage, 294
Congestive heart failure, 153t, 317t, 319–320
Conjunctival icterus, 291, 291f
Contact pallor, 86, 86f
Continuing education, 7
Continuous suture, 229, 229f
Coping, 5
Cornelius, W. P., 367–368
Corrosive poisons, 317t
Corticosteroids, 325, 326t
Cortisone, 325
Cosmetics, 297, 397
Coupling compound system, 116
Covid-19
    Delta variant of, 33
    embalming of bodies with, 465–467
    vaccinations for, 33–34
Crandall, Joel E., 372, 387, 388f, 389, 391, 393
Cranial aspiration, 219
Cranial cavity
    partial autopsy of, 259
    preparation of, 256–259, 257f–259f
Cranial incisions
    closure of, 240, 241f
    description of, 457
Cranial nerve X, 125
Cranial purge, 211
Cranial vault, 241f
Cranium, 212
Creams, 223
Cremated remains, 343
Cremation
    definition of, 409
    water, 97
Crepitation, 93, 176, 232, 332
Cresol, 56
Creutzfeldt-Jakob disease, 35, 433, 436–446
Cribriform plate, 219, 219f
Crusades, 355
Crystalloids, 206
Cudbear, 105
Curry, Gladys, P., 395
Custodial care, 234
Cyanide, 300
Cytotoxic drugs, 325

# D

da Vinci, Leonardo, 354–355
Dead, the
   in ancient Egypt, 3
   public sentiment toward, 4–5
   reverence for, 3–4
   rituals for, 4
   universal customs regarding, 4
Death
   ancient Egyptians' view of, 3
   biological, 83
   body temperature at, 86
   brain, 83
   clinical, 83
   embalming and, postmortem interval between, 152–153, 154t, 277, 297
   finality of, 6
   inexpert tests of, 94
   postmortem cellular, 83
   postmortem changes. *See* Postmortem period
   as process, 83
   psychosocial model of, 5–6
   rituals of, 4
   signs of, 84
   somatic, 83
   tests of, 93–94
   viewing the body after, 6–7
Death pallor, 287
Death rattle, 83
Death struggle, 83
Decay, 31, 91
Deceased donor, 263
De-Ce-Co needle injector, 397
Decedent Care Report form, 18, 25f–26f
Decedent care stations, 65, 66f
Decompose, 31
Decomposition
   advanced protocol, 285–286, 317t
   arterial injection in, 285–286
   autolysis in, 91–92
   of carbohydrates, 92
   catalysts of, 91–92
   color changes associated with, 92–93, 283, 283f
   definition of, 11, 31, 91
   dehydration associated with, 283
   description of, 85t, 176t
   desiccation associated with, 283
   desquamation associated with, 93, 93f
   discolorations caused by, 294
   embalming of body in, 89t, 155t, 284–285
   gas from, 93, 176t, 177, 196, 284, 334
   hypodermic injection in, 285–286
   of lipids, 92
   odor associated with, 93, 283–284
   order of, 92
   purge associated with, 92f, 93, 284
   in refrigerated bodies, 280, 281f
   restricted cervical injection in, 284–285
   sectional arterial embalming in, 285
   signs of, 92f–93f, 92–93
   six-point injection in, 284
   tongue in, 285
   treatment of features in, 285
   vascular changes in, 283
Decontamination, 43
Decubitus ulcers, 152, 156, 175, 297, 321
Deep-link attachments, 5
Defamation of character, 7
Defibrillators, 171, 172f, 230
Dehydrating fluid, 116
Dehydration
   antemortem, 304–305
   arterial embalming affected by, 305
   causes of, 303
   challenges associated with, 305
   description of, 85t, 87–88, 88f
   discoloration caused by, 293
   of fingers, 293
   monitoring of, postmortem, 155t, 157
   post-embalming, 306
   postmortem, 155t, 157, 305
   problems associated with, 305t
   in refrigerated bodies, 282, 301
   skin affected by, 305, 305t
   tissue, 281
   wrinkles caused by, 304f
Delayed embalming
   arterial solution strength and volume in, 278–279
   in decomposition
      color changes associated with, 283, 283f
      dehydration, 283
      embalming protocol, 284–285
      gases, 284
      livor mortis, 283
      odors, 283–284
      purges, 284
      vascular changes, 283
   overview of, 277
   of refrigerated bodies, 280–283, 281f–282f
   restricted cervical injection for, 278
   of rigor mortis bodies, 279t, 279–280
   six-point injection for, 278
   swelling concerns in, 282, 282f
Delayed viewing, 343, 343f, 416–419
Demarcation line, 457
Demisurgery, 389, 390f, 391–392
DeMort-Ology, 391–392
Density, 115
Dental tie, 167
Dentures, 165–166, 232
Department of Defense mortuary standards, 405–409
Dermasurgery, 392
Dermis, 287
Descending abdominal aorta, 129t
Descending colon, 213
Descending thoracic aorta, 129t
Desiccation, 283, 305
Desquamation, 93, 93f, 284, 296–297
Dhona, Charles O., 389, 391–393, 395
Diabetes mellitus, 247f, 247–248, 293, 317t, 321, 327
Diagonal incision, 142, 142f
Dialdehydes, 99–100
Dialysis, 206f, 206–207
Diethanolamine, 56
Diethylene glycol, 56
Differential pressure, 199, 200
Diffusion
   arterial solution, 193, 201–202, 204–205, 205f
      description of, 193, 204–205, 207
      dialysis in, 206f, 206–207
      mechanisms of, 205–207
      osmosis in, 206, 206f
      pressure filtration, 205–206
      schematic diagram of, 206f
      signs of, 201–202
   definition of, 204, 207
Dillinger, John, 393
Dimethylformamide, 56
Direct heart drainage, 148, 188–189
Direct incision method, 218
Discolorations
   abdomen, 283, 283f
   antemortem, 288
   before arterial injection, 204
   ascites, 292
   blood
      antemortem, 288–289
      ecchymosis, 175, 288, 290, 290f, 294
      extravascular, 289–291
      hypodermic treatment for, 290
      intravascular, 289
      livor mortis as, 289
      petechiae, 290, 290f
      postmortem, 289
      postmortem stain as, 291, 300f. *See also* Postmortem stain
      pre-injection fluids for clearing of, 289
      surface embalming for, 290
   of blood, 87t, 89
   from blunt trauma, 297t, 300
   from burns, 297t, 297–298, 298f
   from carbon monoxide poisoning, 289, 297t, 298–299
   "cherry-red," 289, 298f
   classification of, 287–289
   conditions related to, 294–301
   cosmetics for, 297
   decomposition, 294
   definition of, 287, 295
   dehydration, 293
   description of, 175
   diabetes mellitus, 293
   from drownings, 297t, 299
   from electrocution, 297t, 298
   embalming chemicals as cause of, 293–294
   from exsanguination, 297t, 300
   generalized, 287
   from gunshot wounds, 297t, 299–300
   from hanging, 297, 297t
   jaundice, 291–292, 292f
   localized, 287
   from mold, 297t, 301, 343f
   from mutilations, 297t, 300
   nephritis, 292–293
   pathological, 291–293

Discolorations (*Cont.*):
  pharmaceutical, 291
  from poisoning, 297t, 300
  postmortem, 288
  in refrigerated bodies, 297t, 300–301
  of skin, 175
  from strangulation, 297, 297t
  surface, 293
  treatment of, 231
Disease(s)
  infectious, work-related, 432–434
  transmission of, 33
Disinfectants
  characteristics of, 233
  definition of, 43
  topical
    antimicrobial activity of, 451–453
    broad-spectrum, 43
    in preparation room, 43, 45
Disinfection
  of body before arterial injection, 160
  terminal, 43, 233
  terminology associated with, 43
  of work environment, 42
Distal, 128
Distal forearm, 128–129
Distal leg, 135–136, 136f
Distention
  eye, 268
  eyelids, 299–300
  gases that cause, 333t
  treatment of, 231–232
Diverticulum, 213
Documentation, 7–8, 49. *See also* Forms
Dodge, A. Johnson, 371–372, 389, 396
Dodge, George B., 371–372
Dodge, Walter, 372
Dodge Chemical Company, The, 149, 395, 397
Donation. *See also* Organ donation; Tissue donation
  advancements in, 274
  body, 14
  consent process for, 263–264
  federal legislation and regulations, 263
  impact of, 264
  moment of silence process of, 263–264
Dorsalis pedis artery, 136, 136f
Double "T" incision, 142f, 143
Double-curved needles, 74
Drain tube, 189–490
Drainage
  alternate, 190
  in autopsy, 251
  blood, 185, 203
  closed, 186, 191
  concurrent, 190
  direct heart, 148, 188–189, 189f
  disinfection of, 191
  first, 191
  hydrocephalus, 313
  instruments for, 76–78, 77f, 189–190
  intermittent, 190, 191f
  lymphatic, 185f, 185–187
  methods of, 190
  purpose of, 187
  from right atrium, 143, 144f, 148, 187, 187f
  sites for, 187–188
  techniques for improving, 190–191
Drainage forceps, 74, 75f
Drain tubes, 77f, 189
Drains, surgical, 173, 231
Drench shower, 66
Dressing forceps, 73, 73f
Dressing table, 70, 70f
Drownings, 297t, 299
Drug(s)
  antibiotics, 325
  antidiabetic, 326t, 327
  anti-inflammatory, 325
  chemotherapeutic, 152, 323–327, 326t
  corticosteroids, 325, 326t
  embalming affected by, 324–325
  multidrug, 324–325
  opioids, 326–327, 327f
  radioactive isotopes, 326
Drug treatments, 152, 153t
Dry abrasions, 176
Dry gangrene, 291, 317t
Dry skin, 296
Duodenum, 213
Dyes, 105, 106f, 117, 202, 202f
Dying
  antemortem period, 83
  as process, 83
Dyslipidemia, 337

## E

Ebola hemorrhagic fever virus, 433
Ecchymosis, 175, 288, 290, 290f, 294, 324f
ECG. *See* Electrocardiogram
Eckels, Howard S., 373, 389, 390f
Ecuador, 353
Edema. *See also* Ascites
  agonal, 84
  aspiration of, 292f
  burns as cause of, 313
  cellular, 307, 307t
  definition of, 306
  diseases associated with, 306–307
  embalming challenges caused by, 308
  of face, 164, 307t
  of foot, 310f
  generalized, 154t, 308–310
  of hands, 307t
  of legs, 307t, 310
  local treatments for, 310–313
  localized, 306
  lymphedema, 310, 311f
  pitting, 307t, 308
  postmortem, 88
  pulmonary, 307t, 320
  skeletal, 197
  solid, 307t, 307–308
  of trunk, 311
Edema reducing fluid, 117
EDTA, 56, 104

Educational materials, 396–399
EEG. *See* Electroencephalogram
Egyptians
  description of, 3, 347–348
  preparation steps used by, 349–352
EKG. *See* Electrocardiogram
Elderly
  arteriosclerosis in, 245–246
  arthritic conditions in, 245
  cardiac disease in, 247
  diabetes mellitus in, 247f, 247–248
  malignancy in, 246–247
  mouth closure in, 245
  senile purpura in, 246, 246f
Electric aspirator, 67, 211
Electric spatula, 268
Electrocardiogram, 94
Electrocution, 297t, 298
Electroencephalogram, 93
Ellsworth, Elmer, 363
Emaciated features, 461–462
Embalm, 31
Embalmers
  biological hazards for, 34–36
  objectives of, 308
  occupationally acquired infection risks, 34–35
  universal precautions used by, 35
Embalmer's gray, 163, 293
Embalming
  air pollution and, 427
  anatomical, 13–14
  art of, 464–465
  arterial. *See* Arterial embalming
  authorization for, 16, 16f
  burial and, 3–4
  cavity. *See* Cavity embalming
  classifications of, 12–13
  definition of, 3, 11, 31
  delayed. *See* Delayed embalming
  Egyptian practices in, 349–352
  expectations of, 12, 342
  fundamentals of, 14–15
  hypodermic. *See* Hypodermic embalming
  objectives of, 36, 84, 287, 303, 323
  phases of, 159, 278
  practical model of, 7
  during pregnancy, 36
  professional standards for, 8
  professionalism in, 378–379
  purpose of, 464–465
  as restorative process, 11–12
  soft method of, 14
  standards for, 406–409
  steps of, 278
  supplemental. *See* Supplemental embalming
  terminology associated with, 31
  variations in techniques, 157t
  waterless, 114–115
Embalming analysis
  confidentiality during, 149
  definition of, 13, 149
  factors to consider, 149–150, 278, 303

guidelines for, 150
historical methods of, 149, 347–384
information used in, 150–153
post-embalming monitoring and
  treatments, 156–158
postmortem conditions, 149
pre-embalming analysis
  age, 151
  definition of, 149
  drug treatments, 152, 153t
  intrinsic body conditions, 151, 154t
  musculature, 151
  postmortem interval between death and
    embalming, 152–153, 154t
  primary condition, 151
  same basic treatment, 151–152
  surgery, 152
  weight, 151
Embalming and Decedent Care Forms
  Attention Funeral Director, 18, 24f
  Authorization for Minimum Care Services,
    17, 18f
  Authorization for Restorative and
    Cosmetic Care, 17, 17f
  Authorization to Prepare Donation Cases
    for Viewing, 17, 20f
  Decedent Care Report, 18, 25f–26f
  Embalming Authorization, 16, 16f
  Embalming Report, 18, 27f–30f
  Green Funeral Release and
    Indemnification, 17, 21f
  Identification of Remains of the Decedent,
    17, 22f
  Minimum Care Authorization When
    Embalming is Declined, 17, 19f
  Trauma Viewing Without Embalming, 18,
    23f
Embalming and Decedent Care Report, 7–8,
  14, 344
Embalming Authorization form, 16, 16f
Embalming chemicals
  accessory, 118–120
  aldehydes, 99
  aliphatic nitrohydroxy compounds, 99
  antimicrobial activity of, 451–453
  arterial, 111, 111t
  autopsy compounds, 119
  autopsy gels, 118
  cautery chemicals, 118
  components of, 95
  dialdehydes, 99–100
  discolorations, 293–294
  formaldehyde. See Formaldehyde
  formaldehyde-free alternatives, 96
  glutaraldehyde, 99–100
  glyoxal, 99
  hardening compounds, 119
  mold inhibitors, 120
  "one-bottle," 412–414
  packaging of, 95
  paraformaldehyde, 58, 98–99
  phenol, 100, 100f
  preservative formaldehyde, 111–112
  purposes of, 95

sealing agents, 120
solvents, 119
tissue builder, 118–119
trioxane, 99
work practice controls for, 109
Embalming chemistry, 412–414
Embalming fluids
  alcohols in, 101
  anticoagulants in, 103–104
  borates in, 102–104
  buffers in, 102
  carbonates in, 102
  chemical principles of, 97
  in children, 243–244
  coloring agents in, 105–106
  components of, 96f
  description of, 95
  dyes in, 105, 106f, 202
  early patents for, 368
  EDTA in, 104
  emulsified oils in, 103
  essential oils in, 107
  ethylene glycol in, 103
  floral compounds in, 107
  fluorescent dyes in, 202
  formaldehyde. See Formaldehyde
  formaldehyde-free alternatives, 96
  germicides in, 101–102
  glycerine in, 103
  glycols in, 103
  gums in, 103
  humectants in, 102–103
  inorganic salts in, 103
  modifying agents in, 102
  perfuming agents in, 106–107
  pouring of, into embalming machine, 109,
    110f
  preservatives in
    definition of, 97
    description of, 95–96
  propylene glycol in, 103
  quaternary ammonium compounds in,
    102
  salts in, 101
  solvents in, 107
  sorbitol in, 103
  strength of, 243–244
  surface tension of, 104–105
  surfactants in, 104
  water in, 107
Embalming machines, 12, 70–72, 71f, 176t,
  233
Embalming preservative powder, 119
Embalming Report form, 18, 27f–30f
Embalming room
  plumbing in, 38–39
  ventilation in, 36, 38
Embalming schools, 368, 372
Embalming table. See Table
Embalming vessels. See also Arteries;
  Capillaries; Veins
  abdominal aorta, 147
  anterior tibial artery, 147, 147f
  axillary artery, 144–145, 145f

brachial artery, 145, 145f
common carotid artery, 140–141, 141f,
  143
comparison of, 139–140
external iliac artery, 147
facial artery, 144, 144f
incisions in
  for common carotid artery, 140–141,
    141f
  technique for, 142f, 142–143
  types of, 140–141, 141f–142f
inferior vena cava, 148
instruments for working with, 143t
internal iliac artery, 148
internal jugular vein, 143–144
ligature around, 141f, 141–142
locating of, 141–142
popliteal artery, 147
posterior tibial artery, 147
preparing of, 141–142
radial artery, 145, 145f
selection of, 139
thoracic aorta, 147
ulnar artery, 145, 146f
Emboli, 317t
Emergency shower, 66
Emphysema, subcutaneous, 176t, 177, 216,
  232, 332–334
Employee Right-To-Know laws, 38
Employers
  record keeping by, 41
  safety data sheet requirements, 53
  training requirements for, 46
Emulsified oils, 103
Endotracheal tubes, 171, 173f
Engineering controls, for formaldehyde, 48
England, 357
Enucleation, 254, 266
Environmental health and safety standards,
  48–49
Environmental Protection Agency
  formaldehyde classification as
    carcinogen by, 36
Enzymes, 12, 31
Eosin, 106
EPA. See Environmental Protection Agency
Epidermis, 287, 305
Epiploic appendices, 213
Erythrosine, 106
ESCO Review, 303
Esophageal varices, 317t
Essential oils, 107
Ethical performance standard, 7–8
Ethical practice, 7
Ethics, 7
Ethiopian stone, 350
Ethiopians, ancient, 353
Ethmoid bone, cribriform plate of, 219,
  219f
Ethyl acetate, 56
Ethyl alcohol, 56
Ethylene glycol, 57, 103
Ethylene glycol monomethyl ether, 57
Ethylenedichloride, 56

Europe, 379–380, 462–464
Evoked response, 94
Evolution injector, 13
Exanthema, 296
Excoriation, 176
Exposure Control Plan, 38
Exsanguination, 297t, 300
External carotid artery, 124f
External iliac artery
    in adults, 130, 132f, 134f, 147
    in infants, 238
External iliac vein, 130, 133f
External jugular vein, 123
External orthopedic devices, 174–175, 175f
Extravascular resistance, 195f, 195–197, 321–322
Eye(s)
    closure of, 168–171, 169f–170f, 237, 285
    distention of, 268
    donation of, 266f–269f, 266–268
    enucleation of, 254, 266
    inner canthus of, 168
    orbit of, 168
    outer canthus of, 168
Eye caps
    description of, 79, 80f, 170f, 171
    in infants, 237
    placement of, 267f
    removal of, 266f
Eye process, 376
Eye protection, 109
Eye speculum, 266f
Eye wash station, 66
Eyelids
    confluent hemorrhage of, 294
    distention of, 299–300
    edema of, 232
    gases in, 335
    supplemental embalming of, 224–225

## F

Facial artery, 125–126, 144, 144f
Facial edema, 164, 307t
Facial hair, 162f, 162–163, 458–459
Facial trauma, 260, 335–336
Faking of mummies, 352
Falconi, Dr., 361
Febrile disease, 317t
Federal regulation, 37, 378
Federal Trade Commission, 37, 342, 378
Feeding tubes, 173, 173f
Fell, Lynda Cheldelin, 7
Femoral artery
    anatomy of, 134f, 134–135
    arterial embalming uses of, 146, 146f
    in children, 243
    in infants, 238
    split injection using, 182
Femoral triangle, 131, 134f
Femoral vein
    anatomy of, 139
    arterial embalming uses of, 146–147, 180f
    in children, 243
Fentanyl, 326–327, 327f
Fermentation, 92
Field, Jan, 379
Filtration gravitation, 207
Fingernails, 161
First drainage, 191
First-degree burns, 298
Fixative, formaldehyde as, 103
Flaccidity, 90
Flies, 160–161
Fluid diffusion, 193, 207. *See also* Diffusion
Flushing, 293–294
Fogging a mirror, 94
Fontanelles, 242, 242f
Foot
    arteries of, 136, 136f
    edema of, 310f
    veins of, 136, 136f
Foramina, 211
Forensic autopsy, 249–250
Forestus, Peter, 355–356
Formaldehyde
    advantages of, 99
    adverse effects of, on body, 96
    air pollution and, 427
    albumin and, 98
    alternatives to, 96
    applications of, 425–426, 426t
    best management practices for, 109–111, 423–424
    cancer studies on, 428–429
    as carcinogen, 36, 98, 428
    chemistry of, 425
    condensation products of, 99
    consumer safety with, 426–427
    definition of, 425
    dehydration caused by, 303
    disadvantages of, 99
    discovery of, 97
    disinfectant properties of, 98
    disinfection uses of, 96
    "donor" compounds of, 99
    drying effect of, 303–304
    in embalming fluid, 96
    engineering controls for, 48
    exposure to
        description of, 36
        health effects of, 54–55, 98, 428–429
        monitoring of, 46–47
        National Cancer Institute investigations on, 98
        occupational, 419–422
        permissible limit for, 46–47
        respirators for, 47
        short-term level, 47
        studies of, 419–422
        time-weighted average for, 46–47
    as fixative, 103
    formalin, 98–99
    graying of tissue by, 163
    health effects of, 54–55
    humectants' effect on, 102
    industrial uses of, 98
    irritation studies on, 428
    mechanism of preservative action by, 101
    medical applications of, 426
    methylene glycol formation from, 101
    neutralization of, 324
    occupational safety with, 426–427
    odor threshold of, 420
    polymers of, 99
    properties of, 97–98, 425
    protein cross-linking by, 101f
    sodium borate effects on, 103–104
    standard for
        historical, 96
        Occupational Safety and Health Administration, 46–48
        state-required, 96
    supplemental fluids used with, 96
    tissue effects of, 98–99
    tissue retention of, 414–416
    ventilation of, 429
    work practice controls for, 47–48
Formaldehyde burn, 294
Formaldehyde Council, 424–425, 428–429
Formaldehyde gray, 163, 288t, 289–290, 293
Formaldehyde index, 98
Formaldehyde Rule, 98
Formalin, 54, 98–99, 376–377, 419
Formic acid, 57
Forms
    Attention Funeral Director, 18, 24f
    Authorization for Minimum Care Services, 17, 18f
    Authorization for Restorative and Cosmetic Care, 17, 17f
    Authorization to Prepare Donation Cases for Viewing, 17, 20f
    Decedent Care Report, 18, 25f–26f
    Embalming Authorization, 16, 16f
    Embalming Report, 18, 27f–30f
    Green Funeral Release and Indemnification, 17, 21f
    Identification of Remains of the Decedent, 17, 22f
    Minimum Care Authorization When Embalming is Declined, 17, 19f
    Trauma Viewing Without Embalming, 18, 23f
Fourth-degree burns, 298
Fractures, 175–176, 176f
Frederick, Jerome F., 114
Full-thickness skin, 268, 270, 274f
Fumeless cavity fluids, 118
Funeral
    social function of, 5
    world religions' view of, 3–4
Funeral directors
    Federal Trade Commission regulation of, 37
    tuberculosis exposure by, 34
Funeral embalming, 462

## G

Galen, Claudius, 354–355
Gallbladder, 213
Gangrene, 291, 317t–318t, 321, 321f, 333

Gannal, Jean Nicholas, 359f, 359–360, 362, 368
Gas gangrene, 176t, 333–334
Gases
    arterial solution injection affected by, 196–197
    decomposition, 93, 176t, 177, 196, 284, 334
    description of, 176t, 176–177
    distention caused by, 333t
    extravascular resistance caused by, 322
    in eyelids, 335
    in face, 335
    in facial tissues, 335
    in neck, 335
    odors caused by, 284
    in orbital areas, 335
    purge caused by, 329, 332
    removal of, from tissues, 334–335
    subcutaneous emphysema, 332–333
    tissue, 158, 176t, 177, 333–335
    in trunk tissue, 335
    types of, 332
Gels, 223
General solvent, 119
Generalized edema, 154t, 184, 308–310
Germicides, 43, 101–102
Gladstone, William Evart, 4
Gloves, 39, 41f, 109
Glutaraldehyde, 55–56, 99–100, 378
Glycerine, 103
Glycols, 103
Glycosuria, 247
Glyoxal, 99
Gravitation, 88
Gravity bowl, 377
Gravity embalming, 195
Gravity filtration, 207
Gravity fluid injector, 361f
Gravity percolator, 70
Green burial, 96
Green Burial Council, 96
Green Funeral Release and Indemnification form, 17, 21f
Greer, Prince, 367–368
Grief, complicated, 6
Grieving, 5
Grooved director, 78, 78f, 142, 142f, 143t, 189
Guanches, 353
Gums, 103
Gunshot wounds, 297t, 299–300, 318t

# H

Hair
    basics of, 456
    blow drying of, 457–458
    care of, 161–162, 456–459
    cleansing of, 456
    conditioning of, 456–457
    curly, 457
    facial, 162–163, 458–459
    professionally finished, 458
    shampooing of, 161f
    trimming of, 458
Hand, hypodermic injection of, 224
Hand cream, 397
Hand washing, 39
Hanging, 297, 297t, 318t
Hardening compounds, 119
Harlan, Richard, 360–361
Hast, Ron, 3
Hauptmann, Bruno, 393
Hazard communication, 41
Hazard Communication Rule, 45–46
Hazard Communication Standard, safety data sheet requirements in, 50–53
Hazardous chemicals
    accidental release of, 51
    composition of, 50–51
    disposal of, 52
    ecological information about, 52
    examples of, 53–58
    exposure controls for, 51
    fire-fighting measures for fires caused by, 51
    first-aid measures for, 51
    handling of, 51
    identification of, 50
    ingredients in, 50–51
    personal protection for, 51
    physical properties of, 51–52
    properties of, 51–52
    reactivity of, 52
    regulatory information about, 53
    safety data sheets for, 50–53
    stability of, 52
    storage of, 51
    toxicological information about, 52
    transport of, 52–53
Hazardous waste, 49
Head
    arteries of, 121–126, 122f–126f
    injection of, 254
    veins of, 121–126, 122f–126f
Head blocks, 80, 81f, 164
Heart, 319
Heart beat, 94
Heart surgery, 152
Heart valve grafts, 264, 265f
Heat spatula, 268
Hemoglobin, 287
Hemolysis, 89, 300
Hemorrhage, 318t
Hemorrhagic fever viruses, 433
Hemostats, 73, 73f
Hepatitis, 35–36, 433, 447–449
Hepatitis B
    characteristics of, 449
    exposure to, 34
    vaccination for, 39
Herodotus, 348, 352
Hexylene glycol, 57
Hidden suture, 228, 228f
High-index arterial fluid, 116
Hippocratic Oath, 4
*Histoplasma capsulatum,* 338
Histoplasmosis, 338
*History of Embalming,* 360, 362
HIV. *See* Human immunodeficiency virus
Hohenschuh, William Peter, 373
Holding room, 64
Hollow viscera, 210t
Holmes, Thomas, 363–364, 364f
Homo sapiens, 3
Hospital autopsy, 249
Human composting, 97
Human immunodeficiency virus, 35
Human remains. *See also* Body
    cremated, 343
    disinfection standards for, 95–96, 404
    handling of, 8
    nonviewable, 408–409
    pathogenic agents in, 33
    postmortem specimens from, microbiologic evaluation and enumeration of, 453–455
    receiving of, 344, 344f
    safe work practice for working with, 33–34
    secure sheltering of, 343
    shipping of, 343–344
    viewable, 407–408
Humectants, 102–103, 112, 117, 293, 306
Hunter, John, 358–359
Hunter, William, 357–358, 362
Hutton, Frank A., 365
Hydro Chemical Company, 397
Hydroaspirator with vacuum breakers, 66, 67f, 211
Hydrocele, 307t, 308, 312–313
Hydrocephalus, 307t, 308, 313
Hydrogen sulfide, 92, 283
Hydrolysis
    alkaline, 97
    description of, 91–92
Hydropericardium, 307t
Hydrothorax, 197, 307t, 308, 312, 322, 329
Hyperglycemia, 247
Hypertonic solutions, 115, 310f
Hypodermic embalming
    definition of, 13
    description of, 12, 224
    in infants, 239–240, 241f
Hypodermic injection
    in decomposition, 285–286
    in edema, 309
    hypovalve trocar for, 14
Hypodermic syringes, 175
Hypostasis, 85t, 86–87, 87t, 89, 155t, 287, 288t
Hypotonic solutions, 115, 304, 306f
Hypovalve trocar, 76, 77f

# I

Icterus, conjunctival, 291, 291f
Ideal pressure, 200–201
Ideal rate of flow, 200–201
Identification
    description of, 14, 409–412
    viewing of body for, 342
Identification of Remains of the Decedent form, 17, 22f
Ileum, 213
Iliac drain tubes, 77f, 189

Iliofemoral region, 146
Imbibition, 88
Implantable cardioverter-defibrillator, 171, 172f, 230
Inactive dyes, 105, 106f
Incas, 353
Incision(s). *See also specific incision*
   closure of, 226–229, 227f–229f
   common carotid artery, 140–141, 141f
   infection risks, 171
   suturing of, 226
   technique for, 142f, 142–143
   types of, 140–141, 141f–142f
Incision spreaders, 75, 75f
Index
   definition of, 112
   formaldehyde, 98
   high-index arterial fluid, 116
Infant(s)
   arterial embalming in, 239
   autopsied, 238–239, 239f
   body fat in, 237
   body water in, 237
   cavity treatment in, 238
   common carotid artery in, 238
   embalming solution in, 239
   feature setting in, 237–238
   hypodermic embalming in, 239–240, 241f
   nonautopsied, 238
   positioning in, 238
   pre-embalming analysis of, 237–243, 239f–243f
   skin of, 237
   sternum of, 243f
   supplemental embalming in, 239–240, 241f
   surface embalming in, 240
   vessel selection in, 238
Infant trocar, 212
Infectious agents
   exposure to
      attire for, 40f
      work practice controls for, 39
   transmission of, 42t
Inferior vena cava, 148
Influenza pandemic of 1918-1919, 96
Inguinal region, 130–131
Injection
   arterial. *See* Arterial injection
   restricted cervical. *See* Restricted cervical injection
   six-point. *See* Six-point injection
Injection devices
   air pressure machine, 72, 72f
   bulb syringe, 70
   embalming machines, 70–72, 71f
   gravity and bulb syringe, 70
   gravity percolator, 70
   hand pump, 70
Injection point, 140
Injection pressure, 200
Inlays, 223, 240
Inner canthus, 168
Inorganic salts, 103
Instant tissue fixation, 184–185, 268, 278, 299

Instruments
   aneurysm hooks, 73, 73f, 143t
   aneurysm needles, 73, 73f
   arterial tubes, 13, 75–76, 76f, 141f, 143t
   autoclaving of, 42
   bistoury knife, 73
   cavity fluid injector, 79, 79f
   cleaning of, 233
   decontamination of, 42–43
   description of, 72
   disinfection of, 335
   drainage, 76–78, 77f
   drainage forceps, 74, 75f
   early types of, 355–356
   eye caps, 79, 80f
   grooved director, 78, 78f, 142, 142f, 143t, 189
   hemostats, 73, 73f
   hypovalve trocar, 76, 77f
   incision spreaders, 75, 75f
   injection, 75–76, 76f
   ligature thread, 75, 75f
   mouth formers, 79, 80f
   nasal tube aspirator, 78, 78f
   needle injector, 79, 80f
   plastic garments, 80, 81f
   positioning devices, 79–80, 80f–81f
   postmortem suture needles, 74, 75f
   retractors, 75, 75f
   scalpel, 73f–74f, 73–74
   scissors, 74, 74f, 143t
   spring forceps, 74, 75f, 78, 143t
   steam sterilization of, 42
   stopcocks, 76, 77f
   storing of, 234f
   trocar, 78–79, 79f
   Y-tube, 76, 77f
Interlocking suture, 227
Intermittent drainage, 190, 191f
Internal iliac artery, 148
Internal jugular vein
   anatomy of, 121, 123, 125
   blood drainage uses of, 139
   left, 143
   raising of, 144
   right
      description of, 143–144
      one-point injection using, 179, 180f
International Agency for Research on Cancer, 36
Interstitial fluid, 207, 306
Intradermal suture, 228, 228f
Intravascular diseases, 317t–318t
Intravascular pressure, 195, 202, 205
Intravascular resistance, 195f, 195–196, 320
Intravenous catheters, 174
In-use materials, 396–399
Inversion suture, 172f, 228f–229f, 228–229, 242f, 257, 258f
Ireland, 380–381
Irion, Paul, 7
Ischemia, 318t
Isobutane, 57
Isopropyl alcohol, 57

**J**
Jaramillo, Camilio Andres, 381–382
Jaundice, 153t, 184, 291–293, 292f
Jaundice fluids, 96, 116
Jejunum, 213
Jews, 352
Johnson, Edward C., 3, 393, 396, 399f
Judicious counsel, 7
Jugular drain tube, 77f
Jung, Carl, 7

**K**
Karaya, 103
Kennedy, John F., 4–5
Ketosis, 247
*Klebsiella pneumoniae*, 35
Knot, 229, 230f
Known Shipper Program, 343
Kodiak Archipelago, 354
Koninckx, Alain, 379–380

**L**
Labeling, Hazard Communication Rule requirements for, 46
Lacerations, 175–176
Lactic acid, 89
Large intestine, 213
"Laying in" process, 97, 97f
Leakage, 158, 234
Leave-taking, 7
Left atrioventricular valve, 319
Left common carotid artery, 254
Left common iliac artery, 252
L'Engle, Madeleine, 6
Leukemia, 291, 318t
Lewis, E. C., 367
Life expectancy, 245
Lifting, of body, 160
Ligature test, 94
Ligature thread, 75, 75f
Lincoln, Abraham, 365, 368
Lindbergh, Charles A., 393
Lindemann, Erich, 6–7
Linear guide, 121, 125f
Lip(s)
   adhesive glue on, 238
   closure of, 164, 168, 169f, 238
   corner eminences of, 168
   moisture in, 304
   positioning of, 168, 169f
   supplemental embalming of, 224
Lipase, 92
Lipids, 92
Liver, 213, 324
Liver failure, 153t
Living donor, 263
Livor mortis
   clearing of, 289
   in decomposition, 283, 288t
   definition of, 289
   description of, 85t, 87, 87f, 89, 155t, 175, 202, 203
   illustration of, 289f
Local autopsy, 238

Local regulations, 38
Long, Esmond R., 347
Long, Thomas G., 4
Long bone, 272f–274f, 272–274
Longitudinal incision, 143
Loopuypt needle, 74
Lou Gehrig's disease, 245
Lower limbs. *See also* Foot
    arteries of, 130–136, 132f–136f
    injection of, 252–253
    veins of, 130–136, 132f–136f
Luer-lok arterial tube, 76, 76f
Lumen, 140, 196, 321
Lung purge, 211t, 330f, 330–331, 331t
Lyford, Benjamin F., 367
Lymphatic circulation
    drainage of, 185f, 185–187
    schematic diagram of, 185f–186f
Lymphedema, 310, 311f
Lynch, Thomas, 7
Lysosomes, 91

## M

Maggots, 160, 235
Male genitalia, 218–219
Malignancy, in elderly, 246–247
Mandible, securing of, 165f–166f, 165–167
Mandibular suture, 167
Manner of death, 249
Manual aids, 278
Marbling, 283, 294, 294f
Marburg hemorrhagic fever virus, 433
Mastic compounds, 120
Material safety data sheets. *See* Safety data sheets
Mausoleum demolition and disentombment project, 341–342
Mayans, 354
Mayer, Robert G., 399f
Mayer, Sheridan, 395f, 395–396
Mechanical aids, 278
Median sternotomy, 264
Medical autopsy, 249
Medical devices, 171–174, 172f–174f, 230–231
Medical embalming, 462
Medications, 152. *See also* Drug(s)
Medicolegal autopsy, 249–250
Medieval funeral procession, 387f
Melanin, 287
Melanocytes, 287
Meningitis, 291
Methicillin-resistant *Staphylococcus aureus*, 35, 432, 450–451
Methyl alcohol, 57
Methyl ethyl ketone, 57
Methylene chloride, 57
Methylene glycol, 101
Mexico, 354
Microbial contamination, 45t
Microbicides, 43t
Microorganisms
    endogenous invasion of, 88–89
    translocation of, 84, 85t, 88–89
Midline incision, 264, 264f
Military religious campaigns, 355

Mineral spirits, 57
Minimum Care Authorization When Embalming is Declined form, 17, 19f
Misrepresentation, 7
Mites, 160
Mitford, Jessica, 4–5
Mitral valve, 319
Modesty cloth, 160, 161f
Moisture, 303–314. *See also* Dehydration
    edema. *See* Edema
    in lips, 304
    normal body, 303–304
    overview of, 303
Mold, 235, 297t, 301, 343f
Mold inhibitors, 120
Molding plaster, 57
Moniliasis, 338
Morgan, John, 361
Moribund, 83
Mortuary education, 374–375, 379
Mortuary putty, 120
Mortuary science, 374
Mortuary science license, 37
Moustaches, 459
Mouth
    closure of
        in elderly, 245, 246f
        securing of mandible for, 165f–166f, 165–167
        sequence of, 165
    convex curvature of, 168f
    feature setting of, in rigor mortis, 280
    modeling of, 167–168
    supplemental embalming of, 224
Mouth formers, 79, 80f
MRSA. *See* Methicillin-resistant *Staphylococcus aureus*
Multidrug-resistant pathogens, 35
Multipoint injection, 181, 181f, 322
Mummies
    Egyptian, 351–352
    Peruvian, 353
Mummiform coffin, 351, 351f
Musculature suture, 166, 246f
Mutilations, 297t, 300, 318t
*Mycobacterium tuberculosis*, 36
Mycotic infections, 338–339
Myocardial steatosis, 337

## N

Nails, 161
Nasal process, 376
Nasal spine, 166
Nasal tube aspirator, 78, 78f, 212
Nasopharyngeal tubes, 173, 173f
National Archeological Museum, 3
National Cemetery System, 363
National Council on Mortuary Education, 375
National Funeral Directors Association
    environmental health and safety standards, 48–49
    guidelines from, submitted to OSHA, 402–405
    history of, 369

National Institutes of Health, 337
National Organ Procurement and Transplantation Network, 263
Natron, 350
Natural burial, 96
Natural means of preservation, 347
Natural organic reduction, 97
Neanderthals, 3
Neck
    arteries of, 121–126, 122f–126f
    veins of, 121–126, 122f–126f
Necrobiosis, 84
Necrosis, 84
Needle embalming, 376
Needle injector
    description of, 79, 80f
    securing of mandible using, 165f–166f, 165–166
Needlestick injuries, 34
Nephritis, 292–293
Nerves
    arteries versus, 139–140, 140t
    veins versus, 139–140, 140t
New Testament, 3
New York School of Embalming, 392
Nine-region method, 214, 215f
Nitrocellulose, 57
"No-drainage" injection method, 447
Nondehydrating fluid, 116
Nonionic surfactants, 105
Nonionizing radiation, 36
NOR. *See* Natural organic reduction
North American Indians, 354
Nose, supplemental embalming of, 225
N-suture, 220, 231, 231f
Nuance AireTynt cosmetic applicator, 397, 399f
Nysten's law, 91

## O

Obesity, 337
Occupational Safety and Health Administration
    Bloodborne Pathogens Standard
    Formaldehyde Standard, 46–48
    Hazard Communication Rule, 45–46
    hazardous substance standards of, 36
    National Funeral Directors Association Committee guidelines submitted to, 402–405
    preparation room requirements, 61–62
Occupationally acquired infections, 34–35
Odor, decomposition-related, 93, 158, 283–284
Odou, Lina D., 374
Old Testament, 3
Omentum, 238
Omohyoid muscle, 123
One-point injection, 179–181, 180f, 191
Operative aids, 278
Ophthalmoscope, 93
Opioids, 326–327, 327f
OPOs. *See* Organ Procurement Organizations
OPTN. *See* National Organ Procurement and Transplantation Network

Organ, 263
Organ donation
  consent process for, 263–264
  definition of, 263
  impact of, 264
  process of, 263–264
Organ donors
  deceased, 263–264
  incisions in, 264–265
  living, 263
  recovery and preparation of, 264–266, 265f–266f
Organ Procurement Organizations, 263
Orthodichlorobenzene, 57
Orthopedic devices, 174–175, 175f
OSHA. *See* Occupational Safety and Health Administration
Osmosis, 206, 206f
Outer canthus, 168
Overdose death, 259
Oxalic acid, 57

**P**
Paasche Company, 397, 398f
Pacemakers, 171, 172f, 230
Palpation, 127
Pancreas, 213
Paradichlorobenzene, 58
Paraformaldehyde
  description of, 58, 98–99, 425
  in embalming powder, 119
Paralysis, 152
Paratertiary pentyl phenol, 58
Paré, Ambroise, 356
Parker, Bonnie, 393
Parotid gland, 255
Partial autopsy, 218, 238, 250, 259–260
Passive physical transport systems, 193
Passive transport, 205
Pathological discolorations, 291–293
Pathological skin lesion, 295f
Pediculicide, 160
PEL. *See* Permissible exposure limit
Pelvic cavity
  absorbent compound placed in, 242
  aspiration of, 210f, 218
Pelvic viscera, 213
Peptide bond, 91, 101
Peptide linkage, 91, 101
Peptones, 91
Perchloroethylene, 48
Perfuming agents, 106–107
Period of the Anatomists, 347, 354–362
Periodic monitoring, 234–235
Permissible exposure limit, for formaldehyde, 46–47
Perphry, 349
Persians, ancient, 352
Personal hygiene, 233–234
Personal protective equipment
  description of, 33, 39
  illustration of, 40f–41f
  selection of, 109
Peru, 353

Petechiae, 290, 290f
Petroleum jelly, 397
Pettigrew, Thomas Joseph, 361
Pharmaceutical discolorations, 291
Phenol, 55, 100f, 100–101, 118
Phlebitis, 318t
Phycomycosis, 338
Physical anthropology, 396
Pitting edema, 232, 307t, 308
Pityriasis capitis simplex, 457
Pityriasis steatoides, 457
Plastic garments, 80, 81f, 232–234, 233f
Platysma muscle, 122, 144
Pludeman, John, 341
Plumbing, in embalming room, 38–39
Pneumatic collar, 164
Pneumonia, 318t
Poisoning, 297t, 300
Polypeptides, 91
Ponceau, 106
Popliteal artery, 135, 135f, 147
Popliteal fossa, 135
Positioning blocks, 80, 81f
Positioning devices, 79–80, 80f–81f
Post-embalming dehydration, 306
Post-embalming monitoring, 156–158
Post-embalming purge, 332
Post-embalming treatments, 223
Posterior axillary folds, 126–127
Posterior tibial artery, 135–136, 147
Posterior vertical incision, 140, 141f
Posthepatic jaundice, 291
Postmortem caloricity, 89, 89t, 155t, 281
Postmortem cellular death, 83
Postmortem clots, 186
Postmortem coagula, 186
Postmortem dehydration, 305
Postmortem edema, 88
Postmortem hypostasis, 287
Postmortem interval between death and embalming, 152–153, 154t, 277, 297
Postmortem period
  chemical changes in
    body pH, 85t, 89t, 89–90, 155t
    caloricity, 89, 89t, 155t, 281
    causes of, 85
    decomposition. *See* Decomposition
    list of, 85t
    postmortem stain, 85t, 87t, 89, 90f, 155t, 175, 282, 288t, 289, 291, 300f
    rigor mortis, 85t, 89t, 90f, 90–91, 155t
  discolorations in, 288
  physical changes in
    algor mortis, 85t, 86, 86f, 155t
    blood viscosity, 85t, 88
    bruising, 294
    causes of, 84
    dehydration, 85t, 87–88, 88f, 155t, 305
    hypostasis, 85t, 86–87, 87t, 89, 155t
    list of, 85t
    livor mortis, 85t, 87, 87f, 89, 155t, 175, 289
    translocation of microorganisms, 85t, 88–89

Postmortem stain, 85t, 87t, 89, 90f, 155t, 175, 282–283, 288t, 289, 291, 300f
Postmortem suture needles, 74, 75f
Potential pressure, 72, 200
Powders, 225
PPE. *See* Personal protective equipment
Predynastic period, 348
Pre-embalming analysis
  age, 151, 237
  definition of, 149
  drug treatments, 152, 153t
  of infants, 237–243, 239f–243f
  intrinsic body conditions, 151, 154t
  livor mortis, 202
  musculature, 151
  postmortem interval between death and embalming, 152–153, 154t
  primary condition, 151
  same basic treatment, 151–152
  surgery, 152
  weight, 151
Pregnancy, embalming during, 36
Pregnancy Discrimination Act, 36
Pre-injection fluid, 111
Preparation room
  air conditioning in, 68
  body lifts in, 68f, 68–69
  building permits for, 62
  ceiling hoists in, 68, 68f
  ceiling of, 66
  cross-ventilation in, 68
  design of, 62, 62f, 65, 65f
  doors of, 66
  dressing room, 64
  electric aspirator in, 67
  epoxy coatings in, 65–66
  equipment in, 68f–72f, 68–72
  equipment standards for, 63–64
  facility standards for, 63–64
  floor plans for, 62, 62f–63f
  flooring in, 65–66
  holding room, 64
  hydroaspirator with vacuum breakers in, 66, 67f
  injection devices in
    air pressure machine, 72, 72f
    bulb syringe, 70
    embalming machines, 70–72, 71f
    gravity and bulb syringe, 70
    gravity percolator, 70
    hand pump, 70
  instruments in
    aneurysm hooks, 73, 73f
    aneurysm needles, 73, 73f
    arterial tubes, 75–76, 76f
    bistoury knife, 73
    cavity fluid injector, 79, 79f
    description of, 72
    drainage, 76–78, 77f
    drainage forceps, 74, 75f
    eye caps, 79, 80f
    grooved director, 78, 78f, 142, 142f
    hemostats, 73, 73f
    hypovalve trocar, 76, 77f

incision spreaders, 75, 75f
injection, 75–76, 76f
ligature thread, 75, 75f
mouth formers, 79, 80f
nasal tube aspirator, 78, 78f
needle injector, 79, 80f
plastic garments, 80, 81f
positioning devices, 79–80, 80f–81f
postmortem suture needles, 74, 75f
retractors, 75, 75f
scalpel, 73f–74f, 73–74
scissors, 74, 74f
spring forceps, 74, 75f, 78
stopcocks, 76, 77f
trocar, 78–79, 79f
Y-tube, 76, 77f
local ordinances for, 63
location of, 64
Occupational Safety and Health Administration requirements, 61–62
plumbing for, 66–67
purpose of, 61
refrigeration units in, 68
requirements for, 61–64
sinks in, 67
size of, 65
sound insulation in, 66
state codes for, 63–64
tables in
arrangement of, 65
body transfer, 159
description of, 69f, 69–70
topical disinfectants in, 43–45, 44t
transfer boards in, 69
ventilation in, 67–68, 430–432
walls of, 66
water supply in, 67
windows in, 66
Preservation
definition of, 31
long-term, 416–419
Preservative demand
description of, 112–113
for rigor mortis bodies, 279, 279t
Preservatives
definition of, 31
formaldehyde. *See* Formaldehyde
formalin, 98–99
mechanism of action, 101–102
modifying agents in, 102
packaging of, 95
phenol, 55, 100, 100f, 100–101, 118
principles of, 100–101
surface tension of, 104
Preserve, 31
Pressure filtration, 195, 205–206
Pressure sore, 175
Pressure–flow differentials, 199
Primary dilution, 111, 206
Primary disinfection, 43
Primary flaccidity, 90

Primary injection fluids, 116
*Principles of Restorative Act As the Embalmer Should Know Them*, 374, 394, 395f
Prion, 7
Professional practice, competence in, 7
Professionalism, 378–379
Progesterone, 325
Propane, 58
Propylene glycol, 58, 103
Prostate gland, 213
Proteases, 91
Proteins
chemistry of, 323
cross-linking of, 101
definition of, 31
denaturing of, 325
description of, 100–101
reactive centers of, 11
Proteolytic enzymes, 323, 325
Proteoses, 91
Proximal, 128
Prunk, Daniel H., 365–366, 366f
*Pseudomonas aeruginosa*, 35
Psychosocial model of death, 5–6
Ptomaines, 91
Pulmonary edema, 307t, 320
Pulmonary embolism, 259
Pulse, 94
Purge
after drowning, 299
anal, 156, 330–331, 331t
brain, 331, 331t
in cavity embalming, 283
cranial, 211
definition of, 329
description of, 92f, 93, 156–157
embalming solution, 330f, 331–332
gas as cause of, 329
lung, 319, 330f, 330–331, 331t
post-embalming, 332
reaspiration after, 235
skin areas protected from, 330
stomach, 211t, 330, 330f, 331t
treatment of, 231
Purpura, 175, 324f
Purse-string suture, 174, 174f, 220, 221f, 231, 231f
Pustular lesions, 297
Pustules, 176
Putrefaction, 31, 91
Putrescine, 283–284
Pyruvic acid, 89

## Q

Quadrant method, 214, 215f
Quartz, 58
Quaternary ammonium compounds, 58, 102

## R

Radial artery, 128, 128f, 145, 145f
Radiation therapy, 36
Radioactive isotopes, 326
Ramazzini, Bernardino, 362

Rate of flow
in adults, 200
in children, 244
definition of, 244
Razor abrasion, 294, 305
RCI. *See* Restricted cervical injection
Re-aspiration, 220–221, 235
Recipe method, 149
Recompose, 97
Rectum, 213
Recycling, 49
Re-embalming, 343
Refrigerated bodies
arterial preparation in, 282, 282f
cavity embalming, 282–283
challenges associated with, 281f
decomposition in, 280, 281f
dehydration issues in, 282, 301
discolorations associated with, 297t, 300–301
embalming of, 280–283, 281f–282f
frozen tissue in, 283
livor mortis in, 300
rigor mortis in, 282
Refrigeration units, 68
Regulatory agencies
federal, 37
legislative intent, 36–37
local, 38
state, 37
Reichle, Richard G., 399
Remains. *See* Human remains
Renal failure, 153t, 313–314, 336
Rendon Funeral Home, 381–382
Rendon/Rose Hockett guidelines, 114
Renouard, C.A., 369–370, 373, 376, 379, 391
Respiration, 94
Restorative art
definition of, 387
educational materials, 396–399
emerging technology in, 399
history of, 372, 387–400
in-use materials, 396–399
*Restorative Art*, 395
Restricted cervical injection
in decomposition, 284–285
delayed embalming use of, 278
description of, 182–184, 183f, 192, 248
in diabetes mellitus, 321
in eye donation, 267–268
generalized edema managed with, 309f
in jaundice, 292
as primary injection method, 459–461
in rigor mortis, 280
Reticuloendothelial cytomycosis, 338
Retractors, 75, 75f
Reverence for the dead, 3–4
Reverse suture, 220, 231f
Richardson, Clyde E., 393
Right atrium
direct heart drainage from, 148, 188–189, 189f
venous drainage from, 143, 144f, 148, 187, 187f

Right common carotid artery
  anatomy of, 125f
  one-point injection using, 179, 180f
Right common iliac artery, 240f, 252
Right-to-know laws, 38, 62
Rigor mortis
  arterial injection in, 280
  body positioning in, 280
  definition of, 279
  description of, 85t, 89t, 90f, 90–91, 155t
  embalming of bodies in, 279–280
  extravascular resistance caused by, 322
  firming of tissue versus, 203
  physiology of, 279
  preservative demand for, 279, 279t
  in refrigerated bodies, 282
  relieving of, 163, 163f, 203, 279
  restricted cervical injection in, 280
  six-point injection in, 280
  stages of, 279
Rituals, 4, 7
Ruysch, Frederick, 357

## S

Safety data sheets, 45, 48, 50–53, 95, 109
Salafia, Alfredo, 361–362, 387
Salts, 101
Sanitation, 11–12, 31
Sanitizer, 43
Saphenous vein, 273f
Saprophytic bacteria, 91
SARS. See Severe acute respiratory syndrome
SARS-CoV-2, 466. See also Covid-19
Scabies, 160
Scabs, 176
Scaling skin, 296
Scalp disorders, 457
Scalpel, 73f–74f, 73–74
Scarpa's triangle, 131, 134f
Schade, Charles T., 376
Scissors, 74, 74f, 143t
Sealing agents, 120
Secondary dilution, 206
Secondary flaccidity, 90
Second-degree burns, 298, 298f
Sectional arterial embalming, 181, 181f, 285, 300
Sedatives, 326t
Seepage, 234
Segato, Girolamo, 361
Semilunar incision, 140–141, 141f
Semilunar valve, 319
Semipermeable membrane, 115f
Senile purpura, 246, 246f
Separator, 74, 74f, 143t
Serratus anterior muscle, 127
Severe acute respiratory syndrome, 432–433, 465
Shampooing of hair, 161f
Sharps
  disposal of, 15
  handling of, 49
Sharps containers, 74, 74f
Shaving, of facial hair, 162f, 162–163

Shipping of human remains, 234, 343–344
Shock, 318t
Short-term exposure level, for formaldehyde, 47
Siculus, Diodorus, 349
Sigmoid colon, 213
Simmons, Lena, 374, 392
Sinks, 67
Siphonage, 66
Six-point injection
  in decomposition, 284
  delayed embalming use of, 278
  description of, 181f, 181–182
  in rigor mortis, 280
Skeletal edema, 197
Skin
  back, 270f–271f
  broken, 296
  color of, 287
  dehydration effects on, 305, 305t
  donation of, 268–270, 269f–270f
  dry, 296
  full-thickness, 268, 270, 274f
  jaundice, 291–292
  layers of, 287
  scaling, 296
  split-thickness, 268, 270
  torn, 176
  trauma to, 295f
  unbroken but discolored, 296
Skin lesions, 175, 295, 295f
Skin slip, 93, 93f, 176, 284, 296–297, 305
Skin ulcerations, 175
Slip hub arterial tube, 76, 76f
Slocum, Ray E., 149, 395
Sludge, 88
Small intestine, 213
Snyder–Westberg device, 377
Sodium hypochlorite, 58
Sodium pentachlorophenate, 58
Solid edema, 307t, 307–308
Solvents, 48, 119
Somatic death, 83
Sorbitol, 103
South America, 381–382
South East Asia, 379
Spatula, 393, 394f
Special purpose fluids, 95, 313
Specific gravity, 115
Spinal cord autopsy, 250, 251f
Spleen, 213
Split injection, 182, 182f, 192, 461–462
Split-thickness skin, 268, 270
Spriggs, A. O., 394, 397
Spring forceps, 74, 75f, 78, 143t
Squamous epithelium, 204
Squat lift, 160
Squeegee effect, 42
Stabilize, 31
Stallard, Frank, 395
Steam sterilization, 42
Sterilization, 43
Sternocleidomastoid muscle, 122–123
Sternum, 242

Stethoscope, 93
Stimulants, 326t
Stoma, 173–174, 174f, 230
Stomach, 213
Stomach purge, 211t, 330, 330f, 331t
Stopcock, 76, 77f
Strangulation, 297, 297t
Strap line, 141, 141f
*Streptococcus pyogenes*, 432
Stroke, 152, 317t
Strub, Clarence G., 373–374, 374f, 394, 394f
*Study of Mortuary Customs of North American Indians*, 354
Styloid, 128
Subclavian artery, 129t
Subcutaneous emphysema, 176t, 177, 216, 232, 332–333, 334
Sublingual gland, 255
Sublingual suture, 166
Submaxillary gland, 255
Substrate, 31
Sucquet, J. P., 359
Sullivan, Felix Aloysius, 371
*Sunnyside, The*, 364f, 387, 388f, 391, 393
Super adhesive glues, 229, 258–259
Superficial fascia, 131
Superior thyroid artery, 254
Supplemental embalming
  definition of, 13
  of eyelids, 224–225
  hypodermic embalming, 224
  of infants, 239–240, 241f
  of larger areas, 225–226
  of lips, 224
  of mouth, 224
  of nonvisible areas, 225
  of nose, 225
  surface embalming, 223–224
Supplemental fluids
  in adolescents, 244
  co-injection fluid, 111, 117
  definition of, 95
  dyes, 117
  edema reducing fluid, 117
  pre-injection fluid, 111, 116–117
  water corrective fluid, 117
Supplemental hypodermic injection, 255, 255f
Supraclavicular incision, 140, 141f
Surface discolorations, 293
Surface embalming, 13, 199, 223–224, 240, 290
Surface evaporation, 88
Surface tension, 104–105
Surfactants, 104
Surgical cap, 40f
Surgical drains, 173, 231
Suture needles, postmortem, 74, 75f
Suture thread, 75, 75f, 229
Sutures, 227f–228f, 227–229
Suturing, 226
Swammerdam, Jan, 357
Synthetic coloring agents, 105
Synthetic gum, 103
Syphilis, 318t
Syrians, ancient, 352

## T

"T" incision, 142f, 143
Table(s)
    arrangement of, 65
    body transfer onto, 159, 252
    description of, 69f, 69–70
    types of, 69f, 69–70
Talc, 58
Tallon, Glyn, 380–381
Taphonomy, 93
Tardieu spots, 89, 282–283, 290
Task-sharing, 326
TCE. *See* Trichloroethylene
Tepid water, 105
Terminal disinfection, 43, 233, 404
Tetracycline, 325
*Textbook of Facial Reconstruction, A,* 395
Thanatopraxy, 462
Third-degree burns, 298, 298f
Thoracic aorta, 129t, 147
Thoracic cavity
    absorbent compound placed in, 242
    aspiration of, 210f, 218
    partial autopsy of, 259–260
Thorax, 212
Three-dimensional printing, 399
Thrombosis, 318t
Thrush, 338
Thumb, hypodermic injection of, 225f
Till, Emmett, 4
Till-Mobley, Mamie, 4
Time of death, 249
Time-weighted average, 46–47
Tisdale, Sallie, 4
Tissue, formaldehyde retention in, 414–416
Tissue blebs, 310, 311f
Tissue builder, 118–119
Tissue builder solvent, 119, 175
Tissue channeling, 268
Tissue donation
    bone, 270–275, 272f
    connective tissue, 270–275
    definition of, 263
    embalming practices for, 270
    eyes, 266f–269f, 266–268
    skin, 268–270, 269f–270f
    vessels, 270–275, 273f
Tissue firming, 155, 203
Tissue gas, 158, 176t, 177, 333–335
Tissue gas fluid, 116
Tissue reducing spatula, 268
Toltecs, 354
Toluene, 58
Tongue, 254–255
Topical disinfectants
    antimicrobial activity of, 451–453
    applications of, 44t
    broad-spectrum, 43
    in preparation room, 43–45, 44t
Tracheostomy tubes, 173, 173f
Tragacanth, 103
Training, 46
Tranchina, Giuseppe, 359
Tranquilizers, 326t
Transfer boards, 69
Transferring, of body, 160
Transition state, 92
Transmissible spongiform encephalopathies, 437
Transportation Security Administration, 343
Transverse colon, 213, 216, 216f, 218
Transverse incision, 142, 142f
Trauma Viewing Without Embalming form, 18, 23f
Trichloroethane, 58
Trichloroethylene, 48, 58
Tricuspid valve, 319
Trioxane, 99
Triple-base fluid, 100
Trocar
    aspiration using, 217, 217f
    description of, 13, 78–79, 79f, 212
Trocar button, 220, 220f, 377
Trocar button applicator, 79, 79f
Trocar guides, 214, 216
True tissue gas, 176t, 177, 334
Trunk
    arteries of, 129, 129t–131t
    autopsy of, 252f
    edema of, 311
    orifices of, packing the, 171
    veins of, 129, 129t–131t
TSA. *See* Transportation Security Administration
TSEs. *See* Transmissible spongiform encephalopathies
Tuberculosis, 34, 36, 318t, 465–466
Tumors, 318t
Tunica adventitia, 315, 316f
Tunica externa, 315, 316f
Tunica intima, 315, 316f
Tunica media, 315, 316f
TWA. *See* Time-weighted average

## U

U-incision, 264, 265f
Ulcerations
    decubitus ulcers, 152, 156, 175, 297, 321
    treatment of, 231
Ulcerative lesions, 297
Ulnar artery, 128–129, 129f, 145, 146f
Undergarments, plastic, 80, 81f
*Undertaker's Manual, The,* 369, 369f, 376
Uniform Anatomical Gift Act, 264
United Kingdom, 462–464
United Network for Organ Sharing, 263
Universal Precautions label, 35f
UNOS. *See* United Network for Organ Sharing
Upper limbs
    arteries of, 126f–129f, 126–129
    injection of, 253–254
    veins of, 126f–129f, 126–129
Urinary bladder
    anatomy of, 213
    trocar guide for, 216
Urinary catheters, 174

## V

Vagina, 213
Valvular heart diseases, 316, 318–319
Vancomycin-intermediate *Staphylococcus aureus,* 35
Vancomycin-resistant Enterococci, 35, 450–451
Vancomycin-resistant *Staphylococcus aureus,* 35
Vasa vasorum, 140
Vascular considerations
    aortic aneurysm, 316
    arteriosclerosis, 315–316, 317t
    congestive heart failure, 319–320
    valvular heart diseases, 316, 318–319
    vasodilation, 320
Vascular embalming, 194
Vasoconstriction, 318t, 320
Vasodilation, 320
Vegetable gum, 103
Veins. *See also specific veins*
    arteries versus, 139–140, 140t, 316f
    of distal leg, 135–136, 136f
    of foot, 136, 136f
    of head, 121–126, 122f–126f
    layers of, 315, 316f
    of lower limbs, 130–136, 132f–136f
    lumen of, 140
    of neck, 121–126, 122f–126f
    nerves versus, 139–140, 140t
    of trunk, 129, 129t–131t
    of upper limbs, 126f–129f, 126–129
Venous coagula, 320f, 320–321
Ventilation
    cross-ventilation, 68
    in embalming room, 36, 38
    in preparation room, 67–68, 430–432
    systems for, 109, 110f
Vessels. *See* Arteries; Embalming vessels; Veins
Viewing of body
    after death, 6–7, 342
    delayed, 343, 343f
    without embalming, 18, 23f, 342
Viral hepatitis, 447–449
Von Hofmann, Wilhelm, 97
VRE. *See* Vancomycin-resistant Enterococci
VRSA. *See* Vancomycin-resistant *Staphylococcus aureus*

## W

Warburton Act, 359
Wastewater management, 49
Water control unit, 66
Water corrective fluid, 117
Water cremation, 97
Waterless embalming, 114–115
Web-based mortuary science education, 379
Welch's bacillus, 177

Wet abrasions, 176
Wet gangrene, 291
Whip suture, 229, 229f
Wicking, 312, 313f
Wig care, 458
Work environment
　disinfection of, 42
　sanitary, 42f
Work practice controls
　for embalming chemicals, 109
　for formaldehyde, 47–48
　for infectious agents, 39
Worm suture, 228f–229f, 228–229, 257
Worsham, Albert H., 372–373

**Y**
Yarrow, H. C., 354
Yellow to green jaundice, 293
Y-incision, 250, 250f
Y-tube, 76, 77f

**Z**
Z-suture, 220, 231, 231f